DATE DUE

ANNUAL PROGRESS IN CHILD PSYCHIATRY AND CHILD DEVELOPMENT 1990

ANNUAL PROGRESS IN CHILD PSYCHIATRY AND CHILD DEVELOPMENT 1990

Edited by

STELLA CHESS, M.D.

Professor of Child Psychiatry
New York University Medical Center

and

MARGARET E. HERTZIG, M.D.

Associate Professor of Psychiatry
Cornell University Medical College

BRUNNER/MAZEL, *Publishers* ● **New York**

Library of Congress Card No. 68-23452
ISBN 0-87630-602-4
ISSN 0066-4030

Published by
BRUNNER/MAZEL, Inc.
19 Union Square
New York, New York 10003

Manufactured in the United States of America
10 9 8 7 6 5 4 3 2 1

CONTENTS

ANNUAL PROGRESS IN CHILD PSYCHIATRY AND CHILD DEVELOPMENT 1990

Part I

DEVELOPMENTAL STUDIES

The papers in this section reflect many of the major themes of current developmental research. In the first paper, Zeanah, Anders, Seifer, and Stern seek to bridge the gap between developmental research and psychodynamic theory and practice. The findings of a large number of studies of temperament, motivational systems, affect development and regulation, development of the sense of self, infant-caregiver attachment, and continuities and discontinuities in development are summarized. Infants during the first three years of life are depicted as increasingly capable of responding to, interacting with, and actively engaging their environments. These capacities develop in orderly patterns with discrete developmental shifts in levels of function and adaptation that change both the infant's experience and the environment's experience of the infant. This portrait is familiar to those who have followed developmental research over the past 25 years. In addition, the authors approach the issue of continuities and discontinuities in development with the intriguing suggestion that although behavioral discontinuities are observable, they occur within the context of subjective continuity provided by the infant's developing sense of self and the stability of early relationship patterns.

Moving from description to theory building, the authors highlight the importance of considering developmental progressions from the perspective of continuing and mutually reciprocal transactions between individual and environment. The authors propose that a *continuous construction* model can account for the the multi-determined interactive complexities of development and psychopathology. In this model, patterns of internal subjective experience and patterns of relating to others are derived from both past and present relationship experiences. The model allows for continuous change within the context of an overall coherence of an individual's sense of self, personal history, and relationship patterns. Examples of how this approach may inform therapeutic interventions will be of interest to clinicians, many of whom already are aware of the discrepancy between actual practice and more traditional concepts of *fixation and regression*. The success of a theory is measured not only in how well it accounts for already available data, but also in terms of its ability to raise new questions. The heuristic value of this contribution in focusing investigative attention on the developmental course of a sense of self, and a sense of self with others is clearly evident.

The second paper in this section is a methodologically elegant report of a study designed to examine the relationship between an aspect of self-development measured by self-recognition and the expression of fear and embarrassment. Here,

1

Lewis, Sullivan, Stanger, and Weiss provide a clear and concise review of the development of emotional expression and the self system. Fear is considered a "primary emotion" observable under appropriate conditions in children as young as 10 weeks of age, but embarrassment and other so-called "secondary emotions" (empathy and perhaps envy) do not emerge until around the second birthday. Observation of the interdigitating time frames within which self-conscious emotions and the referential self emerge gave rise to the hypothesis that specific cognitive skills are necessary for the emergence of a "secondary emotion" (embarrassment) but not for a "primary emotion" (fear). The investigators use techniques based upon observable behavior to make inferences about the subjective state. Utilizing the mirror-rouge procedure to distinguish between those who showed self-recognition and those who did not, children ages 9-24 months were exposed to experimental situations thought to differentially elicit clearly defined fear and embarrassment behaviors. As anticipated, embarrassment but not fear or wariness was related to self-recognition.

The findings of this study serve as a reminder that despite the propensity of researchers to investigate discrete lines of development—sense of self, emotional expression, cognitive organization, and so forth—development is, in fact, seamless, with simultaneous changes occurring in all areas. Reorganizations among differing developmental trajectories is a continual process, and the authors have taken an important step toward putting "humpty-dumpty together again."

The paper by William Beardslee on the role of self-understanding in resilient individuals places the findings of his study of resilient adolescents whose parents have serious affective disorder (reprinted in the 1989 Annual Progress) in a larger context. In the present paper, the major findings of three separate studies directed toward elucidating dimensions of adaptation are summarized. The investigations were informed by the proposition that the place to begin to study resilient individuals is with what they themselves report about their own lives, especially about what has sustained them. An open-ended life history data-gathering method, developed in the course of interviewing individuals living in the South who had worked in the civil rights movement for more than 15 years, was also used in the study of resilient survivors of childhood cancer and of the children of parents with affective disorder. Subjects in all three studies were encouraged to reflect on their histories as they responded to questions such as: "How do you understand yourself and your situation?" "What keeps you going?" "What are the sources of your strength?" "How have you been able to cope so well?" "What kinds of insights do you have that help you keep going?" "How would you advise others in this situation to best help themselves?" Although patterns of adaptation were found to differ somewhat in relation to the nature of the stressful experience, all subjects identified self-understanding as important to their resilience. Dimensions of self-understanding evident in all three groups included adequate cognitive appraisal, realistic appraisal of the capacity for and consequences of action, and action itself. Among those subjects who were studied longitudinally, self-understanding deepened and became more comprehensive over time.

Beardslee's conclusion that resilient individuals have a total organizing conceptualization of who they are and how they came to be parallels the suggestion made by Zeanah et al., in the first paper in this section, that in therapeutic situations, the establishment of links with the past may be most useful in helping patients appreciate the model that guides current behaviors, and to evaluate more consciously its appropriateness to present situations. Investigative efforts directed toward the study of *how* resilient individuals form their own syntheses of personal experience, understand themselves and integrate family and individual experience, would as Beardslee proposes, further clarify this process.

The paper by Matheny addresses a central issue in developmental research—continuity and discontinuity of behavior over time. A very sophisticated research methodology has been employed to examine the consistency and change of inhibitory behaviors at 12, 18, 24, and 30 months of age in a sample of 130 twins. Ratings of behavior pertaining to inhibition were available from three sources at each age; direct observations obtained in a laboratory setting; direct observations obtained in conjunction with infant mental testing; and a temperament measure from a questionaire completed by parents. In summary, the findings indicate that for individual twins, age to age and situation to situation correlations were in the moderate range, consistent with the findings of other studies. However, when the twins were recombined into twin pairs, within-pair correlations indicated that monozygotic twins (MZ) were more concordant than dizygotic (DZ) twins for each behavior at each age. In addition, the MZ twins were more concordant for the direction and degree of behavioral change from age to age and from situation to situation.

Matheny makes the time-honored interpretation of twin research—greater concordance among monozygotic versus dizygotic twins speaks to genetic contribution for the trait of behavioral inhibition, and more important, to changes with regard to this trait over time. That the degree of coordination between behavioral trajectories representing short-term changes from one observation to another is systematically related to the closeness of the genetic relationship between individuals is of great interest. Matheny proposes that it is just this coordination of MZ twin pair changes in behavioral patterns that makes it possible to begin to identify a consistent "trait" that regulates observable behavioral changes.

Further research is required to define what may be the links between what is conceptualized as personality, and the components of subjective experience that Zeanah et al. have suggested, is what provides continuity in the face of overt behavioral change.

Careful methodology utilizing multi-modal measures over time also characterizes the next paper in this section—a study of psychoendocrine regulation. Gunnar, Mangelsdorf, Larson, and Hertsgaard have examined the relationship of both the quality of attachment (as assessed by the Ainsworth paradigm) and emotional temperament (as assessed by direct observations of children during the administration of the Louisville Laboratory Temperament Assessment, as well as by parental reports and salivary cortisol level). This examination included 66 children who were tested at nine and at 13 months. The complex array of findings are cogently presented and the methodologic issues limiting interpretation are thoroughly discussed. Unlike the responses of nonhuman primate infants, only small elevations of salivary cortisol were noted in response to maternal separation, and adrenocortical activity was not associated with quality of attachment. Nevertheless, at both nine and at 13 months, infants who exhibited greater increases in adrenocortical activity during testing had more negative emotional temperaments. Moreover, at nine months of age, cortisol levels were more closely associated with emotional tone during the testing procedure, which included separation from the mother, than they were with mothers' reports of child temperament. At 13 months, the magnitude of cortisol increases during separation was associated with maternal reports of emotional temperament prior to testing. This pattern is interpreted as suggesting that between nine and 12 months the adrenocortical response may be becoming more sensitive to trait-like as opposed to state-like aspects of infant psychological functioning. These findings begin to clarify both the timing of the emergence of more enduring behavioral characteristics as well as their neuroendocrine correlates.

In the final paper in this section, Jacklin begins her review of issues of gender by pointing out that speculation about differences between males and females is a national preoccupation. Indicating that an exhaustive summary of gender research in developmental psychology would almost completely overlap the entire field, she confines consideration to three areas: the measurement of intellectual abilities; biology and behavior; and socialization. In each of these areas, gender issues are found to be in different stages of empirical and theoretical advance. The chronicle of gender research regarding the measurement of intellectual abilities has followed the progress of the times, with changes in empirical findings over the last two decades having evolved partly as a result of feminist concerns in research and education. In the biology and behavior area, hypothesis formation and testing are in the early stages as new technologies open up new possibilities for populations to study. In the area of socialization, there is both a long history of research and continual revision and generation of new hypotheses. Jacklin characterizes the socialization of gender as a moving target, suggesting that the product we are trying to predict may itself be changing.

Although recognizing the difficulties involved in gender research, Jacklin underscores the need for continued work in this area, as well as changes in the way the media, teachers, parents, and society in general view gender issues. For Jacklin, times are changing—but change is not rapid enough for many boys and girls who are relegated by their gender roles to less than full lives.

1

Implications of Research on Infant Development for Psychodynamic Theory and Practice

Charles H. Zeanah, Thomas F. Anders, and Ronald Seifer

Brown University, Providence

Daniel N. Stern

University of Geneva, Switzerland

Recent research on infant development is reviewed to consider its implications for psychodynamic theory and practice. To address the question of the importance of early experiences for development, research on continuities and discontinuities in development, temperament, motivational systems in infancy, affect development and regulation, development of the sense of self, and infant-caregiver attachment are reviewed. Two major implications emerge, both emphasizing the need for more complexities in our conceptualizations. First, research on infant development underscores the importance of context in development and cautions about the limits of reductionistic thinking and theories. Second, a major paradigmatic shift away from the fixation-regression model of psychopathology and development is indicated. A new model that better fits available data is proposed instead. In this continuous construction model, there is no need for regression, and ontogenetic origins of psychopathology are no longer necessarily tied to specific critical or sensitive periods in development. Implications for psychodynamic treatment are also described. Key Words: psychodynamic theory, infant development, sense of self, fixation-regression.

Reprinted with permission from *Journal of the American Academy of Child and Adolescent Psychiatry,* 1989, Vol. 28, No. 5, 657–668. Copyright © 1989 by the American Academy of Child and Adolescent Psychiatry.

Dr. Zeanah is supported in part by a Research Scientist Development Award from NIMH (MH00691).

5

Freud (1940) described the infant's relationship to his or her mother as "unique, without parallel, established unalterably for a whole lifetime as the first and strongest love object and as the prototype for all later love relations" (p. 188). Following in this tradition, most other psychodynamic theorists have accorded a vitally important role to infancy and early relationship experiences. In the last 25 years, an increasing number of methodologically rigorous studies on infant development have yielded results that contribute significantly to psychodynamic assertions about the nature and consequences of early experiences. Although many important questions remain, and controversies abound, a coherent picture is emerging. In this selective review of research on infant development, we discuss two major themes germane to psychodynamic theory and practice.

The first theme concerns the importance of context in development and emphasizes the continuing and mutually reciprocal transactions between individual and environment. Recognizing the multi-determined interactive complexities of development and psychopathology requires moving beyond reductionistic thinking and theory building. This perspective is particularly important to emphasize during the current period of dramatic advances by neuroscientists and molecular biologists. What has been learned about development from infancy research strongly suggests that searching for the causes of disordered behavior and personality organization in genetic markers and biochemical defects will never provide the complete picture. Whatever contributions the synaptic cleft and the receptor make to psychopathology are more meaningfully considered within the larger contexts in which they are imbedded. From the standpoint of infant development, this theme of contexts highlights the importance of early infant-caregiver relationship experiences.

Research on infant development has led to the second theme, that is, supplanting drive theory's fixation-regression model with a *continuous construction* model of development and psychopathology. Traditionally, psychodynamic theory has considered relationship experiences to be organized by the oral, anal, and phallic libidinal stages or modes of relating. Psychopathology is understood to derive from regression to fixation points, the latter resulting from constitutional vulnerabilities and/or from infantile traumas within certain critical or sensitive periods. This *fixation-regression* model of psychopathology also guides treatment. Psychoanalysis or psychoanalytic psychotherapy prescribes gradually uncovering the original trauma or fixation point so that it may be worked through. In this conceptualization, the ontogenetic origin of psychopathology arises from the particular libidinal stage of development in which there is a trauma or a constitutional weakness.

In the continuous construction model, patterns of internal subjective experience and patterns of relating to others are derived from past relationship experiences but are continuously operating in the present. The model is "continuous" in two senses. First, it alludes to dynamic, ongoing transactions between individual and environment throughout development. Second, continuous refers to the overall coherence of an individual's sense of self and personal history, as well as the coherence of his or her relationship patterns. This coherence implies both repetition of previous patterns and a tendency to resist change.

The shift from a fixation-regression model to a continuous construction model has important implications for the ontogenetic origins of psychopathology and for the conduct of psychotherapy. The most important difference in the continuous construction model and the fixation-regression model is that the former does not specify the point of origin of various forms of psychopathology or link them to particular developmental phases. Instead, it leaves the question of putative origin open, allowing each issue's origin to emerge from each patient's own particular life story. Since the pattern is ongoing, "ingression" (rather than regression) into salient clinical issues in the here and now occurs through the transference relationship.

Since both the fixation-regression model and the continuous construction model imply some degree of continuity between early and later experiences, the concept of development continuities and discontinuities is reviewed. Then, how continuity relates to empirical findings on infant temperament, motivational systems, and affect development is discussed. Next, because the sense of self integrates these domains of development and is closely linked to subjective experience, continuities and discontinuities in the early development of self are reviewed. Specifically, two major theoretical models of self development that have been drawn from infancy research are reviewed and their differing psychodynamic implications are considered. In keeping with the recognition that continuity in infant development is even clearer at the level of relationship patterns, theoretical and empirical work on patterns of infant-caregiver attachment relationships and their implications for the importance of early experience are described. In the concluding section, the implications of these research results for conceptualizing psychopathology and conducting psychotherapy are highlighted.

CONTINUITIES AND DISCONTINUITIES IN DEVELOPMENT

Belief in the importance of early "traumatic" experiences in the formative years of infancy and an interest in identifying individuals at risk for later psychiatric disorder has led investigators to search intensively for significant continuities in development. The medical model of psychopathology led early psychoanalytic theorists to predict that psychological traumas and biological propensities lead to predictable sequelae and consequences. Contrary to expectations, one of the major results of the search for continuities in behavior has been the recognition that discontinuities in early development are far more readily apparent than continuities (Emde and Harmon, 1984; Rutter, 1987). This, coupled with evidence of adequate coping in some resilient children and adults despite adverse early experiences, has led some to ascribe little, if any, significance to experience in the early years (Kagan, 1984a; Clarke and Clarke, 1976).

An initial conundrum for developmentalists interested in continuities has been the widespread recognition that major periods of development reorganization occur during the first two years of life. These *biobehavioral shifts* are rather discrete epochs during which biological, cognitive, affective, and social characteristics of the infant reorganize and subsequently emerge as qualitatively new capacities of greater complexity (Emde et al., 1976; Emde, 1985). These changes have been widely recognized and extensively reviewed elsewhere (McCall et al., 1977; Kagan, 1984b; Emde, 1985; Stern, 1985a). The major features of the biobehavioral shifts are summarized briefly below.

Around 2 to 3 months after birth, a variety of behavioral changes may be observed. Although the total amount of sleep does not change dramatically, a diurnal cycle of sleep/wake appears, with brief waking periods becoming consolidated into longer daytime bouts of wakefulness and sleep periods becoming more prolonged and shifted to the night. Many infants begin for the first time to sleep through the night. Enhanced cognitive abilities are evident by more rapid learning in habituation, classical conditioning, and operant conditioning. Even more striking for parents are the social and affective changes. Soon after crying or "colicky" behavior begins to diminish, infants begin to make prolonged eye-to-eye contact and smile and coo responsively in the presence of a human face (Emde and Harmon, 1972; Emde et al., 1976).

The next period of reorganization occurs at around 7 to 9 months of age. Biological changes permit postural and locomotor advances. In the cognitive domain, infants develop a rudimentary understanding of means-ends differentiation, along with intentionality, object permanence, and a sense of anticipation. Affectively, the consolidation of these advances is accompanied by the onset of a specific attachment to a primary caregiver, manifest in part by separation reactions and stranger wariness.

At 12 to 13 months, more changes appear. Cognitively, infants have a new appreciation of the independence of entities in the world. Mobility is greatly enhanced by the infant's beginning to walk, further contributing to a new sense of the infant as a more autonomous individual. Affective advances are evident by the appearance of social referencing to resolve uncertainty (Campos and Stenburg, 1981). Affects begin to be used instrumentally by the infant (Klinnert et al., 1984), and affect attunement by caregivers provides the infant with a richer experience of empathy (Stern, 1985b).

The final transformation in the first 2 years occurs at 18 to 20 months. Symbolic representation dramatically advances, and language becomes increasingly preferred as a means of communication. For the first time, infants understand consistently that words are an agreed upon means of designating objects and later events. Self-awareness, gender recognition, and the capacity for self-reflection first become evident. Advances in peer relatedness soon follow these other developments.

Each of these developmental transformations leads to qualitative shifts in biological, cognitive, affective, and social organization, changing both how the infant experiences the world and how others experience the infant (Stern, 1985a). Recognition of these developmental discontinuities suggests that simple links between early and later behaviors are unlikely. Development means inevitable changes in both the individual and the environment. The widely accepted transactional model of development (Sameroff and Chandler, 1975) describes the process by which the infant is changed by environmental influences even as he or she influences and changes that environment. The continuing, mutually reciprocal relationship between infant and environment requires an understanding of continuity as a product of this increasingly complex process and underscores the importance of considering infant development within its environmental context. Research reviewed below on temperament, motivational systems, and affect development addresses some of the complexities of early development as they effect continuity as a basic psychodynamic principle. In addition, the review draws attention to important components of subjective experience that provide the foundation for an individual's sense of personal, historical continuity.

Temperament

Investigators of infant temperament initially hoped to describe early, stable manifestations of personality. Following the approach of Thomas, Chess, and colleagues (Thomas et al., 1963), most investigators and theorists have considered temperament to be the style by which individuals behave in different situations over time, attempting to capture the essence of those behaviors that comprise personality. Temperamental dimensions refer to behavioral tendencies rather than discrete behavioral acts (Goldsmith et al., 1987). Typically, temperament has been aligned with the notion of personality traits rooted in an individual's biology (Goldsmith et al., 1987).

Research in behavioral genetics has examined parent-child, sibling, and twin concordances, measured by parental reports. Overall, results indicate a significant contribution of genetic factors to temperament (Plomin, 1987). Several dimensions of temperament appear to have genetic contributions, including emotionality, activity, and sociability (Buss and Plomin, 1984). Interestingly, stability of inherited traits may actually increase with increasing age, pointing to the complexity of gene-environment interaction (Scarr and Kidd, 1983; Plomin, 1987). In a similar manner, studies of behavioral inhibition (shyness) have demonstrated continuity in selected extreme samples from 2 to 6 years of age. A number of biological correlates of this characteristic also have been demonstrated (Kagan et al., 1988).

The major methodologic problem for temperament research has been concern about the adequacy of parental reports for assessing children's temperaments. Parents have been shown to have systematic biases in their ratings based on their social class, race, anxiety level, and mental health status (Sameroff et al., 1982; Vaughn et al., 1987). To a degree, parents also develop preconceived notions even before their children are born as to what their temperaments will be (Zeanah et al., 1985, 1986a; Mebert and Kalinowsky, 1986). Mother-father-observer agreements about temperament are only moderate or less (Hubert et al., 1982; Field and Greenberg, 1982; Zeanah et al., 1986b), perhaps reflecting the generally low (about 0.25) agreement among different informants who have different roles with a particular child (Achenbach et al., 1987). The basic question from these studies remains, is continuity in the infant's behavior or in the perception of the informant?

Clinically, the most important construct to emerge from temperament research is that of infant difficulty (Bates, 1980), although there has been considerable debate about its meaning and measurement (Bates, 1980; Thomas et al., 1982; Bates, 1983; Carey, 1986; Zeanah et al., 1986c). Adverse temperament characteristics in infancy, if stable, provide an opportunity for early identification of individuals at risk for subsequent psychopathology. The problem has been that evidence for continuity of temperamental traits is equivocal at best, especially when measured in infancy (Hubert et al., 1982).

Despite these conceptual differences and shortcomings in assessment, temperament remains a compelling if frustratingly elusive construct. From the clinical standpoint, the major point about temperament is that direct links between temperament types and psychiatric disorders are limited, although there are scattered findings relating both parental reports and laboratory assessments of temperament to some clinical conditions (Rothbart and Goldsmith, 1985; Carey, 1986; Rosenbaum et al., 1988). These links are greatly strengthened when the infant's temperament is considered in context (Graham et al., 1973; Cameron, 1978). Wolkind and DeSalis (1982), for instance, found that 4-month-old infants with difficult temperaments were significantly more likely to be behavior disordered at age 3 years if their mothers were clinically depressed.

All of these results have led to interest in considering temperament in the context of the parent-child relationship. Thomas, Chess, and colleagues (Thomas et al., 1963, 1968) originally formulated the "goodness-of-fit" construct, emphasizing the interaction between parental responses and differing infant temperamental types in the production of disordered behavior. Seifer and Sameroff (1986) expanded this model to integrate more systematically the contextual factors associated with parental responses to and interpretation of differing behavioral styles in young children. As a result, their model highlights the importance of the subjective experiences of parent and infant and emphasizes the importance of context in understanding early development and its disorders. Research on infant temperament underscores the fallacy of theoretical models that attempt to explain development and psychopathology without sufficient attention to context.

Motivational Systems

As a result of infancy research, motivational systems in infancy have been expanded beyond the libidinal and aggressive drives proposed by Freud. One of the domains of motivation that recent infancy research has described compellingly is curiosity. From the moment of birth, infants actively and preemptorily seek stimulation, especially social stimulation (Stern, 1977; Anders and Zeanah, 1984). Since Wolff's (1966) seminal work on the importance of the state of alert inactivity for learning, a host of investigations using paired comparison and habituation paradigms have capitalized on infant preferences for novelty to discover other infant capacities. Stern (1985a) cites evidence from such paired comparison paradigms indicating that under conditions of novelty, even young infants would rather look than eat, underscoring the importance of curiosity as a basic motivational system. Infants posses inborn biases and preferences for certain types of stimulation, along with a tendency to explore, to form and test hypotheses about what is occurring in the world (Brunner, 1977; Kagan et al., 1978; Lamb and Sherrod, 1981; Lipsitt, 1983).

Another closely related area of research on basic motivational systems is mastery motivation. Research on mastery motivation was inspired by White's (1959) theory of effectance motivation, a relatively early divergence from accepted psychoanalytic theory on the nature of drives. White believed that individuals are intrinsically motivated to explore and to master their environmental contexts. His position was congruent with Hunt's (1965) view of infants as motivated, active constructors of their environments. Following in this tradition, Harter (1978) developed a theoretical model that links environmental consequences of mastery behavior with individual differences in self-esteem. Specifically, contexts that encourage and reinforce attempts at mastery are believed to promote positive feelings of self-efficacy and internal perceptions of control.

White, Hunt, and Harter emphasized the universal aspects of mastery motivation as a behavioral characteristic of the species. Yarrow and colleagues (Yarrow et al., 1983) began a series of studies of infants in the first year of life to determine individual differences in the degree and manner in which mastery motivation was expressed. Their strategy for measuring mastery motivation was to present a series of toys that emphasize production of effects, sensorimotor practice, or problem solving to infants, and to assess the degree to which the infants explored and mastered the situation with a minimum of adult guidance. Clear individual differences in attention, persistence, exploration, and task success were demonstrated in these studies (Yarrow et al., 1983; Morgan and Harmon, 1984). Further, these differences have been related to developmental status, handicapping conditions, and interactions with parents (Jennings et al., 1988; Macturk et al., 1985; Yarrow et al., 1982, 1984). In addition, it appears that goal-directed behavior, rather than task success, is related to self-efficacy as manifest in contingent positive affect displays (Macturk et al., 1987).

Some theoreticians, particularly in the field of self psychology, have asserted that the overarching motivational system driving behavior is a feeling of competence (Basch, 1988). In this line of reasoning, competence subsumes curiosity, mastery, effectance, and even sex and aggression as a superordinate construct. Competent behavior is the external goal and self-esteem is the internal goal in this important motivational system.

Sroufe and colleagues have inspired a growing body of research on the development of social competence in infants and toddlers (Sroufe and Waters, 1977; Matas et al., 1978; Waters and Sroufe, 1983). Two major points are emphasized in their work. First, social competence is defined as the flexible and effective use of available personal, social, and physical resources to achieve goals (Waters and Sroufe, 1983). Second, infant behaviors are examined in terms of their organization (Sroufe and Waters, 1977); that is, *patterns* of behavior instead of isolated behaviors are assessed. Crucial is the appreciation, familiar to clinicians, that individual infant behaviors have different meanings in different contexts and at different developmental periods. Behaviors are considered intimately tied to the important relationships of the child in various contexts and in different developmental periods. Meaningfully organized patterns of behavior are more stable and predictive than individual behaviors alone (Sroufe and Waters, 1977; Waters, 1978; Sroufe, 1983).

Two year olds' effective use of social support is an important ingredient in their ability to function competently in problem solving tasks. This includes seeking help when needed and at times rebuking unnecessary interference by adults. Individual differences in dyadic interaction in this regard are readily demonstrable (Matas et al, 1978) and are predictive of later peer relationships (Sroufe, 1983).

Recent investigations have taken a more integrative approach to studying mastery and competence in infancy. Frodi et al. (1985) have found that security of attachment at 1 year predicts mastery behavior 8 months later. Maternal control styles and sensitivity also affected mastery behavior of 1-year-old infants (Grolnick et al., 1984). Following these leads, Seifer et al. (in press) have developed a model of social competence in toddlers that emphasizes the integration of security of attachment, mastery motivation, affect expression, modulation and self-control, and task success.

The most important psychodynamic implication of these research findings concerns the maintenance of self-esteem. Research in this area points to infants' motivation by curiosity and the desire to explore, by the urge to master, and by the desire for competence to behave in ways that maintain self-esteem. In other words, evidence suggests a variety of behaviors that are more usefully explained by other motivational systems rather than as discharges of excess psychic energy. And maladaptive behaviors can be explained in terms other than compromise solutions to conflict situations.

Affect Development and Regulation

Research on infants and adult-infant relationships indicates that throughout development, emotions regulate behavior, internal processes, and social interactions (Barrett and Campos, 1987). For example, much as Freud speculated, fear helps the individual avoid dangerous situations, activate the fight-flight response, and alert others to the presence of danger. This research also supports traditional psychodynamic theory about the role of emotions in personality formulation and about their importance in clinical treatment (Emde, 1988a, b).

The impetus for research on affect development comes from demonstrations of ontogenetic changes in facial expressions and the recognition of seven discrete emotions—joy, sadness, anger, fear, surprise, disgust, and interest—in extensive cross-cultural studies (Izard, 1971; Ekman et al., 1972). The implication of this work is that parents and infants are biologically predisposed to display and to interpret certain emotional expressions in one another and to interact on the basis of these interpretations.

Further work demonstrates that facial expressions of emotions show regularity in their form and time of emergence. Both parents and objective observers reliably recognize facial expressions in infants in the first year of life (Emde, 1985, 1988a). In fact, interest, disgust, and physical distress are readily demonstrable at birth and have specifiable elicitors and predictable interactional consequences (Izard and Malatesta, 1987). In the first 7 months of life, the maturation of surprise, sadness, anger, and fear appear to be primarily biologically programmed, although social experiences may have great influence as early elicitors and contingent reinforcers of these actions.

Emotional expressions are especially important motivators and regulators of social behavior. In early infancy, caregiver responses are differentially influenced by infant expressions of emotions (Malatesta, 1981), and infants are in turn influenced by the caregiver's affective expressions (Tronick et al., 1986). With the maturation of higher order central nervous system inhibitory mechanisms and the development of more complex cognitive abilities, emotional expressions become increasingly subject to control. They also become increasingly useful as a means of regulating the behavior of others. Although many caregivers already may interpret infant affect expressions as intentional in neonates (Kaye, 1982), they still recognize a qualitative change towards the latter part of the first year as they begin to perceive infants using their emotional expressions instrumentally to obtain desired goals (Klinnert et al., 1984).

The importance of the emotional availability of caregivers to their infants has been stressed by many psychodynamic theorists and investigators (Bowlby, 1969/1982; Mahler et al., 1975; Ainsworth et al., 1978; Emde and Easterbrooks, 1985; Sroufe, 1988). Recent research with 1-year-olds has demonstrated that in situations of uncertainty, infants look to their caregivers for help in evaluating their emotional reaction to the uncertainty. This form of emotional signaling has been termed social referencing (Campos and Stenberg, 1981; Klinnert et al., 1982). Social referencing, which occurs at a time when the infant might have more difficulty with evaluating the safety and consequences of his or her own actions and the new meanings of a variety of environmental events, appears to be an important precursor of real self-awareness (Emde, 1985).

Infants begin to label their own feeling states towards the end of the second year of life (Bretherton and Beeghly-Smith, 1982). Together with capacities for self-awareness, this period marks the initial appearance of an observing ego. The child can have one feeling and simultaneously think about another feeling and deal with it symbolically, opening up new possibilities for complexity and for conflict between internal experience and external expression. There is substantial evidence that infants can learn to deny emotional expression of ongoing feelings, thus dissociating expression and feelings (Barrett and Campos, 1987; Izard and Malestesta, 1987).

The significance of continuity of emotional development has been stressed most explicitly by Emde (1985). He suggests that it is an individual's emotional experiences that give a sense of identity throughout development. Being able to access our own feelings consistently gives us a sense of familiarity about who we are despite many changes over time. Further, because this "affective core" is rooted in biology, it provides a means by which we are able to appreciate the feelings of others and to relate to others empathically. In other words, the affective domain provides an important component of the continuous construction model. Whether affect deserves *the* central or merely an important place in memory and the subjective sense of continuity is controversial (Stern, 1988), but few would disagree that one of the most compelling continuities posited is an individual's sense of self.

DEVELOPMENT OF THE SENSE OF SELF

Development of the sense of self is fundamental to a discussion of infant development because it is in the individual's identity that the domains of temperament, motivational systems, competence, and affect become integrated. There is an increasing consensus that organizational features of the sense of self give coherence and continuity to individual experience (Damon and Hart, 1986). Although Horney (1951), Kohut (1977), Kernberg (1975), and other psychoanalytic theorists have described the sense of self from the adult perspective, infancy research has fostered new and important theories about the early *development* of the sense of self. Rather than reviewing in detail the voluminous research with infants bearing on self development, we present a review instead of the two major conflicting theoretical perspectives, Mahler's (Mahler et al., 1975) theory of separation-individuation and Stern's (1985a) theory of self development. These theories share a central focus on the infant's sense of self and on the overarching clinical issues of being alone and being with others as fundamental human concerns. Nevertheless, their implications for psychodynamic theory and practice lead us in different directions. The theory of separation-individuation is fully compatible with drive theory's fixation-regression model, but the self development theory of Stern illustrates the continuous construction model. As a result, they necessarily provide different and incompatible views of the course of self development, the origins of psychopathology, and the strategies of psychotherapy.

Compatible with empirical findings that self-awareness develops at about 18 months (Lewis and Brooks-Gunn, 1979) is the influential theoretical work on self development that began with Mahler and her colleagues (Mahler et al., 1975). Based on extensive, longitudinal observations of a small sample of middle-class mothers and children, together with clinical experiences with older psychotic children, Mahler and her colleagues elaborated a widely known theory of self development. They proposed that an infant's psychological birth is a gradual process that extends throughout the first 2 years after physical birth. The gradual discovery of self-awareness and independence from the mother was described as the process of separation-individuation. For the first 2 months, infants are in a *normal autistic phase,* in which physiological processes are dominant over psychological processes. From 2 to 6 months, in the *normal symbiotic phase,* the infant "behaves and functions as though he and his mother were an omnipotent system—a dual unity within a common boundary" (Mahler et al., 1975, p. 44).

Following this phase, the process of separation-individuation begins. During the initial phase of *differentiation,* the infant "hatches" out of the "symbiotic orbit" and begins to make initial tentative moves away from the mother. These moves are increased during the next *phase of practicing,* as the infant's burgeoning motor abilities and increased interest in the object world lead to longer periods of time playing away from the mother. With cognitive advances in the middle of the second year, infants' awareness of separateness grows. This dawning awareness of separateness and loss of omnipotence that characterize the *rapprochement crisis* are accompanied by an affective shift in the infant from joyous intoxication to increased petulance and sadness. Infant ambivalence about fusion and separateness during this period is inferred from the well-described behavioral patterns of "shadowing" the mother and alternately "darting away" from her. Following resolution of the rapprochement crisis, infants begin to accept their separateness in the phase designated *on the way to object constancy.*

Despite the richness of Mahler's descriptions, the lack of methodological rigor has left unanswered the question of whether the observations merely confirmed investigator biases or critically tested specific hypotheses (Minde, 1981, 1982). The theory of separation-individuation also appears both to overestimate *and* to underestimate the capacities of infants in the first 2 years of life (Horner, 1985; Stern, 1985a; Horner, 1988). A wealth of research has established the infant's active engagement with the world immediately after birth, which is incompatible with Mahler's connotations of "autistic" disinterest in, or avoidance of, human contact (Peterfreund, 1978; Lichtenberg, 1983; Horner, 1985; Stern, 1985a). Mahler's description of symbiosis too readily ascribes to infants capacities for symbolic functioning (i.e., those necessary for hallucinatory wish-fulfillment) that are well beyond anything that has been demonstrated in infants at this age and also ignores what is known about capacities for differentiation (Horner, 1985; Stern, 1985a). Feeling omnipotent is also incompatible with infants' everyday perceptual experiences (Horner, 1985) and requires sophisticated reality-distorting capacities in the subjective experience of very young infants. Contrary evidence suggests that in infancy the reality principle precedes the pleasure principle, meaning that defensive operations, in the psychodynamic sense, require cognitive capacities beyond those available to 4-month-old infants (Stern, 1985a).

Finally, because of its derivation from the psychopathology of older psychotic children, the theory of separation-individuation is fundamentally pathomorphic. The attribution to normal infants of characteristics of later psychopathology fits with the fixation-regression model of psychopathology, but is highly problematic in explaining normal development (Bowlby, 1969/1982; Peterfreund, 1978; Klein, 1980; Horner, 1985; Stern, 1985a).

In striking contrast to Mahler's theory, Stern's (1985a) theory of self development suggests that infants never subjectively experience undifferentiation; in fact, in his view they are not capable of this since "only an observer who has enough perspective to know the future course of things can even imagine an undifferentiated state" (p. 46). Instead, Stern envisions the infant as experiencing five relatively distinct senses of self, each of which emerges in conjunction with the new capacities that accompany the biobehavioral shifts described earlier.

Stern has proposed that in the first 2 months of life, infants repeatedly experience the process of relating diverse objects and experiences in order to identify their invariant properties. Research indicates that some of this capacity for relating is innate, as infants' apparently possess a capacity for a model representation that allows them to "match" stimulation across different sensory modalities. Other means of relating are quickly learned, as networks of perceptions become organized and integrated.

Stern designates this sense of experiencing the coming into being of organization, the sense of *emergent self.*

Following the first biobehavioral shift at 2 to 3 months, another sense of self is added to the first. The *core sense of self* is the physical self that is experienced as a coherent, willful, bounded physical entity with a unique affective life and history belonging to it. Stern cites a wealth of empirical support for the infant's capacity for self-agency, self-coherence, self-affectivity, and self-history necessary for a core sense of self. The infant quickly learns that regulation of his or her emotional states is dependent upon others (adult caregivers), but even self-with-other experiences still belong entirely to the infant's own self.

After the second and third biobehavioral shifts, the infant's new capacities for sharing attention, intentions, and affective states with an other (all of which have ample empirical support) ushers in the *subjective sense of self.* With this addition to the emergent sense of self and the core sense of self, the infant experiences a dramatic advance in relatedness. For the first time, the infant is aware of his or her ability to match and to mismatch mental states with an other.

The *verbal sense of self* emerges after the onset of the final biobehavioral shift in the first 2 years. This new sense of self involves the ability to reflect on oneself and to use language to communicate about oneself to others. The advantages of the verbal sense of self in vastly expanding the infant's experiences and relatedness are obvious, but Stern also points out a darker side of this new sense of self. The infant experiences the limitations of language in rendering experiences, particularly those experienced in the domains of the other three senses of self. "Language forces a space between interpersonal experience as lived and as represented. And it is exactly across this space that the connections and associations that constitute neurotic behavior may form" (Stern, 1985a, p. 182).

In the third or fourth year of life, the infant begins to use language for more than objectifying and labeling. For the first time, the infant demonstrates an ability to narrate his or her own life story. This momentous achievement marks the beginning of an ability to change how one views oneself that is essential for psychodynamic psychotherapy. The *narrative sense of self* describes the new domain of experience that constructs a story from a variety of elements (e.g., actor, action, intentions, instrumentality, and context) drawn from other senses of self (Stern, 1989a, b). The narrative self requires a qualitatively different mode of thought from problem solving or other kinds of talking. Although it is not yet clear why or how children begin to construct an autobiographical history, it is clear that this history becomes the life story that an adult patient initially presents to a therapist.

Unlike most other developmental theories that involve sequential phases or stages, Stern's suggests that, once formed, the senses of self operate continuously and simultaneously. None of them is necessarily dominant at any time in development nor is any one necessarily linked to a particular clinical issue. Furthermore, subjective experience throughout development is organized not by phase-specific clinical issues such as orality, attachment, or mastery, but instead by the emergent, core, subjective, verbal, and narrative senses of self. Regression is unnecessary in this conceptualization, because of the continuing presence and growth of each of the five senses of self throughout the lifespan. This is precisely the continuity implied by the continuous construction model.

These two major theories of self development agree about the importance of the individual's subjectivity and the centrality of the sense of self in any attempt to understand development. Both conceptualizations address the fundamental human problem of being with others and being alone, and they view this problem as a central organizer of human experience. They also share much agreement about salient clinical issues such as autonomy and what it feels like to be with an other. Nevertheless, the nature of the individual's subjectivity is radically different in the two systems. In addition to vastly different conceptualizations of individual experience, the theories of Mahler and Stern also understand the origins of psychopathology differently. Mahler's work illustrates the fixation-regression model of psychopathology, with later problems understood as repetitions of infantile traumas. Further, the form of later pathology is determined by the sensitive period of self development in which the trauma occurred. Stern's conceptualization, on the other hand, illustrates the continuous construction model, in which there is no regression but only ingression into an ongoing sense of self that is appropriate to a particular clinical issue. The form of later pathology is not necessarily related to the developmental period in which it occurred originally. Since the self emerges in the context of the parent-infant relationship, a fundamental issue for both models is the degree to which early relationships experiences become internalized within the self during development.

INTERNAL REPRESENTATIONS AND RELATIONSHIP PATTERNS

Another domain in which continuity has been recognized amidst change is in patterns of relationships between infants and their caregivers (Sroufe and Fleeson, 1986). A central tenet of virtually all psychodynamic theories has been the notion that adults recreate early relationship experiences in subsequent relationships. The "compulsion to repeat" was originally described by Freud (1920) in the context of neurotic repetitions of maladaptive behaviors. The degree to which the childhood experiences of an individual are important influences on that individual's subsequent parenting behavior, and the factors that increase or decrease the likelihood of repetition, are of enormous clinical relevance. Relationship continuity and repetition imply some capacity in infants to internalize and carry forward relationship patterns. Recent research has attempted to operationalize the construct of internal representations of relationship experiences in order to explain how infants experience and reenact relationship patterns.

Internal representations are essentially memory structures that re-present a version of lived experience to an individual. Stern (1985a) has outlined the process by which they are formed. The infant lives a particular experience, and, when it is over, the experience is instantaneously transformed into a memory. After the infant has lived a number of similar experiences, each of which has been transformed into a particular memory, the infant abstracts an average version of the experience. This abstract average of related memories of experiences is an internal representation. This is analogous to the development of natural categories of objects in memory that has been described by Rosch et al. (1976) and of generalized event representations described by Nelson and Gruendel (1981).

There is an increasing consensus that internal representations are organized hierarchically from small units reflecting subjective experience to increasingly large networks reflecting more global appraisals (Stern, 1985a, 1989a, b; Bretherton, 1985, 1987). These large networks, termed "working models" by Bowlby (1969/1982), not only re-present lived experience, but also are presumed to perceive and interpret incoming information selectively, to generate anticipations, and to guide behavior in relationships. They are not merely passive filters of experience but contribute towards an individual's active recreations of relationship experiences (Zeanah and Anders, 1987). This assumes a constructive, narrative view of memory and recall, consistent with recent research in cognitive psychology (Reiser et al., 1985).

Relationship Patterns in Infants

The cross-model perceptual capacity in young infants described earlier implies that a primitive representational capacity exists even at birth. Other evidence supports the notion that infants "internalize," or retain patterns of experience, in the first few months of life. During one phase of face-to-face interactions with their 3-month-old infants, mothers were instructed to "look depressed" (Cohn and Tronick, 1983). Infants became disorganized and distressed in response and, interestingly, they continued to exhibit distressed behavior for a period of time after their mothers resumed normal interaction with them. Further, when infants of clinically depressed mothers were compared to infants of nondepressed mothers in the same interactional paradigm, the infants of nondepressed mothers became significantly more distressed during the "look depressed" phase of interaction (Field, 1984). This suggests that the depressed appearance of the nondepressed mothers was a greater violation of expectation than the depressed appearance of the clinically depressed mothers.

Other empirical support relevant to the construct of internal representations and the intergenerational transmission of relationships has come from investigations of attachment in infants and adults (Sroufe and Fleeson, 1986). Inspired by the ethologic-attachment theory of Bowlby (1969/1982, 1973, 1980), Ainsworth et al. (1978) developed the most widely used assessment of attachment relationships, a laboratory paradigm known as the Strange Situation. This procedure involves a series of increasingly stressful episodes for 11- to 20-month-old infants. On the basis of the organization (rather than the content) of the infant's reunion behavior with respect to the caregiver following a brief separation, it is possible to classify the infant's pattern of attachment to that caregiver.

According to attachment theory, infants should use their attachment figures as a secure base to explore the novel environment provided by the Strange Situation. Following the caregiver's return, an infant should seek to reestablish interaction with the caregiver and, if distressed, should seek comfort from the caregiver. When infants behave in this manner, they are classified as *securely* attached to that caregiver. In contrast, some infants seem surprisingly undistressed by their caregivers' leaving and actively avoid them on return, ignoring the caregiver's bid for interaction and attending instead to toys. The relationship between these infants and caregivers is termed *avoidant*. Other infants protest vigorously when their caregiver leaves the room during the Strange Situation procedure, but they behave ambivalently when their caregivers return, alternately demanding contact and then resisting it. Relationships characterized by this pattern are termed *ambivalent*.

What is being classified is not simply a temperamental trait of the infant, as some have suggested (Chess and Thomas, 1982; Chess, 1984; Kagan et al., 1987). If infants are assessed in the Strange Situation with different caregivers, they behave differently depending on the quality of attachment to the caregiver with whom they are assessed (Main and Weston, 1981; Belsky et al., 1984; Grossman et al., 1985). Independence of Strange Situation classifications of the same infant with different caregivers emphasize that attachment classifications are relationship specific. Obviously, this does not preclude the possibility that temperamental traits exert indirect effects on attachment classification, through effects on caregivers' sensitivity and responsiveness, for example. Nevertheless, Strange Situation classification apparently reflects the infant's view of his or her relationship with a specific caregiver at a particular point in time (Hinde, 1982).

Strange Situation classifications are preceded by characteristic patterns of caregiver interactive behavior at home during the preceding year. The most consistent finding is that caregivers who are sensitive and responsive (i.e., consistently nurturant, attentive, and nonintrusive while interacting with their infants) have secure attachment relationships with them at 1 year (Ainsworth et al., 1978; Egeland and Farber, 1984; Belsky et al., 1984; Grossman et al., 1985). Because Strange Situation classifications are preceded by certain interactive patterns at home, they may be understood as "summary outcome scores" of infants' relationship experiences with primary caregivers in the first year of life. The working hypothesis of attachment theory is that these summary scores reflect the infant's internal representation of the relationship with a particular caregiver.

Infant attachment classifications derived from behavior during the Strange Situation procedure are apparently stable. Under conditions of low stress and adequate support, the infant's classification with the caregiver remains stable between 12 and 18 months (Waters, 1978; Main and Weston, 1981; Belsky et al., 1984). When attachment classification changes from secure to insecure, it is related to an increase in stresses or a decrease in supports (Vaughn et al., 1979; Thompson et al., 1982). In other words, factors that would be expected to disrupt caregiver-infant relationships and therefore to change infant representations of those relationships have been demonstrated to affect them in predictable ways.

In support of psychodynamic assertions about carrying forward relationship patterns, attachment classification of infants predicts subsequent psychosocial adaptation (Sroufe, 1988). Infants who are securely attached to their primary caregivers at 12 months of age are more autonomous at age 2 years (Matas et al., 1978), have more advanced symbolic play development (Slade, 1987), are more socially competent with peers and more ego-resilient (flexible, self-reliant, curious, involved) in preschool and kindergarten years (Arend et al., 1979; Waters et al., 1979; Troy Sroufe, 1987; Oppenheim et al., 1988). School-aged children previously classified as securely attached demonstrate more competent overall functioning (Main et al., 1985), higher self-esteem (Cassidy, 1988), and less psychopathology (Lewis et al., 1984; Erickson et al., 1985) than those previously classified as insecurely attached.

Internal Representations in Adults

Believing that individual differences in internal representations of attachment ought to be measurable in adults as well as infants, Main and her colleagues provided a second major conceptual and methodological advance in attachment research. George et al. (unpublished manuscript) developed a measure to classify adults' description of their own childhood attachment relationships. The Adult Attachment Interview inquires about early relationships, separations, losses, and other attachment-relevant experiences. Scoring relies not on the content of the adult's descriptions, but rather on the organization of thoughts and feelings, and qualitative aspects of descriptions. Thus, whether an adult describes early experiences and relationships as good or bad is less important than the degree to which the adult has integrated these experiences, as reflected in having access to memories and feelings regarding significant attachment figures and experiences and coherently describing these early events and experiences.

Following the attachment classification system of the Strange Situation for infants, adults are classified as *dismissing* of attachment (corresponds to avoidance in infants), *autonomous* with respect to attachment (corresponds to secure in infants), or *preoccupied* by past attachments (corresponds to ambivalence in infants). Adults classified as autonomous value relationships, maintain a balanced view of their role in relationships and a tolerance for imperfection in themselves and others and are coherent in describing early experiences. Adults classified as dismissing or preoccupied lack these qualities. The dismissing group describes attachment relationships as unimportant or claims to be unaffected by them and often have difficulty remembering early experiences. The specific memories they do recall often contradict their idealized global descriptions of experiences. The preoccupied group still seems dependent upon and overly concerned with their families and early experiences are are often still struggling to please family members. This group generally exhibits considerable difficulty providing a coherent depiction of relationships or experiences.

Intergenerational Continuity

If the Strange Situation measures the "infant side" of the attachment relationship and the Adult Attachment Interview measures the "adult side" of the attachment relationship, then psychodynamic assertions about intergenerational transmission lead us to expect convergence in the measures. Indeed, as Main and Goldwyn (1984, 1989) have pointed out, there are striking parallels in the patterns of infant behavior in the Strange Situation procedure and the patterns of adult patterns of language, thought, and memory in the interview. For instance, adults classified as dismissing turn their attention away from attachment relevant information during the Adult Attachment Interview, while simultaneously asserting their independence. They emphasize the normalcy of their experiences and minimize adversity or the effects of adversity. In similar fashion, infants classified as avoidant turn their attention away from their caregiver in the Strange Situation, as if they are dismissing the importance of the parent, their relationship to the parent, and their own need for comfort. Infants classified ambivalent are either angrily inconsolable or passively ineffective during the reunion episodes of the Strange Situation, and adults classified preoccupied are angrily engaged in an unsuccessful struggle to please their parents or passively incoherent about poorly defined childhood experiences.

Recent investigations with the Adult Attachment Interview have examined the agreement between adults' classifications in the Adult Attachment Interview and their children's classification to that adult in the Strange Situation. In a preliminary investigation, Main et al. (1985) found a 76% agreement between mothers' AAI classification and their children's Strange Situation classification measured 5 years previously. Eichberg (1987), who interviewed mothers 6 to 12 months after their infants were observed in the Strange Situation, found an 82% exact agreement between mothers' attachment classifications and the classification of their infants' relationships to them. Results from these investigations and the parallels in infant and adult behavior described above imply that the caregivers and infants share similar patterns of processing attachment information and of affective arousal; in other words, similar internal representations of their relationship. These similarities in how caregivers and their young children represent their relationship provide valuable preliminary insights into the process by which relationship patterns may be carried forward across generations.

Mothers' attachment classifications are overwhelmingly more insecure in clinical populations (Crowell and Feldman, in press; Benoit et al., in press) and are related to their interactive behaviors with their young children (Crowell and Feldman, in press). These findings provide preliminary evidence that internal representations of attachment in adults may be meaningful indices of how they relate as caregivers to their children. In terms of the continuous construction model, internal representations occupy a pivotal position between internal subjective experience and outward interactional behavior. As such, they become a major focus of treatment.

DISCUSSION

The foregoing review highlights significant areas of research demonstrating that infants in the first 3 years of life are well organized to respond to, interact with, and actively engage their environment. These capacities develop in orderly patterns with discrete developmental shifts in levels of function and adaptation that change both the infant's experience of the environment and the environment's experience of the infant. Discontinuity in individual behaviors occurs within the subjective continuity of the infant's developing sense of self and the stability of early relationship patterns. But what are the implications of these findings for current theory and practice?

The transactional model of development has provided an understanding of psychopathology that takes us beyond the linear causality of nature-nurture dualism. Current research in infancy has substantiated the view that reductionistic approaches to understanding behavior are not likely to be successful. Development requires both nature and nurture, and it is the context in which these experiences interact that requires understanding in order to predict subsequent psychopathology. Even with continuities in developmental processes that are obvious, such as the social deficits in autistic children, it is the fit between continuously present markers, biological and environmental, that contributes substantially to outcome. Contexts are especially important in infancy, when psychiatric disorders are less clearly localized within an individual and more appropriately within an infant's specific important relationships (Anders, 1989). These relationships provide the initial organizing context in which the fit between individual subjective experience and environmental demands occurs.

From the psychodynamic perspective, the question is not merely whether biological propensities or environmental stressors lead to maladaptive behavior, but, also, are the disturbances fixed, or can they be altered by therapy or by other forms of treatment? Emde (1988b) has called the discrepancy between the fixed rigidity of neurotic character pathology on the one hand, and the paucity of demonstrable behavioral continuities in individual infants on the other, the central developmental paradox. The key to understanding this paradox is in the recognition that continuities are at the level of subjective experience and relationship patterns rather than individual behaviors. An infant who avoids his or her mother after a brief separation at 12 months of age will be more dependent on the preschool teacher and more likely to victimize classmates. This same infant is also at increased risk for subsequent psychopathology (Sroufe, 1983; Erickson et al., 1985; Troy and Sroufe, 1987). Continuity in this case is clearly not at the level of individual behaviors in the infant but in the relationship pattern with the primary caregiver and the internal insecurity that colors his or her subjective experience.

A related question with origins in early psychoanalytic theory asks whether single traumatic early experiences inexorably alter subsequent behavior. There is increasing evidence from the research literature that massive psychological and/or physical trauma experienced by individuals at any age have long-lasting effects on behavior (Eth and Pynoos, 1985). Nevertheless, especially in early infancy, single traumatic events have limited effects. More important are the ongoing contexts in which these traumatic events occur. Early, brief separations from caregivers and abrupt weanings, for instance, are considered far less traumatic for development than disordered relationships involving the infant in a pattern of insensitive caregiving. Context provides the arena in which environmental stresses interact with individual biological propensities to shape individual personalities with unique vulnerabilities and invulnerabilities.

As described in this review, current research in infancy also supports a paradigm shift away from the fixation-regression model and toward the continuous construction model of development and psychopathology. Various clinical issues may originate at any point in development and exert their influence on self experience or relationship experiences. Emphasis is on the individual's ongoing dynamic patterns of internal representations and interpersonal relationships. This conceptualization has important implications for treatment, as well.

If a patient's major conflictual themes are no longer tied to specific phases of development but instead are derived from the reconstructed "moments" that emerge in the patient's reported life story, then psychotherapy with adults must become more individualized (Stern, 1985a). Preconceived formulations concerning ontogenetic origins of psychopathology are no longer valid. For example, control conflicts no longer imply inevitable anal trauma. Furthermore, recovering the putative origins of clinical trauma is useful only to the extent that it enables the individual to make changes in the here and now, to challenge representational distortions, and to gain some conscious control over current behavior. The link with the past may be most useful in helping the individual appreciate the model that guides his or her current behavior and to evaluate more consciously its appropriateness in the present, especially as regards intimate relationships and providing for the young. In treating children, the focus is less on retracing origins and meanings of specific symptomatic behaviors and more on changing current environmental contexts that support the maladaptive behavior or symptomatology.

Since the crucible for early experiences is actually the context of primary relationships, the construct of relationship psychopathology has become the focus of therapeutic attention. The transference relationship both with the therapist and with significant others in the individual's life continues to be the model for this process. The characteristics that underlie the primary attachment relationship, namely emotional availability, dependability, empathic attunement, sensitivity to developmental needs, and provision of comfort and security, are also prerequisites of the therapeutic relationship (Peterfreund, 1983). The therapist's presence, availability, and sensitivity provide opportunities for intense relationship experiences that provide a context for understanding the individual's current internal representation of intimate relationships.

The complexities of human development are mirrored in the complexities of psychotherapy. Just as there is no single determinant of psychopathological behavior, there is also no single therapy that can resolve every disorder. Multiple therapeutic approaches are frequently necessary, depending upon the particular psychopathology. Infancy research, however, supports the psychodynamic assertion that amelioration of relationship pathology requires therapeutic relationship experiences, with particular strengths implicit in the transference relationship as a major potential vehicle for change.

Whether the psychotherapeutic process can foster significant changes in those aspects of personality and psychopathology that derive from internal representations, or whether psychotherapy merely provides understanding of individual patterns of vulnerability and invulnerability remains controversial. Psychotherapy with children and families has demonstrated how difficult it is, even at an early age, to induce significant characterologic changes. Even removing young children from extremely pathological environments and placing them in more optimal settings does not provide magical transformations of personality or behavior. Simplistic therapeutic interventions are as limited as unitary etiologic formulations. Complex, multidetermined problems in development require complex, multimodal solutions. The contribution of psychodynamic psychotherapy seems best suited to recreating the context of early development in order to reset the level of vulnerability and invulnerability for disordered behavior.

REFERENCES

Achenbach, T. M., McConaugh, S.H., & Howell, C. T. (1987), Child/adolescent behavioral and emotional problems. *Psychol. Bull.,* 101:213–232.

Ainsworth, M. D. S., Blehar, M., Waters, E., & Wall, S. (1978), *Patterns of Attachment.* Hillsdale, N.J.: Lawrence Erlbaum.

Anders, T. F. (1989), Toward a nosology of relationship disorders. In: *Relationships and Relationship Disorders,* ed. A. J. Sameroff and R. N. Emde. New York: Basic Books.

Anders, T. F. & Zeanah, C. H. (1984), Early infant development from a biological point of view. In: *Frontiers of Infant Psychiatry II,* ed. J. D. Call, E. Galenson, and R. L. Tyson. New York: Basic Books.

Arend, R., Grove, F. L., & Sroufe, L. A. (1979), Continuity of individual adaptation from infancy to kindergarten. *Child Dev.,* 50:950–959.

Barrett, K. C. & Campos, J. J. (1987), Perspectives on emotional development II. In: *Handbook of Infant Development,* ed. J. D. Osofsky. New York: John Wiley & Sons.

Basch, M. (1988), *Understanding Psychotherapy.* New York: Basic Books.

Bates, J. E. (1980), The concept of difficult temperament. *Merrill-Palmer Quarterly,* 26:299–319.

Bates, J. E. (1983), Issues in the assessment of difficult temperament. *Merrill-Palmer Quarterly,* 26:299–319.

Belsky, J., Rovine, M., & Taylor, D. (1984), The Pennsylvania infant and family development project III. *Child Dev.,* 55:718–728.

Benoit, D., Zeanah, C. H., & Barton, M. L. (1989), Maternal attachment disturbances in failure to thrive. *Infant Mental Health Journal* (in press).

Bowlby, J. (1969/1982), *Attachment.* New York: Basic Books.

Bowlby, J. (1973), *Separation.* New York: Basic Books.

Bowlby, J. (1980), *Loss.* New York: Basic Books.

Bretherton, I. (1985), Attachment theory: retrospect and prospect. In: *Growing Points in Attachment Theory and Research,* ed. I. Bretherton and E. Waters. SRCD Monographs, Vol. 49, No. 6, Serial no. 209.

Bretherton, I. (1987), New perspectives on attachment relations. In: *Handbook of Infant Development,* ed. J. D. Osofsky. New York: Wiley.

Bretheron, I. & Beeghley-Smith, M. (1982), Talking about internal states. *Developmental Psychology,* 18:906–921.

Brunner, J. S. (1977), Early social interaction and language acquisition. In: *Studies in Mother-Infant Interaction,* ed. H. R. Schaffer. London: Academic Press.

Buss, A. H. & Plomin, R. (1984), *Temperament: Early Developing Personality Traits.* Hillsdale, N.J.: Lawrence Erlbaum.

Cameron, J. R. (1978), Parental treatment, children's temperament, and the risk of childhood behavioral problems 2. *Amer. J. Orthopsychiat.* 48:140–147.

Campos, J. J. & Stenburg, C. (1981), Perception, appraisal and emotion. In: *Infant Social Cognition,* ed. M. Lamb & L. Sherrod. Hillsdale, N.J.: Erlbaum.

Carey, W. (1986), Interactions of temperament in clinical conditions. *Advances in Developmental and Behavioral Pediatrics,* 6:83–115.

Cassidy, J. (1988), Child-mother attachment and the self in six-year-olds. *Child Dev.* 59:121–134.

Chess, S. (1984), What does behavior in the Strange Situation tell us? *Behavioral and Brain Sciences,* 7:148–149.

Chess, S. & Thomas, A. E. (1982), Infant bonding: mystique and reality. *Amer. J. Orthopsychiat.,* 52:213–222.

Clarke, A. M. & Clarke, A. D. B. (1976), *Early Experience: Myth and Evidence.* London: Open Books.

Cohn, J. F. & Tronick, E. Z. (1983), Three month old infants' reactions to simulated maternal depression. *Child Dev.,* 54:185–193.

Crowell, J. & Feldman, S. (1988), The effects of mothers' internal models of relationships and children's behavioral and developmentat status on mother-child interaction. *Child Dev.,* 59:1273–1285.

Damon, W. & Hart, D. (1986), Stability and change in children's self-understanding. *Social Cognition,* 4:102–118.

Egeland, B. & Farber, E. A. (1984), Infant-mother attachment. *Child Dev.,* 55:753–771.

Eichberg, C. G. (1987), Quality of infant-parent attachment. Paper presented to the Biennial Meeting of the Society for Research in Child Development.

Ekman, P., Friesen, W. V., & Ellsworth, P. (1972), *Emotion in the Human Face.* New York: Pergammom Press.

Emde, R. N. (1985), The affective self: continuities and transformations from infancy. In: *Frontiers of Infant Psychiatry,* ed. J. Call, E. Galenson, and R. Stimston, Vol. 2. New York: Basic Books.

Emde, R. N. (1988a), Development terminable and interminable I. *Int. J. Psychoanal.,* 69:23–42.

Emde, R. N. (1988b), Development terminable and interminable II. *Int. J. Psychoanal.,* 69:283–296.

Emde, R. N., & Easterbrooks, M. A. (1985), Assessing emotional availability in early development. In: *Early Identification of Children at Risk,* ed. W. K. Frakenberg, R. N. Emde, & J. W. Sullivan. New York: Plenum Press.

Emde, R. N., Gaensbauer, T., & Harmon, R. J. (1976), Emotional expression in infancy. *Psychological Issues,* Monograph 37. New York: International Universities Press.

Emde, R. N., & Harmon, R. J. (1972), Endogenous and exogenous smiling systems in early infancy. *J. Am. Acad. Child Psychiatry,* 11:177–200.

Emde, R. N. & Harmon, R. J. (1984), Entering a new era in the search for developmental continuities. In: *Continuities and Discontinuities in Development,* ed. R. N. Emde and R. J. Harmon. New York: Plenum Press.

Erickson, M. F., Sroufe, L. A., & Egeland, B. (1985), The relationship between quality of attachment and behavior problems in preschool in a high risk sample. In: *Growing Points in Attachment Theory and Research,* ed. I. Bretherton and E. Waters. SRCD Monographs Vol. 49, No. 6, Serial no. 209.

Eth, S. & Pynoos, R. (1985), *Posttraumatic Stress Disorder in Children.* Washington, D.C.: American Psychiatric Association Press.

Field, T. (1984), Early interactions between infants and their postpartum depressed mothers. *Infant Behavior and Development,* 7:527–532.

Field, T. & Greenburg, R. (1982), Temperament ratings by parents, teachers of infants, toddlers and preschool children. *Child. Dev.,* 53:160–163.

Freud, S. (1920), *Beyond the Pleasure Principle.* In: *The Complete Works,* Vol. 18. London: Hogarth Press.

Freud, S. (1940), *An Outline of Psychoanalysis.* In: *The Complete Works,* Vol. 23. London: Hogarth Press.

Frodi, A., Bridges, L., & Grolnick, W. (1985), Correlates of mastery-related behavior. *Child Dev.,* 56:1291–1298.

Goldsmith, H. H., Buss, A. H., Plomin, R., Rothbart, M. K., Thomas, A., Chess, S., Hinde, R. A., & McCall, R. B. (1987), Roundtable: what is temperament? four approaches. *Child Dev.,* 58:505–529.

Graham, P., Rutter, M. & George, S. (1973), Temperamental characteristics as predictors of behavior disorders in children. *Amer. J. Orthopsychiat.,* 43:328–339.

Grolnick, W., Frodi, A., & Bridges, L. (1984), Maternal control style and the mastery motivation of one-year-olds. *Infant Mental Health Journal,* 5:72–82.

Grossman, K., Grossman, K. E., Spangler, G., Suess, G., & Unzner, L. (1985), Maternal sensitivity and newborns' orientation responses as related to quality of attachment in northern Germany. In: *Growing Points in Attachment Theory and Research.* ed. I. Bretherton and E. Waters. SRCD Monographs, Vol. 49, No. 6, Serial no. 209.

Harter, S. (1978), Effectance motivation reconsidered. *Human Develop.,* 21:34–64.

Hinde, R. A. (1982), Attachment: some conceptual and biological issues. In: *The Place of Attachment in Human Behavior,* ed. C. M. Parkes and J. Stevenson-Hinde. New York: Basic Books.

Horner, T. M. (1985), The psychic life of the young infant. *Amer. J Orthopsychiat.,* 55:324–344.

Horner, T. M. (1988), Rapprochement in the psychic life of the toddler. *Amer. J Orthopsychiat.,* 58:4–15.

Horney, K. (1951), *Neurosis and Human Growth.* New York: Norton.

Hubert, N. C., Wachs, T. D., Peters-Martin, P., & Gandour, M. J. (1982), The study of early temperament. *Child Dev.,* 53:571–600.

Hunt, J. M. (1965), Intrinsic motivation and its role in psychological development. In: *Nebraska Symposium on Motivation,* Vol. 13, ed. D. Levin. Lincoln, Nebraska: University of Nebraska Press.

Izard, C. E. (1971), *The Face of Emotions.* New York: Appleton-Century-Crofts.

Izard, C. E. & Malatesta, C. Z. (1987), *Perspectives on Emotional Development I.* New York: Wiley.

Jennings, K. E., Connor, R. E., & Stegman, C. E. (1988), Does a physical handicap alter the development of mastery motivation during the preschool years? *J. Am. Acad. Child Adolesc. Psychiatry,* 27:312–317.

Kagan, J. (1984a), Continuity and change in the opening years of life. In: *Continuities and Discontinuities in Development,* ed. R. N. Emde and R. J. Harmon. New York: Plenum Press.

Kagan, J. (1984b), *The Nature of the Child.* New York: Basic Books.

Kagan, J., Kearsley, R. B., & Zelazo, P. R. (1978), *Infancy: Its Place in Human Development.* Cambridge, Mass.: Harvard University Press.

Kagan, J., Reznick, J. S., & Snidman, N. (1987), Temperamental variation in response to the unfamiliar. In: *Perinatal Development: A Psychobiological Perspective,* ed. N. A. Krasnegor, E. M. Blass, M. A. Hofer, and W. P. Smotherman. Orlando, Fla.: Academic Press.

Kagan, J., Reznick, J. S., & Snidman, N. (1988), Biological bases of childhood shyness. *Science,* 240:167–171.

Kaye, K. (1982), *The Mental Life of Babies.* Chicago: University of Chicago Press.

Kernberg, O. (1975), *Borderline Conditions and Pathological Narcissism.* New York: Aronson.

Klein, M. (1980), On Mahler's autistic and symbiotic phase. *Psychoanalysis and Contemporary Thought,* 4:69–105.

Klinnert, M. D., Campos, J. J., Sorce, J. F., Emde, R. N., & Svejda, M. (1982), Emotions as behavior regulators. In: *Emotions in Early Development,* ed. R. Plutchik and H. Kellerman. New York: Academic Press.

Klinnert, M. D., Sorce, J. F., Emde, R. N., Stenberg, C., & Gaensbauer, T. (1984), Continuities and change in early emotional life. In: *Continuities and Discontinuities in Development,* R. N. Emde and R. J. Harmon. New York: Plenum.

Kohut, H. (1977), *Analysis of the Self.* New York: Aronson.

Lamb, M. E. & Sherrod, L. R. (1981), *Infant Social Cognition.* Hillsdale, N.J.: Lawrence Erlbaum.

Lewis, M. & Brooks-Gunn, J. (1979), *Social Cognition and the Acquisition of Self.* New York: International Universities Press.

Lewis, M., Feiring, C., McGuffog, C., & Jasher, J. (1984), Predicting psychopathology in six-year-olds from early social relation. *Child Dev.,* 55:123–126.

Lichtenberg, J. D. (1983), *Psychoanalysis and Infant Research.* Hillsdale, N.J.: Analytic Press.

Lipsitt, L. P. (1983), *Advances in Infancy Research,* Vol. 2. Norwood, N.J.: Ablex.

Macturk, R. H., Hunter, F. T., McCarthy, M. E., Vietze, P. M., & McQuiston, S. (1985), Social mastery motivation in Down syndrome and nondelayed infants. *Topics in Early Childhood/Special Education,* 4:93–109.

Macturk, R. H., McCarthy, M. E., Vietze, P. M., & Yarrow, L. J. (1987), Sequential analysis of mastery behavior in 6 and 12 month old infants. *Developmental Psychology,* 23:199–203.

Mahler, M., Pine, F., & Bergman, A. (1975), *Psychological Birth of the Human Infant.* New York: Basic Books.

Main, M. & Goldwyn, R. (1984), Predicting a mother's rejection of her infant from representations of her own childhood experiences. *International Journal of Child Abuse and Neglect,* 7:203–217.

Main, M. & Goldwyn, R. (1989), Interview based adult attachment classification. *Developmental Psychology* (in press).

Main, M., Kaplan, N., & Cassidy, J. (1985), Security of attachment in infancy, childhood, and adulthood. In: *Growing Points in Attachment Theory and Research,* ed. I. Bretherton & E. Waters. SRCD Monographs, Vol. 49, No. 6, Serial no. 209.

Main, M. & Weston, D. (1981), Security of attachment to mother and to father. *Child Dev.,* 52:932–940.

Malatesta, C. Z. (1981), Infant emotion and the vocal affect lexicon. *Motivation and Emotion,* 5:1–23.

Matas, L., Arend, R. A., & Sroufe, L. A. (1978), Continuity of adaption in the second year. *Child Dev.,* 49:547–556.

McCall, R. B., Eichorn, D., & Hogarty, P. (1977), *Transitions in Early Mental Development,* SRCD Monographs 42 (1177).

Mebert, C. J. & Kalinowsky, M. F. (1986), Parents' expectations and perceptions of infant temperament. *Infant Behavior and Development,* 9:321–334.

Minde, K. K. (1981), Review of *The Selected Papers of Margaret Mahler,* New York: Jason Aronson. *Journal of the American Academy of Child Psychiatry,* 20:426–428.

Minde, K. K. (1982), Dr. Minde replies to Dr. Mahler. *J. Am. Acad. Child Psychiatry,* 21:94–95.

Morgan, G. A. & Harmon, R. J. (1984), Developmental transformations in mastery motivation. In: *Continuities and Discontinuities in Development,* ed. R. N. Emde and R. J. Harmon. New York: Plenum Press.

Nelson, K. & Gruendel, J. (1981), Generalized event representations. In: *Advances in Developmental Psychology,* Vol. 1, ed. M. E. Lamb and A. L. Brown. Hillsdale, N.J.: Lawrence Erlbaum.

Oppenheim, D., Sagi, A., & Lamb, M. (1988), Infant-adult attachments on the kibbutz and their relation to socioemotional development 4 years later. *Developmental Psychology,* 24:427–433.

Peterfreund, E. (1978), Some critical comments on psychoanalytic conceptualizations of infancy. *Int. J. Psychoanal.,* 59:427–441.

Peterfreund, E. (1983), *The Process of Psychoanalytic Therapy.* Hillsdale, N.J.: Lawrence Erlbaum.

Plomin, R. (1987), Developmental behavioral genetics and infancy. In: *Handbook of Infant Development,* ed. J. D. Osofsky. New York: Wiley.

Reiser, B. J., Black, J. B., & Abelson, R. P. (1985), Knowledge structures in the organization and retrieval of autobiographical memories. *Cognitive Psychology,* 17:89–137.

Rosch, E., Mervis, C. B., Gray, W. D., Johnson, D. M., & Boyes-Braem, P. (1976), Basic objects in natural categories. *Cognitive Psychology,* 8:382–439.

Rosenbaum, J. F., Biederman, J., Gersten, M., Hirschfield, D. R., Meminger, S. R., Herman, J. B., Kagan, J., Reznick, S., & Snidman, N. (1988), Behavioral inhibition in children of parents with panic disorder and agoraphobia: *Arch. Gen. Psychiatry,* 45:463–470.

Rothbart, M. K., & Goldsmith, H. H. (1985), Three approaches to the study of infant temperament. *Developmental Review,* 5:237–260.

Rutter, M. (1987), Continuities and discontinuities from infancy. In: *Handbook of Infant development*, ed. J. D. Osofsky. New York: Wiley.

Sameroff, A. J. & Chandler, M. J. (1975), Reproductive risk and the continuum of caretaking casualty. In: *A Review of Child Development Research,* Vol. 4. Chicago: University of Chicago Press.

Sameroff, A. J., Seifer, R. & Elias, P. K. (1982). Sociocultural variability in infant temperament ratings. *Child Dev.,* 53:164–173.

Scarr, S. & Kidd, K. K. (1983), Developmental behavior genetics. In: *Handbook of Child Psychology,* 4th ed., ed. P. H. Mussen. New York: Wiley.

Seifer, R. & Sameroff, A. J. (1986), The concept, measurement, and interpretation of temperament in young children. In: *Advances in Developmental and Behavioral Pediatrics,* 7:1–43.

——Vaughn, B. E., Lefever, G. & Smith, C. (in press), Relationships among mastery motivation and attachment within a general model of competence. In: *Perspectives on Mastery Motivation in Infants and Children,* ed. P. M. Vietz & R. H. Macturk.

Slade, A. (1987), Quality of attachment and early symbolic play. *Developmental Psychology,* 23:78–85.

Sroufe, L. A. (1983), Individual patterns of adaptation from infancy to preschool. In: *Development and Policy Concerning Children with Special Needs. Minnesota Symposium on Child Psychology,* Vol. 16, ed. M. Perlmutter. Hillsdale, N.J.: Lawrence Erlbaum.

Sroufe, L. A. (1988), The role of infant-caregiver attachment in development. In: *Clinical Aspects of Attachment,* ed. J. Belsky and T. Nesworski. Hillsdale, N.J.: Lawrence Erlbaum.

Sroufe, L. A. & Fleeson, J. (1986), Attachment and the construction of relationships. In: *The Nature and Development of Relationships,* ed. W. W. Hartup and Z. Rubin. Hillsdale, N.J.: Lawrence Erlbaum.

Sroufe, L. A. & Waters, E. (1977), Attachment as an organizational construct. *Child Dev.,* 48:1184–1199.

Stern, D. N. (1977), *The First Relationship: Infant and Mother.* Cambridge, Mass.: Harvard University Press.

Stern, D. N. (1985a), *The Interpersonal World of the Infant.* New York: Basic Books.

Stern, D. N. (1985b), Affect attunement. In: *Frontiers of Infant Psychiatry II,* ed. J. Call, E. Galenson, and R. L. Tyson. New York: Basic Books.

Stern, D. N. (1988), Affect in the context of the infant's lived experience. *Int. J. Psychoanal.,* 69:233–238.

Stern, D. N. (1989a), The representation of relational patterns. In: *Relationships and Relationship Disorders,* ed. A. J. Sameroff and R. N. Emde. New York: Basic Books.

Stern, D. N. (1989b), Crib narratives from a psychoanalytic perspective. In: *Narratives From The Crib,* ed. K. Nelson. Cambridge, Mass.: Harvard University Press.

Thomas, A., Chess, S., Birch, H. G., Hertzig, M. E., & Korn, S. (1963), *Behavioral Individuality in Early Childhood.* New York: New York University Press.

Thomas, A., Chess, S., & Birch, H. G. (1968), *Temperament and Behavior Disorders in Children.* New York: New York University Press.

Thomas, A., Chess, S., & Korn, S. J. (1982), The reality of difficult temperament. *Merrill-Palmer Quarterly,* 28:1–20.

Thompson, R. A., Lamb, M. E., & Estes, D. (1982), Stability of infant-mother attachment and its relationship to changing life circumstances in an unselected middle class sample. *Child Dev.,* 53:144–148.

Tronick, E. Z., Cohn, J. E., & Shea, E. (1986), The transfer of affect between mothers and infants. In: *Affective Development in Infancy,* ed. M. Yogman and T. B. Brazelton. Norwood, N.J.: Ablex.

Troy, M. & Sroufe, L. A. (1987), Victimization among preschoolers. *J. Am. Acad. Child Adolesc. Psychiatry,* 26:166–172.

Vaughn, B. E., Bradley, C. F., Joffe, L. S., Seifer, R., & Barglow, P. (1987), Maternal characteristics measured prenatally predict ratings of temperamental difficulty on the carey infant temperament questionnaire. *Developmental Psychology,* 23:152–161.

Vaughn, B., Egeland, B., Sroufe, L. A., & Waters, E. (1979), Individual differences in infant-mother attachment at twelve and eighteen months: stability and changes in families under stress. *Child Dev.,* 50:971–975.

Vaughn, B. E., Taraldson, B. J., Crichton, L., & Egeland, B. (1981), The assessment of infant temperament. *Infant Behavior and Development,* 4:1–17.

Waters, E. (1978), The reliability and stability of individual differences in infant-mother attachment. *Child Dev.,* 49:483–494.

Waters, E. & Sroufe, L. A. (1983), Social competence as a developmental construct. *Developmental Review,* 3:79–97.

Waters, E., Wippman, J., & Sroufe, L. A. (1979), Attachment, positive affect, and competence in the peer group. *Child Dev.,* 54:821–829.

White, R. W. (1959), Motivation reconsidered: the concept of competence. *Psychological Review,* 66:297–333.

Wolff, P. (1966), *The Causes, Controls, and Organization of Behavior in the Neonate,* Monograph 17. New York: International Universities Press.

Wolkind, S. N. & DeSalis, W. (1982), Infant temperament, maternal mental state and child behaviour problems. In: *Temperamental Differences in Infants and Young Children* (Ciba Foundation Symposium 89). London: Pitman Books Ltd.

Yarrow, L.J., Morgan, G. A., Jennings, K. D., Harmon, R. J., & Gaiter, J. L. (1982), Infants' persistence at tasks. *Infant Behavior and Development,* 5:131–141.

Yarrow, L., McQuiston, S., Macturk, R. H., Klein, R. P., & Vietze, P. M. (1983), Assessment of mastery motivation during the first year of life. *Developmental Psychology,* 19:159–171.

Yarrow, L. J., Macturk, R. H., Vietze, P. M., McCarthy, M. E., Klein, R. P., & McQuiston, S. (1984), Developmental course of parental stimulation and its relationship to mastery motivation during infancy. *Developmental Psychology,* 20:492–503.

Zeanah, C. H. & Anders, T. F. (1987), Subjectivity in parent-infant relationships. *Infant Mental Health Journal,* 8:237–250.

Zeanah, C. H., Keener, M. A., & Anders, T. F. (1986a), Adolescent mothers' prenatal fantasies and working models of their infants, *Psychiatry,* 49:193–203.

Zeanah, C. H., Keener, M. A., & Anders, T. F. (1986b), Developing perceptions of temperament and their relation to mother and infant behavior. *J. Child Psychol. Psychiatry,* 27:499–512.

Zeanah, C. H., Kenner, M. A., Anders, T. F., & Levine, R. (1986c), Measuring difficult temperament in infancy, *J. Dev. Behav. Pediatr.,* 7:114–119.

Zeanah, C. H., Keener, M. A., Stewart, L., & Anders, T. F. (1985), Prenatal perception of infancy personality. *J. Am. Acad. Child Psychiatry,* 24:204–210.

2

Self Development and Self-Conscious Emotions

Michael Lewis, Margaret Wolan Sullivan,
Catherine Stanger, and Maya Weiss
Institute for the Study of Child Development, Robert Wood Johnson
Medical School, University of Medicine and Dentistry of New Jersey

In each of 2 studies, the mirror-rouge technique was used to differenti-
ate children into those who showed self-recognition and those who did
not. In Study 1, 27 children (aged 9–24 months) were observed in 2
experimental situations thought to differentially elicit fear and embar-
rassment behaviors. In Study 2, 44 children (aged 22 months) were seen
in the situations of Study 1 and 3 additional contexts thought to elicit
embarrassment behavior. The results of both studies indicate that
embarrassment but not wariness was related to self-recognition.

This article explores the relation between self development as measured by self-recognition and the expression of fear and embarrassment. Fear, but not embarrassment, has been considered a primary emotion (Tomkins, 1963). Our general hypothesis is that specific cognition skills are necessary for the emergence of the secondary emotions, although they are not necessary for the primary emotions. In particular, self-referential behavior is not necessary for the emergence of fear but is necessary for the emergence of embarrassment.

The current literature on emotions in the first 2 years focuses on the appearance of what has been called the fundamental or primary emotions (Lewis & Michalson, 1983). These emotions are characterized both by their early appearance and by having prototypic and universal facial expressions. Beyond the appearance of these early emotions, the emergence of other emotions remains relatively uncharted,

Reprinted with permission from *Child Development*, 1989, Vol. 60, 146–156. Copyright © 1989 by the Society for Research in Child Development, Inc.

This research is supported from a grant by W. T. Grant Foundation to Michael Lewis and by HD 17205 to Margaret W. Sullivan.

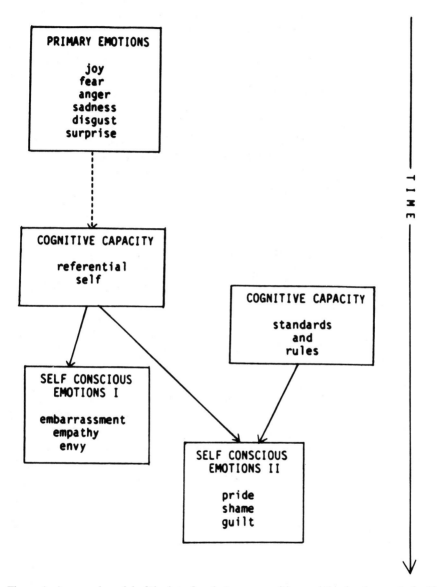

Figure 1. A general model of the interface between cognition and the development of self-conscious emotions.

although some empirical work on pride and guilt, especially within an achievement situation, has recently appeared (Geppert & Kuster, 1983; Heckhausen, 1984).

Theories regarding the origins of the secondary emotions and their dynamics and relation to one another are largely untested, perhaps because measurement methods, operational definitions, and a catalog of possible emotions are not well developed. The appearance of some emotions after the emergence of the primary ones has led to their classification as secondary or derived emotions (Lewis & Michalson, 1983; Plutchik, 1970). The use of the terms primary, secondary, or derived promotes a number of alternative views regarding the course of emotional development. One model presumes that these later emotions are derived from the earlier ones and are composed of combinations of the primary emotions, as all colors are composed from the three primary ones (Plutchik, 1970). Another model considers that these secondary emotions follow the primary ones but are not constructed from these earlier ones (Izard, 1977). Still another model holds that emotions are tied to cognitive processes; those needing the least cognitive support emerge first, and those needing more emerge later (Lewis & Michalson, 1983). To the degree that the earlier, primary emotions contribute to cognitive development, it can be said that they are indirectly related to the secondary or derived emotions (Lewis, Sullivan, & Michalson, 1984).

Although the sequence of emergence of primary emotions has yet to be fully articulated, it seems that by 12 months of age, they all have appeared. Even so, it is not until the middle of the second year that the secondary emotions are observed (Borke, 1971; Lewis & Brooks-Gunn, 1979a; Stipek, 1983). More elaborate cognitive abilities either are necessary for, or occur prior to, the emergence of this new class of emotions—abilities that appear between the end of the first year and the middle of the second year of life.

Figure 1 presents a general developmental model. In Stage 1, the primary emotions appear. The timing of the emergence of particular primary emotions is undetermined as yet; interest, joy, physical distress, and disgust expressions appear to be present at or shortly after birth (Izard, 1977).[1] Anger expressions have been observed as early as 4 months (Stenberg, Campos, & Emde, 1983), surprise by 6 months (Charlesworth, 1969), and given the appropriate eliciting circumstances, surprise, anger, fear, and sad expressions can be observed in 10-week-old infants (Sullivan & Lewis, in press).

In Stage 2, self-referential behavior emerges, although the self system has been undergoing development over the first 2 years of life. Self-other differentiation appears first, followed by object permanence, which appears around 8 months, even

---

[1]The distinction between emotional state, expression, and experience has been made (Lewis & Michalson, 1983; Lewis & Rosenblum, 1974). Here we refer to emotional states and expressions. Emotional experiences require more elaborate cognitive ability (Lewis & Brooks-Gunn, 1979b; Lewis & Michalson, 1983).

though permanence is not consolidated until 18 months or so (Piaget, 1954). Self-referential behavior has a developmental course and appears between 15 and 24 months of age (Bertenthal & Fischer, 1978; Lewis & Brooks-Gunn, 1979b).

The appearance and consolidation of these cognitive skills provide the underpinning for the emergence of Stage 3, the first class of secondary emotions. Self-conscious emotions are characterized by self-referential behavior and include embarrassment, empathy, and perhaps envy. These emotions appear before or around the second birthday. At the same time, children learn about other aspects of their social world, including emotional scripts (Michalson & Lewis, 1985) and rules of conduct that allow them to evaluate their own production and behavior (Kagan, 1981). This leads to the second class of self-conscious emotions—self-evaluative emotions, such as guilt, shame, and pride. Self-evaluative emotions emerge after the self-conscious emotions since they require more cognitive capacity.

In order to observe the relation between self-referential behavior and these secondary emotions, it is necessary (1) to observe the development of two classes of emotion, one associated with primary, the other with self-conscious emotions, and (2) to study their relation to self-referential behavior. The primary emotion of fear (or wariness) will appear early and not require self-referential behavior, while embarrassment should emerge with or following self-referential behavior.

STUDY 1

Method

Subjects

The subjects were 27 infants divided into three age groups: nine were between 9 and 12 months ($\overline{X}$ age: 10.5 months); 10 were aged 15–18 months ($\overline{X}$ age: 17 months); and eight were aged 21–24 months ($\overline{X}$ age: 22.5 months). Data from three additional subjects were omitted from analysis because of an uncooperative child, a videotape problem, and failure of the mother to follow instructions.

Apparatus and Procedure

Each subject was given a Bayley Test of Mental Maturity in addition to the three experimental conditions, the order of which was counterbalanced across all subjects. All conditions were videotaped.

Facing the stranger. The child was seated in a high chair while the mother sat close by in a laboratory room (3 × 4 m). At a signal, an unfamiliar woman appeared in the door and slowly walked toward the child, taking about 15 sec to reach the infant, whereupon she touched the subject's hand, turned, and left the room.

Facing the mirror. The same infants received two different procedures using a mirror. In both situations, the infant was placed in front of a one-way mirror (46 × 89 cm) mounted on a large (1.22 × 2.44 cm) sheet of plywood behind which a videocamera was placed.

In the first procedure, on the experimenter's signal the infant was placed in front of the mirror by the mother. The child's facial and gestural response in front of the mirror was obtained from the videotape. In the second procedure, nonscented rouge was applied to the infants' noses by their mothers, who pretended to wipe their child's face. The children were placed in front of the mirror and their behavior toward the marked nose was observed (see Lewis & Brooks-Gunn, 1979a, for a more specific description).

Measures

Self-recognition. Mark-directed behavior (touching of the spot on the nose) during the mirror-rouge episode has been found to be the most reliable indicator of self-recognition in numerous studies (Lewis & Brooks-Gunn, 1979a), and served as the index of self-referential behavior. Nose touching was scored from videotape for all subjects by two coders; reliability was 100%. Coding of self-recognition was carried out independently of coding the emotions and was done by different codes.

Fear/wariness. The prototypic situation for studying fear in young children has been the approach of a stranger. The appearance of full-blown fear or distress reactions to the stranger approach is not a universal reaction (Rheingold & Eckerman, 1973); however, mild negative reactions and inhibited behavior have been noted and termed wariness (Lewis & Rosenblum, 1974).

Wariness was defined as an attentive look characterized by a neutral or sober facial expression accompanied by a sudden inhibition of ongoing vocal or other behavior and was followed by gaze aversion. All three components were required to be present in the designated sequence in order for wariness to be scored. Whenever they occurred, fear expressions and crying were coded. A fear face was defined as it is described in the MAX coding system (Izard & Dougherty, 1982). Crying also was scored. Interobserver reliability, the number of agreements over number of agreements plus number of disagreements, was (90%) fear, (92%) wariness, and (98%) cry.

Embarrassment. Darwin (1872/1965) was the first to describe self-conscious emotions, including the phenomenon of blushing, although he used self-conscious emotion terms somewhat interchangeably. Izard (1977) and Tomkins (1963) treated shame and embarrassment as behaviorally identical. Embarrassment has been defined to include blushing (originally identified by Darwin in 1872) and a "silly smile" and/or laughter, particularly giggling (Buss, 1980). Hand gestures and body movements also have been implicated as components of embarrassment and serve to distinguish it from amusement (Edelman & Hampson, 1981; Geppert, 1986).

A prototypical eliciting situation does not exist for embarrassment. Buss (1980) has discussed several situations, including breaches of privacy, public self-consciousness, and overpraise. Public self-consciousness, which may be a quite useful procedure with young children, may be elicited by viewing the self in a mirror as others watch. Although it may seem counterintuitive to expect a mirror to elicit embarrassment (it is not a social situation, for example), viewing oneself in a mirror is an attentional manipulation, and one which can direct attention to specific aspects of the self. Amsterdam (1972), Dixon (1957), and Schulman and Kaplowitz (1977) all reported instances of self-conscious behavior in young children viewing themselves in mirrors.

The behavioral criteria for embarrassment were selected by relying primarily on the descriptions of Buss (1980), Edelman and Hampson (1981), and Geppert (1986). The behaviors necessary to score embarrassment were a smiling facial expression followed by a gaze aversion and movement of the hands to touch hair, clothing, face, or other body parts. These hand gestures appear to capture the nervous movements previous investigators state are characteristic of embarrassment. Such body touching could accompany smiling/gaze avert, or follow it immediately. All three behaviors were required for a person to be scored as having shown embarrassment, although very similar findings as those to be reported were found when only smiling and gaze aversion were used as the criteria. Blushing was not used as a criterion for embarrassment since it appears to be an infrequent response, even in older preschool children (Buss, 1980). Interobserver reliability for embarrassment was 85%.

TABLE 1
Distribution of Subjects at Each Age Who Exhibit Various Emotional Behaviors during Stranger Approach and Before a Mirror

AGE (in Months)	N	Cried (n)	Fear (n)	Wary (n)	Embarrassed (n)
Stranger:					
9–12	9	7	1	7	1
15–18	10	1	3	10	1
21–24	8	1	1	6	0
Total	27	9	5	23	2
Mirror:					
9–12	9	2	1	0	2
15–18	10	0	0	0	3
21–24	8	0	0	0	5
Total	27	2	1	0	10

Results

A dichotomous (yes/no) score for self-recognition, crying, fear, wariness, and embarrassed faces was obtained. Table 1 presents these data by age and condition.

Stranger condition. Few subjects cried or showed a fear face, although most showed a wary face. There was a significant difference between wary (and cry) and embarrassed faces ($Z = 4.83, p < .01$) and cry and embarrassed faces ($Z = 5.00, p < .01$). While there were no age differences in wary face, there were age differences in the cry face, $\chi^2(2) = 12.02, p < .01$, with the younger subjects showing the most cry.

Mirror condition. No subjects showed wariness (two showed crying), but 10 subjects showed embarrassment (Wilcoxon $T = 2.00, p < .005$). Nine subjects cried and five showed a fear face in the stranger approach, but only two subjects cried, and one showed a fear face in the mirror condition ($Z = 4.89, p < .01, Z = 3.77, p < .01$, respectively). While 10 subjects showed embarrassment in the mirror condition, only two showed it in the stranger approach ($Z = 2.74, p < .01$). The number who showed embarrassment increased with age, $\chi^2(2) = 9.90, p < .01$.

Self-recognition behaviors. Ten of 27 children showed mark-directed behavior. None touched their noses either during the non-rouge mirror situation or the stranger condition. Age changes were significant, $\chi^2(2) = 5.5, p < .01$, and consistent with prior findings (Lewis, Brooks-Gunn, & Jaskir, 1985).

Relationship between Self-Recognition and Emotional Expression

A chi-square analysis was conducted to determine the relation of both wariness and embarrassment to self-recognition. Yates's corrected chi squares for the total sample ($n = 27$) and Fischer's exact probability, when the data for the 15–24-month-olds were examined ($n = 18$), were used. Wariness was not significantly associated with self-recognition; touchers and nontouchers were equally likely to exhibit wariness, 80% versus 82%, respectively. Embarrassment was more likely to occur for subjects who touched their noses than for those who did not, $\chi^2(1) = 5.32, p < .02$.[2] Of these subjects who showed embarrassment, 80% also touched their noses. Thus, despite the low level of embarrassment exhibited in the study, almost all subjects who exhibited embarrassment touched their noses.

---

[2]When the 15–24-month-olds were combined in an attempt to unconfound age, which is related both to self-recognition and embarrassment, embarrassment was associated with recognition (Fischer's exact probability, $p < .02$).

Relationship between Self-Recognition, Emotional Expression, and General Cognitive Ability

The significant relation between self-recognition and embarrassment and the lack of relation between self-recognition and wariness might be due to a third factor, that is, the child's general cognitive ability. To test for this, we examined children's scores on the Bayley Scales of Infant Development and found no relation between the MDI scores and their performance on any of the three tasks.

Discussion

Infants' responses to the stranger approach situation were consistent with the literature (Rheingold & Eckerman, 1973). Infants showed wariness more than fear. Wariness was expressed when infants faced a stranger and not when they were exposed to a mirror. Wariness, like fear, theoretically need not involve a referential self, although it does require detection of the familiar versus novel and possibly self-other discrimination.

Embarrassment was seen in the mirror, but not in the stranger situation. Mirrors direct the child's attention to itself and result in embarrassment (Amsterdam, 1972). The relatively moderate frequency of embarrassment may be attributable to the situation used to elicit it. Even so, embarrassment in the older two age groups (15–24-month-olds) was moderately high; 44% of the subjects exhibit this behavior.

The relation between self-recognition ability and embarrassment but not wariness was supported. The overwhelming number of subjects who showed embarrassment also touched their noses in self-recognition. No evidence was found for a relation between recognition and wariness or the effects of general cognitive ability on these associations.

STUDY 2

A second study was undertaken to further pursue these results. Besides seeking to replicate the findings, Study 2 addressed some of the specific issues raised. Age changes in self-recognition and embarrassment may have produced a spurious association between self-referential behavior and embarrassment. Use of more subjects all of the same age would not confound the age variable. Although other variables may affect the relation between self-recognition and embarrassment, the results of Study 1 indicate that general cognitive ability is not one of these factors.

The use of more than one situation to elicit embarrassment provides an opportunity to explore situations likely to elicit this emotion. Since Buss (1980) has suggested that exposure and overpraise may elicit embarrassment, we chose, besides the mirror situation, to look at three other conditions likely to lead to embarrassment. Moreover, looking at four situations as elicitors of embarrassment permits an assessment of the amount of embarrassment each child shows by looking at the number of times the child exhibited this emotion.

Method

Subjects

The subjects were 44 children, 19 females and 25 males, who were part of a short-term longitudinal study of emotional development. The mean age of the sample was 22 months ($\pm$ 2 weeks).

Procedures

Each subject received five emotion-eliciting situations administered in a random order. Each was videotaped, and close-up views of the child's face and upper body were obtained. The situations were as follows.

The stranger situation. The situation was conducted as in Study 1 except that a small table and chair were used in lieu of the high chair. An unfamiliar female other than the experimenter served as the stranger during the approach sequence.

The mirror situation. The mirror procedure was the same as in Study 1 and included two segments—one without rouge, which served as the embarrassment situation, and one with rouge, which provided the index of self-referential behavior.

Overcompliment situation. The experimenter initiated interaction with the child, during which she lavishly complimented the child in an effusive manner. A series of four to five compliments were made about the child or his or her appearance. For example, the child was told he was smart, cute, had beautiful hair, and had lovely clothes, etc.

Request-to-dance situations (mother and experimenter). In these two situations, the experimenter handed the mother a small tambourine and asked the mother to coax the child to dance, or did so herself. They each said, "Let's see you dance, dance for me, I'll sing 'Old MacDonald' [or a song familiar to the child]." The dance situation was utilized since conspicuousness is thought to be an elicitor of embarrassment (Buss, 1980). The episode terminated either when the child complied and danced, or upon direct refusal.

Measures

Fear, cry, wariness, and embarrassment, along with self-recognition, were defined and coded as in Study 1. Interobserver reliabilities were fear face

(92%), wariness (92%), cry (95%), embarrassment (87%), and self-recognition (100%).

Results

Table 2 presents the numbers and percentage of subjects by sex showing fear face, crying, wariness, and embarrassment for each of the five conditions. Given the frequencies, only wariness and embarrassment were analyzed. Wariness showed an overall condition effect (Cochran Q test, $Q = 30.15, p = <.001$) such that wariness is more likely in the stranger situation than in any of the others: stranger versus mirror, $\chi^2(1) = 50.22, p < .001$; stranger versus compliment, $\chi^2(1) = 17.3, p < .001$; stranger versus dance/m, $\chi^2(1) = 60.00, p < .001$; stranger versus dance/e, $\chi^2(1) = 22.38, p < .01$. Wariness, rather than embarrassment, was seen in the stranger condition ($Z = 4.08, p < .01$).

Embarrassment also shows an overall condition effect (Cochran Q test, $Q = 14.04, p < .01$) and was less likely to occur in the stranger situation than in any of the others: stranger versus mirror, $\chi^2(1) = 5.78, p < .02$; stranger versus compli-

TABLE 2
Emotional Expression by Experimental Condition

			EXPRESSION					
		Wary		Fear		Cried		Embar-rassed
Condition	N	n	%	n	%	n	%	n	%
---	---	---	---	---	---	---	---	---	---
Stranger:									
Total	44	24	55	0	0	2	5	2	5
Males	25	19	76	0	0	2	8	2	8
Females	19	5	26	0	0	0	0	0	0
Mirror:									
Total	44	2	5	2	5	4	9	11	25
Males	25	1	4	1	5	3	12	6	24
Females	19	1	5	1	4	1	5	5	26
Compliment:									
Total	41	4	10	0	0	1	2	13	32
Males	22	4	18	0	0	0	0	5	23
Females	19	0	0	0	0	1	5	8	42
Dance for mother:									
Total	43	0	0	0	0	4	9	10	23
Males	22	0	0	0	0	3	12	3	13
Females	19	0	0	0	0	1	5	7	37
Dance for experimenter:									
Total	41	2	5	0	0	2	5	13	32
Males	23	2	9	0	0	0	0	4	17
Females	18	0	0	0	0	1	5	9	50

ment, $\chi^2(1) = 8.99$, $p < .003$; stranger versus dance/m, $\chi^2(1) = 4.92$, $p < .025$; stranger versus dance/e, $\chi^2(1) = 8.99$, $p < .003$. Embarrassment did not differ by condition.

Self-Recognition and Emotional Behavior

Across conditions, an aggregate count of the number of subjects who showed a range of behavior was obtained (see Table 3). This range varies from never showing the emotion on any of the four conditions to showing the emotion on each condition.[3] Table 4 presents by condition the number and percentage of subjects who showed wary and embarrassment behavior as a function of self-recognition. It was

TABLE 3
Number of Times Embarrassment and
Wariness Were Observed
Over the Situations Used to Elicit Them

	EMBARRASSMENT (Mirror, Compliment, Dance-M, Dance-E Conditions)				
	0	1	2	3	4
Total	20	9	7	5	3
Males............	14	6	2	2	1
Females	6	3	5	3	2
Touchers	7	7	6	4	2
Nontouchers	13	2	1	1	1

	WARINESS (Stranger Condition)	
	0	1+
Total............	17	27
Males............	4	21
Females	13	6
Touchers........	10	16
Nontouchers......	7	11

---

[3]Table 3 also shows the aggregate score for wary behavior. However, since wariness was exhibited so seldom in the other conditions, the aggregate scores of more than 1 occurred for only five subjects, and we have combined them into the 1 + category

predicted that while there would be no difference between touchers and non-touchers for wary behavior, touchers would show significantly more embarrassed behavior than nontouchers.

The first analysis looked at the numbers of subjects who did and did not show the two emotions across conditions as a function of self-recognition. Of the touchers, seven did not show any embarrassment, while 19 showed embarrassment on at least one condition. Likewise, there were 13 nontouchers who showed no embarrassment, while there were only five nontouchers who showed embarrassment, a significant difference, $\chi^2(1) = 8.08$, $p < .005$. Of those subjects who showed at least one occasion of embarrassment, approximately 80% touched their noses. Moreover, 32 out of 44 subjects showed the predicted relation between embarrassment and self-recognition. Observation of the number who showed wary behavior as a function of self-recognition revealed no significant differences; only self-recognition is related to embarrassment.

A condition analysis (see Table 4) revealed that for the stranger condition, there was no significant difference in wariness as a function of self-recognition, while there were several significant (or near significant) effects for embarrassment. Subjects who showed self-recognition also exhibited more embarrassment in the compliment (Fischer's exact, $p < .055$), dance/m (Fischer's exact, $p < .11$), and

TABLE 4
For Total Sample, Those Who Have Attained Self-Referential Behavior (Touchers) and Those Who Have Not (Nontouchers)

| | % OF SUBJECTS SHOWING WARY OR EMBARRASSMENT | | | | | | | | | |
| | Stranger | | Mirror | | Compli-ment | | Dance-Exp | | Dance-Mother | |
	W	E	W	E	W	E	W	E	W	E
Total............	55	5	5	25	10	32	5	32	0	23
Touchers........	54	8	4	31	4	42	8	44	0	27
Nontouchers.....	56	0	6	17	18	18	0	13	0	18
	NO. OF SUBJECTS SHOWING WARY OR EMBARRASSMENT									
	Stranger		Mirror		Compli-ment		Dance-Exp		Dance-Mother	
	W	E	W	E	W	E	W	E	W	E
Total............	24	2	2	11	4	13	2	13	0	10
Touchers........	14	2	1	8	1	10	2	11	0	7
Nontouchers.....	10	0	1	3	3	3	0	2	0	3

dance/e (Fischer's exact, $p < .02$) conditions. Thus, the overall effect was replicated by observing each of the conditions individually.

Sex Differences

Two classes of sex differences can be observed: first, sex differences in embarrassment and wariness independent of self-recognition; and second, sex differences in the relation between self-recognition and embarrassment. Table 3 allows us to observe these effects. With respect to wariness, four males showed none, while 21 subjects showed at least one occasion of wariness, while for females the numbers were 13 versus six, respectively, $\chi^2(1) = 10.32, p < .002$. Across all four conditions, females showed more embarrassment than males. For males, 15 showed none, while 10 showed at least one occasion of embarrassment, while for females the numbers were 6 versus 13, respectively, $\chi^2(1) = 2.60, p < .10$. Of the subjects who showed two or more occasions of embarrassment, 20% of males and 52% of females showed this effect ($p < .001$). When the same analysis is performed by condition, similar findings appear, especially for the conditions on which there was a high degree of wariness observed. For the stranger and compliment conditions, there is a significant sex difference, with males showing more wariness than females, $\chi^2(1) = 10.74, p < .005; \chi^2(1) = 3.84, p = .05$, respectively. Sex differences in embarrassment by condition indicated that females showed more embarrassment than males for the dance/e condition, $\chi^2(1) = 3.57$, $p < .05$.

Observation of the relation between embarrassment and self-recognition by sex indicates that both sexes show a strong relation between this cognitive milestone and emotional development. Of males who showed embarrassment, 10 out of 11 touched their noses, while of the females who showed embarrassment, nine of 13 touched their noses. Likewise, there was no relation between wariness and self-recognition for either sex.

Discussion

The general discussion will consider three issues: (1) situations eliciting emotions and measures, (2) the interface of cognition and emotion, and (3) individual and sex differences in the development of embarrassment.

Situations and Measures

The data from both studies agree, even though Study 1 varied age. Embarrassment, but not wariness, was related to self-recognition when observed either by looking at age changes in the ability to recognize oneself in the mirror or by looking at individual differences in this ability during the period of time when it is being acquired.

The approach of a stranger has long been used as a situation to elicit fear, although wariness rather than fear is usually observed (see Lewis & Rosenblum, 1974). Embarrassment is elicited by situations that produce exposure of the self, although Buss (1980) describes embarrassment also as being elicited by impropriety or lack of social competence, as well as conspicuousness. There are many situations that might be used to elicit this emotion, and we found that four were successful: viewing oneself in the mirror (in both studies), being complimented, and being asked to perform (to dance). Self-conspicuousness is the central feature of these situations. While these situations are different in terms of the amount of embarrassment elicited, they did not produce much wariness/fear. Likewise, few subjects showed embarrassment during stranger approach. These situations, therefore, are adequate to observe embarrassment.

Although the measurement of wariness/fear has been well established, the measurement of embarrassment has received less attention, although since Darwin (1872/1965) it has been described and seen in young children (Amsterdam, 1972; Dixon, 1957; Lewis & Brooks-Gunn, 1979a; Schulman & Kaplowitz, 1977). In this study, the measurement approach used provides an easy criteria for observing its presence.

One problem with using nervous touching as part of the criteria is that this is a behavior also used in the self-recognition measure. In order to eliminate any confusion, we limited our definition of embarrassment to smiling and gaze averting, a procedure used by some (Buss, 1980). Using this new measure to compare embarrassment with self-recognition resulted in findings quite similar to those when nervous touching is included. Under this measurement procedure, many more subjects would be said to show embarrassment. For example, in Study 1, 21 rather than 10 subjects showed embarrassment. Although the numbers of subjects increase, the percentage of subjects who show embarrassment, without using nervous touching as a criteria, and who show self-recognition is 78%, while 22% show embarrassment and no self-recognition. These figures are similar to the findings using nervous touching; thus, there is no reason to believe that our definition of embarrassment affects the results reported.

The Role of Cognition and Affect

We have suggested that in order for all secondary emotions, both self-conscious and self-evaluative, to emerge, a referential self is necessary. It is important to note that a self system and its development consists of several features (Lewis & Brooks-Gunn, 1979b). While details of this system are still being worked out (see, e.g., Pipp, Jennings, & Fischer, 1987), self-other differentiation, self-permanence, and the ability to consider the self as a separate entity are some of the features of this system. The ability to consider one's self—what has been called self-awareness or referential self—is one of the last features of self to emerge, occurring in the last half of the second year of life. The ability to consider one's self rather than the ability to differentiate or discriminate self from other is the cognitive capacity that allows for all self-conscious emotions such as embarrassment and empathy, although the development of standards is also needed for self-conscious evaluative emotions such as shame, guilt, and pride. Self-referential behavior has been defined operationally as the ability of the child to look at its image in the mirror and to show, by pointing and touching its nose, that the image in the mirror *there* is located in space *here* at the physical site of the child itself. In the results reported in both studies, embarrassment, in general, does not occur unless self-referential behavior exists.[4]

While a third factor may be related to our findings, given the observed relation between embarrassment, but not wariness, and self-referential behavior, it would seem that self-recognition behavior represents an important milestone in the child's development of a self system and in its general cognitive and emotional development.

The relation between the primary emotions and the development of the self has been suggested (Lewis et al., 1985; Schneider-Rosen & Cicchetti, 1984; Stern, 1985), but little empirical work has been conducted relating these two systems. The mother-child relationship has been proposed to affect the development of self, but only two studies have shown any relation (Lewis et al., 1985; Schneider-Rosen & Cicchetti, 1984). While it appears likely that socioemotional behavior and its socialization affect the child's developing self system, there is only weak evidence to indicate any direct effect of early emotional life on the referential self. Nevertheless, the development of the self system impacts on the child's subsequent emotional life.

---

[4]The relation between embarrassment display and self-referential behavior is not perfect. In both studies, a very few subjects showed embarrassment but did not show self-referential behavior. We cannot explain why this occurred, except to point out that very few subjects did so and that the measurement systems, for either self-recognition or embarrassment, are not perfect. It may be the case that a child was scored as embarrassed and was not, or the child did not touch their noses during the test for some reason and should have, given that they possess self-referential ability. The latter seems more likely, since we had only one situation of self-recognition but four situations in which to measure embarrassment. In fact, in Study 2 there were five children who showed embarrassment but did not touch their noses. Review of their behavior before the mirror indicates that four of the five can be said to have recognized themselves. One subject labeled her image by name. The utterance was unintelligible but apparently was accepted by the mother as her name. Three other children showed concern over the rouge on their noses and appeared to be upset by its appearance. Although those four subjects did not touch their noses when they looked in the mirror, they appeared to recognize themselves since they complained about the rouge on their noses. If this is so, then of the subjects who showed embarrassment ($n = 24$), 96% had some type of self-referential behavior.

Sex Differences

While males are more wary than females in the stranger approach situation, females are more embarrassed than males. Sex differences in fear/wariness, when they appear, indicate that females are more wary than males (Maccoby & Jacklin, 1974). For embarrassment, there are still fewer data, unless we look to variables such as sociability or shyness, where there is some evidence that at adolescence females are more shy and less sociable than males (see Crozier, 1979; Gould, 1987). It is difficult to determine exactly why these sex differences appear. Differential socialization practices might account for differences in emotional expressivity (Brooks-Gunn & Lewis, 1982; Malatesta & Haviland, 1982). Although there are few studies in this regard, data from the classroom indicate that teachers are more apt to direct their comments pertaining to the self's action (how well or poorly a problem was handled) to boys than to girls, while they are more apt to direct comments pertaining to the self (good or bad child) to girls than to boys (Cherry, 1975). Differential socialization may produce these sex differences.

Individual differences were determined by obtaining a total score of embarrassment over four conspicuous situations. While most children exhibited either no embarrassment or one embarrassment over the four situations, there were eight children who showed embarrassment 75% or more of the time. Maternal reports confirm that these children are most easily embarrassed. Data collected on these same children at 3 years indicate that these eight children remain easily embarrassed (Lewis, Stanger, & Sullivan, in press). The etiology of individual differences in embarrassment has not been studied; some have suggested, however, that besides differences in parental behavior, temperament differences might play some role (Kagan, Garcia-Coll, & Reznick, 1984; Zimbardo, 1977; Jones, Check, & Briggs, 1986; Zimbardo, 1977). Clearly, more work, both on individual as well as sex differences, needs to be undertaken. Given an adequate measurement system and situations now available to elicit these emotions, such an undertaking is possible.

REFERENCES

Amsterdam, B. K. (1972). Mirror self image reactions before age two. *Developmental Psychology, 5*, 297–305.

Bertenthal, F. I., & Fischer, K. W. (1978). The development of self-recognition in the infant. *Developmental Psychology, 11*, 44–50.

Borke, H. (1971). Interpersonal perception of young children: Egocentrism or empathy. *Developmental Psychology, 5*, 263–269.

Brooks-Gunn, J., & Lewis, M. (1982). Affective exchanges between normal and handicapped infants and their mothers. In T. Field & A. Fogel (Eds.), *Emotions and early interaction* (pp. 161–188). Hillsdale, NJ: Erlbaum.

Buss, A. H. (1980). *Self-consciousness and social anxiety.* San Francisco: W. H. Freeman.

Charlesworth, W. R. (1969). The role of surprise in cognitive development. In D. Elkind & J. H. Flavell (Eds), *Studies in cognitive development: Essays in honor of Jean Piaget* (pp. 257–314). London: Oxford University Press.

Cherry, L. (1975). The preschool child-teacher dyad: Sex differences in verbal interaction. *Child Development,* **46**, 532–535.

Crozier, W. R. (1979). Shyness as anxious self-preoccupation. *Psychological Reports,* **44**, 959–962.

Darwin, C. (1965). *The expression of emotion in animals and man.* Chicago: University of Chicago Press. (Original edition 1872)

Dixon, J. C. (1957). The development of self-recognition. *Journal of Genetic Psychology,* **91**, 251–256.

Edelman, R. J., & Hampson, S. E. (1981). The recognition of embarrassment. *Personality and Social Psychology Bulletin,* **7**, 109–116.

Geppert, U. (1986). *A coding system for analyzing behavioral expressions of self-evaluative emotions.* Munich: Max-Planck Institute for Psychological Research.

Geppert, U., & Kuster, U. (1983). The emergence of "wanting to do it oneself": A precursor of achievement motivation. *International Journal of Behavioral Development,* **6**, 355–370.

Gould, S. J. (1987). Gender differences in advertising response and self-conscious variables. *Sex Roles,* **5/6**, 215–225.

Heckhausen, H. (1984). Emergent achievement behavior: Some early developments. In J. Nicholls (Ed.), *The development of achievement motivation* (pp. 1–32). Greenwich, CT: Jai.

Izard, C. E. (1977). *Human emotions.* New York: Plenum.

Izard, C. E., & Dougherty, L. M. (1982). Two complementary systems for measuring facial expressions in infants and children. In C. E. Izard (Ed.), *Measuring emotions in infants and children* (pp. 97–126). New York: Cambridge University Press.

Jones, W. H., Check, T. M., & Briggs, S. R. (Eds). (1986). *Shyness.* New York: Plenum.

Kagan, J. (1981). *The second year. The emergence of self-awareness.* Cambridge, MA: Harvard University Press.

Kagan, J., Garcia Coll, C., & Reznick, J. S. (1984). Behavioral inhibition in young children. *Child Development,* **55**, 1005–1019.

Lewis, M., & Brooks-Gunn, J. (1979a). *Social cognition and the acquisition of self.* New York: Plenum.

Lewis, M., & Brooks-Gunn, J. (1979b). Toward a theory of social cognition: The development of self. In I. Uzgiris (Ed.), *New directions in child development: Social interaction and communication in infancy* (pp. 1–20). San Francisco: Jossey-Bass.

Lewis, M., & Brooks-Gunn, J., (1985). Individual differences in early visual self-recognition. *Developmental Psychology,* **21**, 1181–1187.

Lewis, M., & Michalson, L. (1983). *Children's emotions and moods: Developmental theory and measurement.* New York: Plenum.

Lewis, M., & Rosenblum, L. (1974). (Eds.). *The origins of fear.* New York: Wiley.

Lewis, M., & Rosenblum, L. (1978). Introduction: Issues in affect development. In M. Lewis & L. Rosenblum (Eds.), *The development of affect: The genesis of behavior* (Vol. 1, pp. 1–10). New York: Plenum.

Lewis, M., Stanger, C., & Sullivan, M. W. (in press). Deception in three year olds. *Developmental Psychology.*

Lewis, M., Sullivan, M. W., & Michalson, L. (1984). The cognitive-emotional fugue. In C. E. Izard, J. Kagan, & R. B. Zajonc (Eds.), *Emotions, cognition and behavior* (pp. 264–288). London: Cambridge University Press.

Maccoby, E. E., & Jacklin, C. N. (1974). (Eds.). *The psychology of sex differences.* Stanford, CA: Stanford University Press.

Malatesta, C. Z., & Haviland, J. M. (1982). Learning display rules: The socialization of emotional expression in infancy. *Child Development, 53,* 991–1003.

Michalson, L., & Lewis, M. (1985). What do children know about emotions and when do they know it? In M. Lewis & C. Saarni (Eds.), *The socialization of emotions* (pp. 117–140). New York: Plenum.

Piaget, J. (1954). *The origins of intelligence in children* (M. Cook, trans.). New York: Norton.

Pipp, S., Jennings, S., & Fischer, K. W. (1987). Acquisition of self and mother knowledge in infancy. *Developmental Psychology, 23,* 86–96.

Plutchik, R. (1970). Emotions, evolution and adaptive processes. In M. Arnold (Ed.), *Feelings and emotion* (pp. 384–402). New York: Academic Press.

Rheingold, H. L., & Eckerman, C. O. (1973). Fear of the stranger: A critical examination. In H. Reese (Ed.), *Advances in child development and behavior* (Vol. 8, pp. 186–223). New York: Academic Press.

Schneider-Rosen, K., & Cicchetti, D. (1984). The relationship between affect and cognition in maltreated infants: Quality of attachment and the development of visual self-recognition. *Child Development, 55,* 648–658.

Schulman, A. H., & Kaplowitz, C. (1977). Mirror-image response during the first two years of life. *Developmental Psychology, 10,* 133–142.

Stenberg, C., Campos, J., & Emde, R. (1983). The facial expression of anger in seven-month-old infants. *Child Development, 54,* 178–184.

Stern, D. N. (1985). *The interpersonal world of the infant.* New York: Basic.

Stipek, D. J. (1983). A developmental analysis of pride and shame. *Human Development, 26,* 42–54.

Sullivan, M. W., & Lewis, M. (in press). Emotion and cognition in infancy: Facial expressions during contingency learning. *International Journal of Behavioral Development.*

Tomkins, S. S. (1963). *Affect, imagery and consciousness: Vol. 2. The negative affect.* New York: Springer.

Zimbardo, P. G. (1977). *Shyness: What it is, what I do about it.* New York: Addison-Wesley.

3

The Role of Self-Understanding in Resilient Individuals: The Development of a Perspective

William R. Beardslee

Children's Hospital, Boston, Massachusetts

Three studies are reviewed in which an in-depth life-history approach was used, and in which a strong connection was demonstrated between self-understanding and resilience. Subjects were civil rights workers in the South, survivors of childhood cancer, and adolescents whose parents had serious affective disorders. Dimensions of the concept of self-understanding which are evident in all three investigations are explored, and the study of resilience as part of an integrative approach to the understanding of human behavior is outlined.

There is increasing awareness of the need for health promotion and disease prevention as a complement to the more traditional approach in which disorders are dealt with only after their appearance (Richmond & Kotelchuk, in press). Interest has grown in ways of characterizing the range and complexity of healthy or adaptive, as opposed to psychopathological, behavior. A major factor contributing to this interest has been the research dealing with youngsters at risk due to a parent's mental disorder, parental divorce, or similar family stress. Despite the expectation that most, if not all, subjects would fare poorly, these risk studies have had in common the finding that significant numbers of youngsters are resilient and manifest highly adaptive behavior. Another contributing factor has been the observation in many longitudinal studies (Kohlberg, Lacrosse, & Ricks, 1972; Vaillant & Vaillant, 1981) that good psychological functioning in childhood and adolescence is the best predic-

Presented at a symposium in honor of Leon Eisenberg at the Harvard Medical School, Boston, November 1987. Reprinted with permission from *American Journal of Orthopsychiatry,* 1989, Vol. 59, No. 2, 266–278. Copyright © 1989 by the American Orthopsychiatric Association, Inc.

Support for this work was provided by a William T. Grant Foundation Faculty Scholar Award to the author and by the Overseas Shipholding Group, Inc.

tor of good adult outcome. Thus, from a developmental point of view, adequate characterization of the dimensions of adaptation is crucial.

As yet no consensus exists with regard to the conceptual framework that would be most useful in assessing healthy behavior, and certainly none with regard to the instruments that would best serve that purpose. Much progress has been made in the refinement of criteria and the construction of standard interview instruments to assess diagnostic categories of psychopathology, but no such comparable effort exists for the measurement of adaptive behavior or resiliency. Part of the problem is that the researcher or clinician must define health or adaptation as a prerequisite to examining it, and there is no agreement on a definition. Indeed, as Offer and Sabshin (1984) have observed, widely divergent definitions exist, ranging from health as normative behavior to health as an ideal state. Further, the range of behavior and inner states that may be adaptive is broader than that used to define a specific disorder or pathology. A wide range of behavior and functioning must be examined. This makes precise definition more difficult.

Investigators who have examined individuals at high risk have begun to characterize adaptation. Moreover, they also have provided examples of resiliency—unusually good adaptation in the face of severe stress. Studies of youngsters at risk that have identified resilient individuals include: *1*) longitudinal examinations of youngsters at risk because of diminished economic resources, minority status, or other factors (Werner & Smith, 1982); *2*) epidemiologic investigations that have included distressed or disadvantaged populations (Rutter, 1979, 1981); *3*) descriptions of response to particular stressful circumstances such as medical illness (Cohen & Lazarus, 1983); and *4*) the experience of growing up in a home with a schizophrenic or affectively disordered parent (Kauffman, Grunebaum, Cohler, & Gauer, 1979; Watt, Anthony, Wynne, & Rolf, 1984).

Since ratings in these studies are based on observed and reported behavior, rather than inferred processes, it has been possible to achieve reliability of ratings. Investigators concur that description of the subject's current behavioral functioning is the first essential step in assessing resiliency and overall adaptation (Beardslee, 1986). The presence of a close, confiding relationship has commonly been found in the early life of resilient individuals; such relationships appear to be protective against the effects of future stressful occurrences (Eisenberg, 1979; Lieberman, 1982; Rutter, 1986). Constitutional factors, for example certain temperaments, are also present in those who become resilient (Porter & Collins, 1982). Also important are inner psychological characteristics and the individual's modes of thought, response, and action. These are expressed in certain coping styles, in positive self-esteem and a sense of being effectual and in control of one's surroundings (Garmezy, 1983; Rutter, 1986). Within this range of ways of coping or responding fits self-understanding, the central focus of the present report.

The author's interest in self-understanding arose from the conviction that the place to begin in studying resilient individuals is with what they themselves report about their own lives, especially about what has sustained them. This is in part because standardized instruments for measuring resiliency do not exist and in part because the individuals studied—civil rights workers, survivors of cancer, and children of parents with affective disorder—lived and worked in life situations that were unusual and not well described. An open-ended, life history data-gathering method was developed. This was applied first to the study of civil rights workers who had stayed in the movement more than 15 years (Beardslee, 1983a, 1983b). Insights and concepts from that study were subsequently applied to the study of the survivors of cancer (Beardslee, 1981) and then to the resilient children of parents with affective disorder (Beardslee & Podorefsky, 1988) systematically identified from a larger study.

The work represents an evolution in both conceptual and experimental terms from an initial study of a few remarkable men and women to a more quantitative approach for identification and description of adaptive behavior. It is based on an inductive approach that builds from individual life experience toward a more general concept of self-understanding. All three studies started with the gathering of detailed information about the many facets of individual lives of resilient young people faced with unusual stress. This paper provides the opportunity to reflect on the commonalities in the role of self-understanding in three rather different groups of resilient individuals.

As an orientation, self-understanding was defined in these studies as an internal psychological process through which an individual makes causal connections between experiences in the world at large and inner feelings. The process of self-understanding leads to an explanatory and organizing framework for the individual. This organizing framework develops over time and eventually becomes a stable part of the individual's experience. Self-understanding requires not only the presence of thought and reflection about oneself and events, but also action congruent with such reflection. In mature self-understanding there is an emotional importance tied to the organizing framework that has evolved: the individual believes that self-knowledge is valuable, takes the process of self-understanding seriously, and devotes time and effort to it.

STUDY METHODS

In the initial study, the author interviewed individuals who had lived in the South and worked in the civil rights movement for more than 15 years, and presented 11 of their life histories in depth. Six years later, 10 of the 11 were reinterviewed; all were found to be working in the same geographic areas, and all had maintained their commitments (Beardslee, 1983a; Beardslee, 1983b). In the second study, the author worked with the principal investigators of a long-term quantitative psychosocial outcome study of survivors of childhood cancer, conducted at the Dana-Farber Cancer Institute (Beardslee, 1981). The study of survivors was undertaken to explore the role of self-understanding in a context very different than that of the civil rights movement, not self-chosen and not under the control of the individual. Indeed, denial of the event and its consequences was expected to be more salient. Three resilient individuals from three different stages of the life cycle—early adolescence, early adulthood, and mid-adulthood—were described. The third study drew on a larger investigation of children of parents with affective disorders, involving 275 youngsters from 143 families, of which the author was principal investigator at the Massachusetts General Hospital (Beardslee & Podorefsky, 1988). By means of over-all adaptive function ratings, the 20 individuals with best functioning in high-risk families were selected. Two and one-half years after the initial assessment, 18 were reinterviewed with a shortened, but standard, assessment of adaptive functioning and psychopathology and by means of the in-depth life history.

The method of data collection was similar in all three endeavors. It involved an in-depth interview with two main components: an open-ended history, starting with the individual's current situation and eventually including both current and past experience, and a focus on the subject's understanding of himself or herself. The interviewer asked specific questions about the individual's history and current situation, and then put questions such as: "How do you understand yourself and your situation?" "What keeps you going?" "What are the sources of your strength?" "How have you been able to cope so well?" "What kinds of insights do you have that help you keep going?" "How would you advise others in this situation to best help themselves?"

The aim throughout was to describe the conscious perceptions and self-understanding of the subject. There was no attempt to interpret unconscious processes or to place the interviewer in the position of being able to make such inferences. The reasons for the study and for their selection were made clear to the subjects from the beginning. Every effort was made to establish and maintain rapport in the interviews.

The analysis of the interviews was done by repeated readings of the verbatim accounts, leading to the identification of common themes, then reanalysis of the interviews to see whether the themes identified appeared in all the histories. In the first two studies, all of the interviewing and the common theme recognition was done by the author. In the third (Beardslee & Podorefsky, 1988), a colleague did all of the interviewing and the common themes were identified by both investigators. Thus, it has been possible to train others in the method.

FINDINGS

Civil Rights Workers

The first main theme in the civil rights workers' accounts was a description of the common stresses they faced in their lives as organizers. They also spoke repeatedly about having to contain, over a long period of time, anger generated by the slow pace of change in the system and the death and disfigurement of so many of the workers. Another theme among the civil rights workers was their shared experience in joining the movement; they were aware of being gripped by and part of something new and strange and good.

Central to their being able to sustain themselves was their closeness to others. Their relationships in the movement involved deep, personal intimacy and superseded all other relationships in their lives. For example, almost all of their marriages reflected a shared commitment to the civil rights movement and almost all of their close friends were movement organizers. The way out of the intense segregation of Southern society led to deep and lasting changes in the personal relationships of those who got involved. These relationships had two dimensions: first, the organizers became dependent on and shared with the other organizers with whom they worked; second, their organizing led to new relationships with people in the communities in which they worked. Both were sustained over time. Also, at least in the workers' accounts, the continual close relationships facilitated major changes in their lives and within themselves; they became organizers and leaders and were able to sustain their endeavors over many years.

Over time, a sense of worth and a belief in what they were doing came to characterize them. Taking action, being organizers, was the visible expression of a new inner consciousness. This new belief came to be integrated, either with a belief system about political organization or a belief system within a religious framework. Gradually, the workers became aware of what they could and could not do and were able to specify more limited goals for themselves. They also tied their current experiences and their psychological identities to their past experience. As one said:

> My roots are here where I started in the Movement. Being in the
> Movement was the start of another life-style for me. Here I came open
> to another way of hope . . . This is the place where I found myself.
> (Beardslee, 1983)

They reported that self-understanding was an essential dimension of their being able to function effectively. This understanding involved an external dimension—an ability to perceive changes in the world and respond to them—and an internal dimension—a means of gauging their capacity to respond to situations and to follow through as required. From a psychological point of view, these few individuals underwent lasting change through the movement. They developed new or significantly altered identities. John Lewis, now a Congressman from Atlanta's Fifth District, offered a clear description of the process:

> Being involved tended to free you. You saw segregation, you saw discrimination, and you had to solve the problem, but you also saw yourself as the free man, as the free agent, being able to act . . . After what Martin Luther King, Jr., had to say, what he did . . . as an individual you couldn't feel alone again. It [being in the Movement] gave a new sense of pride, it was a sense of new identity, really. You felt a sense of control over what was happening and what was going to happen. (Beardslee, 1983b)

From a longitudinal perspective, the identities of these individuals as activists and organizers became a stable part of their lives.

Survivors of Childhood Cancer

Somewhat surprisingly, the cancer survivors had detailed, in-depth memories of what had happened to them and of their medical treatments (Beardslee, 1981). They believed relationships were key in their adjustment. They felt that self-understanding played an important role. Part of their understanding consisted in realistic appraisal of the likelihood of the recurrence of cancer. Putting the event of having cancer into perspective in relation to other events also was important. As an example, one of the survivors had had an amputation and had developed a career as a counselor, helping others with disabilities. His experience in understanding himself in relation to cancer contributed substantially to success in his occupation.

The importance of a developmental perspective was emphasized by examining the three individuals at different stages of the life cycle. Each described his understanding as evolving over time. The developmental life stage defined to some extent the challenges the subject faced; e.g., a high school student expressed concern about athletics, friends, and school, while a man in mid-life was concerned with employment prospects and his children.

Children of Parents with Affective Disorder

The study of adolescent offspring of parents with affective disorders involved two assessments, both employing standard quantitative measures; the later assessment, two and one-half years after the first, included an open-ended interview as well (Beardslee & Podorefsky, 1988). Fifteen of the 18 youngsters were functioning well at both points. At the second assessment, when their average age was 19, these young men and women had developed intimate and rewarding relationships with others; were achievers and problem solvers; were outstanding in school and related activities; and almost all were heavily involved in caring for their ill parents. They were deeply and uniformly aware of parental illness; they described their experience in terms of changes in parental behavior or outlook, such as parents' irritability, sadness, lack of energy, and excessive drinking; they focused on the loneliness of their parents' lives and the disruption of their own lives, rather than distancing themselves through diagnostic categorizing of their parents.

Self-understanding and understanding of their parents' illness were evident in many ways among the 15 individuals who were coping well. They were able to reflect on changes over time in themselves and in their parents' behavior; they were clearly able to distinguish between their own experiences and their parents' illnesses; they were able to talk about parental difficulties and, in many cases, be saddened by them and empathetic, yet not overwhelmed. Most importantly, they were clearly able to think and act independently of their parents' illness; in all cases, they were aware that something was wrong with their parents and had concluded that they were not the cause of their parents' problem. They claimed that the realization that it was not their fault was crucial to understanding what was happening and to their capacity to deal with the experience of having an ill parent.

Dimensions of Self-Understanding

The findings reviewed above suggest five dimensions of self-understanding common to all three studies. Three dimensions involve aspects of the definition of self-understanding which can be applied either cross-sectionally or longitudinally, while the other two can only be understood from a longitudinal perspective.

1. *Adequate cognitive appraisal.* The life situations the individuals faced were complex and changed over time in all three groups. In all three, the individuals were able to describe the major dimensions of the stresses and how they themselves changed. The appraisal of the stresses allowed the individuals to focus their energies and take appropriate action. For example, the focus for the civil rights workers, early in the movement, was the need to draw local people into the struggle, to lead them in demonstrations, and to help them form organizations. The workers' accounts of their early involvement reflected this. In the late sixties and into the seventies, those who stayed had to develop managerial and fund-raising skills, and to assume leadership positions. Some ran for public office. They had to appraise correctly the shifting political and social landscape in order to find opportunities for small projects. Appraisals of the changing circumstances, and of the need for concomitant change within themselves, were crucial components in their long-term commitment to being organizers.

For the children of parents with affective disorder, the course of the parental illness and their life situations changed. Some parents underwent hospitalization and recovered. Some parents experienced chronic insidious disorder from which there was no recovery and which came to color and change their perception of the world. Some families underwent divorce, and relationships with their fathers were lost to the youths, while in other families this did not occur. In some families, extreme economic hardship was experienced and, indeed, the youngsters themselves became wage earners. In some instances, youngsters actually got their parents into treatment for their disorders. Each of the different aspects of parental disorder and the attendant life disruptions had to be identified and responded to separately. The set of issues to be dealt with changed over time; it was essential for the youngsters to recognize what they were dealing with and to change their strategies. Their accounts reflected this.

For the survivors of cancer, their actual medical disorder and its intensive treatment were in the past and had not recurred. The consequences, however, had somewhat different meanings to each, and each individual's awareness changed over time.

Quantitative evidence exists on the connection between stressful life events and short-term illness outcomes (Elliott & Eisdorfer, 1982) and on the importance of cognitive appraisal in managing specific stresses such as hospitalization (Lazarus & Folkman, 1984). This aspect of the changing nature of stress over the long term and the need for the individual to alter his or her appraisal in response, which has not received nearly as much attention, is emphasized by the experiences of these resilient individuals.

2. *Realistic appraisal of the capacity for and consequences of action.* This dimension has two main components: *1)* the individual's assessment of personal capacity for action and *2)* the individual's assessment of the effects of personal actions. Perhaps most striking in this regard were the civil rights workers, who had dreams of transforming the society in which they lived. This vision was vital to their work. Nonetheless, those who stayed in the movement were also able to focus on limited, achievable goals, such as the election of a black county commissioner or the organization of a successful economic boycott. More and more they came to direct their energies to what they could do and learned not to blame themselves for dreams that were not realized. They shaped what they expected of themselves to their capacities and to their assessments of what could be done.

The children of parents with serious affective disorder, who wished to cure their parents, came to understand that this was not possible. At the same time, they realized that their own lives would not be forfeit, and that they could be of great help to their parents in limited ways. This, too, involved realistic appraisal. A sense of identity and of continuity is necessary for an individual to be able to exercise this capacity. A sense of control over one's surroundings, the knowledge that the locus of control resides within oneself, has been shown to be important in a variety of other stressful situations (Lefcourt, 1981; Rotter, 1966). The value of a broad sense of control coupled with the capacity to recognize one's limits is underscored by the accounts of the study subjects.

3. *Action.* In all three studies the individuals who proved to be resilient were those who engaged in actions in the world in addition to having an inner understanding. Children of parents with affective disorders saw themselves as active problem solvers and took a tremendous amount of pride in that. Civil rights workers defined themselves by the actions that they took.

4. *Developmental perspective.* The individuals' self-understanding in all three studies underwent change over time. Adolescents generally described somewhat different issues and had somewhat different concerns than did adults, and their perspectives on themselves were also different. Many of the civil rights workers were in late adolescence when first involved with the movement. They described their concerns at the time primarily in terms of successful actions, such as registering people to vote. At first interview, many had young children; by the second interview many had children entering adolescence. Much of the involvement of the workers now centered on teaching their children and others of their children's age about the movement, passing on what they knew. Thus, as their lives and family situations changed, their perspective changed. Among the survivors of cancer, a similar development of perspective was evident. One man had concerns about fertility because of the radiation treatment he had received. These concerns became prominent in his mind only when he became a young adult and thought of marrying. Another man, who was a father at the time of assessment, spent much time in describing and thinking through how to present his illness to his children.

As the individuals grew older, their understanding of themselves deepened and became more comprehensive. It came to include more elements. This was most explicit in the lives of the civil rights workers, for whom understanding the connections between life experiences prior to the movement and their roles and selves within the movement was essential. They came to recognize crucial continuity in themselves and in their actions and to tie their activism, their new selves as leaders, to their pasts. Each was able to remember a strong parental figure who, in one way or another, opposed segregation and supported the quest for racial justice to which they had dedicated their lives. One of the workers from Mississippi said that her mother always taught her that "black was honest." She indicated that this had been, and remained, very important for her in her activism and leadership (Beardslee, 1983b).

5. *Understanding as a protective factor.* Since self-understanding was seen by all the study subjects as important to their resilience, it is worth exploring the role that the achievement of understanding played in their adaptation to subsequent stress. Although resolving this question is impossible when only cross-sectional data are available, there is enough evidence from the retrospective reports and some longitudinal data to begin to address the issue.

In studying all the life histories, the author was aware that he was tapping into an ongoing process of understanding which had been present for a long time and would continue into the future. The study of the civil rights workers involved a longitudinal component; they were assessed at two points in time, six years apart. The presence of self-understanding at the first point was highly associated with continued self-understanding and continued good functioning at the later assessment. All had remained committed activists. The youngsters whose parents had serious affective disorder were also assessed at two points in time. Their adaptive functioning was relatively stable. Although their self-understanding was not assessed the first time, retrospectively, they reported considerable understanding which had characterized them in the years prior to being interviewed.

Over time, as all these individuals gradually came to find some certainty and predictability in their world and in their sense of themselves, they were able to build on their past experiences to anticipate future experiences. For example, among the youngsters whose parents had serious affective disorders, initial responses to the unanticipated illnesses of their parents were reactive. Eventually, however, the young men and women were able to deal with the various setbacks, hospitalizations, and difficulties of parental illnesses. They learned how to cope with them. That is, they anticipated both the stresses and their own responses; in fact, in coming to understand their responses they were better able to manage the stresses. This was true of the civil rights workers, as well. They initially entered the movement with great intensity and commitment. Through their work they found relationships with others and took actions that made a real and large difference in the rights and the ability of black people to participate in the nation's political process. As these initial experiences became consolidated within the individuals, they were able to change and adapt to the shifting circumstances of the movement, particularly the very difficult times of the late sixties and early seventies. Their sense of themselves, once established, was not altered by subsequent negative events. Part of this was due to fundamental changes in confidence and self-esteem which allowed them to view the future with hope, albeit a "troubled" hope (Beardslee, 1983b). It was almost as if they expected, from time to time, sudden sharp turnings in the course they had been following. Central to their functioning was the ability not to be immobilized by these sudden turnings, but to assess them and then take action.

The survivors of cancer did not anticipate, at least not consciously, having cancer again. They learned what had helped them cope with the illness experience—close personal relationships, for example—and were able to apply this awareness to situations that came up subsequently. In this sense, elements of the individuals' self-understanding can be seen as common across the three studies, although the resilience manifested may be rather different for a person coping with cancer than it is for a civil rights worker who stays in the movement for 15 years.

The factor of past experience was also important in some aspects of these individuals' resiliency, particularly in relationships. In all three studies, those who coped best emphasized the importance of relationships. The capacity to experience relationships in depth, to have intimate and confiding relationships, evolved over time and, to some extent at least in these lives, was heavily dependent on having had good relationships in the past. All of the resilient individuals interviewed in these studies were able to talk not only about sound current relationships but about sound past relationships, as well.

Group Differences

While there are important similarities in the behavior of the three types of resilient individuals studied, there are also notable differences. Perhaps most crucial is the centrality of the stressful experience in the individuals' lives. The civil rights workers' psychological identities were bound up completely with their choice of vocation. That choice influenced much of the subsequent course of their lives, and was an essential element in their understanding of themselves. For the survivors of cancer, the events connected to the disease and its treatment were very important during the course of the illness. After they had recovered, much of their energy was spent in returning to regular functioning and in putting those experiences behind them. For most, the experience of illness did not determine the future course of their lives. Children of parents with affective disorders, on the other hand, underwent the experience of parental illness at a vulnerable stage in their emotional development. Their experience during childhood and adolescence had profound influence on how they later saw themselves within their families and on the leadership roles they adopted within those families. The extent to which this early experience will continue to be a crucial determinant in their lives as they grow up and move outside the sphere of family influence remains to be seen.

DISCUSSION

Conceptual Framework

The method of study reported has been inductive, building from the individual life experience to three main definitional components of understanding and the recognition of two other fundamental concepts: that understanding is a process of development and that it appears to function as a protective factor. The perspective on self-understanding delineated in this paper may relate to several theoretical and conceptual traditions. The first of these is psychoanalytic ego psychology. Following Hartman's (1958) fundamental observation that there are a large number of internal psychological processes which are not defensive and do not rest on conflict, but perform functions in the larger sense of adaptation, control, and integration, a fruitful elaboration of such processes has taken place (Blank & Blank, 1979). In this context, self-understanding can in part be conceptualized among the higher level, complex integrative ego functions. A sense of self is necessary for self-understanding. Recent explorations of the meaning and role of self in psychoanalytic theory may have some relevance in furthering the conceptualization of self (Pine, 1986; Stechler & Kaplan, 1980).

Secondly, Erikson's (1950) concept of a series of life stages, each with its own particular developmental challenge, is relevant to the way that long-term stresses were responded to by the resilient individuals in these studies. In Erikson's terms, the central task of late adolescence is identity formation. At least for the civil rights workers, understanding themselves and what had happened to them became integrated into a sense of identity. In fact, the identity was made clear through the understanding manifest in language in the interviews. Thus, in these resilient individuals, the development, over time, of a capacity to understand themselves both helped them form psychological identities and allowed them to communicate these identities to others.

Within psychology, stemming from the fundamental observations of Jean Piaget, developmental frameworks have been described that demonstrate a series of stages in the evolution and growth of moral development (Kohlberg & Colleagues, 1987) and the capacity to conceive of and enter into the world of the other, i.e., friendship and peer and family relationships (Selman, 1980). Of particular importance within this framework is the capacity for mutuality in adolescence (Beardslee, Schultz, & Selman, 1987). Following a similar theoretical framework, Damon and associates (Damon & Hart, 1982, 1986; Shorin & Hart, 1988) have articulated four increasingly complex and differentiated stages of self-understanding that apply to all youngsters—from early childhood, to middle and later childhood, through early adolescence, and into late adolescence. Dimensions of the self in each of these stages are explored in four main spheres—physical attributes, active attributes, moral or personal choices, and overarching belief systems. As in Selman's work, Damon and associates' theoretical observations are grounded in empirical evidence and the application of these principles to clinical work has begun (Shorin & Hart, 1988). Their work is concerned with describing a universal process and provides an important conceptual framework for the development of self-understanding in individuals.

Whether in the interpersonal negotiation framework of Selman or in the self-understanding framework of Damon, the approach has demonstrated a growth in the cognitive capacity of the developing individual to conceive of the world in increasingly complex terms over time; that is, what is measured is the capacity to think in increasingly differentiated levels. The present author's study of resilient individuals involves subjects who not only have the cognitive capacity to conceive of complex levels of relationships or of self-understanding, but who have taken actions or manifested beliefs consistent with that capacity; that is, they have achieved intimate relationships or have taken action reflecting their understanding. In this sense, two components often separated in more traditional developmental research—theoretical understanding and an action orientation—are both present in the study of these resilient individuals.

The Nature of Self-Understanding

The aim of the interviews and of the studies was to be comprehensive in allowing the individuals to describe the breadth and nature of their world view and their understanding of themselves and their capacities. Family influence, broader social forces or cultural influences, difficulties they had experienced and strengths they had identified were all inquired about in detail. At each point, opportunity was provided for the individuals to comment on what weight the particular factor had in determining how they developed and how they understood themselves.

Given both the in-depth nature of the interviews and the longitudinal perspective, the resulting concept of self-understanding is broad. It is complex, involving many perceptual, cognitive, and affective responses. This approach has not aimed at demonstrating the validity of a larger theory, but rather at examining the proposition that resilient individuals have a total organizing conceptualization of who they are and how they came to be. Furthermore, the way this organizing framework, or self-understanding, contributes to their resiliency has been explored. This comprehensive view yields different insights than does the study of individual component processes of understanding.

Limitations of the Concept

It is important to emphasize that this article has dealt with self-understanding in resilient individuals in particular life circumstances in which identification of stresses and reflection appear to help in adaptation.

Self-understanding was certainly important in the lives of the civil rights workers. It guided their choice to become involved in and then to remain in the movement. Furthermore, they were public figures, involved in leadership. They were able to use their understanding of themselves and their situations to guide others. Their own experiences, their own life stories, were a part of what they shared, of who they were, and of why they were able to be effective leaders. Self-understanding may thus have been of particular importance because they were leaders and organizers. It is possible that in certain other life situations, processes of reflection and self-understanding are less prominent or less meaningful—for example, in performing certain clearly defined tasks, such as coping with an extreme physical environment.

A more general theory of the role of understanding would have to involve study of its application to all individuals, not just those who are resilient. Self-understanding may be particularly strongly associated with resiliency in the face of certain intense stresses, but not so important in general adaptation to living in groups of people in general.

In all three groups of individuals, there had been sufficient time, and the event or stressors had been sufficiently large, for reflection to take place. Focusing on the role of understanding in general problems of adaptation or living would require a somewhat different strategy. The level of understanding that could be expected to be developed within a short time in response to a new stressor remains to be described.

This is not an examination of the etiology of self-understanding or of resiliency. These studies do not deal directly with genetic factors or constitutional ones, such as temperament, which undoubtedly are important at least in laying the groundwork for later resiliency. For example, the children of parents with affective disorder who were resilient were free of medical illness, had relatively high scores on measures of intelligence (average IQ 112), and did not have a history of learning disability or developmental delays. Many youngsters in the overall risk sample who were without physical illness and had high intelligence were not among the resilient, but the coming together of these three characteristics suggests that, on average, the resilient youths probably had some constitutional factors that contributed to their strength.

There is a strong element of judgment inherent in this work, both in the way the interviewers elicited the information and in the recognition and identification of common themes. This may be tempered somewhat by the knowledge and skill of the interviewers. The author had considerable personal experience and had worked in depth in all of the areas investigated. The co-investigator in the third study was experienced in work with children of parents with affective disorder. Still, there is a subjective element in the studies and their findings.

The concentration on the connection between resiliency and self-understanding does not address the issue of how much understanding there is in individuals who do not cope as well in the face of such stresses. For example, the role of understanding in depressed children of parents who had serious affective disorder was not investigated; children who became depressed were not studied because they did not fully manifest resiliency. Furthermore, a means of gauging partial or incomplete self-understanding would have been required, and quantitative instruments to do this are not yet available.

Research Implications

The robustness of the finding of the connection between self-understanding and resiliency in three separate studies, each with more rigorous selection methods and quantitative assessment of adaptive behavior, strongly suggests that self-understanding is an important inner psychological process in resilient individuals. The connection between resiliency and self-understanding in these three nonclinical samples emphasizes the role of self-understanding as a general process in individuals' mastery of difficult situations.

Much more study of the concept of resiliency is indicated. It should involve exploration of genetic and constitutional dimensions and environmental influences, as well as much more detailed characterizations of the components of resiliency. Refinements in the quantitative measurement of self-understanding are also needed. Some recent work indicates that self-understanding can be reliably and validly measured in relation to other ego functions (Beardslee, Jacobson, Hauser, Noam, & Powers, 1986).

In terms of assessment, the life history method has value primarily when used in combination with quantitative measures. What the life history method does provide is a comprehensive approach to describing the stresses that individuals have faced. Furthermore, it presents a rich opportunity for the generation of hypotheses about factors that may contribute to resiliency which may not be captured by existing instruments. The use of the life history method in the study of understanding allows descriptions of individual lives and individual responses. It also permits the investigator to recognize many other qualities, such as courage, personal identity and integrity, and empathy for others, which are distinct from self-understanding but linked in the accounts. Above all, it allows the investigator to probe the comprehensive organizing framework through which an individual makes sense of life experience, and to learn how the individual assesses the influence of that framework.

From a clinical perspective, the work emphasizes the individuality of experience in response to a common stressor, whether it be having cancer or having a parent with serious illness. Clinicians working with individuals who have undergone similar stresses should inquire in as much detail as possible about the response to stresses such as hospitalization of parents, changes in family structure, etc. Attention to the definitional components of self-understanding separately is likely to be useful, as intervention may be directed at any, or all, of them.

This work also suggests that another fruitful area for exploration is the study of ways to enhance individuals' understanding. The success of cognitive therapies and cognitive stress management techniques (Meichenbaum & Jaremko, 1983) indicates that, in a more limited and clearly defined area related to understanding, these approaches have great merit. One approach to prevention of disorder is the description of resiliency, so that what is *in vivo* protective to youngsters can be characterized and used as a model in identifying dimensions to be encouraged in all youths at risk. The development of self-understanding, particularly the dimensions of adequate cognitive appraisal and of ability to take action, appears to help individuals deal with future stresses. This perspective may be usefully instilled in a variety of preventive intervention programs (Beardslee, in press).

Recently, much attention has been given to the need for integrative concepts of behavior that bridge the biological and the environmental or psychologically-based explanations. Rutter (1986) and Eisenberg (1986) have addressed this theme with particular cogency. One promising approach to this conceptual integration may be found in the study of how resilient individuals form their own syntheses of personal experience. The ways in which they understand themselves, the process by which they integrate family and individual influences with other factors, may point the way toward bringing about a synthesis of these different kinds of explanations of human behavior.

REFERENCES

Beardslee, W. R. (1981). Self-understanding and coping with cancer. In G. Koocher & J. O'Malley (Eds.), *The Damocles syndrome: Psychosocial consequences of surviving childhood cancer.* New York: McGraw-Hill.

Beardslee, W. R. (1983a). Commitment and endurance: A study of civil rights workers who stayed. *American Journal of Orthopsychiatry, 53,* 34–42.

Beardslee, W. R. (1983b). *The way out must lead in: Life histories in the civil rights movement* (rev. 2nd ed.). Riverdale, NY: Lawrence Hill and Co.

Beardslee, W. R. (1986). Need for the study of adaptation in the children of parents with affective disorder. In M. Rutter, C. Izard, & P. Read (Eds.), *Depression in young people: Developmental and clinical perspectives.* New York: Guilford Press.

Beardslee, W. R. (in press). The development of a preventive intervention for families in which parents have serious affective disorder: Clinical issues. In G. Keitner (Ed.), *Depression and families: Recent advances.* Washington, DC: American Psychiatric Press.

Beardslee, W. R., Jacobson, A. M., Hauser, S. T., Noam, G. V., & Powers, S. (1986). An approach to evaluating adolescent adaptive processes: Validity of an interview-based measure. *Journal of Youth and Adolescence, 15,* 355–375.

Beardslee, W. R., & Podorefsky, D. (1988). Resilient adolescents whose parents have serious affective and other psychiatric disorders: Importance of self-understanding and relationships. *American Journal of Psychiatry, 145,* 63–69.

Beardslee, W. R., Schultz, L., & Selman, R. (1987). Level of social-cognitive development, adaptive functioning, and DSM-III diagnoses in adolescent offspring of parents with affective disorders: Implications of the development of the capacity for mutuality. *Developmental Psychology, 23,* 807–815.

Blank, G., & Blank, R. (1979). *Ego psychology II: Psychoanalytic developmental psychology.* New York: Columbia University Press.

Cohen, F. & Lazarus, R. (1983). Coping and adaptation in health and illness. In R. Mecham (Ed.), *Handbook of health, health care, and the health professions.* New York: Free Press.

Damon, W., & Hart, D. (1982). The development of self-understanding from infancy through adolescence. *Child Development, 52,* 841–864.

Damon, W., & Hart, D. (1986). Stability and changes in children's self-understanding. *Social Cognition, 4,* 102–118.

Eisenberg, L. (1979). A friend, not an apple, a day will help keep the doctor away. *American Journal of Medicine, 66,* 551–553.

Eisenberg, L. (1986). Mindlessness and brainlessness in psychiatry. *British Journal of Psychiatry, 148,* 497–508.

Elliott, G. R., & Eisdorfer, C. (Eds.). (1982). *Stress and human health: Analysis and implications of research* (A study by the Institute of Medicine, National Academy of Sciences). New York: Springer.

Erikson, E. (1950). *Childhood and society.* New York: Norton.

Garmezy, N. (1983). Stressors of childhood. In N. Garmezy & M. Rutter (Eds.), *Stress, coping and development in children.* New York: McGraw-Hill.

Hartman, H. (1958). *Ego psychology and the problem of adaptation.* New York: International Universities Press.

Kauffman, C., Grunebaum, H., Cohler, B., & Gamer, E. (1979). Superkids: Competent children of psychotic mothers. *American Journal of Psychiatry, 11,* 1398–1402.

Kohlberg, L., & Colleagues (1987). *Child psychology and childhood education: The cognitive-developmental view.* New York: Longman.

Kohlberg, L., Lacrosse, J., & Ricks, D. (1972). The predictability of adult mental health from childhood behavior. In B. Wolman (Ed.), *Manual of child psychopathology.* New York: McGraw-Hill.

Lazarus, R., & Folkman, S. (1984). *Stress, appraisal and coping.* New York: Springer.

Lefcourt, H. (1981). *Research with the locus of control construct, Vol. 1: Assessment methods.* New York: Academic Press.

Lieberman, M. (1982). The effects of social supports on response to stress. In L. Golberger & S. Breznitz (Eds.), *Handbook of stress: Theoretical and clinical aspects.* New York: Free Press.

Meichenbaum, D., & Jaremko, M. (Eds.). (1983). *Stress reduction and prevention.* New York: Plenum Press.

Offer, D., & Sabshin, M. (Eds.). (1984). *Normality and the life cycle: A critical integration.* New York: Basic Books.

Pine, F. (1985). *Developmental theory and clinical process.* New Haven: Yale University Press.

Porter, R., & Collins, G. (Eds.). (1982). *Temperamental difference in infants and young children* (Ciba Foundation Symposium 89). London: Pitman.

Richmond, J.B., & Kotelchuck, M. (in press). Coordination and development of strategies and policy for public health promotion in the United States. In W. W. Holland, E. G. Knox, & R. Detels (Eds.), *Textbook of public health* (Vol. 2). Oxford: Oxford University Press.

Rotter, J. (1966). Generalized expectancies for internal versus external control of reinforcement. *Psychological Monographs: General and Applied, 80* (Whole No. 609).

Rutter, M. (1979). Protective factors in children's response to stress and disadvantage. In R. Kent (Ed.), *Primary prevention of psychopathology, Vol. III: Social competence in children.* Hanover, NH: University Press of New England.

Rutter, M. (1981). Stress, coping and development: Some issues and some questions. *Journal of Child Psychology and Psychiatry, 22,* 323–356.

Rutter, M. (1986). Meyerian psychology, personality development and the role of life experiences. *American Journal of Psychiatry, 143,* 1077–1087.

Selman, R. L. (1980). *The growth of interpersonal understanding.* New York: Academic Press.

Shorin, M. Z., & Hart, D. (1988). Psychotherapeutic implications of the development of self-understanding. In S. Shirk (Ed.), *Cognitive development and child psychotherapy.* New York: Plenum Press.

Stechler, G., & Kaplan, S. (1980). Development of the self. *Psychoanalytic Study of the Child, 35,* 85–105.

Vaillant, G., & Vaillant, C. (1981). Natural history of male psychological health, X: Work as a predictor of positive mental health. *American Journal of Psychiatry, 138,* 1433–1440.

Watt, N., Anthony, J., Wynne, L., & Rolf, J. (Eds.). (1984). *Children at risk for schizophrenia: A longitudinal perspective.* New York: Cambridge University Press.

Werner, E., & Smith, R. (1982). *Vulnerable but invincible: A longitudinal study of resilient children and youth.* New York: McGraw-Hill.

4

Children's Behavioral Inhibition Over Age and Across Situations: Genetic Similarity for a Trait During Change

Adam P. Matheny, Jr.

University of Louisville School of Medicine

Ratings of behaviors pertaining to inhibition were observed for 130 twins participating in a longitudinal study. Ratings were available for four ages (12, 18, 24, and 30 months) and from three sources at each age: direct observations obtained in a laboratory setting, direct observation obtained in conjunction with infant mental testing, and a temperament measure from a questionnaire completed by parents. For the individual twins, the age-to-age correlations were in the moderate range (.26 to .64). The situation-to-situation correlations were generally in the same range (.17 to .64). When the twins were recombined into twin pairs, within-pair (intraclass) correlations indicated that monozygotic (MZ) twins were more concordant than dizygotic (DZ) twins for each of the behaviors at each of the ages. Also, the MZ twins were more concordant for the direction and degree of behavioral change from age to age or from situation to situation. These data provide additional evidence for the biological influence on behavioral inhibition, a characteristic that has been studied in temperament and personality research. The results suggest that the trait of behavioral inhibition and a change in the trait are genetically conditioned. In addition, it is suggested that the concept of trait be expanded to include the person-centered biological regulation of change.

Reprinted with permission from *Journal of Personality,* 1989, Vol. 57, No. 2, 215–235. Copyright © 1989 by Duke University Press.

This report was supported in part by U.S. Public Health Service Grants HD 03217, HD 14352, and HD 22637, the National Science Foundation Grant BNS 76–17315, and by a grant from the John D. and Catherine T. MacArthur Foundation. The assistance of R. Arbegust, J. Henry, M. Hinkle, J. Lechleiter, B. Moss, S. Nuss, D. Sanders, and A. Thoben is gratefully acknowledged.

In recent years there has been a resurgence of interest in reformulating models of personality development to include biological determinants. This change may have been fostered by the advances in genetics and particularly behavior genetics. The identification of a variety of behaviors that earmark infant individuality, however, may be credited with some revamping of strong environmentalistic positions. Individual differences among infants' experiences have accounted for individual differences in some behaviors, but explanations based on experience alone often have faltered. When environmental conditions seemed remarkably similar, such as found in newborn nurseries, behavioral differences among infants seemed to beg for explanations that included inherent biological factors, including genetics. As Escalona observed, "The same environmental conditions are likely to have a different impact upon infants who differ in a biological characteristic" (1968, p. 58).

The studies of individual behavioral differences among infants took shape within the framework of temperament, a construct that has had a synonymous connection with personality, or has been considered as a more biological facet of personality (e.g., Buss & Plomin, 1975; Eysenck, 1981; Gray, 1971). Temperament has been used to refer to innate characteristics, presumably more stable over time, and more isolable among the behaviors of the young human and other mammals. For the study of children, the New York Longitudinal Study (Thomas, Chess, Birch, Hertzig, & Korn, 1963) staked the ground for temperament research as an endeavor apart from personality research.

Berger (1982) has outlined the bridge between the conceptual domains of temperament and personality by suggesting that among children some early appearing behavioral features, such as activity, sociability, and emotionality, provide a common link with similar characteristics among adults. The link could be semantic only, but Berger argued that these behavioral features were shared because there was evidence of behavioral stabilities within and between the two domains. He pointed out, however, that the issue of behavioral stability is a problem. Because behavioral instability has created difficulties for personality traits (Mischel, 1969), it also creates difficulties for temperament traits. Moreover, by implication, behavioral instabilities create difficulties for bridging temperament and personality. Obviously, the isolation of stable temperament characteristics becomes just as important to temperament research as it is to personality research.

Unfortunately, children's temperament as measured in the first years of life has not been found to be markedly stable over time or across situations (for a review, see Hubert, Wachs, Peters-Martin, & Gandour, 1982). Some investigators see this problem as due to the lack of refined temperament measures and have taken steps to create scales and methods of observation that could improve stabilities (e.g., Bates, Bennett-Freeland, & Lounsbury, 1979; Matheny & Wilson, 1981; Rothbart, 1981). Others see instability as an inevitable consequence of the influence of situational or age-related changes. Whatever view prevails, as long as temperament correlations across ages or across situations are relatively low, the evidence for temperament traits is hardly compelling.

Matheny and Dolan (1975) examined the issue of the stability of temperament traits from a different perspective. They studied twins who were assessed for a temperament characteristic—adaptability—extracted from playroom observations and ratings of behaviors during mental testing at five ages between 9 and 30 months. In the playroom, adaptability was represented by a composite of ratings of the child's distress to the departure of a parent, the degree to which the child adjusted to the departure, and the degree to which the child was involved with play activities. In the test-taking situation, adaptability was represented by a composite of ratings on three scales from Bayley's (1969) Infant Behavior Record: social orientation to the examiner, cooperation, and emotional tone. At each of the five ages, there were low-order correlations (rs from .26 to .42) between the two sets of ratings, indicating that the rank ordering of the twins' adaptability scores was not markedly preserved from one situation to the other. Yet, when the patterns of ratings, generated from one situation to the next, were compared for pairs of twins, the identical twin pairs' patterns were more congruent than the fraternal twins' patterns. In effect, while the rank ordering of adaptability for individuals changed across situations, the change was synchronized for two individuals according to their genetic similarity.

The study by Matheny and Dolan (1975) was provocative because it suggested that the concept of trait could include systematic change as well as stability. If regularities of change could be demonstrated from one situation to the next or from one age to the next, then trait manifestations could include both the flow and stasis of behavior.

The present study was undertaken to extend Matheny and Dolan's approach by employing twins to examine a general behavioral characteristic previously identified in studies of temperament and personality as having a strong genetic basis. The behavioral characteristic, inhibition, represents the organism's tendency to approach or withdraw (Thomas et al., 1963) when confronted with the unfamiliar or unexpected. This characteristic in one form or another is considered to be a primary feature of infants' responses to novel persons, objects, and events. Among children, individual differences have been identified by the following: the categories of inhibited versus uninhibited (Garcia-Coll, Kagan, & Reznick, 1984; Kagan, Reznick, & Snidman, 1988); general and specific features of visual novelties (Bronson, 1970; Scarr & Salapatek, 1970); social interaction anxiety versus spontaneity (Kagan & Moss, 1962), and apprehension (Plomin & Rowe, 1979). Similar features have been considered as essential features of adult personality (e.g., Cattell, Eber, & Tatsuoka, 1970; Eysenck & Eysenck, 1985; Gray, 1982; Tellegen, 1985) and have provided developmental links between childhood and the adult years (Kagan & Moss, 1962; Tuddenham, 1959).

During the early years of childhood, this characteristic pertains to individual variations in reactions to unfamiliar objects, people, or events as evidenced by crying, withdrawal, inhibition of activity, shyness, fearfulness, and wariness, in contrast with positive affect, spontaneity in engagements with people or objects, and an outgoing, uninhibited manner. These same contrasts can be found among descriptions of older children's and adults' personalities and figure prominently in the broad distinctions made between introversion and extroversion.

Genetic studies of aspects of inhibition have been conducted for children and adults (Cattell et al., 1970; Daniels & Plomin, 1985; Freedman & Keller, 1963; Goldsmith & Campos, 1986; Goldsmith & Gottesman, 1981; Matheny, 1980, 1983; Matheny & Dolan, 1976; Phillips, Fulker, & Rose, 1987; Rose & Ditto, 1983; Rose, Miller, Pogue-Geile, & Cardwell, 1981; Torgersen & Kringlen, 1978). The evidence indicates that among infants, children, adolescents, and adults there is a strong genetic influence on individual differences found for sensitivity to threat, fears, shyness, and inhibition when confronted with novelty. Few of the studies cited have focused on the developmental change, if any, of behavioral inhibition, particularly during early childhood when individual differences are not as likely to remain stable over time.

For the present study, behavioral inhibition was investigated by a multimethod, longitudinal approach. To map behavioral inhibition, we chose three sources of ratings: emotional tone—from direct observations obtained in a laboratory setting; fearfulness—from direct observations obtained in conjunction with infant mental testing; and approach/withdrawal—from a temperament questionnaire completed by parents. Ratings from all three sources were available for twins followed in a longitudinal study when the twins were 12, 18, 24, and 30 months of age.

METHOD

Subjects

The twins in this study were recruited as part of a longitudinal study of temperament (Wilson & Matheny, 1986). From the larger longitudinal sample, twin pairs with complete longitudinal data at 12, 18, 24, and 30 months were selected. The twins were from families representing the entire socioeconomic range found in the Louisville, Kentucky, metropolitan area. According to the occupations of head of household (Reiss, 1961) about 30% of the families were in the lowest two deciles of the rating scales of occupation, and the remaining families were distributed in roughly equal proportions among the remaining eight deciles.

Zygosity was established for the same-sex twin pairs by determining the match for 22 or more antigens tested from blood-typing. A lack of match on any of the antigens classified a twin pair as fraternal. For practical reasons, the twins were not blood-typed until they were at least 3 years of age. As a consequence, all of the data had been collected prior to an objective determination of zygosity.

The data to be reported were obtained from 130 twins who came from 33 pairs of identical twins and 32 pairs of fraternal twins. The fraternal twin pairs consisted of 19 same-sex pairs and 13 opposite-sex pairs.

Behavior During Laboratory Observations

The laboratory observations were made when infants visited the laboratory at 12, 18, 24, and 30 months. During the visits, the infants were engaged in a standard set of specific activities organized in a prearranged sequence in a playroom. The activities, called vignettes, took place with and without the presence of the infants' mothers, with each twin infant engaged alone with a staff member when the other twin was given Bayley testing, and with both twin infants together but engaged individually with two staff members. All vignettes were scheduled in a sequence exactly duplicated for all infants; videotapes of the vignettes were made according to a timed format carefully organized to yield one hour of videotape representing a morning visit at the laboratory. The organization of the visits, schedule and description of the vignettes, and format for videotaping have been provided elsewhere (Matheny & Wilson, 1981); for illustration, however, several of the vignettes employed at the specified ages are described below.

Cuddling (12 months). The infant is picked up and held by the interactionist in an upright position with the infant's head resting on the interactionist's shoulder. The interactionist's free arm provides support for the infant's back. (After the infant is placed in this position, the degree to which the infant's body stiffens, pushes away, or yields to cuddling is noted.) As the infant is held, the interactionist turns around slowly so that the infant's postural adjustment can be videotaped from several angles. The routine is carried out with the infant held at least once in the left arm and at least once in the right. (Time allotted, 2 minutes.)

Visible Barrier (12 months). This vignette is based on a test item from the Cattell Infant Intelligence Scale (1960). The infant is seated in a feeding table which has a large tray in front, and the infant is given an attractive small toy. When the infant holds the toy and proceeds to play with it, the toy is taken from the infant and moved away, but within reach. As the infant reaches for the toy, a transparent plexiglass screen is placed upright between the infant and the toy. If the infant does not attempt to obtain the toy, the screen is removed and the same or another toy is given to the infant. If the toy evokes interest, the procedure is repeated. (Time allotted, 2 minutes.)

Cobbler Bench (18, 24, and 30 months). The infant is seated in front of a small wooden bench with pegs inserted in holes in the bench. The infant is shown how to hit the pegs with a wooden hammer in order to drive the pegs from one side to another. The infant is encouraged to attempt and then continue the procedure. (Time allotted, 2 minutes.)

Super-Brix (18, 24, and 30 months). Large, lightweight cardboard blocks are placed in front of the infant who is encouraged or helped to build a tall structure. Once the structure is completed, the infant is given a ball and encouraged to knock down the structure. The staff member creates a lot of excitement about the structure being torn down. (Time allotted, 2 minutes.)

Trick-Box (18, 24, and 30 months). Two boxes, identical in size and appearance, are placed in front of the infant. Each box has a lid at the top and a door at the side. One "ordinary" box is completely empty inside; the other—"trick"—box has a mirror inside that gives the illusion of the box being completely empty when, in fact, only part of the interior is visible. The infant is shown an attractive toy being placed in the top of the "ordinary" box and shown how to obtain the toy by opening the side door. On repeated trials, when the infant can retrieve the toy without being shown, the toy is placed in the top of the trick box and, as before, the infant is asked to find the toy. The exercise is repeated. (Time allotted, 2 minutes.)

Other vignettes provided opportunities for a twin to respond to an imitative game, role-play with a doll and a puppet, look at a book of pictures, and engage in play with a mechanical dog that barks while moving toward the twin. In total, there are 15 vignettes provided to the twins at each age. Several of the vignettes were conducted with both twins together, but the largest number were conducted with each twin separated from parent and co-twin. The schedule of videotaped vignettes included 18 minutes for each twin separately, 12 minutes for both twins together, but with parent absent, and 12 minutes for an orientation session and a finale that included the parent. About half of the vignettes were conducted by one team of interactionists and about half by a different team. Therefore, an interactionist did not participate with the same twin throughout the entire visit.

The rating scales used in the laboratory playroom were emotional tone, activity, attentiveness, social orientation, and vocalizing. Previous factor analyses incorporating these scales indicated that the core temperament factor, composed of emotional tone, attentiveness, and social orientation, was anchored by the scale emotional tone (Matheny, Wilson, & Nuss, 1984; Wilson & Matheny, 1983, 1986); therefore, emotional tone was used to represent inhibition in the playroom. This scale refers to the child's principal emotional state rated along a 9-point scale: 1 = extremely upset, crying vigorously; 3 = upset, but can be soothed; 5 = bland, no apparent reaction; 7 = contented, happy; 9 = excited, animated.

Ratings of emotional tone were made by having raters—who had not interacted with the twins—independently view a videotape and then rate emotional tone for each successive 2-minute period. The ratings for all of the 2-minute periods were condensed by obtaining an average rating that represented each twin's predominant emotional tone for the succession of experiences in the laboratory playroom. Interrater reliability for emotional tone has been found to be .92 (Wilson & Matheny, 1983).

Behavior During Mental Testing

During a portion of the visit to the research center, each twin accompanied by a parent was taken to a room adjacent to the laboratory playroom. There the twin was given the Bayley Scales of Infant Development (Bayley, 1969), a developmental test which includes the Infant Behavior Record (IBR). The IBR consists of rating scales that represent a wide variety of behaviors observed during Bayley testing, and is filled out after the test is completed. From the rating scales, the scale fearfulness was selected for this study because it refers to the degree of fear, caution, or inhibition of actions observed throughout developmental testing. The highest rating of 9 represents a strong indication of a fear of the strange; the lowest rating of 1 represents no evidence of fear, caution, or inhibition. Interrater reliability for fearfulness was determined for 172 infants and found to be .78.

Behavior From the Temperament Questionnaire

The mother's report of the child's temperament at each age was assessed by having the mother complete the Toddler Temperament Scale (Fullard, McDevitt, & Carey, 1984), a questionnaire based on the nine characteristics of temperament formulated by the New York Longitudinal Study (Thomas et al., 1963). The 97 items comprising the questionnaire refer to behaviors associated with specific activities and events at home. Each item is rated on a 6-point scale ranging from 1 = almost never, to 6 = almost always typical of the child. Twelve items pertain to approach/withdrawal, the temperament characteristic that refers to the child's tendency to move toward or withdraw from persons, events, and situations. In accord with the study by Garcia-Coll et al. (1984), this characteristic was selected to represent the mother's report of the twins' behavioral inhibition. The average rating of the 12 items was calculated so that a lower score represented more withdrawn or inhibited behaviors. One-month, test-retest reliability for 47 children has been reported to be .89 for approach/withdrawal (Fullard et al., 1984).

In summary, ratings representing twins' tendencies to be inhibited or uninhibited were available as part of the behavioral assessments for three situations—the standardized set of activities in a laboratory playroom, the structured set of activities during mental testing, and the relatively unstructured activities and events within the home setting—for four ages: 12, 18, 24, and 30 months.

RESULTS

Behavioral Stability

The stability of individual differences was evaluated by computing the age-to-age correlations[1] for the three temperament measures obtained at the four ages. The results are shown in Table 1.

The age-to-age correlations were moderate and generally comparable for intervals of 6 months. Quite obviously, the longer intervals, such as 12 to 30 months, produced the lowest correlations, especially for the measure fearfulness. In the main, all three temperament measures provided significant stability coefficients; nevertheless, the moderate level of the stability coefficients indicated that the rank ordering of the twins' scores for each temperament measure was changing from one age to the next.

TABLE 1
Age-to-Age Correlations for Temperament Measures Obtained at 12,
18, 24, and 30 Months

| Age-to-age interval (months) | Temperament measures (source) | | |
	Emotional tone (lab)	Fearfulness (test)	Approach (parent)
12 to 18	.48	.26	.58
12 to 24	.30	.20	.49
12 to 30	.28	.01	.27
18 to 24	.56	.61	.62
18 to 30	.48	.28	.48
24 to 30	.51	.50	.64

[1]For the computation of correlations among measures from the individual twins, including both twins in every pair introduces dependencies in the data set. Randomly selecting one twin from each pair would remove the dependencies, but the sample size would be halved. To retain the original sample size, another approach was taken. The data set was divided into identical and fraternal pairs, then these sets were further divided into two sets each: twins in each pair whose given names were first alphabetically (Twin A) and twins in each pair whose given names were second alphabetically (Twin B). The correlations were then computed for the four sets: identical twin A, identical twin B, fraternal twin A, fraternal twin B. The correlations for the four sets were transformed to Fisher's *z* coefficients, averaged, and then converted to the correlations shown in Tables 1 and 2.

Convergent Validity

Table 2 provides the concurrent correlations among the temperament measures for each of the four ages. The relations were modest, with the majority of the correlations being found in a range from .32 to .64 (average $r = .45$).

Evidently, at each age there was a convergence among the three temperament measures: laboratory playroom, mental testing, and parental report. Despite the differences in settings, instruments employed, and observers, a common feature of the twins emerged. The feature at one extreme represented a child who tended to be emotionally distraught, fearful, or inhibited in the presence of "strange" activities, and withdrew from novel events, persons, or situations. At the other extreme, the feature represented a child who tended to be positive in emotional tone, not fearful, and less inhibited or withdrawn in the face of novelty. This feature, as defined by the rating scales employed, is akin to the distinction between inhibited-uninhibited children described by Garcia-Coll et al. (1984).

TABLE 2
Concurrent Correlations Among Temperament Measures Obtained
at 12, 18, 24, and 30 Months

Age and measures	Temperament measures (source)		
	Emotional tone (lab)	Fearfulness (test)	Approach (parent)
12 Months			
Emotional tone	—	.51	.36
Fearfulness		—	.43
Approach			—
18 Months			
Emotional tone	—	.64	.42
Fearfulness		—	.44
Approach			—
24 Months			
Emotional tone	—	.63	.34
Fearfulness		—	.42
Approach			—
30 Months			
Emotional tone	—	.56	.32
Fearfulness		—	.17
Approach			—

Note. Correlations $> .18$, significant at $p < .05$, $N = 130$.

Twin Analyses

The next question concerned the degree of genetic influences on the three temperament measures for each of the four ages. This question was addressed by comparing the pair (intraclass) correlations for identical or monozygotic (MZ) twin pairs with the pair correlations for fraternal or dizygotic (DZ) twin pairs. Therefore, the individual twins were reconstituted into 33 pairs of MZ twins and 19 pairs of same-sex DZ twins. Opposite-sex DZ pairs were excluded from the twin analyses because behavioral contrast within girl-boy pairs might contribute to lower DZ correlations.

The pair correlations for the MZ and DZ twins are presented in Table 3. Regardless of age or measure, the magnitude of the MZ correlations was higher than that of the DZ correlations. With the exception of measures of emotional tone and fearfulness at 12 months and approach at 24 months, the differences between the MZ and DZ correlations were significant. The negative correlations for the measure of approach of fraternal pairs do not fit a genetic model for fraternal correlations, and may represent either parental reports exaggerating contrasts within fraternal pairs, or error from the small sample of DZ pairs. Nevertheless, the consistent pattern of the differences argues for a strong genetic influence on each of the aspects of behavioral inhibition from 12 to 30 months.

Synchrony of Changes

Over age. From Table 2, the age-to-age stability correlations of each of the temperament measures indicated that the individual twins were undergoing relative changes over time. With these stability correlations as background, the pattern of

TABLE 3
Twin Correlations for Temperament Measures

Measure	Zygosity	Age			
		12 months	18 months	24 months	30 months
Emotional tone (lab)	Identical	.59	.83*	.87*	.79*
	Fraternal	.27	.28	.26	.25
Fearfulness (test)	Identical	.76	.77*	.80*	.63*
	Fraternal	.48	.02	.20	− .09
Approach (parent)	Identical	.67*	.83*	.15	.48*
	Fraternal	− .21	− .07	− .16	− .18

Note. Number of pairs: 33 identical, 19 same-sex fraternal.
*$p < .05$ for R identical $> R$ fraternal.

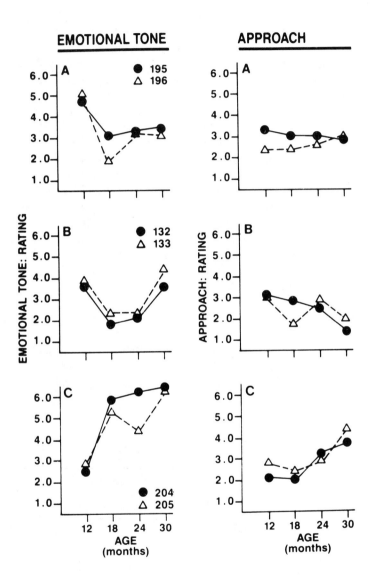

Figure 1. Illustrative Curves for Ratings of Emotional Tone and Approach for Three Monozygotic Twin Pairs

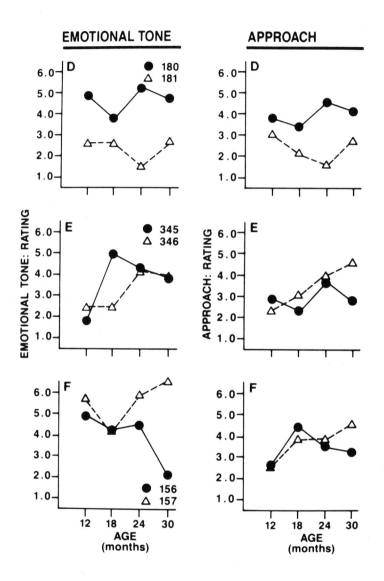

Figure 2. Illustrative Curves for Ratings of Emotional Tone and Approach for Three Dizygotic Twin Pairs

the MZ/DZ correlations in Table 3 suggested that when age-to-age changes occurred, MZ twin pairs were more concordant than DZ twin pairs for such changes. If that were the case, age-to-age changes can be attributed to a genetically influenced, systematic effect, rather than to other unidentified sources, including measurement error. The systematic effect would simply be shown by the evidence that the MZ twin pairs share a more similar pattern of change over ages than the DZ twin pairs.

To illustrate, the ratings of emotional tone and approach for three MZ twin pairs were plotted for ages 12 to 30 months and the resultant curves are presented in Figure 1. Each data point represents each twin's rating for emotional tone or approach, with lower ratings representing either more distress or more withdrawal. One MZ pair, the bottom pair depicted in panel C, became more positive and approachful over age; the top pair in panel A became less positive and more withdrawn over age; and the middle pair in panel B showed a decrease and then increase in positive emotionality but a gradual decrease in approach for one twin contrasted with a zigzag change for approach as measured for the other twin. In general, with some divergence within a twin pair at some ages, the pattern for one MZ twin was matched by that of the other MZ twin.

For contrast, similar plots of emotional tone and approach were made for three DZ pairs, and these curves are presented in Figure 2. In these pairs, the divergence within each pair is evident. For example in the bottom DZ pair (panel F) the twins diverged markedly for emotional tone so that by 30 months one twin was considerably more positive than the other. The DZ twins in panel D also diverged markedly for emotional tone and approach, and stood in sharp contrast with the DZ pair depicted in panel E.

TABLE 4
Twin Concordance for Temperament Profiles: Across Age or Across Measures

Measure (over 12, 18, 24, 30 months)	Pair correlations	
	Identical	Fraternal
Emotional tone (lab)	.79*	.26
Fearfulness (test)	.75*	.21
Approach (parent)	.53*	− .15
Age (over emotional tone, fearfulness, approach at same age)		
12 months	.69*	.31
18 months	.79*	.08
24 months	.68*	.12
30 months	.66*	.00

$*p < .05$ for R identical $> R$ fraternal.

These trends in the curves generated by the MZ and DZ pairs were expressed for the entire sample by computing pair (intraclass) correlations. The pair correlations for these profiles take into account both the elevation of the scores within each pair and the matching of the profile of age-to-age changes within each pair (Wilson, 1979). Prior to the computations, the total variance of the scores for the set of MZ pairs and the set of DZ pairs was compared. There was no significant difference between the two sets.

The correlations for the profile analyses applied to emotional tone, fearfulness, and approach over the four ages are provided in Table 4. The pair correlations for the MZ pairs were significantly higher than those for the DZ pairs, indicating that the age-to-age changes in the twins' behavior were synchronized more closely within MZ pairs.

Across situations. The same analytic strategy applied to find the profile similarity of age-to-age changes for each behavior was appropriate for the analyses of twin similarity across situations at each age. Again, prior to computing the pair (intraclass) for the MZ and DZ pairs, the total variance for each set of twins was compared. No significant differences were found between the two sets.

The MZ and DZ pair correlations for profile similarity across situations at each age are presented in Table 4. Here again, the MZ pairs were significantly more concordant than the DZ pairs. Thus, at any age, whatever behavioral changes were represented by the ratings obtained from the three situations, the MZ pairs were yoked together more closely than the DZ pairs for such changes.

Composite score: Behavioral inhibition. The sequence of steps of the analyses, whose results are shown in Tables 1 to 4, was provided to show how each measure contributed to the trait and to the twin analyses for the trait. A further logical step was to construct a composite score of behavioral inhibition for each twin by adding standardized scores of the three measures obtained for each twin of each of the four ages. The composite of the three temperament measures presumably represents three items of a single scale representing the trait at each age. The age-to-age corre-

TABLE 5
Twin Correlations for Composite Scores of Behavioral Inhibition

Age	Pair correlations	
	Identical	Fraternal
12 months	.71*	.25
18 months	.90*	.08
24 months	.81*	.11
30 months	.73*	.03
Profile: 12 to 30 months	.79*	.13

$*p < .05$ for R identical $> R$ fraternal.

lations for the composite scores were the following: 12 to 18 months, .51; 12 to 24 months, .37; 12 to 30 months, .18; 18 to 24 months, .61; 18 to 30 months, .53; 24 to 30 months, .64. The MZ and DZ pair correlations for the composite scores of behavioral inhibition at each age and the profile correlations across ages are shown in Table 5.

DISCUSSION

The results from this study, with multimeasure, multi-occasion data, affirm the identification of a temperament characteristic that characterizes some children's tendencies to be vigilant, still, less active, upset, shy, or withdrawn when faced with doubtful, unfamiliar, or unexpected occurrences. The contrasting tendencies of other children represent the bolder, less guarded, more outgoing and positive aspects of encounters with the same environmental conditions. Garcia-Coll et al. (1984) refer to children represented by the first set of behaviors as inhibited and the children represented by the second set as uninhibited, a distinction that she and her colleagues established clearly when extreme groups were identified. Other investigators (e.g., Bronson, 1970; Kagan & Moss, 1962; Plomin & Rowe, 1979; Tuddenham, 1959) have focused on essentially the same childhood behaviors; the labels attached to the contrasting features have differed somewhat, however. At the moment the choice of labels is arbitrary, but it is clear that in a variety of ambiguous or unfamiliar situations, some children are more negative, guarded, or hesitant even to the point that they will withdraw or, given advance warning, avoid such situations entirely. Among adults, similar behavioral tendencies to be shy, cautious, timid, or restrained are classified as qualities of introversion (Eysenck & Eysenck, 1985) and represent a dimension of inhibitory control (Tellegen, 1985). In one fashion or another, at one age or another, at least the outlines of a temperament/personality trait seem to be established.

The stability of behavioral inhibition also supports a trait notion. In the present study, the age-to-age correlations for each behavioral feature obtained from each of the situations indicated a modest level of stability over half-year intervals. Bronson (1970) has found that fear as represented by crying at 4 to 9 months was correlated (.56) with shyness between 2 and 3 years. From the Fels longitudinal data, Kagan and Moss (1962) have reported that behavioral inhibition during the first 3 years, as represented by anxiety concerning social interactions, predicted similar characteristics during a subsequent 3-year period. Children who were extremely inhibited during the first 3 years were more likely to disengage or refrain from peer interactions during the second 3-year period. Tuddenham (1959) found stability from 14 to 33 years for individuals characterized along a dimension representing inhibition—spontaneity.

The data from the present study as well as other studies of children (Daniels &

Plomin, 1985; Freedman & Keller, 1963; Goldsmith & Campos, 1986; Goldsmith & Gottesman, 1981; Matheny, 1980, 1983; Matheny & Dolan, 1976; Torgersen & Kringlen, 1978) provide mounting evidence that there is a consistent and strong genetic influence on inhibitory behaviors. The present study extends the evidence considerably by characterizing the trait by several methods over several occasions and then demonstrating evidence of MZ > DZ correlations for either method or occasions.

The present evidence for a trait must be qualified, however, because the sample sizes are small. Moreover, the correlations for the individual twins observed across methods (situations) were modest. In fact, the correlations derived for individual twins measured by the three methods at each age are subject to the criticisms raised by Berger (1982). In the present study, for example, situation-to-situation correlations ranged from .17 to .64. In addition, if one considers age differences as representing loosely defined changes in situations, the age-to-age correlations (ranging from .01 to .64) reflect the same limitations. Therefore, the empirical results simply add to a collection of similar correlations now accumulating for temperament traits (Hubert et al., 1982).

By now the problem of the consistency and stability of personality—the relative importance of traits or situations for determining behavior—has been reviewed extensively (e.g., Jackson & Paunonen, 1980; Kendrick & Funder, 1988). The discussions have varied, with suggestions encompassing an appeal that behavioral aggregates will improve measures of the behavioral stability or consistency of traits (Epstein, 1980; Paunonen, 1984), proposals for analyses incorporating interactions between traits and situations (e.g., Magnussen & Endler, 1977; Thomas & Chess, 1980), and reminders that literal consistency or stability may not be as important as the identification of coherence among different behaviors (Kagan, 1980; Magnusson & Endler, 1977).

Among these suggestions, the recommendation for behavioral aggregates to improve trait stability is particularly germane to the present study. The measure of emotional tone in the laboratory is an aggregate of ratings across a variety of activities spanning about a 3-hour visit. Approach/withdrawal as rated by the parents is an aggregate of 12 items presumably reflecting the parents' distillation of observations across a wide variety of activities during 6-month intervals. By and large, these two measures were more reliable and more stable than the measure of fearfulness which was obtained from a single rating representing an examiner's distillation of a testing interval of about an hour. Moreover, an additional aggregate, created by a composite score of all three measures, provided somewhat improved age-to-age stabilities of the trait examined in this study.

The trait model that has been subject to much criticism assigns the primary determinants of behaviors to internal dispositions that maintain behavioral consistencies from situation to situation. It is not necessary for consistency to be demonstrated by the preservation of equivalent levels of a specified trait among individuals from one situation to the next. Consistency is demonstrated by the maintenance of rank ordering of individuals even when the absolute levels of the trait change from situation to situation or from time to time. In terms of variance, the percentage of variance attributed to trait consistency must overshadow the percentage of variance attributed to some other source(s). At the moment, it is fashionable to consider the other source(s) as situations.

Unfortunately, situations may be defined conceptually in such a way that they can vary continuously and their numbers can be increased limitlessly. In effect, the variance attributed to situations can be increased to a considerable degree.[2] Given the flexibility of defining situations and the requirement that a trait must be consistent, one can liken situations to the bellows of an accordion and a trait to a note or chord that must be played repeatedly but not necessarily in the same octave. Changes in the note or chord played are attributed to movements of the accordion's bellows, even if the musical composition was written in such a way that other keys could or should be played.

The present twin study and two previous twin studies (Dworkin, 1979; Matheny & Dolan, 1975) suggest that one can demonstrate strong person-centered consistencies even when there are modest correlations for persons across situations. Dworkin (1979) required adult twins to complete questionnaires that asked for reports of reactions pertaining to anxiety or dominance for various situations. These imagined or projected measures of anxiety or dominance were then used to compare MZ and DZ correlations. For anxiety, but not dominance, the MZ correlation exceeded the DZ correlation, suggesting that the cross-situational profile was genetically influenced. Dworkin's study called upon imagined responses to situations, and one might speculate that the MZ twins were more concordant than DZ twins for the cognitive activities underlying imagination; the results could be simply an indirect effect from genetic influences on cognition. Nevertheless, the previously described study by Matheny and Dolan (1975) and the present study do not depend on twin subjects' reporting how they might respond in various situations.

The evidence for a genetic influence on the patterning of changes of temperament and personality traits assessed for twins is gradually accumulating and has been reviewed elsewhere (e.g., Plomin, 1986; Rowe, 1987). Although the congruences among patterns of twins' temperament or personality measures have not been as high as the congruence for intelligence (Wilson, 1978), the genetically influenced synchronization of the patterns is clearly apparent. The behavioral trajectories representing short-term changes from one observation to the other seem to be coordinated systematically for genetically related individuals. It is this coordination of the

---

[2]It is also true that the variance for traits can be made larger (e.g., Bowers, 1973; Golding, 1975).

MZ twin pairs' changes in the behavioral patterns that informs us that there is a semblance of a trait that regulates behavior.

REFERENCES

Bates, J. E., Bennett-Freeland, C. A., & Lounsbury, M. L. (1979). Measurement of infant interactions. *Child Development, 50*, 794–803.

Bayley, N. (1969). *Bayley scale of infant development.* New York: Psychological Corporation.

Berger, M. (1982). Personality development and temperament. In R. Porter & G. M. Collins (Eds.), *Temperamental differences in infants and young children* (pp. 176–187). London: Pitman.

Bowers, K. S. (1973). Situationism in psychology: An analysis and a critique. *Psychological Review, 80*, 307–336.

Bronson, G. (1970). Fear of visual novelty: Developmental patterns in males and females. *Developmental Psychology, 2*, 33–40.

Buss, A. H., & Plomin, R. (1975). *A temperament theory of personality development.* New York: Wiley.

Cattell, P. (1960). *The measurement of intelligence of infants and young children* (rev. ed.). New York: Psychological Corporation.

Cattell, R. B., Eber, H., & Tatsuoka, M. M. (1970). *Handbook for the Sixteen Personality Factor Questionnaire (16PF).* Champaign, IL: IPAT.

Daniels, D., & Plomin, R. (1985). Origins of individual differences in infant shyness. *Developmental Psychology, 21*, 118–121.

Dworkin, R. H. (1979). Genetic and environmental influences on person-situation interactions. *Journal of Research in Personality, 13*, 279–293.

Epstein, S. (1980). The stability of behavior: II. Implications for psychological research. *American Psychologist, 35*, 790–806.

Escalona, S. (1968). *Roots of individuality.* Chicago: Aldine.

Eysenck, H. J. (1981). *A model for personality.* Berlin: Springer-Verlag.

Eysenck, H. J., & Eysenck, M. W. (1985). *Personality and individual differences.* New York: Plenum.

Freedman, D. G., & Keller, B. (1963). Inheritance of behavior in infants. *Science, 140*, 196–198.

Fullard, W., McDevitt, S. C., & Carey, W. B. (1984). Assessing temperament in one to three year old children. *Journal of Pediatric Psychology, 9*, 205–217.

Garcia-Coll, C., Kagan, J., & Reznick, J. S. (1984). Behavioral inhibition in young children. *Child Development, 55*, 1005–1019.

Golding, S. L. (1975). Flies in the ointment: Methodological problems in the analysis of the percentage of variance due to persons and situations. *Psychological Bulletin, 82*, 278–288.

Goldsmith, H. H., & Campos, J. J. (1986). Fundamental issues in the study of early temperament: The Denver Twin Temperament Study. In M. E. Lamb, A. Brown, & B. Rogoff

(Eds.), *Advances in developmental psychology* (pp. 231–283). Hillsdale, NJ: Lawrence Erlbaum.

Goldsmith, H. H., & Gottesman, I. (1981). Origins of variation in behavioral style: A longitudinal study of temperament in young twins. *Child Development, 52*, 91–103.

Gray, J. A. (1971). *The psychology of fear and stress.* New York: Plenum.

Gray, J. A. (1982). *The neuropsychology of anxiety.* Oxford: Oxford University Press.

Hubert, N. C., Wachs, T. D., Peters-Martin, P., & Gandour, M. J. (1982). The study of early temperament: Measurement and conceptual issues. *Child Development, 53*, 571–600.

Jackson, D. N., & Paunonen, S. V. (1980). Personality structure and assessment. *Annual Review of Psychology, 32*, 503–551.

Kagan, J. (1980). Perspectives on continuity. In O. G. Brim & J. Kagan (Eds.), *Constancy and change in human development* (pp. 26–74). Cambridge, MA: Harvard University Press.

Kagan, J., & Moss, H. A. (1962). *Birth to maturity.* New York: Wiley.

Kagan, J., Reznick, J. S., & Snidman, N. (1988). Biological bases of childhood shyness. *Science, 240*, 167–171.

Kendrick, D. T., & Funder, D. C. (1988). Profiting from controversy: Lessons from the person-situation debate. *American Psychologist, 43*, 23–34.

Magnussen, D., & Endler, N. S. (1977). *Personality at the crossroads: Current issues in interactional psychology.* Hillsdale, NJ: Lawrence Erlbaum.

Matheny, A. P., Jr. (1980). Bayley's Infant Behavior Record: Behavioral components and twin analysis. *Child Development, 51*, 1157–1167.

Matheny, A. P., Jr. (1983). A longitudinal study of stability of components from Bayley's Infant Behavior Record. *Child Development, 54*, 356–360.

Matheny, A. P., Jr., & Dolan, A. B. (1975). Persons, situations, and time: A genetic view of behavioral change. *Journal of Personality and Social Psychology, 32*, 1106–1110.

Matheny, A. P., Jr., & Dolan, A. (1976). Twins: Within-pair similarity on Bayley's Infant Behavior Record. *Journal of Genetic Psychology, 28*, 263–270.

Matheny, A. P., Jr., & Wilson, R. S. (1981). Developmental tasks and rating scales for the laboratory assessment of infant temperament. *JSAS Catalog of Selected Documents in Psychology, 11*, 81 (Ms. No. 2367).

Matheny, A. P., Jr., Wilson, R. S., & Nuss, S. M. (1984). Toddler temperament: Stability across settings and over ages. *Child Development, 55*, 1200–1211.

Mischel, W. (1969). Continuity and change in personality. *American Psychologist, 24*, 1012–1018.

Paunonen, S. V. (1984). Optimizing the validity of personality assessments: The importance of aggregation and item content. *Journal of Research in Personality, 18*, 411–431.

Phillips, K., Fulker, D. W., & Rose, R. J. (1987). Path analysis of seven fear factors in adult twin and sibling pairs and their parents. *Genetic Epidemiology, 4*, 345–355.

Plomin, R. (1986). *Development, genetics, and psychology.* Hillsdale, NJ: Lawrence Erlbaum.

Plomin, R., & Rowe, D. C. (1979). Genetic and environmental etiology of social behavior in infancy. *Developmental Psychology, 15*, 62–72.

Reiss, A. J. (1961). *Occupations and social status.* New York: Free Press of Glencoe.

Rose, R. J., & Ditto, W. B. (1983). A developmental-genetic analysis of common fears from early adolescence to early adulthood. *Child Development, 54*, 361–368.

Rose, R. J., Miller, J. Z., Pogue-Geile, M. F., & Cardwell, G. F. (1981). Twin-family studies of common fears and phobias. In L. Gedda, P. Parisi, & W. E. Nance (Eds.), *Twin research 3: Intelligence, personality and development* (pp. 169–174).

Rothbart, M. K. (1981). Measurement of temperament in infancy. *Child Development, 52*, 569–578.

Rowe, C. D. (1987). Resolving the person-situation debate: Invitation to an interdisciplinary dialogue. *American Psychologist, 42*, 218–227.

Scarr, S., & Salapatek, P. (1970). Patterns of fear development during infancy. *Merrill-Palmer Quarterly of Behavior and Development, 16*, 53–90.

Tellegen, A. (1985). Structures of mood and personality and their relevance to assessing anxiety, with an emphasis on self-report. In A. H. Tuma & J. D. Maser (Eds.), *Anxiety and the anxiety disorders* (pp. 681–706). Hillsdale, NJ: Lawrence Erlbaum.

Thomas, A., & Chess, S. (1980). *The dynamics of psychological development.* New York: Brunner/Mazel.

Thomas, A., Chess, S., Birch, H. G., Hertzig, M., & Korn, S. (1963). *Behavioral individuality in early childhood.* New York: New York University Press.

Torgersen, A. M., & Kringlen, E. (1978). Genetic aspects of temperamental differences in infants: A study of same-sexed twins. *Journal of the American Academy of Child Psychiatry, 17*, 433–444.

Tuddenham, R. D. (1959). The constancy of personality ratings over two decades. *Genetic Psychology Monographs, 60*, 3–29.

Wilson, R. S. (1978). Synchronies in mental development: An epigenetic perspective. *Science, 202*, 939–948.

Wilson, R. S. (1979). Analysis of longitudinal twin data. *Acta Geneticae Medicae et Gemellologiae, 28*, 93–105.

Wilson, R. S., & Matheny, A. P., Jr. (1983). Assessment of temperament in infant twins. *Developmental Psychology, 19*, 172–183.

Wilson, R. S., & Matheny, A. P., Jr. (1986). Behavioral genetics research in infant temperament: The Louisville Twin Study. In R. Plomin & J. Dunn (Eds.), *The study of temperament: Changes, continuities, and challenges* (pp. 81–97). Hillsdale, NJ: Lawrence Erlbaum.

5

Attachment, Temperament, and Adrenocortical Activity in Infancy: A Study of Psychoendocrine Regulation

Megan R. Gunnar

Institute of Child Development, University of Minnesota

Sarah Mangelsdorf

University of Michigan

Mary Larson and Louise Hertsgaard

Institute of Child Development, University of Minnesota

Examined the relations among adrenocortical stress reactivity, infant emotional or proneness-to-distress temperament, and quality of attachment in 66 infants tested at 9 and at 13 months. Performed the Louisville Temperament Assessment at 9 months and conducted the Strange Situation at 13 months. Adrenocortical activity was not associated with attachment classifications. Emotional temperament at 9 months was strongly correlated with emotional temperament at 13 months. There was also evidence that at both ages infants who were more prone to distress experienced greater increases in adrenocortical activity during the laboratory tests. Significantly, however, although both the Louisville Temperament Assessment and the Strange Situation involve maternal separation (a potent stimulant of the adrenocortical system in nonhu-

Reprinted with permission from *Developmental Psychology,* 1989, Vol. 25, No. 3, 355–363. Copyright © 1989 by the American Psychological Association, Inc.

This research was supported by National Institute of Child Health and Human Development Grant HD-16494 to Megan R. Gunnar. Portions of these data were presented at the meeting of the Society for Research in Child Development, Baltimore, April 1986.

We would like to thank all those who helped in this research, including Debra Andreas, Joan Connors, Jill Isensee, Sarah Lang, and Roberta Kestenbaum. Special appreciation is expressed to Michael Steffes, Kay Gornik, and Linda Nelson for their work in establishing the salivary cortisol assay, and to Adam Matheny and the late Ron Wilson for their generosity in providing training tapes and data for the Louisville Assessment.

man primate infants), we noted only small elevations in cortisol, and
these elevations were significant only at 9 months.

The past few years have seen a renewed interest in the study of the interplay between psychological and physiological processes during normal development. This renewed interest can be traced to (a) increased awareness of the intimate linkages between central and peripheral physiological systems (e.g., Cernic & Pennington, 1987; Kandel & Schwartz, 1981; Locke et al., 1985), (b) renewed interest in the study of temperament and its physiological basis among developmental psychologists (Goldsmith et al., 1987), and (c) improved measurement techniques allowing assessment of brain activity and neuroendocrine activity, in addition to autonomic nervous system activity, in both normal and atypical populations of infants and children (e.g., Fox & Davidson, 1987; Gunnar, 1987; Kagan, Reznick, & Snidman, 1987; Nelson & Salapatek, 1986).

Activity of the adrenocortical system and linkages between this neuroendocrine system and emotion systems near the end of the first year form the focus of this article. The adrenocortical system has long been of interest to researchers concerned with stress reactivity and the regulation of stress reactions in human adults and animals (Mason, 1968). In addition to physical trauma, psychological events are known to produce elevations in cortisol, the primary hormonal product of this system in humans (Mason, 1968). Currently, there is controversy over whether negative emotional states or collative variables associated with novelty, uncertainty, and strangeness characterize the psychological factors that trigger the adrenocortical stress response (Gunnar, Mangelsdorf, Kestenbaum, Lang, Larson, & Andreas, in press; Gunnar, Marvinney, Isensee, & Fisch, in press; Levine, 1985; Rose, 1980; Tennes & Mason, 1982). Under circumstances in which negative emotions are the normative response to novel, uncertain, or strange events, however, these two perspectives cannot be distinguished. Both would predict positive correlations between emotional distress and elevations in cortisol. Such positive correlations have been found in studies examining newborns (Anders, Sachar, Kream, Roffwarg, & Hellman, 1970; Gunnar, 1986; Tennes & Carter, 1973) and older infants (Tennes, Downey, & Vernadakis, 1977). What has not been examined is whether a stable, temperament-like disposition of proneness to distress in uncertain situations is associated with the magnitude of the adrenocortical response. We examined this in the present study.

We used maternal separation as the uncertain event. In nonhuman primate infants, maternal separation triggers large and prolonged elevations in cortisol (e.g., Levine, Wiener, Coe, Bayart, & Hayashi, 1987). There is also evidence that the magnitude of the response is associated with characteristics of the mother-infant relationship. Infants from more balanced, harmonious relationships show greater increases in cortisol upon separation than infants from more imbalanced, disharmonious relationships (Gunnar, Gonzales, Goodlin, & Levine, 1981). In the only study of cortisol and maternal separation in human infants, Tennes, Downey, and Vernadakis (1977) failed to find significant increases in urinary cortisol excretion following a 1-hour home separation among 12-month-old infants. The familiar home environment, however, may have helped to buffer the response. Nonetheless, as in the nonhuman primate data, Tennes et al. did find that babies who were more responsive when their mothers returned showed higher cortisol excretion rates than babies who were ambivalent or avoidant using Ainsworth's scales. They also found that babies who were more distressed during the separation had higher cortisol excretion rates. These data, then, raise the possibility that cortisol elevations during separation might be linked both to the infant's temperamental proneness to distress in response to uncertain situations and to the quality of the mother-infant attachment relationship. Specifically, infants who are more prone to distress and who have secure relationships with their mothers may be more stressed by separation, as indexed by adrenocortical activity, than babies who are either less prone to distress or who are from insecure relationships. According to Belsky and Rovine's (1987) recent argument, this would suggest that infants receiving Ainsworth's B3 and B4 classifications should exhibit higher cortisol concentrations than infants in other attachment classification groups because they are viewed as being both securely attached and prone to distress. Conversely, Ainsworth's A (avoidant) babies should exhibit the least increase in cortisol during separations because they are viewed as being neither securely attached nor prone to distress. We examined the linkages between adrenocortical activity during separation and both prone-to-distress temperament and quality of attachment.

A third focus of our research was methodological. The development of techniques to measure cortisol in small samples of free-flowing saliva, as opposed to earlier techniques requiring urine or blood, has opened the door to measurement of this neuroendocrine system in normal infants and children. Currently, there are a number of research projects underway in the United States, Europe, and Scandinavia in which salivary cortisol is being measured to index stress in infants and children. Those doing this work, however, are still operating largely in the dark with regard to the events that will trigger increases, developmental changes in the cortisol response, the factors influencing basal activity, when to sample, and what to expect with regard to individual differences. Therefore, we also examined some of these questions.

In order to examine these questions, we tested infants at 9 and, again, at 13 months. Infant temperament was assessed in four ways: First, at 9 months we observed the infant in the home and obtained measures of social and emotional behavior under low-challenge conditions. Second, at 9 months we conducted the Louisville Laboratory Temperament Assessment (Matheny & Wilson, 1981). This assessment involves two long maternal separations (19 and 30 min). The Louisville Assessment was chosen because measures of emotional tone (*high distress to glee-*

ful) derived from it have been shown to (a) correlate with maternal reports of infant temperamental reactions to novelty and strangeness, (b) correlate at 9 and 24 months with neonatal measures of irritability, and (c) reflect genetic influence (Matheny, 1984; Matheny, Riese, & Wilson, 1985; Matheny, Wilson, & Nuss, 1984; Riese, 1987). The length of the assessment (1 hr), the fact that it was conducted in an unfamiliar laboratory setting, and the duration of separation (49 min total) also allowed us to examine whether separation would trigger elevations in cortisol under conditions and at an age that would seem optimal for triggering an adrenocortical response. Third, at 13 months the mothers completed the Toddler Temperament Scale (Fullard, McDevitt, & Carey, 1984), and we analyzed the three dimensions shown by Matheny (1984) to correlate with the Louisville Temperament measures (i.e., approach, adaptability, and mood). Finally, we assessed quality of attachment at 13 months using the Strange Situation (Ainsworth & Wittag, 1969).

METHOD

Subjects

The subjects were 75 infants who were 9 months (± 2 weeks) at first testing. Of these, 35 girls and 31 boys completed the 13-month assessments and constituted the sample analyzed here. Average paternal education was 15.5 years (range = 12–20 years), and average maternal education was 15.4 years (range = 10–20 years). Approximately half of the subjects (56%) were firstborn and only children. At 9 months, 82% of the babies were not in any form of day care (including a nanny in the home). Seven infants were in day care for less than 20 hr a week, and 5 were in day care for more than 20 hours a week. According to maternal report, those not in day care were with babysitters for an average of between two and four times a month.

Procedure

Parents were contacted by telephone using a file from the Institute of Child Development at the University of Minnesota of families interested in participating in research. The general procedures were described and an appointment was made for the initial home visit.

Nine-month home visit. We scheduled home visits (60–75 min) in the morning hours at the parents' discretion, with the restriction that we observe a normal feeding. The purpose of the visit was to teach the mother to obtain measures of salivary cortisol and to observe mother-infant feeding and play interaction. The observer obtained a salivary cortisol sample shortly after arriving at the home (see description of salivary sampling below). The Egeland Feeding and Play Scales were then completed (Egeland, Deinard, Taraldson, & Brunnquell, 1975). In most cases, one observer visited the family, but, for 15 families, two observers were present to obtain estimates of agreement. On the basis of previous reports (Vaughn, Taraldson, Crichton, & Egeland, 1980), we chose seven infant scales for analysis of infant home temperament. (Maternal data will be reported elsewhere.) The key variable was a 9-point scale labeled *Baby's Temperament,* a scale of the infant's emotional tone during the home observations. The actual range in our sample was from 4 (between Point 3, *moody, inconsistent,* and Point 5, *content, neutral*) to 9 (*pleasant and cheerful, seems almost always in a pleasant mood and often responds with glee and pleasure*). The other measures were as follows: crying at beginning of observations (0/1); looks at mother during feeding (9 points); social behavior of baby (7 points); general activity level (6 points); satisfaction with play (9 points); and poor attentiveness during play (distribution in our sample was from 5 = *balanced attention,* to 9 = *highly distractible*).

Observer agreement within one scale point ranged from 73% to 100% ($M = 90\%$), and Cohen's kappas ranged from 0.50 to 0.92. The low agreement was for looks at mother, and discrepancies on this item appeared to be due to difficulty in positioning both observers so that each could see the infant's face. The infant scales were summed according to the sign of their correlation coefficient with the Baby Temperament scale to produce a Home Emotional Temperament score. Item-total correlations were as follows: 0.81 for emotional temperament, 0.73 for social behavior, 0.48 for satisfaction with play, 0.30 for looks at mother, -0.55 for poor attention, and -0.52 for crying. (The correlation for activity level was negligible.)

Nine-month Louisville Assessment. Within 1 week of the home observation, the mother and infant came to the University for the Louisville Temperament Assessment. First, we obtained an initial salivary sample. The experimenter then took 6 min to explain the assessment to the mother and to help the mother and infant feel comfortable. This 6-min warm-up period was videotaped. The mother then left the room, and the experimenter began the Louisville Assessment vignettes (see Matheny & Wilson, 1981). The infant experienced two sets of vignettes, each set conducted by a different experimenter. Between sets there was a 5-min reunion period with the mother. The first set of vignettes consisted of seven 2-min task periods that were videotaped for later scoring and one 5-min free-play period that was not scored (19 min total). The second set of vignettes included nine 2-min task periods and two 6-min free play periods that were not scored (30 min total). In all, infants who completed the entire assessment were separated from their mothers for a total of 49 min. If an infant became upset, the experimenter stopped administering the task/vignette and began a standardized soothing sequence. If the baby could not be soothed, that set of vignettes was terminated, and the mother returned to the room. If the first set of vignettes was terminated, the second set was attempted.

One coder scored all of the Louisville tapes for the key variable *emotional tone,* the principal emotional state during each 2-min scoring period (1 = *extremely upset, wailing, protest*, 3 = *momentary upset, short verbal protest*, 5 = *bland, undifferentiated emotionally*, 7 = *sustained smile, approachful and reactive during part of the interval*, and 9 = *highly excited, gleeful, or animated*). A second coder scored a subset of the tapes for agreement (Cohen's $_k$ = 0.85). In addition, Matheny and Wilson provided several videotapes and scoring sheets that were used during training to ensure similarity in interpretation between research groups. We computed separate scores for each of the four sections of the assessment (i.e., warm-up, Vignettes 1, reunion, and Vignettes 2). Emotional tone was prorated for sessions that were terminated early because of distress. Prorating was done within each section of the assessment. Thus, if Vignettes 1 had to be terminated early, the score for emotional tone during Vignettes 1 was prorated, but the score for the next section, reunion, was based on infant behavior during reunion. As noted, the second set of vignettes was always attempted, even when the first set had to be terminated early. This allowed all infants to be scored for emotional tone in all sections of the assessment.

Thirteen-month Toddler Temperament Scale. As a means of examining the stability of emotional temperament in our sample, the mothers were mailed the Toddler Temperament Scale (Fullard et al., 1984) several weeks prior to the 13-month assessment. Three items shown by Matheny (1984) to be highly correlated with emotional tone from the Louisville assessment were chosen for analysis. They were Approach (high scores reflect withdrawal), Adaptability (high scores reflect poor adaptability and problems in management; e.g., the child accepts being dressed and undressed without protest, the child can be coaxed out of a forbidden activity, etc.), and Mood (high scores reflect negative mood). Because of a clerical error, nearly one-third of the questionnaires were missing several pages, and, thus, each scale was missing items. The alpha coefficients, especially for the Approach scale (0.86), have been shown to be good for infants of this age (Prior, Sanson, Oberklaid, & Northan, 1987). Nonetheless, we calculated all results reported for these scales both with and without subjects with incomplete questionnaires. None of the results differed significantly, and results are reported for the entire sample.

Thirteen-month attachment assessment. At 13 months (±2 weeks), the infants and their mothers returned to the University for the Strange Situation assessment (Ainsworth & Wittig, 1969). Immediately on entering the testing room and prior to performing the Strange Situation test, a salivary sample was obtained. The Strange Situation was videotaped and subsequently coded following procedures described in Ainsworth, Blehar, Waters, and Wall (1978). (The primary coder, Debra Andreas, and the reliability coder, Sarah Mangelsdorf, were trained by L. Alan Sroufe.) Intercoder agreement was 90% for subclassifications. Three infants were classified as D because they showed a combination of avoidant and resistant behavior. Of the remaining 63 infants, 16% (n = 10) were avoidant (A), 58% were secure (B; 16 were B1 or B2, and 21 were B3 or B4), and 25% were resistant (n = 16). Others have reported similar distributions for comparable samples (e.g., Belsky & Rovine, 1987). In addition to quality of attachment coding, a second coder, blind to the classifications, scored all the tapes using the Emotional Tone scale. Emotional Tone was scored every minute and averaged within each 3-min Strange Situation period. Agreement estimates (Cohen's $_k$ = 0.81) for the scoring of Strange Situation emotional tone were obtained with the coder who scored the 9-month Louisville videotapes.

Independence of coders and experimenters. All assessments were completed by coders and experimenters who were blind to the infants' behavior in other assessments.

TABLE 1
Salivary Cortisol Collection Periods With Means and Standard Deviations of Sampling Times

Sample	Time		Purpose
	M (a.m.)	SD (min)	
			9 months
Observer Home	8:30	26	Teach mother to collect saliva and obtain early morning base
Parent Home	9:45	52	Obtained on a "normal" day within 1 week of laboratory test as a baseline against which to judge the laboratory preseparation concentrations
Initial Laboratory	10:00	43	Obtained as a baseline against which to judge the response to laboratory testing; taken as soon as the infant got to the laboratory; expected that coming to a new place might elevate cortisol
Post Laboratory	10:56	46	Obtained at the end of the Louisville assessment; duration of testing varied with infant distress; correlation between duration of testing and delta cortisol (post–initial) was $-.25$ ($p = .06$), with distress controlled, $r = .05$
			13 months
Parent Home	9:24	48	As at 9 months
Initial Laboratory	9:20	47	As at 9 months
Post Laboratory	9:52	49	Obtained at the end of Strange Situation testing; duration of testing varied with infant distress; correlation with delta cortisol was $-.04$ (NS)

Note. Correlations between time of sampling and cortisol corrected for number of tests were all *ns*. One correlation was greater than .20 (Initial Laboratory at 13 months). There were no differences in sampling times or in average duration between Initial and Post samplings among attachment groups.

Salivary cortisol. We sampled saliva for cortisol determination seven times during the study. Samples were obtained by swabbing the mouth and having the infants chew or suck on a cotton dental roll. Wetted sections of the cotton roll were then placed in a needleless syringe, and clear saliva was expressed into a vial and stored briefly (i.e., less than 36 hours) in a standard freezer section of a refrigerator. Samples were then placed at $-20°C$ until assayed. Whenever possible, 500µl of clear saliva were collected. At least a sample of 250 µl was needed for duplicate assay. To encourage sucking and stimulate saliva production, the cotton roll was dipped in sweetened Kool-Aid crystals. Use of the cotton roll has the advantage of being simple and efficient, but also has the disadvantage of slightly altering the cortisol values. Pilot testing with adults showed that concentrations of cortisol were approximately 0.05 µg/dl higher with the cotton roll; however, values calculated with and without the cotton roll were highly correlated ($r > .90$).

The seven collection periods are described in Table 1 along with the mean time of collection. All testing was conducted in the morning hours, and care was taken to schedule infants at approximately the same time of morning at both the 9- and 13-month assessments. Because of schedule conflicts, however, the testing at 13 months occurred approximately 40 min earlier than the testing at 9 months. Within subjects, home and laboratory baselines at each age were obtained, on average, within 20 min of the same time, although on different days. Within subjects across age, home baselines were obtained within 20 min (on average) of the same time, and laboratory baselines were obtained within 40 min (on average) of the same time.

Salivary samples were assayed in batches, with all samples for the same infant in the same batch to control for interassay variation. We determined cortisol using a modification of the Amersham International, Amerlex Cortisol RIA kit (University of Minnesota Hospital, 1987). The interassay coefficient of variation was 7.1%, and the intraassay coefficient was 4.1%. Samples were assayed in duplicate. The results at 9 months indicated that neither height, weight, nor ponderal index (measured in the laboratory) was significantly correlated with any of the four cortisol samples obtained at 9 months (*r*s ranged from $-.14$ to .17).

RESULTS

Salivary Cortisol

We initially examined the cortisol values for outliers that were potentially due to sampling close to a pulse of adrenocortical activity. Outliers were defined as those values greater than three standard deviations above the mean, as determined separately for each sampling period. Three subjects had only one value in that range; however, there were 5 babies who had multiple extreme values. These 5 infants were sorted into a separate group, and their data were analyzed separately. For the remaining subjects, cortisol values were transformed (log 10) to help normalize the distributions.

Intercorrelations among cortisol values. Next, we examined the correlations among the cortisol values (see Table 2). At 9 months, the values obtained by the observer in the home were significantly associated with all the other 9-month cortisol measures. At both 9 and 13 months, the associations among the Parent Home, Laboratory Initial, and Laboratory Post values were similar; the two baseline measures were significantly associated with each other, and neither baseline measure was associated with the Laboratory Post values at either age. We then computed correlations across age. None of the baseline measures were associated across age (*ps* > .10). However, the correlation between the two Laboratory Post measures approached significance: $r(57) = 0.23, p = .08$.

Response to test situations and associations with quality of attachment. The cortisol data were then prepared for a 2 (sex) × 4 (attachment: A, B1–B2, B3–B4, and C) × 2 (age × 3 (trials: Parent Home, Laboratory Initial, and Laboratory Post) analysis of variance (ANOVA), with repeated measures on the last two factors. Because missing values require a listwise deletion of data, we examined the number of subjects missing one or more values. Eighteen infants (30%) had missing data and were disproportionately represented in the insecure groups (As = 40%, Cs = 46%, Ds = 33%, Total Insecure = 46%, and Total Secure = 20%), χ^2 (1, $N =$

TABLE 2
Correlations Among Salivary Cortisol Measures Within Age

Measure	1	2	3	4
9 months				
1. Observer Home	—	.43*	.39*	.44*
2. Parent Home		—	.65*	.18
3. Initial Laboratory			—	.16
4. Post Laboratory				—
13 months				
1. Observer Home	—			
2. Parent Home		—	.47*	.09
3. Initial Laboratory			—	.15
4. Post Laboratory				—

Note. *df*s ranged from 48 to 59.
* $p < .01$.

66) $= 3.58, p < .10$. For this reason, the repeated-measures analysis was performed without the attachment factor.

The results yielded a significant effect of trials, $F(2, 88) = 11.19, p < .001$ (with the Greenhouse-Geisser correction, $dfs = 1, 40$, and $p < .01$). Post-hoc analyses were performed using paired t-tests to reduce the problem of listwise deletion of subjects. On average, only 7% of the cases were missing during any one sampling period. The means and standard deviations for all sampling periods, including the Observer Home sample, are shown in Table 3. At both 9 and 13 months, the Laboratory Initial values were significantly lower than the Parent Home values: at 9 months, $t(50) = 4.8, p < .01$, and at 13 months, $t(57) = 2.6, p < .05$). At both ages the Laboratory Post values were not significantly different from the Parent Home values. However, at 9 months the Laboratory Initial value, $t(58) = 3.5, p < .01$. At 13 months the difference was in the same direction but did not achieve significance, $t(50) = 1.6$.

We examined the effect of attachment quality (A, B1–B2, B3–B4 and C) using one-way ANOVAs. None of the analyses for any of the time periods or for the delta or difference scores achieved significance. Similar null results were obtained when separate t-tests were performed for secure versus insecure groupings and for the suggested molar temperament groupings (A1 to B2 vs. B3 to C2).

Behavioral Analyses

First, we examined the relations among emotional tone measures in similar contexts within age for the purpose of data reduction. Infant emotional temperament at home was modestly associated with emotional tone during the warm-up period in the laboratory at 9 months, $r(56) = .23, p < .10$, as was infant emotional tone during Episodes 2 (mother and baby) and 3 (mother, baby, and stranger) of the Strange

TABLE 3
Salivary Cortisol Means and Standard Errors

Age	Observer Home		Parent Home		Initial Laboratory		Post Laboratory	
	M	SE	M	SE	M	SE	M	SE
9 months	0.59	0.02	0.53	0.03	0.42	0.03	0.51	0.02
13 months	—		0.57	0.03	0.50	0.02	0.55	0.02

Note. Ns ranged from 52 to 61. Values are based on log-transformed distributions and have been reconverted for purposes of presentation. Values are expressed as μg/dl.

Situation at 13 months, $r(58) = .31, p < .05$. At each age these nonseparation measures of emotional tone were standardized and averaged. Within age, emotional tone scores during separation periods were highly correlated: at 9 months, emotional tone during Vignettes 1 was correlated with emotional tone during Vignettes 2, $r(59) = .67, p < .01$. At 13 months, the intercorrelations of emotional tone during the three separation periods of the Strange Situation ranged from .64 to .71 ($ps <$ .01). Two Separation Emotional Tone scores were computed by averaging emotional tone during separation periods within age (Separation 9 and Separation 13). Emotional tone was correlated across the two reunion episodes of the Strange Situation, $r(56) = 0.58$, and one measure of Reunion Emotional Tone was constructed at 13 months. (Note that at 9 months there was only one reunion period during the Louisville testing.)

Finally, the three measures from the Toddler Temperament Scale were intercorrelated, $rs(58) = 0.33$ to 0.53, $ps < .05$, therefore, one Questionnaire Temperament summary scale was computed by averaging these measures. Item-total correlations for the summary scale were .86 for Approach, .83 for Adaptability, and .67 for Mood. Because the Toddler Temperament scales were scored in a negative direction (i.e., withdrawal, nonadaptability, and negative mood), the summary Questionnaire Temperament scale was reversed so that higher values would reflect positive responses and match the direction of the Emotional Tone scoring system. The intercorrelations of these measures were then examined (see Table 4).

To reduce the emotional tone data further, we computed factor analyses on the emotional tone data at each age. One factor was identified at each age, accounting for 47.7% and 41.9% of the variance at 9 and 13 months, respectively. We used the

TABLE 4
Intercorrelations of Emotional Temperament Measures

Measure	9 months			13 months			
	1	2	3	4	5	6	7
1. Nonseparation (9 months)	—	.36***	.42***	.27**	.40***	.41***	.22*
2. Separation (9 months)		—	.59***	.28**	.54**	.24*	.41***
3. Reunion (9 months)			—	.26**	.49***	.32***	.37***
4. Nonseparation (13 months)				—	.33**	.41***	.22*
5. Separation (13 months)					—	.68***	.28**
6. Reunion (13 months)						—	.19
7. Questionnaire Temperament							—

Note. *df*s ranged from 54 to 59.
* $p < .10$.   ** $p < .05$.   *** $p < .01$.

factor weights to create summary Emotional Temperament scores. The weights for Nonseparation, Separation, and Reunion Emotional Tone were 0.51, 0.71, and 0.81 at 9 months, and 0.50, 0.79, and 0.84 at 13 months. At 13 months, the weight for Questionnaire Temperament was 0.31. These factor-weighted summary variables, Emotional Temperament 9 and Emotional Temperament 13, were correlated, $r(59)$ = 0.57, $p < .001$.

Temperament and Salivary Cortisol

On the basis of the pattern of salivary cortisol correlations noted earlier (see Table 2), we computed two summary measures of cortisol at each age. One measure was the average of the Parent Home and Initial Laboratory values (Basal 9 and Basal 13), and one measure (Delta 9 and Delta 13) indicated the increase in salivary cortisol during the course of the laboratory testing (Laboratory Post minus Laboratory Initial). These four summary measures were used in analyses of the relations between salivary cortisol and emotional temperament. We analyzed the Observer Home value separately because of its different pattern of correlations with the other cortisol measures and because it was obtained earlier in the morning.

The relations between temperament and the summary salivary cortisol values are shown in Table 5. Only one of the correlations with baseline cortisol achieved statistical significance. The pattern with delta cortisol was stronger. Overall, infants with

TABLE 5
Correlations Between Emotional Temperament and Salivary Cortisol

Emotional temperament at	Observer Home	Basal 9 months	Basal 13 months
	Basal cortisol measures		
9 months	−.13	.15	.10
13 months	−.16	.06	.33*
	Delta cortisol measures		
Emotional temperament at		9 months	13 months
9 months		−.30**	−.16
13 months		−.24*	−.25*

Note. *df*s ranged from 54 to 59.
* $p < .05$.   ** $p < .01$.

more positive emotional temperaments showed less of an increase in salivary cortisol during testing at 9 and 13 months. We examined the relations between delta cortisol and temperament further using stepwise multiple regression. At each age the separate indices of emotional tone were used to predict concurrent increases in cortisol during testing. The results showed that at 9 months only Separation Emotional Tone contributed uniquely to the prediction of changes in cortisol concentrations during the Louisville testing, $R = -.37$, $F(1, 54) = 8.4$, $p < .01$. At 13 months, only the mothers' reports of temperament made a unique contribution to the prediction of changes in cortisol concentrations during the Strange Situation, $R = -.31$, $F(1, 53) = 5.57$, $p < .05$. The zero-order correlation between Separation Emotional Tone and Delta Cortisol in the Strange Situation was $-.14$, *ns*.

Because the Questionnaire Temperament summary scale was composed of scores for 3 dimensions of temperament, we examined the contribution of these dimensions to the prediction of delta cortisol at 13 months in order to specify the nature of the emotional temperament contribution further. A stepwise multiple-regression analysis indicated that, once the Mood Scale was removed from the equation, the multiple correlation of .33 achieved significance, $F(2, 53) = 3.16$, $p < .05$. Because both the Approach and Adaptability scales loaded highly and similarly on the summary scale, any attempt to distinguish their individual unique contributions to the prediction of delta cortisol was considered inappropriate.

Cortisol Intercorrelations Reassessed

Given the associations between temperament and delta cortisol, we reassessed the pattern of correlations between baseline cortisol and postsession cortisol. Partial correlations were computed controlling for the summary temperament variables. Following this analysis, similar partial correlations were computed controlling for emotional tone during separation. (The results are shown in Table 6.) At both 9 and 13 months, Parent Home baseline concentrations were not significantly associated with Laboratory Post values when temperament or separation emotional tone were controlled. However, at both ages, an association emerged between Laboratory Initial and Post values once either temperament or emotional tone during separation was controlled.

Infants With Extreme Cortisol Values

Finally, we examined the data for the 5 infants with extreme cortisol concentrations. Neither sex, attachment classification, nor emotional temperament clearly differentiated these 5 infants: 2 were female, 2 were securely attached, and 3 were insecure-resistant attached. We weighted their emotional tone scores using the factor weights to yield summary temperament scores. We then converted these scores to *z* scores using the means and standard deviations for the total sample. The *z* scores ranged from 0.9 to −0.8 for the 5 infants at 9 months, and from −1.9 to 1.4 at 13 months. Although the scores at 13 months were more extreme, the range from very negative emotional tone to very positive does not suggest a consistent temperamental reason for these infants to have extremely high cortisol concentrations. There was sufficient saliva left to examine salivary albumin concentrations for 1 of these 5 infants. This infant did have elevated concentrations (greater than 1.0 mg/dl), suggesting the possibility of an oral wound, perhaps from teething.

DISCUSSION

In both Old and New World monkeys, separation from mother results in large elevations in adrenocortical hormones (see review by Coe, Wiener, Rosenberg, & Levine, 1985). As noted, Tennes and her colleagues (1977) failed to find similar elevations among 1-year-old human infants using urinary measures of cortisol and a home separation. The first question that we addressed here was whether elevations in salivary cortisol would be observed in response to the Louisville Assessment at 9 months or the Strange Situation Assessment at 13 months—assessments that both involved maternal separation. The results left the answer ambiguous. Compared with home baselines, we did not note significant elevations in cortisol at either age. Compared with laboratory baselines, we noted a significant elevation in response to the Louisville Assessment at 9 months, but the response to the Strange Situation at 13 months was not statistically significant.

Ignoring for the moment the baseline measure obtained by the home observer at 9

TABLE 6

Partial Correlations Among Salivary Cortisol Baseline and Response Measures Within Age Controlling for Infant Temperament

	Variable partialed out of correlation at			
	9 months		13 months	
Baseline measure	Temperament 9	Separation Emotional tone	Temperament 13	Separation Emotional tone
Observer Home	.35***	.29**	—	—
Parent Home	.16	.20	.19	.14
Initial Laboratory	.25*	.26**	.37***	.33***

*Note. df*s range from 47 to 58. Observer Home value obtained only at 9 months.
* $p < .10$. ** $p < .05$. *** $p < .01$.

months, the pattern of intercorrelations among cortisol measures suggests that the initial laboratory concentrations provided the best baseline estimates. At both ages, the infant's salivary cortisol concentrations at home predicted their concentrations when they entered the laboratory. The initial laboratory concentrations should reflect activity of the adrenal cortex during the trip into the laboratory. Thus, infants with higher concentrations at home maintained higher relative concentrations while traveling to the university for testing. At both ages, neither home nor initial laboratory concentrations, however, predicted postassessment cortisol levels. This pattern of correlations suggests that both basal and stress activity of the infant adrenocortical system were being assessed. This conclusion was supported further by the following two results: (a) There was modest stability in postassessment cortisol concentrations across age despite substantial differences in the duration of separation in the two assessments. (b) When individual differences in emotional response to separation were controlled statistically, a significant correlation between initial and postassessment cortisol concentrations emerged. Thus, the difference between postassessment and initial laboratory concentrations would seem to reflect a change from basal to stress regulation of the infant pituitary-adrenal system. However, the size of the response was quite small in comparison with responses shown by monkey infants to maternal separation.

Perhaps the most striking cortisol results were what seemed to be significant reductions in cortisol concentrations between Parent Home and Laboratory Initial samples at both ages. It is unclear why these declines occurred. One possibility is that drowsiness or reduced activity (or both) induced during transit to the laboratory produced transient decreases in basal pituitary-adrenocortical activity. Being strapped into a car seat would, by necessity, restrict activity, and parents commonly report that riding in the car makes babies drowsy and sleepy. The possibility that drowsiness or lowered activity produced a decline in basal activity is consistent with a report by Tennes and Vernadakis (1977) of lower urinary cortisol levels following naps as compared with active-awake periods during the day among 12-month-olds. It is inconsistent with recent conclusions that an adult-like, circadian rhythm in adrenocortical activity develops by 3 months of age (e.g., Francis et al., 1987). With the exception of postprandial increases in circulating cortisol (Quigley & Yen, 1979, as cited in Riad-Fahmy, Read, & Hughes, 1983), transient fluctuations in basal activity have not been reported for human adults. Indeed, among adults it appears to take 10 days to 2 weeks for the adrenocortical circadian rhythm to readjust following even major shifts in sleep–wake patterns (Anders, 1982). Additional work is clearly needed to understand the factors influencing basal activity of the infant pituitary-adrenocortical system. At this point it seems possible that, perhaps as with sleep–wake patterns, basal adrenocortical regulatory processes are not fully mature in infancy, even though they may have matured to the point of producing the adult-like single early morning peak in cortisol secretion.

The second major question that we addressed was whether either basal or stress-induced activity of the adrenocortical system is related to emotional functioning during infancy. We assessed two aspects of the emotion system: the quality of attachment and emotional temperament. We found no evidence that quality of attachment was related to adrenocortical activity. Neither basal, postassessment, nor delta cortisol values at either 9 or 13 months varied as a function of any combination of Strange Situation classifications. Nonetheless, the problem of proving the null hypothesis aside, it would be premature to conclude that quality of attachment is unrelated to adrenocortical activity in infancy for two reasons.

First, the postassessment cortisol measure at 13 months was obtained immediately following the conclusion of the Strange Situation. This meant that only 30 min had elapsed from the time the Initial Laboratory sample was obtained and less than 25 min had elapsed since the beginning of the first separation in Episode 4. This may have been too brief a time interval for detecting the full adrenocortical response. Although the salivary time course in infancy has not been established, it is typically assumed that 15 to 30 min may elapse between the onset of stimulation and the production of a substantial cortisol response in plasma. Because it should take even longer for this response to be seen in saliva, it is possible that the post-Strange Situation saliva sample was obtained too early. It should be noted that 6 infants whose postassessment saliva collections were delayed for technical reasons appeared to have somewhat higher postsession concentrations. If the 13-month postsession sample was obtained too early, then these data may not provide an adequate test of the attachment–cortisol relationship. Second, even if the security of the attachment relationship is unrelated to the adrenocortical response in situations involving separation, it may be related to the adrenocortical stress response when the attachment figure is present to act as a source of security. Of course, data from the present study do not address this question.

In contrast to quality of attachment, the results provided clear support of a relation between stress-induced activity of the adrenocortical system and emotional temperament in infancy. At both 9 and 13 months, infants who exhibited greater increases in adrenocortical activity during testing had more negative emotional temperaments. At 9 months, delta cortisol was most closely associated with emotional tone during separation, a finding consistent with the idea that state changes in negative affect serve to regulate the adrenocortical stress response (Mason, 1968). However, at 13 months distress responses during the Strange Situation were not correlated significantly with delta cortisol. Instead, delta cortisol was associated with maternal reports of emotional temperament obtained prior to testing. This latter finding suggests that between 9 and 12 months the adrenocortical response may be becoming sensitive more to trait-like than to state-like aspects of infant psychological functioning.

This conclusion is consistent with the argument that negative emotions do not activate the pituitary-adrenocortical stress response; instead, factors regulating this neuroendocrine system overlap with those that influence affect (Gunnar et al., in press; Levine, 1985). Collative variables such as novelty, discrepancy, and strangeness (Hennessy & Levine, 1979; Rose, 1980), along with loss and lack of control that may also increase uncertainty (Levine, 1985), have been identified as important in triggering and regulating stress-related adrenocortical activity. These same factors are also involved in regulating emotional behavior during infancy (e.g., Gunnar, 1980; Lewis & Rosenblum, 1974).

In our own work, the emphasis on novelty and uncertainty, as opposed to negative emotions, is based on evidence that elevations in cortisol are sometimes positively and sometimes negatively correlated with crying and other indices of emotional distress (see review by Gunnar et al., in press). We have also noted that among children highly familiar with the stressor (e.g., blood sampling among children with phenylketonuria), developmental increases in distress were not associated with increases in cortisol. Instead, increases in uncertainty about controlling expressions of distress in this group were associated with large increases in cortisol over baseline concentrations (Gunnar et al., 1988 in press). These data, data from others that have shown both rapid adaptation of the adrenocortical response on repeated or prolonged exposure to stressors, and evidence that intense behavioral distress can continue long after cortisol has returned to baseline concentrations (see review by Rose, 1980), have all led to the argument that novelty, uncertainty, and strangeness, rather than emotional distress, are the primary psychological triggers of the adrenocortical system (Gunnar et al., in press; Levine, 1985).

Infants may differ in their sensitivity to novelty and reactivity to uncertainty (Gunnar, 1980; Rothbart & Derryberry, 1981). These differences may, in part, underlie individual differences in emotional temperament as measured in the present study. Being sensitive and reactive to novelty and uncertainty may be the temperamental characteristic influencing both hormonal and emotional responses to separation in infancy. This possibility is supported by the fact that the Approach and Adaptability scales were the temperament dimensions associated with delta cortisol. The questions on the Approach scale deal primarily with wary reactions to strangers and strange places. Questions on the Adaptability scale deal with resistance to caregiving activities and the capacity to adapt to novel and uncertain situations. It is unlikely that these factors are the only ones involved in determining infant affective reactions to stressful events, nor are they likely to be the sole determinants of the adrenocortical stress response. This is consistent with the modest size of the correlations obtained at both ages in this study.

It is also consistent with the data on the 5 infants with extremely high salivary cortisol concentrations. None of these infants were at the extremes of the temperament distributions at 9 months; however, this was the age when 4 of the 5 infants exhibited extreme cortisol concentrations. Just why these infants had such high salivary cortisol levels cannot be determined from these data. None of them showed physical symptoms that would lead one to suspect central nervous system or peripheral target lesions. With the exception of one subject whose mother questioned whether he was ill, none appeared to be sick, although subclinical infections cannot be ruled out. It is also possible that these extreme concentrations were the result of cortisol entering the salivary pool directly from plasma through oral lesions. The salivary albumin concentrations on the 1 subject with sufficient saliva remaining for assay were consistent with this hypothesis. Clearly it would be wise to check infants for teething in future studies. Finally, psychosocial factors involving disruptions in family functioning may also have contributed to high concentrations. This seems possible for at least 2 of the infants: 1 whose mother stated that she had "multiple sclerosis brought on by stress," and 1 whose grandfather had just died. If elevations to these concentrations can result from psychosocial stressors in infancy, then we would certainly be dealing with physiologically significant effects.

Until such data are available, it is more conservative to conclude that the adrenocortical system, although responsive to stimulation during infancy, appears almost buffered or dampened in its reactivity to psychological stressors. It may be a relief to know that infants who appear to be behaviorally very stressed by separation and strangers may not be as physiologically stressed as their behavior suggests. At the same time, it is also a challenge to our understanding of the development of psychoendocrine regulation. On the one hand, small increments in responding, such as those in the present study, may merely underscore the importance of novelty in the activation of the adrenocortical system (Rose, 1980). By 9 months, infants in our culture have had repeated experience with separation and strangers. On the other hand, these data may reflect the operation of intervening processes that serve to buffer the adrenocortical response to stressful events during normal development. Data currently being gathered by numerous research groups should soon provide an indication of which of these possibilities is the most likely.

REFERENCES

Ainsworth, M. D. S., Blehar, M., Waters, E., & Wall, S. (1978). *Patterns of attachment: Observations in the stranger situation at home.* Hillsdale, NJ: Erlbaum.

Ainsworth, M. D. S., & Wittig, B. A. (1969). Attachment and the exploratory behavior of one-year-olds in a strange situation. In B. M. Foss (Ed.), *Determinants of infant behavior* (Vol. 4, pp. 113–136). London: Methuen.

Anders, R. (1982). Biological rhythms in development. *Psychosomatic Medicine, 44,* 61–72.

Anders, T., Sachar, E., Kream, J., Roffwarg, H., & Hellman, L. (1970). Behavioral state and plasma cortisol response in the human newborn. *Pediatrics, 46*(4), 532–537.

Belsky, J., & Rovine, M. (1987). Temperament and attachment security in the strange situation: An empirical rapprochement. *Child Development, 58,* 787–795.

Cernic, L. S., & Pennington, B. F. (1987). Developmental psychology and the neurosciences: An introduction. *Child Development, 58,* 533–538.

Coe, L. C., Wiener, S. G., Rosenberg, L. T., & Levine, S. (1985). Endocrine and immune responses to separation and maternal loss in nonhuman primates. In M. Reite & T. Field (Eds.), *The psychology of attachment* (pp. 163–199). New York: Academic Press.

Egeland, B., Deinard, A., Taraldson, B., & Brunnquell, D. (1975). *Manual for feeding and play observation scales.* Unpublished manuscript, University of Minnesota, Minneapolis.

Fox, N. A., & Davidson, R. J. (1987). Electroencephalogram asymmetry in response to the approach of a stranger and maternal separation in 10-month-old infants. *Developmental Psychology, 23,* 233–240.

Francis, S. F., Walker, R. F., Riad-Fahmy, D., Hughes, D., Murphy, J. F., & Gray, O. P. (1987). Assessment of adrenocortical activity in term newborn infants using salivary cortisol determinations. *Journal of Pediatrics, 111,* 129–133.

Fullard, W., McDevitt, S. C., & Carey, W. B. (1984). Assessing temperament in one- to three-year-old children. *Journal of Pediatric Psychology, 9,* 205–216.

Goldsmith, H., Buss, A. H., Plomin, R., Rothbart, M. K., Thomas, A., Chess, S., Hinde, R. A., & McCall, R. B. (1987). Roundtable: What is temperament? Four approaches. *Child Development, 58,* 505–529.

Gunnar, M. R. (1980). Control, warning signals, and distress in infancy. *Developmental Psychology, 16,* 281–289.

Gunnar, M. R. (1986). Human developmental psychoneuroendocrinology: A review of research on neuroendocrine responses to challenge and threat in infancy and childhood. In M. E. Lamb, L. A. Brown, & B. Rogoff (Eds.), *Advances in developmental psychology* (Vol. 4, pp. 51–103). Hillsdale, NJ: Erlbaum.

Gunnar, M. R. (1987). Psychobiological studies of stress and coping: An introduction. *Child Development, 58,* 1403–1407.

Gunnar, M., Gonzales, C., Goodlin, B., & Levine, S. (1981). Behavioral and pituitary-adrenal responses during a prolonged separation period in infant rhesus macaques. *Psychoneuroendocrinology, 6,* 66–75.

Gunnar, M., Mangelsdorf, S., Kestenbaum, R., Lang, S., Larson, M., & Andreas, D. (in press). Stress and coping in early development. In D. Cicchetti (Ed.), Process and psychopathology. Hillsdale, NJ: Erlbaum.

Gunnar, M. R., Marvinney, D., Isensee, & Fisch, R. O. (in press). Coping with uncertainty: New models of the relations between hormonal, behavioral, and cognitive processes. In D. Palermo (Ed.), *Coping with uncertainty.* Hillsdale, NJ: Erlbaum.

Hennessy, J., & Levine, S. (1979). Stress, arousal and the pituitary-adrenal system: A psychoendocrine model. In J. Sprague & A. Epstein (Eds.), *Progress in psychobiological and physiological psychology* (Vol. 8, pp. 133–178). New York: Academic Press.

Kagan, J., Reznick, J. S., & Snidman, N. (1987). The physiology and psychology of behavioral inhibition in children. *Child Development, 58,* 1459–1473.

Kandel, E. R., & Schwartz, J. H. (1981). *Principles of neural science.* New York: Elsevier/North-Holland.

Levine, S. (1985). A definition of stress? In G. P. Moberg (Eds.), *Animal stress* (pp. 51–69). Bethesda, MD: American Physiological Society.

Levine, S., Wiener, S. G., Coe, C., Bayart, F. S., & Hayashi, K. T. (1987). Primate vocalization: A psychobiological approach. *Child Development, 58,* 1408–1419.

Lewis, M., & Rosenblum, L. A. (1974). *The origins of fear.* New York: Wiley.

Locke, S., Ader, R., Besedovsky, H., Hull, N., Solomon, G., & Strom, T. (1985). *Foundations of psychneuroimmunology.* New York: Aldine.

Mason, J. W. (1968). A review of psychoendocrine research on the pituitary-adrenal cortisol system. *Psychosomatic Medicine, 30,* 576–608.

Matheny, A. P. (1984). Twin similarity in the developmental transformations of infant temperament as measured in a multi-method, longitudinal study. *Acta Geneticae Medicae Gemellologiae, 33,* 181–189.

Matheny, A. P., Riese, M. L., & Wilson, R. S. (1985). Rudiments of infant temperament: Newborn to 9 months. *Developmental Psychology, 12,* 486–494.

Matheny, A. P., & Wilson, R. S. (1981). Developmental tasks and rating scales for laboratory assessment of infant temperament. *JSAS Catalog of Selected Documents in Psychology, 11* (Ms. No. 2367).

Matheny, A. P., Wilson, R. S., & Nuss, S. (1984). Toddler temperament: Stability across settings and over ages. *Child Development, 55,* 1200–1211.

Nelson, C. A., & Salapatek, P. (1986). Electrophysiological correlates of infant recognition memory. *Child Development, 57,* 1483–1497.

Prior, M., Sanson, A., Oberkaid, F., & Northan, E. (1987). Measurement of temperament in one- to two-year-old children. *International Journal of Behavioral Development, 10,* 121–132.

Riad-Fahmy, D., Read, G. F., & Hughes, I. A. (1983). Corticosteroids. In C. H. Gray & V. H. T. James (Eds.), *Hormones in the blood* (Vol. 4, pp. 285–315). New York: Academic Press.

Riese, M. L. (1987). Temperament stability between the neonatal period and 24 months. *Developmental Psychology, 23,* 216–222.

Rose, R. M. (1980). Endocrine responses to stressful psychological events. Advances in psychoneuroendocrinology. *Psychiatric Clinics of North America, 3,* 251–276.

Rothbart, M. K., & Derryberry, D. (1981). Development of individual differences in temperament. In M. E. Lamb & A. L. Brown (Eds.), *Advances in developmental psychology* (Vol. 1, pp. 37–86) Hillsdale, NJ: Erlbaum.

Tennes, K., & Carter, D. (1973). Plasma cortisol levels and behavioral states in early infancy. *Psychosomatic Medicine, 35,* 121–128.

Tennes, K., Downey, K., & Vernadakis, A. (1977). Urinary cortisol excretion rates and anxiety in normal one-year-old infants. *Psychosomatic Medicine, 39,* 178–187.

Tennes, K., & Mason, J. (1982). Developmental psychoendocrinology: An approach to the study of emotions. In C. Izard (Ed.), *Measuring emotions in infants and children* (pp. 21–37). Cambridge, England: Cambridge University Press.

Tennes, K., & Vernadakis, A. (1977). Cortisol excretion levels and daytime sleep in one-year-old infants. *Journal of Clinical Endocrinology and Metabolism, 44,* 175–179.

University of Minnesota Hospital. (1987). Cortisol in saliva by radioimmunoassay. Unpublished manuscript. Minneapolis: Author.

Vaughn, B., Taraldson, B., Crichton, L., & Egeland, B. (1980). Relationships between neonatal behavioral organization and infant behavior during the first year of life. *Infant Behavior and Development, 3,* 47–66.

6

Female and Male: Issues of Gender

Carol Nagy Jacklin

University of Southern California

Our culture's preoccupation with gender differences is reflected in the importance developmental psychologists have placed on gender-related issues. In this article, three areas of research where gender is or has been a primary focus of research are discussed: measurement of intellectual abilities, biology and behavior, and socialization processes. Policy implications of the research are suggested.

Speculation about differences between females and males is a national preoccupation. In our culture, people care whether there are fundamental differences between girls and boys, and we place more emphasis on the possibility of such differences than on other kinds of distinctions that could be made. For example, we rarely wonder whether blue-eyed and brown-eyed or short and tall children differ from one another in intellectual abilities or personality.

Psychologists' interest in gender issues has varied over time. In the earliest days of the publication of journals by the American Psychological Association, there was some interest in gender (Hollingworth, 1914, 1916, 1918; Woolley, 1910, 1914), but it did not become a widely used variable in psychological research until the mid-1960s. Developmentalists have had a more continuous interest in gender issues than have psychologists working in other areas. There are two possible reasons for this: First, developmental psychologists were historically more likely than other researchers to use both male and female subjects in their studies, and second, more women have been trained in developmental psychology than in other areas of psychology. Both of these factors bear directly on the issues selected for study within a subject area (Jacklin, 1987).

Reprinted with permission from *American Psychologist,* 1989, Vol. 44, No. 2, 127–133. Copyright © 1989 by the American Psychological Association, Inc.

I want to thank Barrie Thorne, Mary Hayden, Ann Gamsa, Myra H. Strober, Zella Luria, and Aletha Huston for their careful reading of this article. I would also like to thank Jane E. Wilson for general help and Richard Scott Caputo for several careful readings of the article.

Because most current research with children uses both girls and boys as subjects, and investigators typically carry out at least perfunctory tests for sex differences, an exhaustive summary of gender research in developmental psychology would now almost completely overlap the field of developmental psychology as a whole. In this article, I will examine only a few of the current and emerging areas within developmental psychology where gender is important. These areas are measurement of intellectual abilities, biology and behavior, and socialization processes. Although this set of topics represents only a small subset of the possible areas that could be addressed, I have chosen them because they illustrate different stages of empirical and theoretical development within the field. In addition, in these three areas issues of gender are particularly salient.

MEASUREMENT OF INTELLECTUAL ABILITIES

The Math Controversy

In the early 1980s, Benbow and Stanley (1980, 1982, 1983) published a series of articles that caused a stir in both the popular press and academia. They described the scores on a standardized test of mathematical ability for a large population of bright boys and girls. In every study, the boys scored higher than the girls. What was particularly important about these results was that the authors speculated about the biological causes of their findings. As these speculations were exaggerated in the popular media, they became the overriding message of the studies.

Seemingly, Benbow and Stanley's studies supported the popular myth about gender differences in math ability. It is interesting, however, that although Benbow and Stanley speculated about biological causes for their results, they had no biological data. Furthermore, many aspects of their studies were criticized in professional journals. For example, the results were reported as ratios of girls to boys at the highest scores, an analysis that exaggerates the actual group differences in scores. The Benbow and Stanley studies also failed to take into account the children's differential math-related experiences, assuming that enrollment in equal numbers of math classes would equate for this factor (see Eccles & Jacobs, 1986, and Lips, 1988, for reviews of this criticism).

During the time the Benbow and Stanley studies were published, and the associated media blitz occurred, Eccles and her colleagues were collecting data for a large-scale study of mathematics course taking and achievement in seventh through ninth graders. Thus, these researchers had a unique opportunity to record how the media's presentation of a scientific study affects the attitudes of people directly concerned with the subject matter of the study (Eccles & Jacobs, 1986).

The conclusions of the larger, primary study were that math anxiety, gender-stereotyped beliefs of parents, and the perceived value of math to the student account for the major portion of sex differences in mathematical achievement (Eccles, Adler, & Kaczala, 1982; Eccles et al., 1983; Eccles & Jacobs, 1986; Eccles, Kaczala, & Meece, 1982). In addition, Eccles and her colleagues have found that students' attitudes about mathematics are most strongly related to their mothers' beliefs concerning the difficulty of mathematics for their children. Mothers' beliefs were also important in that they directly and strongly influenced their children's math anxiety. Similar results have also been reported for younger children (Entwisle & Baker, 1983).

The related research on the effects of the popular reports of the Benbow and Stanley results compared the attitudes of parents who were aware of the Benbow and Stanley work as reported in the media ("misinformed" parents) with those of parents who had not heard about the work ("uninformed" parents). Briefly, Eccles and Jacobs (1986; see also Jacobs & Eccles, 1985) found that uninformed mothers believed that the mathematics ability of their sons and daughters was equivalent, whereas misinformed mothers of girls felt that math was more difficult for their children than did mothers of boys. Thus, the media campaign had a direct effect on the same attitudes of parents that have a direct effect on children's mathematics course taking and achievement. Clearly, the effects were deleterious to girls. As mothers came to believe that mathematics was much more difficult for girls than boys, their daughters become less likely to take additional math courses.

Another dimension to the mathematics controversy is the relationship of mathematics ability to other seemingly related skills. The relationship between mathematics, science, and spatial ability has been assessed by Linn and Petersen (1985, 1986), who examined the nature, magnitude, and age of first appearance of gender differences in these three domains. After an extensive analysis, they concluded that there is no consistent pattern of gender differences either between or within these ability areas. Indeed, mathematics, science, and spatial abilities are themselves shown not to be unitary ability domains independent of the issue of gender.

Declines in Gender Differences in Intellectual Abilities Over Time

Earlier reviews of studies comparing male and female performance on intellectual tasks found sex differences in verbal behavior (Maccoby & Jacklin, 1974; Sherman, 1971), but current research does not (see Hyde & Linn, 1988, for a review). In addition, it appears that this ability difference has in fact disappeared over time. In their comparison of verbal-ability scores of girls and boys, Hyde and Linn (1988) found that the differences between the sexes has been reduced across the last decades.

Similar decreases in gender differences over the last two decades have been shown in a variety of other intellectual abilities (Feingold, 1988; Rosenthal & Ruben, 1982). Using meta-analysis (a statistical technique for estimating the size of effects and comparing large numbers of studies), Rosenthal and Ruben (1982) concluded that they could not pinpoint a cause for this change. They stated, "we can say that whatever the reason, in these studies females appear to be gaining in cognitive skill relative to males rather faster than the gene can travel!" (p. 711). Most of the subjects tested in the studies included in the Rosenthal and Ruben meta-analysis were of college age, but similar changes have been documented in high school students (Feingold, 1988).

One possible source of change in the relative scores of males and females is efforts to make test items gender neutral (Hyde & Linn, 1988). Such attempts began at least as early as the first edition of the Stanford-Binet Scale of Intelligence. In 1916, the results of the Stanford-Binet were evaluated for gender bias and were judged as not yet gender fair. A discussion of this history and of the myriad ways tests themselves produce gender-related differences is given by Dwyer (1979).

In summary, tests of intellectual abilities have differentiated girls and boys less and less over the last decades. The only exception to this trend is at the highest end of the mathematics-ability continuum, where the ratio of boys outscoring girls has remained constant over the years (Feingold, 1988). One of the mothers in the Eccles and Jacobs (1986) study was quoted as saying, "Perhaps society has encouraged boys in math more than girls. I hope it is changing" (p. 380). Yet change was countered by media reports that emphasized prevailing societal biases about differential male and female abilities. As Eccles and Jacobs (1986) concluded, "passive nondiscrimination" in educational policy and practice is not adequate to counter stereotyped attitudes. More active intervention is needed to make parents' expectations and teachers' behavior gender fair. If such societal fairness were achieved, then tests of differences in intellectual abilities of males and females at all levels could be made equitably.

BIOLOGY AND BEHAVIOR

Male Vulnerability

One important biological fact that distinguishes the sexes is that males are more physically vulnerable than females. This differential vulnerability is particularly pronounced at the beginning and end of the life span.

Many more males than females are conceived, but many more males than females die before birth (e.g., see McMilen, 1979; Novitski, 1977). More males than females experience difficulties during the birth process, resulting in more males than females with birth defects. Even in unproblematic deliveries, the births of male offspring take an average of an hour longer than the births of females (Jacklin & Maccoby, 1982). The length of labor, in turn, has been shown to be more predictive of later problems in infants' and young children's behavior than the drugs a mother receives during labor and delivery (Kraemer, Korner, Anders, Jacklin, & Dimicelli, 1985).

In a review article chronicling greater male vulnerability across the life span, Gualtieri and Hicks (1985) hypothesized an immunoreactive theory of selective male affliction. They suggested there is "something about the male fetus that evokes an inhospitable uterine environment" (p. 427). Simply stated, they believed that the mother's body is stimulated to produce a kind of antibody against a male fetus (but not against a female fetus that is genetically more similar to her) and that these antibodies lead either directly or indirectly to fetal damage. This view has caused considerable controversy, as indicated by the 23 peer commentaries published with their article.

Unlike many of the elusive differences claimed to exist between the sexes, the fact of male vulnerability is well established. This biological difference appears to be a likely candidate for further research into related behavioral development. The concept of risk, especially in infancy, and the eventual outcomes for infants who are at risk have been the subjects of considerable research and discussion (see Kopp & Kaler, this issue). Rarely has this research treated the interesting issue of particular risks to males and their ramifications in later behavior. This area deserves increased research attention in the testing of hypotheses about the role of male vulnerability in behavioral predispositions.

Hormones and Behavior

When differences are found between boys and girls, biological causes are often postulated. An example is the mathematics-achievement differences discussed earlier. Hormonal differences, particularly sex-steroid hormones, are among the most common biological causes given for behavioral sex-related differences. This propensity to suppose sex steroids are causing differences in behavior may be due to the results of early studies with animals. Research with rats and primates has indeed linked levels of sex-steroid hormones and male and female differences in hormone concentrations to some sex-related behaviors such as aggression (see Maccoby & Jacklin, 1974, 1980, for reviews).

In the last decades, considerable advances have been made in studying hormone-behavior linkages directly. Technological developments have made work with human populations much less difficult. It is now possible to obtain reliable measures of sex-steroid and other hormones from saliva. Because these procedures are nonintrusive, subject recruitment has become easier.

Many of the recent hormone studies have been carried out on normal populations of children, particularly adolescents, measuring endogenous (i.e., normally circulating) hormone levels. The emphasis on studies of normal populations rather than selected groups known to have hormonal abnormalities is a clear advance. Through this work, enough data on the association between endogenous hormone levels and behavior are beginning to be amassed to try to come to some tentative summaries, if not conclusions, about hormonal influences on gender-related behavior.

Exactly how hormones affect and are affected by human behavior is still not well understood. The working theory about how the system works has been derived from animal research. Briefly, the theory posits two types of effects: sensitization and activation. Sensitization is believed to occur during the prenatal period, when circulating hormones act to program the fetal brain in a number of ways. This early sensitization may itself affect later behavior. During and after puberty, circulating hormones then activate or interact with the sensitized brain to produce behavioral effects.

It is still very difficult to obtain hormone measures in humans before birth. Thus, studies to test for sensitization effects in normal humans have had to rely on hormone measures taken from the umbilical cord blood at birth. One recent study of intellectual abilities in young children provided support for the sensitization theory. In this study, the amount of androgens (testosterone and androsteindione) from the umbilical cord blood was found to be negatively related to girls' spatial abilities at age six (Jacklin, Wilcox, & Maccoby, 1988). That is, girls with high levels of androgens in their blood at birth had lower scores on tests of spatial ability when they entered school than did girls with low levels of androgens at birth. Unfortunately, circulating hormone measures were not available when the children were tested at six years of age; thus, it was not possible to determine whether prenatal hormones actually sensitized the brain, resulting in differential cognitive abilities. An alternative hypothesis is that hormone levels at birth are related to hormone levels throughout childhood, and the circulating hormones themselves influence cognitive development.

More data are available linking emotional behaviors and hormones. Briefly, findings with young children testing the possible effects of sensitization include a relationship between neonatal hormones and fear and timidity in boys but not in girls (Jacklin, Maccoby, & Doering, 1983) and a relationship between positive moods for boys and girls and different combinations of hormones (Marcus, Maccoby, Jacklin, & Doering, 1985).

Circulating sex-steroid hormones are currently being collected in at least three large-scale studies of adolescents. In these studies, extensive cognitive testing as well as measures of emotions are being taken (Eccles et al., 1988; Susman et al., 1987; Udry, 1988). Although these studies are still in progress, and no firm findings can yet be obtained concerning the role of circulating hormones on adolescent cognitive abilities or emotional responses, early results highlight the complexity of the research. For example, results to date indicate that (a) daily variation in hormone measures is substantial, (b) the variability itself is a stable individual difference, and (c) the variability of an individual's hormone levels may be more important to behavioral outcomes than the absolute amounts of circulating hormones. No firm findings as yet exist as to the role of circulating hormones in adolescence on cognitive abilities.

In research on adolescent emotional behavior, relations have been found between high variability of circulating testosterone and anger in both boys and girls (Susman & Chrousos, 1988). That is, children whose circulating levels of testosterone vary widely from day to day are more likely to show anger. It is the changeability or variability that predicts anger, not the mean level of testosterone.

In summary, one persistent finding in the studies with young children is that a particular hormone is often related to behavior in different ways for girls and boys. That is, if a behavior is correlated positively with a hormone for one sex, it is likely not to be related to that behavior for the other sex. In some cases one finds a positive relation between a hormone measure and behavior for one sex and a negative relation for the other sex.

In the studies of circulating hormones and behavior with adolescent populations, one finds unexpected complexity as well. Daily fluctuations of hormones may be more important than absolute levels. And again, as seen with young children, the effects of a particular hormone may occur only for one sex or may show opposite effects for girls and boys (also see Jacklin, Maccoby, Doering, & King, 1984).

The simple models of hormone-behavior relationships that were developed from animal research are not adequate to explain the data from normal human populations. The relationship between hormones and behavior is normal children and adolescents is complex. New models for explaining the relationship between hormones and normal human behavior are needed.

A word of warning: Correlations between hormones and behavior are typically interpreted as cases in which the biological causes the psychological. It fits our predispositions to assume that hormones cause behavioral outcomes. The hormone system is an open system. Much more empirical work is needed before the direction of the causal arrows are understood.

SOCIALIZATION PROCESSES

The processes by which children grow into adults are of central interest to developmental psychologists. Questions about how and how much parents can influence their children's attitudes and behaviors have always been an important part of developmental psychology.

The development of sex role behavior has similarly been of long-standing interest. How do girls and boys acquire cultural information about sex roles? How does their behavior become aligned with our expectations for female and male children? These questions are even more salient during a time of general questioning of sex role stereotypes for children and adults. Knowing how socialization works would help parents to raise a nonsexist child in a sexist society.

Several theories have been advanced to explain the development of sex role behavior. The three most important theories have come from psychoanalytic, social learning, and cognitive developmental approaches. Very little empirical work exists to support psychoanalytic theory, although it has had some revival and revision in the theoretical work of Chodorow (1978) and Lerman (1986). Social learning theory and cognitive developmental theory, on the other hand, have been the focus of much continuing interest and research in the last decades.

Social learning theory as it describes the learning of gender-related behavior was articulated by Mischel (1966). Briefly, from the very beginning of life, parents and other caretakers treat boys and girls differently. That is, little girls are rewarded for certain behaviors and punished for other behaviors, and these are not the same sets of behaviors for which little boys are rewarded or punished. Children are also believed to choose to imitate models of the same sex (often their parents, but also other children, other adults, and even characters from print or visual media). By and large, social learning depicts the child as a somewhat passive recipient of culturally transmitted information.

Cognitive developmental theory as it describes the learning of gender-related behavior was articulated by Kohlberg (1966; Kohlberg & Ullian, 1974). According to this idea, children cannot understand generalized concepts such as their own sex and its accompanying gender-role expectations until their cognitive abilities are sufficiently developed to a stage or level at which they can understand the constancy of gender. Kohlberg believed gender development was analogous to the Piagetian theory of physical constancy (Piaget, 1954). One of the hallmarks of cognitive developmental theory is the role of the child as an active processor of culturally transmitted information.

Much research has been carried out to test the assumptions of both of these theories (see Maccoby & Jacklin, 1974, for a review). One body of evidence shows that social learning indeed occurs; however, there also appear to be large gaps in its explanatory powers. For example, parents are often observed to treat their young girls and boys similarly, yet the children show a great deal of sex-stereotyped knowledge and behavior. Similarly, considerable evidence both supports and disconfirms cognitive developmental theory. For example, it has been shown that children know much about their own sex-appropriate behavior and attitudes well before a stage theory would predict they should have this knowledge. The current wisdom in trying to decide between these theories may be that no decision is required.

Some current work blurs the line between the two theories; this work will be highlighted here. In work with nursery school children, Fagot (1985a, 1985b) has shown that children certainly do respond to reinforcement patterns, but they respond selectively. Reinforcement is not effective when given by some groups, and it is very effective when given by others. For example, girls respond to the reinforcement given by female and male teachers and by other girls but not to the reinforcement given by boys. Boys respond to the reinforcement given by other boys, but they do not respond to that given by teachers or by girls. In a similar example with parents, Eisenberg and her colleagues (Eisenberg, Wolchik, Hernandez, & Pasternack, 1985) found children are not influenced by parents' positive reinforcement of play choices but instead by parents' own toy choices. Thus, reinforcement may or may not change behavior, depending on the active cognitive processing of the child.

Similarly, research into the effects of modeling shows that children do model the behavior of same-sex adults, but not when the adult is doing something different from other adults. Imitation may be "alive and well" as the authors say (Bussey & Bandura, 1984; Perry & Bussey, 1979), but so is selective cognition and probability assessment by the children.

A more sophisticated variant of cognitive developmental theory and social learning theory is gender schema theory (Bem, 1981, 1983, 1985; Liben & Signorella, 1980, 1987; Martin & Halverson, 1981, 1983). A schema is a set of ideas that helps an individual organize information. Schemas are changing and evolving networks of associations that people use to organize new information and perhaps even to filter information when deciding what they will and will not process.

Gender schemas develop from all the diverse information a child acquires that has anything to do with gender. Included in this information can be modes of behavior, properties of objects, attitudes, and even feeling states. (The background of this theory in memory research, and its current use in gender socialization is given by Archer & Lloyd, 1982.)

A distinct advantage of gender schema theory is that it deals with the primacy the gender concept has for our culture over other possible organizing concepts (Bem, 1983). The theory also deals with the subtle ways information is processed differentially for boys' and girls' behavior. "Adults in the child's world rarely notice or remark upon how strong a little girl is or how nurturant a little boy is becoming, despite their readiness to note precisely these attributes in the 'appropriate' sex" (Bem, 1983, p. 604).

There is a considerable body of research findings documenting the existence of gender schemas, even though this is a very new area of research (e.g., see Bem, 1981, 1985; Liben & Signorella, 1987). Gender schema research will no doubt continue to dominate the research agenda about gender socialization and may change our understanding of socialization in general.

One additional area of research on the socialization of gender is being done outside of developmental psychology by psychological anthropologists. In a landmark study, Whiting and Edwards (1988) have reanalyzed the historic six-culture sample by gender and have added five new cultures. This research by Whiting, Edwards, and their colleagues, adds an important cross-cultural perspective to issues surrounding the socialization of gender.

Eleven cultures have been analyzed for differences by sex in dyadic interactions of adults with children and children with children of different ages. The authors concluded that we are the company we keep. That is, the individuals we interact with, if they are infants, peers, or individuals older than we are, elicit particular behaviors from us. If an individual spends his or her time with an infant, the infant itself seems to bring forth nurturing responses. If that individual spends enough time with infants, he or she will become a nurturer. According to Whiting and Edwards, for example, in many cultures, but not all, young girls are given child-care responsibilities, whereas young boys are not. As a function of those responsibilities, girls are more likely to become nurturant.

The conclusion that we are the company we keep is an intriguing one. It does not explain why girls are more likely to be given one kind of responsibility than another, but it does explain other notions. For example, it has been claimed that people change over their life span (Nash & Feldman, 1981). One of the determinants of such change may be through the company they keep. This notion that we are the company we keep is also congruent with the idea Maccoby termed *self-socialization* (Maccoby & Jacklin, 1974). Certainly, one of the choices individuals have (and have more frequently with age) is the company they keep. Self-socialization does not answer the question of why one makes particular choices, but combined with the company-we-keep notion, it does help to explain why the product differs. This perspective deserves further exploration.

ISSUES OF GENDER IN DEVELOPMENTAL RESEARCH

In this article, I have examined gender issues in three central areas of research in developmental psychology. The quantity of empirical and theoretical work differs greatly in these three areas. As a consequence, our understanding of the psychological processes involved in these areas, and especially of the centrality of gender to this understanding, also differs greatly.

In the first of these areas, measurement of intellectual abilities, there is a long history of interest in gender differences and a large accumulation of empirical findings. What can be concluded from these data is that gender is not an important variable in the measurement of intellectual abilities. One would expect to find less and less focus on gender in future research in this area as reports of sex differences in abilities become less frequent. Although gender issues have been central to the study of intellectual abilities in the past, they should no longer have this emphasis, given the current findings of a lack of gender differences.

In the second area, biology and behavior, it is clear that gender differences exist, but their importance in children's behavioral development is not yet known. Males are physically more vulnerable than females, but little is known about the relationship between vulnerability and other factors. Much work needs to be done before there is a large enough empirical base to reach any conclusions about the phenomena involved. We do not know why males are more physically vulnerable than females, and we do not yet know whether vulnerability does or does not have behavioral and psychological implications. In research on how hormones affect behavior and how behavior affects hormones, the empirical data collection necessary to answer basic questions about sex differences has also just begun. Work has proceeded only far enough to reveal that we have not always been asking the right questions, an important first step. To date, the gender focus in psychological studies in this area of research has served to complicate rather than elucidate. It is now evident that the simple animal models of the influence of hormones on behavior are inadequate to understand normal human behavior. It has been established, for example, that daily variability in hormone levels is a stable individual characteristic and is more highly correlated with adolescent behavior than the absolute level of some sex-steroid hormones.

Studies of socialization processes constitute the area where a focus on gender has generated the most theory. Many empirical studies both support and refute current theoretical positions, and new constructs continue to be proposed and tested. This area continues to be rich both in empirical studies and theory generation. The focus on gender-role learning may serve as the basis for a more general understanding of socialization processes.

Thus, in each of the three research areas discussed here, gender issues are in different stages of empirical and theoretical advance. In one area, measurement of intellectual abilities, the chronicle of gender research has followed the progress of the times. That is, the changes in empirical findings across the last 2 decades have come partly as a result of feminist concerns in research and education. In the biology and behavior area, particularly the studies of male vulnerability and hormones and behavior, hypothesis formation and testing are in the early stages, as new technologies open new populations for study. Gender issues are central to much of the interest in this research, but the actual role of gender has not been well defined.

In the third area, socialization, there is a long history and much research, but also continual revision and generation of new hypotheses. Socialization of gender may be a moving target. The product we are trying to predict may itself be changing.

Working in a subject area like gender, in which issues of immediate personal and political importance are raised, has its challenges and rewards. The fact that one's work is relevant makes it more important and perhaps more fun, but the immediacy itself may make the work more difficult. Moving targets are harder to hit.

PUBLIC POLICY IMPLICATIONS

Many of the gender-related research findings described here have implications for public policy.

Sex Role Stereotypes and the Media

Much of the information that parents have about children is brought to them by the media. But, as we have seen, the media may misinform parents. For example, misinformation about gender and mathematics was disseminated, which limited parents' expectations of their children and directly limited the children's achievement. Nonstereotypic findings and complex findings do not seem to make good copy, but the media has a responsibility to update the public about these issues.

Education and Psychology

Teachers and parents, by and large, do not know the power of expectations in mathematics learning. This is a symptom of a larger problem. Current findings in psychology are not prominent in the education of teachers. Similarly, nationally organized parents groups like the Parent-Teacher Association (PTA) could, but do not currently, bring this kind of information to parents.

Interdisciplinary Research

Public policy issues are multidimensional. It is unlikely that solutions from one discipline will solve these problems. We have seen one example of the fruitfulness of a combination of psychological and anthropological research in the notion that we are the company we keep. There is a need to combine psychology and anthropology, psychology and economics, and other disciplines in the search for solutions to societal problems.

Child Care

Gender roles and the division of labor may play a strong role in causing gender differences. If interacting with infants and children brings forth nurturance in the caregivers, and there is considerable evidence that it does, then we need to rethink who does the child care in our society. Currently women and girls do most of this care while men and boys may even be discouraged from doing it. Why should nurturance be encouraged in only one sex? Nurturing may be an antidote for violence.

Changes are needed in the way the media, teachers, parents, and society view gender issues. Changes are also needed in the way researchers view working with other disciplines and working on public policy issues.

The times are changing. Change may be occurring too quickly for some, but change is not occuring quickly enough for many girls and boys limited by their gender roles to less than full lives.

REFERENCES

Archer, J., & Lloyd, B. (1982). *Sex and gender.* London: Cambridge University Press.

Bem, S. L. (1981). Gender schema theory: A cognitive account of sex-typing. *Psychological Review, 88,* 354–364.

Bem, S. L. (1983). Gender schema theory and its implications for child development: Raising gender-aschematic children in a gender-schematic society. *Signs, 8,* 598–616.

Bem, S. L. (1985). Androgyny and gender schema theory: A conceptual and empirical integration. In T. B. Sonderegger (Ed.), *Nebraska Symposium on Motivation: Psychology of gender* (pp. 179–226). Lincoln: University of Nebraska Press.

Benbow, C. P., & Stanley, J. C. (1980). Sex differences in mathematics ability: Fact or artifact? *Science, 210,* 1262–1264.

Benbow, C. P., & Stanley, J. C. (1982). Consequences in high school and college of sex differences in mathematical reasoning ability: A longitudinal perspective. *American Educational Research Journal, 19,* 598–622.

Benbow, C. P., & Stanley, J. C. (1983). Sex differences in mathematical reasoning ability: More facts. *Science, 222,* 1029–1031.

Bussey, K., & Bandura, A. (1984). Influence of gender constancy and social power on sex-linked modeling. *Journal of Personality and Social Psychology, 47,* 1292–1302.

Chodorow, N. (1978). *The reproduction of mothering: Psychoanalysis and the sociology of gender.* Berkeley: University of California Press.

Dwyer, C. A. (1979). The role of tests in producing sex-related differences. In M. A. Wittig & A. C. Petersen (Eds.), *Sex-related differences in cognitive functioning: Development issues* (pp. 335–353). New York: Academic Press.

Eccles (Parsons), J., Adler, T. F., Futterman, R., Goff, S. B., Kaczala, C. M., Meece, J. L., & Midgley, C. (1983). Expectations, values, and academic behaviors. In J. T. Spence (Ed.), *Achievement and achievement motivation* (pp. 75–146). San Francisco: W. H. Freeman.

Eccles, J., Adler, T. F., & Kaczala, C. M. (1982). Socialization of achievement attitudes and beliefs: Parental influences. *Child Development, 53,* 310–321.

Eccles, J. S., & Jacobs, J. E. (1986). Social forces shape math attitudes and performance. *Signs, 11,* 367–389.

Eccles, J., Kaczala, C. M., & Meece, J. L. (1982). Socialization of achievement attitudes and beliefs: Classroom influences. *Child Development, 53,* 322–339.

Eccles, J. S., Miller, C., Tucker, M. L., Becker, J., Schramm, W., Midgley, C., Holmes, W., Pasch, L., & Miller, M. (1988, March). *Hormones and affect at early adolescence.* Paper presented at the biannual meeting of the Society for Research on Adolescence, Alexandria, VA.

Entwisle, D. R., & Baker, D. P. (1983). Gender and young children's expectations for performance in arithmetic. *Developmental Psychology, 19*(2), 200–209.

Eisenberg, N., Wolchik, S. A., Hernandez, R., & Pasternack, J. F. (1985). Parental socialization of young children's play: A short-term longitudinal study. *Child Development, 56*, 1506–1513.

Fagot, B. I. (1985a). Beyond the reinforcement principle: Another step toward understanding sex role development. *Developmental Psychology, 21*, 1097–1104.

Fagot, B. I. (1985b). Changes in thinking about early sex-role development. *Developmental Review, 5*, 83–98.

Feingold, A. (1988). Cognitive gender differences are disappearing. *American Psychologist, 43*, 95–103.

Gualtieri, T., & Hicks, R. E. (1985). An immunoreactive theory of selective male affliction. *The Behavioral and Brain Sciences, 8*, 427–441.

Hollingworth, L. S. (1914). Variability as related to sex differences in achievement. *American Journal of Sociology, 19*, 510–530.

Hollingworth, L. (1916). Sex differences in mental traits. *Psychological Bulletin, 13*, 377–385.

Hollingworth, L. (1918). Comparison of the sexes in mental traits. *Psychological Bulletin, 25*, 427–432.

Hyde, J. S., & Linn, M. C. (1986). *The psychology of gender: Advances through meta-analysis.* Baltimore: The John Hopkins University Press.

Hyde, J. S., & Linn, M. C. (1988). Are there sex differences in verbal abilities?: A meta-analysis. *Psychological Bulletin, 104*(1), 53–69.

Jacklin, C. N. (1987). Feminist research and psychology. In C. Farnham (Ed.), *The impact of feminist research in the academy* (pp. 95–110). Bloomington: Indiana University Press.

Jacklin, C. N., & Maccoby, E. E. (1982). Length of labor and sex of offspring. *Journal of Pediatric Psychology, 7*, 355–360.

Jacklin, C. N., Maccoby, E. E., & Doering, C. H. (1983). Neonatal sex-steroid hormones and timidity in 6–18 month-old boys and girls. *Developmental Psychobiology, 16*, 163–168.

Jacklin, C. N., Maccoby, E. E., Doering, C. H., & King, D. R. (1984). Neonatal sex steroid hormones and muscular strength of boys and girls in the first three years. *Developmental Psychobiology, 17*, 301–310.

Jacklin, C. N., Wilcox, K. T., & Maccoby, E. E. (1988). Neonatal sex-steroid hormones and intellectual abilities of six year old boys and girls. *Developmental Psychobiology, 21*, 567–574.

Jacobs, J. E., & Eccles, J. S. (1985). Gender differences in math ability: The impact of media reports on parents. *Educational Researcher, 14*, 20–25.

Kohlberg, L. (1966). A cognitive-developmental analysis of children's sex-role concepts and attitudes. In E. E. Maccoby (Ed.), *The development of sex differences* (pp. 82–173). Stanford, CA: Stanford University Press.

Kohlberg, L., & Ullian, D. Z. (1974). Stages in the development of psychosexual concepts and attitudes. In R. C. Friedman, R. M. Richart, & R. L. Vande Wiele (Eds.), *Sex differences in behavior* (pp. 209–222). New York: Wiley.

Kraemer, H. C., Korner, A. F., Anders, T., Jacklin, C. N., & Dimicelli, S. (1985). Obstetric drugs and infant behavior: A reevaluation. *Journal of Pediatric Psychology, 10,* 345–353.

Lerman, H. (1986). *A mote in Freud's eye: From psychoanalysis to the psychology of women.* New York: Springer.

Liben, L. S., & Signorella, M. L. (1980). Gender-related schemata and constructive memory in children. *Child Development, 51,* 11–18.

Liben, L. S., & Signorella, M. L. (Eds.). (1987). *Children's gender schemata.* San Francisco: Jossey-Bass.

Linn, M. C., & Petersen, A. C. (1985). Emergence and characterization of sex differences in spatial ability: A meta-analysis. *Child Development, 56,* 1479–1498.

Linn, M. C., & Petersen, A. C. (1986). A meta-analysis of gender differences in spatial ability: Implications for mathematics and science achievement. In J. S. Hyde & M. C. Linn (Eds.), *The psychology of gender: Advances through meta-analysis* (pp. 67–101). Baltimore: The Johns Hopkins University Press.

Lips, H. M. (1988). *Sex and gender: An introduction.* Mountain View, CA: Mayfield Publishing.

Maccoby, E. E., & Jacklin, C. N. (1974). *The psychology of sex differences.* Stanford, CA: Stanford University Press.

Maccoby, E. E., & Jacklin, C. N. (1980). Sex differences in aggression: A rejoinder and reprise. *Child Development, 51,* 964–980.

Marcus, J., Maccoby, E. E., Jacklin, C. N., & Doering, C. H. (1985). Individual differences in mood: Their relation to gender and neonatal sex steroids. *Developmental Psychobiology, 18,* 327–340.

Martin, C. L., & Halverson, C. F., Jr. (1981). A schematic processing model of sex-typing and stereotyping in young children. *Child Development, 52,* 1119–1134.

Martin, C. L., & Halverson, C. F., Jr. (1983). The effects of sex-typing schemas on young children's memory. *Child Development, 54,* 563–574.

McMilen, M. M. (1979). Differential mortality by sex in fetal and neonatal deaths. *Science, 204,* 89–91.

Mischel, W. (1966). A social-learning view of sex differences in behavior. In E. E. Maccoby (Ed.), *The development of sex differences* (56–81). Stanford, CA: Stanford University Press.

Nash, S. C., & Feldman, S. S. (1981). Sex role and sex-related attributions: Constancy and change across the family life cycle. In M. Lamb & A. Brown (Eds.), *Advances in developmental psychology* (Vol. 1, pp. 1–35). Hillsdale, NJ: Erlbaum.

Novitski, E. (1977). *Human genetics.* New York: Macmillan.

Perry, D. G., & Bussey, I. (1979). The social learning theory of sex differences: Imitation is alive and well. *Journal of Personality and Social Psychology, 37,* 1699–1712.

Piaget, J. (1954). *The construction of reality in the child.* New York: Basic Books.

Rosenthal, R., & Rubin, D. B. (1982). Further meta-analytic procedures for assessing cognitive gender differences. *Journal of Educational Psychology, 74,* 708–712.

Sherman, J. A. (1971). *On the psychology of women.* Springfield, IL: Charles C. Thomas.

Susman, E. J., & Chrousos, G. P. (1988, March). *Physiological reactivity and emotional development in young adolescents.* Paper presented at the biannual meeting of the Society for Research on Adolescence, Alexandria, VA.

Susman, E. J., Inoff-Germain, G., Nottelmann, E. D., Loriaux, D. L., Cutler, G. B., & Chrousos, G. P. (1987). Hormones, emotional dispositions, and aggressive attributes in young adolescents. *Child Development, 58,* 1114–1134.

Udry, R. J. (1988, March). *Biological and social determinants of behavior change in early adolescent boys.* Paper presented at the biannual meeting of the Society for Research on Adolescence, Alexandria, VA.

Whiting, B. B., & Edwards, C. P. (1988). *Children of different worlds: The formation of social behavior.* Cambridge, MA: Harvard University Press.

Woolley, H. T. (1910). A review of recent literature on the psychology of sex. *Psychological Bulletin, 7,* 335–342.

Woolley, H. T. (1914). The psychology of sex. *Psychological Bulletin, 11,* 353–379.

Part II

EPIDEMIOLOGICAL STUDIES

Michael Rutter has chosen the occassion of the 25th aniversery of the initiation of the Isle of Wight studies of educational, psychiatric, and physical disorders of children as a focal point for a thorough and systematic review of epidemiologic investigation in child psychiatry over the past quarter of a century. Rather than "revisiting" the Isle of Wight, Rutter has chosen to focus upon topics and issues not addressed in that investigation, including the study of behavioral disturbance in preschool children and specific child psychiatric diagnoses.

The methodology of the Isle of Wight investigations can be thought to have set the standard for subsequent investigations. Multiple data sources were used to survey an entire geographically defined population. A two-stage research strategy was employed so that a multiple source screen was used to identify children who were likely to have one of the disorders germane to the investigation. Children so identified were then studied in detail using a range of approaches including standardized interviews with parents, teachers as well as the children themselves, together with standardized neurodevelopmental and medical examinations and systematic individual psychological testing of the children. Diagnoses were based on behavioral features, and social impairment was utilized as a criterion of severity. Longitudinal research strategies were employed to examine risk factors prospectively, neurologic findings were related to psychiatric measures, and the ways in which non-responders differed from subjects for whom data was available was assessed. Rutter cites subsequent advances in epidemiological methodology including the further elaboration of longitudional study designs, the discriminating use of high-risk samples to test particular causal hypotheses, and the development of a range of standardized interview measures likely to give replicable diagnoses for most of the broader diagnostic categories.

Not only does this paper provide references to most of the important epidemiological investigations of the past 25 years, but it also includes a distinguished psychiatric epidemiologist's prescription for the future of his science. In elaborating his "wish list" for epidemiologically based studies of the future, Rutter urges going beyond the establishment of "true" prevalence figures for the complete range of psychiatric disorders. Although such data would be useful, their value would be limited because some diagnostic entities are of uncertain validity and there is no direct connection between prevalence and service needs. To address this question, information regarding social impairment, duration response to treatment, and acceptability of intervention is also required. Instead, Rutter calls attention to the importance of a developmental perspective, urging the careful elucidation of age-trends as well as the need for studies of comorbidity, situation specificity, and continuities and discontinuities between childhood and adult life.

The Kauai longitudional study by Werner is one of the largest interdisciplinary investigations of the roots of resiliency in vulnerable children. A multi-racial cohort of 698 children born in 1955 on the island of Kauai, Hawaii have been followed into the third decade of life. The study has monitored the impact on development of a variety of biological and psychosocial risk factors, stressful life events, and protective factors in early and middle childhood and late adolescence and adult life. Werner's paper, "High-risk Children in Young Adulthood" provides an overview of the research strategy and the principal findings derived from this enormously rich data base.

When the developmental course of high-risk children is examined, three types of protective factors emerge that distinguish those who were resilient from those who had developed significant learning or behavioral problems before the age of 18: (1) dispositional attributes of the individual, such as activity level and sciability, at least average intelligence, competence in communication skills, and an internal locus of control; (2) affectional ties within the family that provide emotional support in times of stress; and (3) external support systems, in school, at work or church, that serve to reward the individual's competencies and determination and provide a belief system by which to live.

From a longitudional perspective, Werner reports that the relative impact of risk and protective factors changed from infancy through early and middle childhood to late adolescence and adulthood. At each developmental stage there was a shifting balance that heightened individual vulnerability and protective factors enhancing resilience, which changed, not only with increasing age,but also with the gender of the individual. Werner challenges future investigators to clarify the chain of direct and indirect linkages between various protective factors over time so as to more effectively foster the escape from adversity for vulnerable children.

The focus of the report by Offord, Boyle, and Racine, which is one of a series deriving from the Ontario Child Health Study, is on the correlates of disorder. The findings have major implications both for our understanding of the nature of psychiatric disorders in children and our methods for studying them. The data derive from an interview survey of 1,869 families including 3,294 children in the Province of Ontario carried out in 1983. Four childhood psychiatric disorders were investigated: conduct disorder, hyperactivity, emotional disorder in children 4–11, and these three combined with somatization disorder in adolescents 12–16 years of age. Parents, teachers and adolescents completed a Survey Diagnostic Instrument. Consistent with the findings of other studies, case ascertainment to a large extent was dependent upon who provided the information upon which the diagnosis was based.

The lack of agreement among informants regarding individuals who exhibit clinically important symptomatology found in this study adds to our awareness that the identification of childhood psychiatric disorder is influenced by the perception of informants and the contexts in which assessments are done. Moreover, in addition to disagreements among informants, correlates of disorder—such as low income, parents treated for nerves, parental arrest records, and chronic medical illness—showed evidence of having a different relationship with disorder, depending on the informant. The combining of information from various sources, a common procedure in epidemiologically based studies, must be undertaken with caution as such practices can affect inferences about associated features of disorder in unknown ways. Offord et al. propose that childhood disorder be studied as a contextual phenomenon, and not as a unitary attribute that is an essential component of the child's personality.

Ritvo, Jorde, Mason-Brothers, Freeman, Pingree, Jones McMahon, Petersen, Jenson and Mo offer the final paper in this section.

This report is based on data derived from an epidemiologic survey of autism in the state of Utah. The focus is on recurrence risk estimates and their implications for genetic counseling. The survey employed a four-level system of ascertainment, utilizing DSM-III criteria and a team of experienced clinicians who conducted blind diagnostic evaluations throughout the state. The prevalence of autism was found to be 4 per 10,000 in the general population with a sex ratio of 4 males to 1 female. Estimates of the risk of recurrence were based on 233 autistic children from 207 families. The overall recurrence risk estimate—the chance that each sibling born after an autistic child will develop autism—is 8.6%; if the first autistic child is a male the recurrence risk estimate is 7, and if a female 14.5%.

Ritvo et al. have interpreted these data as suggesting that there may be a subtype of autism that is genetically influenced. It is, as these workers also indicate, most likely that more than one etiological factor and pathological process will be found that can produce the syndrome. Furthermore, the low frequency of occurrence in the general population limited the size of the sample upon which these estimates of recurrence were based. Nevertheless, as the report stresses, this information should be made available to all individuals who have autistic children and who are interested in family planning.

7

Isle of Wight Revisited: Twenty-five Years of Child Psychiatric Epidemiology

Michael Rutter

Institute of Psychiatry, London, England

Child psychiatric epidemiology over the last 25 years is reviewed in terms of conceptual and methodological issues arising out of substantive findings. The Isle of Wight surveys undertaken in the mid-1960s are briefly described to establish a starting point, and progress since then is reviewed in terms of topics not originally covered—especially problems in preschool children and specific psychiatric disorders. The use of epidemiology to study causal hypotheses is considered, methodological advances are noted, and challenges for the future are discussed. Key Words: child psychiatric disorders, epidemiology, causal relationships, sampling, measures.

The first systematic wide scale epidemiological study in the field of child psychiatry was the Buffalo study undertaken by Lapouse and Monk (1958, 1959, 1964; Lapouse, 1965a, b) in the mid-1950s. The findings were most important in indicating the high frequency of emotional and behavioral problems among 6- to 12-year-old children; in showing that many of these problems lessened with increasing age; and in drawing attention to the discrepancy between mother and child reports for some symptoms. The survey was limited from the psychiatric perspective, however, in that diagnoses were not made and in that child interviews were available only in a separate convenience sample rather than in the main study.

Several other surveys undertaken at about the same time, or a little later, added to our knowledge on the epidemiology of children's problems (reviewed in Rutter et al.,

Reprinted with permission from *Journal of the American Academy of Child and Adolescent Psychiatry,* 1989, Vol. 28, No. 5, 633–653. Copyright © 1989 by the American Academy of Child and Adolescent Psychiatry.

1970b), but perhaps the first large scale epidemiological investigation with a child psychiatric focus was provided by the British series of epidemiological studies of educational, psychiatric and physical disorders undertaken on the Isle of Wight during the mid-1960s (see Rutter et al., 1970a, b, 1976; Rutter 1979a). During the quarter of a century since those studies, child psychiatric epidemiology has both burgeoned and strengthened (see Earls, 1980a, b, 1982; Gould et al., 1980; Graham 1977, 1979, 1980; Links, 1983; Offord and Boyle, 1986; Rutter, 1988c; Rutter and Sandberg, 1985; Schmidt and Remschmidt, 1983; Verhulst and Althaus, 1988; Vikan, 1985; Yule, 1981), and it seems an appropriate time to review progress and to assess the key issues for future research in this area. That is the purpose of this paper, the aim being to use empirical findings to discuss some of the key conceptual and methodological issues that face child psychiatric epidemiologists today and which are pertinent for clinicians' understanding and interpretation of the research data stemming from epidemiological surveys.

ISLE OF WIGHT STUDIES

Before considering progress over the last 25 years it is necessary briefly to outline the Isle of Wight studies in order to establish a starting point. The 1964 survey covered intellectual and educational retardation in the entire population of about 3,500 9- to 11-year-old children living on the island (an intrinsic part of England situated just off the south coast, having a total population of some 100,000 in all); psychiatric disorder and physical handicap were surveyed in the same cohort a year later; and comparable conditions were reexamined in the same cohort in 1969 when the children were aged 14 to 15 years. The entire population of 5- to 15-year-old children (some 11,000 in all) was also screened for neuroepileptic disorders (Rutter et al., 1970a). A further survey of 10-year-old children was undertaken in 1969 in order to make direct comparisons with a 1970 survey of the same age group in an inner London borough (Berger et al., 1975; Rutter et al., 1975a, b). In addition, a more limited range of studies were undertaken with infant school children (aged 5 to 7 years).

The studies involved several methodological innovations. First, multiple data sources were used to survey the entire population. These included parent and teacher questionnaires; school records; psychiatric clinic and hospital records; and pediatric records. Second, a two-stage research strategy was employed. Thus, the multiple source screen was used to identify children who were likely to have one of the disorders being studied; then, these children were studied in detail using a range of approaches that included standardized interviews with parents, children and teachers, together with standardized neurodevelopmental and medical examinations and systematic individual psychological testing of the children. Third, the interviews used with both parents and children differed from those used previously in being both clinically orientated and standardized (with systematic testing of reliability and validity). Many clinicians and researchers had hitherto assumed that it was not possible (or, if possible, not useful) to ask children direct questions about their psychopathology; rather, indirect projective or play techniques were needed. Lapouse and Monk had shown that children could report on emotional and behavioral symptoms and the Isle of Wight data confirmed the utility of direct interviews with children and adolescents. Fourth, psychiatric disorders were diagnosed using social impairment as a criterion of severity together with symptom pattern as a criterion of type. Contrary to most psychiatric practice of that era, diagnoses were based purely on behavioral features rather than on assumptions about etiology or intrapsychic mechanisms (see Murphy 1986 for a discussion of changing philosophies regarding "assumptive diagnoses"). However, the criteria used fell far short of the research diagnostic criteria pioneered later by Feighner et al. (1972). Fifth, longitudinal research strategies were used to divide disorders according to age of onset, to examine risk factors prospectively, and to examine the course of disorders over time. Sixth, epidemiological research strategies were used to test causal hypotheses with respect to risk factors that included organic brain dysfunction, family discord and reading difficulties (Rutter, 1981a). Seventh, standardized neurodevelopmental assessments were used to relate neurological findings to psychiatric measures. Eighth, use was made of longitudinal/epidemiological data to determine the ways in which nonresponders differed from subjects for whom data were available (Cox et al., 1977).

The Isle of Wight studies, of course, produced many empirical findings; here, attention will be drawn only to those that opened up issues or raised questions that are currently important. First, because there was separate measurement of symptoms and of social impairment it was possible to determine which specific behaviors were of greatest clinical significance. The findings showed that poor peer relations and inattention/overactivity stood out as behaviors with a strong association with psychiatric disorder. Few children were diagnosed as suffering from a hyperkinetic disorder according to the prevailing U.K. diagnostic criteria (which were much narrower than those for the U.S. concept) but many children showed the symptoms of inattention and overactivity. Most of these also showed conduct disturbance and were diagnosed accordingly. The finding raised questions on how hyperkinetic/ attention deficit disorders should be defined and on how disorders involving both conduct problems and hyperactivity should be diagnosed. So-called "neurotic traits of childhood" such as nail-biting and thumb-sucking were found to be very common and to have only a weak association with disorder.

Second, depressive symptoms and disorders were found to be much more frequent at age 14 to 15 years than at 10 to 11 years; this raised questions on why affective problems became more frequent during adolescence. Also, however, it was striking that the adolescents reported much higher rates of affective symptomatology than evident from parental reports. The observation underlined the importance of interviewing children/adolescents as well as parents, but also raised a query regarding the clinical significance of depressive problems reported by young people but not noted by the adults who interacted with them. It was also notable that depressive symptoms were common in all types of psychiatric disorder and were frequently present in youths with a conduct disorder. This raised questions about the meaning of comorbidity between depression and conduct disorder but also it highlighted important differences between depressive and anxiety/phobic symptoms. Unlike depressive conditions, the latter did *not* show an association with conduct problems. Anxiety and depression frequently co-occur but it seemed that they function in rather different ways and therefore require to be differentiated, even though the distinction may be difficult in individual cases.

Third, the data showed relatively low agreement between parent and teacher reports of children's deviant behavior, and the interview findings suggested that this was, at least in part, a function of children behaving differently in different situations. The observation underlined the need to obtain reports from both teachers and parents and also suggested the potential value of differentiating pervasive from situation-specific disorders—a differentiation that was shown to be useful in the case of hyperactivity.

Fourth, the findings indicated the importance of taking into account regression effects in the measurement of specific reading retardation, and provided a means of doing so. A distinction between specific reading retardation (i.e., reading that was retarded in relation to a person's age and IQ) and general reading backwardness (i.e., reading that was low for chronological age but not necessarily out of keeping with mental age) was shown to be of value in terms of both different correlates and different prognosis.

Fifth, there was a specific focus on patterns of comorbidity and exploration of the possible reasons for associations between disorders (the survey was initially prompted by a concern to check whether the association between poor physical health and psychological/educational problems found in the 1920s in the U.K. still applied in the 1960s). As part of that comorbidity focus, a major overlap was found between specific reading retardation and conduct disorders. Because the overlap group (i.e., those with both) had more in common with the "pure" reading retardation group (in terms of pattern of correlates) than the "pure" conduct disorder group, it was inferred that some cases of conduct disturbance may have arisen on the basis of reading failure or factors associated with it. The strength of the comorbidity between reading difficulties and conduct disturbance emphasized the need for the association, and the reasons for it, to be investigated further.

Sixth, it was also noted that there was a substantial group of children who showed a pattern of disturbance that constituted a mixture of emotional and conduct symptoms. This comorbidity pattern was not studied in the same detail but it was noted that the overlap, or mixed, group seemed to have more in common with the pure conduct disorder group than the pure emotional group. The finding highlighted the need for more systematic study of patterns of comorbidity within the field of child psychiatric disorders.

Seventh, the psychiatric disorders in adolescence with an onset after age 10 were found to have a different set of correlates from those with an onset in earlier childhood. In particular, the later onset disorders did *not* have an association with either reading difficulties or chronic psychosocial adversity. It seemed that greater attention needed to be paid to age of onset as a means of subdividing disorders and, in particular, a focus on disorders with an onset in adolescence was required to elucidate possible causal factors.

Finally, the epidemiological data suggested a causal role for both family adversity and organic brain dysfunction in the genesis of child psychiatric disorders, but doubt was cast on the validity of a concept of a behaviorally distinctive syndrome of "minimal brain dysfunction."

TOPICS NOT COVERED IN THE ISLE OF WIGHT STUDIES

Preschool Children

Although quite extensive in coverage, the Isle of Wight surveys left out many psychiatric topics. Most obviously, they did not cover younger children (except at questionnaire and psychometric level)—an important gap well filled by Richman et al.'s (1982) London study, as well by Earls' Martha's Vineyard Child Health Survey (Earls, 1980a, b; Garrison and Earls, 1985b), Wolkind's (1985) London study (Wolkind, 1985; Wolkind and Kruk, 1985), and Minde and Minde's (1977) Canadian survey. The Richman et al. London study was particularly notable for its inclusion of a follow-up from age 3 to 8 years. The longitudinal data were crucial in showing that some three-fifths of disorders at 3 years of age persisted over the next 5 years. The finding was important in showing that many disorders in preschool children were *not* transient and benign as hitherto commonly supposed. Longitudinal data were also essential in demonstrating that psychosocial adversity (as shown, for example, by maternal depression or family discord) at 3 years of age predicted the development of disorder by age 8 in children without disorder at 3. The prospective predictive association provided strong support for the hypothesis that some aspect of the adversity was *causally* influential in the development of psychiatric disorder (although the data did not delineate the mechanisms involved). However, it was also notable that improvements in family functioning did not necessarily result in remissions in the children's disorders. This important negative finding could mean either that a greater degree of environmental change is needed to bring about remission; or that, once a disorder is established, factors within the child lead to a degree of self-perpetuation; or that the factors leading to onset of disorder differ from those influencing course. This remains an important issue requiring further research.

Longitudinal data were crucial, again, in the demonstration that speech and language delay at 3 years of age predicts the development of emotional and behavioral disorders over the next 5 years in children without disorder at 3 (Stevenson et al., 1985). The association between developmental disorders of speech/language and psychiatric disturbance has now been shown in several epidemiological/longitudinal studies (Beitchman et al., 1986, 1987; Stevenson, 1984; Silva, 1987), as well as by various clinical investigations (Cantwell and Baker, 1987; Howlin and Rutter, 1987). It seems clear that the association is not an artifact and the longitudinal findings strongly suggest that it reflects causal mechanisms. However, the processes involved remain obscure and the frequent persistence of associated social problems into early adult life many years after conversational fluency has been obtained (Mawhood, unpublished data) suggests that the psychiatric disturbance is not simply a secondary reaction to communication difficulties. Again, the elucidation of the causal processes involved remains a research task for the future.

The Martha's Vineyard study confirmed the tendency of preschool problems to persist (54% over a period of 3 years), but it emphasized the low level of consistency between maternal and teachers' reports (Garrison and Earls, 1985a). It was also important in showing the strength of associations between temperamental difficulty and psychiatric disorder (Earls and Jung, 1987). The Quebec epidemiological/longitudinal study (Maziade et al., 1985) added to knowledge on this association by showing that temperamental difficulty at age 7 years was strongly predictive of psychiatric disorder at age 12 years. The psychiatric risk was particularly great when there was the combination of a dysfunctional family and temperamental adversity; superior family functioning largely mitigated the effects of a difficult temperament. Similar findings (over a 1-year time period) derived from the epidemiological/longitudinal study of a high risk group, children reared by mentally ill parents (Graham et al., 1973). That study also showed that temperamentally difficult children tended to elicit negative reactions from their caregivers (Rutter, 1978). Thus, epidemiological findings have both confirmed the reality of the psychiatric risk associated with a difficult temperament and also suggested that temperament does not usually lead directly to disorder; rather it is necessary to take into account the interactions between children and their families. However, major questions remain unanswered. As yet, there is no epidemiological study that has longitudinal data over a period of several years that includes both temperamental and psychiatric data at both time points, together with other variables that may relate differently to temperament and psychiatric disorder. This design is crucial in order to rule out the possibility that the temperamental risk for psychiatric disorder simply reflects early subclinical manifestations that may serve as precursors of disorder. In other words, it is necessary to determine whether temperamental variation and psychiatric disorder have different determinants (such as genetic contributions or psychosocial adversity); and to test whether having differentiated temperament from disorder, temperament still predicts the later development of psychiatric problems. Longitudinal data on parent-child (and teacher-child and peer-child) interactions are also needed to determine the extent to which the psychiatric risk is mediated by the effect of difficult temperamental characteristics in eliciting maladaptive styles of interaction.

Specific Psychiatric Disorders

For the most part, the Isle of Wight data were applied to the rather broad psychiatric groupings of emotional and conduct disorders, rather than to the more specific diagnostic categories of psychiatric classification systems such as *DSM-III-R* (American Psychiatric Association, 1987) and ICD-10 (World Health Organization, in press). However, the limited data relevant to specific categories raised some important issues.

Affective Disorders

First, the follow-up from age 10 to 15 years showed a marked increase in affective disorders over this age period (Rutter et al., 1976a; Rutter, 1979a). The measurement of depressive symptomatology was rather primitive by present day standards but the better data from the Yale high risk study (Weissman et al., 1987a), as well as from other studies (Angold, 1988a, b; Costello, 1989a; Rutter, 1988a; Rutter et al., 1986a) seem to confirm that major affective disorders become substantially more frequent over the adolescent age period. Possibly, too, the female preponderance seen in adult life may also become apparent only at or after adolescence. Data on attempted (Hawton and Goldacre, 1982) and completed suicide (Shaffer, 1986; Shaffer et al., 1988) also show a massive increase in frequency over the teenage years. The findings are provocative and important but numerous questions remain. To begin with, we still lack good epidemiological data across the child to adult age period using comparable standardized measures. It seems clear that not all aspects of dysphoric mood increase in adolescence (Shepherd et al., 1971) and, although the data are limited, it seems that anxiety disorders also do not show this increase (Costello, 1989a; Moreau and Weissman, in press; Orvaschel and Weissman, 1986). Moreover, we lack understanding of *why* affective disorders become more prevalent during adolescence (if further epidemiological studies confirm that they do). Age is an ambiguous variable (Rutter, 1989b) and the increase may reflect mechanisms as diverse as the effects of hormonal change, an increase in life stressors or a diminution in social supports, greater cognitive maturity or the age-dependent expression of a genetic vulnerability (Masten, in press; Peterson, 1988; Rutter, 1988b). Good epidemiological data using designs appropriate for the purpose, are needed to differentiate these postulated mechanisms.

Anxiety Disorders

Until recently, anxiety disorders in childhood have constituted a rather neglected diagnostic group, with few epidemiological data available (Orvaschel and Weissman, 1986). However, recent studies of pediatric primary care (Costello, 1989b; Costello et al., 1988) and general population samples (Anderson et al., 1987; Bird et al., 1988, 1989; Kashani and Orvaschel, 1988; Velez et al., 1989) using structured interview assessments, have shown their frequency. Costello (1989a) concluded that separation anxiety disorders occurred in 3.5% to 5.4% of children, overanxious disorders in 1.6% to 2.9%, and phobias in 2.3% to 9.2%. However, these figures are based on disorders associated with substantial social impairment and the rates are very much higher if diagnoses are based only on symptom constellations. Thus, Kashani and Orveschel (1988) found that 17% of 14- to 16-year-olds met the criteria for one or more anxiety diagnoses (8.7% were identified as "cases" on the basis of impairment). Similarly, Velez et al. (1989) reported that 19% of 9- to 12-year-olds exhibited overanxiety and 26% separation anxiety disorders. The rates in 13- to 18-year-olds were about half as high. There appears to be considerable overlap between the supposedly different types of anxiety disorder and substantial comorbidity with depression. There also is comorbidity with *DSM-III* diagnoses of attention deficit disorder (Anderson et al., 1987; Bird et al., 1988). Stressful life events and low social status appear associated with anxiety disorders (Costello et al., 1988; Velez et al., 1989) but, on the whole, much less is known about the risks associated with environmental disorders, of any type, than those with conduct and hyperkinetic disorders.

Hyperkinetic Disorders

A further condition for which the Isle of Wight studies provided limited data was the hyperkinetic (or attention deficit) syndrome (Schachar et al., 1981). The findings were nevertheless striking in showing (i) that the correlates of pervasive hyperactivity differed from those of situational hyperactivity; (ii) that pervasive hyperactivity showed a strong association with cognitive impairment; and (iii) that pervasive hyperactivity in association with other forms of disturbance carried a poor prognosis for the persistence of psychiatric disorder. The "Cambridge" epidemiological/longitudinal study of boys living in inner London (Farrington et al., in press) and the Stockholm epidemiological/longitudinal study (Magnusson, 1988; Magnusson and Bergman, in press) have both subsequently confirmed that the presence of hyperactivity/inattention in combination with conduct disturbance indicates a more severe disorder with a worse prognosis. The Dunedin longitudinal study also confirmed the association with learning problems (Anderson et al., 1989; McGee and Share, 1988). However, all these studies are limited by their lack of clinical diagnostic data. Subsequent epidemiological studies by Taylor et al. in London (Taylor, 1989; Taylor et al., 1988), by Offord et al. (1987; Offord and Boyle, 1989) in Ottawa, by Boudreault et al. (1988) in Quebec, and by Shen et al. (1985) in China have remedied that gap. All the studies have confirmed the very marked male preponderance for this diagnostic category and the two latter studies have also shown that it is more frequent in geographical areas with a high rate of psychosocial adversity (isolated mountain areas in China and urban areas in Canada). The London investigation also confirmed (with much better data) the association with cognitive deficits; in addition it showed an association with laboratory-measured attentional problems. The Quebec study finding confirmed that pervasive attention deficit disorders differed from situational varieties in the association with verbal deficits and reading difficulties. Taken in conjunction with the findings from clinical investigations, the data suggest that a distinctive syndrome is provided by a pattern of pervasive hyperactivity/inattention, not part of generalized anxiety, with an onset in the preschool years and which tends to be associated with neurodevelopmental delays and neonatal adversity (Rutter, 1989c; Taylor, 1989; Taylor et al., 1988). However, although the evidence suggests that neurodevelopmental impairment is important in the initial genesis of the condition, psychosocial adversity seems to influence its perpetuation into later childhood.

Specific Reading Retardation

The Isle of Wight studies argued for the need to differentiate between specific reading retardation (SRR) and general reading backwardness (GRB) (Rutter and Yule, 1975) and reaffirmed Thorndike's (1963) demonstration that multiple regression procedures were needed to determine whether children's reading skills were discrepant from those expected on the basis of their general intelligence. The argument for the value of differentiating SRR was based on three main sets of findings: (i) correlates that differed from those found with general reading backwardness; (ii) an outcome that similarly differed; and (ii) a "hump" at the bottom of the distribution so that the prevalence of serious underachievers was greater than that expected on statistical grounds. Van der Wissel and Zegers (1985) pointed out the possible biasing effects of floor and ceiling effects in testing the hump hypothesis, but Stevenson (1988) has confirmed that the hump occurs for reading and spelling in 11- and 13-year-olds (but not at age 7 years on group tests), although the hump has not been apparent in other studies (Rodgers, 1983; Share et al., 1987). The crucial test of the SRR hypothesis, however, does not depend on the presence or absence of a hump in the distribution but rather on whether the correlates and outcome of SRR serve to differentiate the syndrome from GRB. A key need in that connection is to include spelling deficits in the concept of SRR in view of their great importance in older age groups (Yule, 1973)—a need that has not been met adequately in any of the investigations, including the Isle of Wight studies. Nevertheless, the weight of evidence from the New Zealand and Australian epidemiological studies suggests that SRR is distinctive from GRB in showing a very marked male preponderance, in being less likely to be accompanied by general neurodevelopmental impairment, and in being particularly associated with speech and language disabilities (Jorm et al., 1986a, b; Silva et al., 1985). Possibly, too, the pattern of association with behavioral problems may be somewhat different in the two types of reading difficulties (McGee et al., 1986). It remains uncertain whether the reading processes per se in SRR differ from those in general backwardness (Frith, 1985; Fredman and Stevenson, 1988).

From a psychiatric perspective, the strong association between reading difficulties and emotional/behavioral disturbance (especially conduct problems) remains a key issue. The strength of the association and its importance for prognosis has been shown (Maughan et al., 1985), but the elucidation of the mechanisms involved remains a task for the future, with the evidence available so far contradictory and open to different interpretations (Rutter and Giller, 1983).

Enuresis

The Isle of Wight study showed that the prevalence of enuresis dropped with increasing age and that male preponderance became evident after age 5 years; the availability of longitudinal data also brought out the important point that many children become wet between the age of 5 and 7 years having previously acquired continence (Rutter et al., 1973). Many enuretic children show no evidence of emotional or behavioral disturbance but an association with such disturbance is evident in older enuretics, particularly in those who also show daytime wetting. Enuresis is more frequent in children from socially disadvantaged backgrounds and in those experiencing psychosocial adversity. All these findings have been well replicated in epidemiological studies both before and after the Isle of Wight study (Douglas, 1973; Essen and Peckham 1976; Kaffman and Elizur, 1977; Miller et al., 1960, Oppel et al., 1968; Stein et al., 1965; Verhulst et al., 1985); unfortunately it cannot be claimed that the findings have thrown much light on the mechanisms involved in this common, but troublesome, problem.

Anorexia Nervosa

Monosymptomatic disorders, such as enuresis, require screening measures that focus on specific behaviors rather than rely on high questionnaire scores that tap a wide range of psychopathology. Similar needs apply to disorders that involve either relatively rare symptoms (such as obsessive-compulsive phenomena) or symptoms that occur in patterns that are different from the broad run of emotional and conduct disorders (such as anorexic or bulimic problems). Progress has been made in this area but there are problems in deciding the extent to which subclinical manifestations parallel the clinical syndrome. Thus, there have been several surveys of anorexic symptoms in adolescent girls (e.g., Crisp et al., 1976; Button and Whitehouse, 1981; Johnson-Sabine et al., 1988; Abraham et al., 1983; Garner et al., 1983; Szmuckler, 1985). These all show that anorexic-type eating disorders are considerably more common (approximately 3%) than overt anorexia nervosa (for which psychiatric case registers suggest a sex-age specific rate of about 4 to 8 per 100,000 females aged 15 to 34 years [Kendell et al., 1973]), with abnormal eating behaviors even more prevalent (occurring in some 1 in 5 adolescent girls). The epidemiological data show that extreme dieting and preoccupations with body shape peak in the postpubertal years in girls, as does anorexia nervosa, but the mechanisms involved and the connections between subclinical and clinical anorexia nervosa have still to be established.

Failure to Thrive

Nonorganic growth retardation and failure to thrive in preschool children has only very recently been subjected to epidemiological enquiry (Dowdney et al., 1987; Heptinstall et al., 1987). The findings have shown a prevalence of about 2%, the affected children predominantly coming from a socially disadvantaged background and tending to show general developmental retardation. Again, the mechanisms remain obscure (although negative family interactions at mealtimes seem important), and it is evident that this is a group requiring further investigation using prospective epidemiological/longitudinal research strategies.

Recurrent Abdominal Pain

It has long been appreciated that recurrent abdominal pain is common in young children and that often it is associated with psychological disturbance (Apley, 1975). However epidemiological data has been sparse. A recent British survey of 6-year-olds showed that one in four had experienced at least three episodes; of these a majority showed some form of emotional or behavioral disturbance but the type followed no clear pattern, although hyperactivity was common (Faull and Nicol, 1986). A general practice survey of 3-year-old children in a London suburb found that, according to maternal reports, 3% had recurrent headache and 9% recurrent stomachache (Zuckerman et al., 1987). Both groups had a much increased rate of emotional/behavioral disturbance; recurrent pain was also associated with maternal depression, and stomachache with marital problems.

Obsessive-Compulsive Disorders

There has been a recent resurgence of interest in obsessive-compulsive disorders arising in childhood. There are particular problems in using lay interviewers to assess these conditions in view of their infrequency and the lack of agreement between lay and professional concepts (Anthony et al., 1985; Breslau, 1987). The Baltimore findings from the Epidemiologic Catchment Area study showed a 1-month prevalence of 0.3% for adults when psychiatric evaluations were used. However, the overall 1-month prevalence from the five ECA sites was 1.3% when data from the structured Diagnostic Interview Schedule were used (Karno et al., 1988). The only systematic epidemiological study in adolescence to use as an appropriate focussed screening measure (the Leyton Obsessional Inventory) (Cooper, 1970; Berg et al., 1988) is that by Flament et al. (1988) of about 5,500 high school students in the ninth to twelfth grades. Those with high scores on the Inventory (plus a low score comparison group) were interviewed by clinicians. A minimum prevalence rate of 0.35% was obtained, the age of onset varying from 7 to 18 years (mean = 12.8 years). Three quarters of the adolescents with OCD also had some other psychiatric condition, usually some form of depressive or anxiety disorder. Only 4 of the 20 subjects had been under psychiatric care, emphasizing the repeated finding that only a minority of young people with psychiatric problems receive psychiatric care. Little is known on the risk factors for OCD.

Pervasive Developmental Disorders and Psychoses

There are few psychiatric disorders for which it can be assumed that the great majority come to psychiatric or pediatric attention but that assumption can be made for psychoses and for autism and the pervasive developmental disorders. Gillberg et al. (1986) used Swedish clinic records to identify psychotic disorders in 13- to 19-year-olds. The overall prevalence figure was 8 per 10,000 with a steady rise from 1 per 10,000 at 13 years to 18 per 10,000 at 18 years; males predominated in the schizophrenic group and females in the affective psychoses. A fifth of psychoses was considered to be substance-induced.

The first general population survey of autism was conducted by Lotter (1966) with additional surveys by Brask (1967), Wing and Gould (1979), Bohman et al. (1983), McCarthy et al. (1984), Gillberg (1984), Steinhausen et al. (1986), Steffenberg and Gillberg (1986), Burd et al. (1987), and Bryson et al. (1988). The findings are in reasonably good agreement in showing an incidence of about 4 per 10,000 for autism as traditionally diagnosed but with partial syndromes much more common, usually being found in severely retarded children. If these are included, the rate rises to some 20 per 10,000. The male:female ratio is about 3 to 1. Pre- and perinatal complications are somewhat raised in frequency (Deykin and MacMahon,

1979a) but do not account for many cases. Epileptic seizures develop in adolescence in about a quarter to a fifth of cases (Deykin and MacMahon, 1979b), especially when autism is associated with severe mental handicap—indicating the importance of organic brain dysfunction. The findings on associations between autism and the fragile X anomaly are contradictory with some surveys showing high rates (e.g., Gillberg and Wahlstrom, 1985) but others quite low ones (see Folstein and Rutter, 1987). It is unclear at present whether the inconsistencies stem from differences in the diagnosis of autism or in the identification of fragile sites or both.

Suicide and Attempted Suicide

Attempted suicide is perhaps the only other condition that usually gives rise to some form of medical care. Epidemiological surveys (based on clinic attendance) show that attempted suicide becomes much more frequent during the adolescent age period, rising to a peak in late adolescence in females and in early adult life in males (Hawton and Goldacre, 1982; Platt et al., 1988). As already noted, suicide also rises sharply in frequency during adolescence, being almost unknown before the age of 10 years, but not reaching a peak until old age (Haim, 1974; Shaffer et al., 1988). Until very recently, epidemiological data on suicidal behavior in interviewed community samples have been lacking, but two recent studies have begun to fill that gap. Velez and Cohen (1988) found a sharp rise in reported suicide attempts at 13 to 14 years of age but surprisingly, a drop in later adolescence. Monck and Graham (1988) reported that 12% of 15- to 19-year-old girls had experienced suicidal ideas; three fifths of these exhibited some form of psychiatric disorder, a rate three times that in girls without suicidal ideation. Both surveys found that mothers were often unaware of their children's suicidal feelings, or even behavior.

Syndromes of Minimal Brain Dysfunction

For a long time there was much psychiatric interest in so-called syndromes of minimal brain dysfunction and there have been several surveys designed to assess their prevalence and correlates (e.g., Gollnitz et al., 1983; Schmidt et al., 1983, 1987; Gillberg et al., 1982; Nichols and Chen, 1981; Shen et al., 1985). The main conclusion from these studies is that the postulated syndrome lacks coherence. That is, there are only weak associations between pre- and perinatal complications, neurophysiological abnormalities, neuropsychological abnormalities and behavioral features (such as hyperactivity) thought to reflect organic brain malfunction. Interest remains in the role of brain damage as an etiological factor (see below) but the concept of a homogeneous brain dysfunction syndrome (minimal or maximal) has fallen into disrepute as a result of the consistent empirical evidence against the concept.

STUDIES OF CAUSAL RELATIONSHIPS

All researchers are taught the important caution that "correlation does not prove causation." Nevertheless, epidemiological data have been important both in noting associations that might be of causal significance and in testing causal hypotheses (Rutter, 1981a). The approaches that have been followed may be exemplified by considering a few specific risk factors.

Risk Factors

Organic Brain Dysfunction. The Isle of Wight studies showed strong associations between overt neuroepileptic conditions and psychiatric disorder (Rutter et al., 1970a). The first test of the causal hypothesis involved attempts to rule out possible third variables, such as mental handicap or physical crippling, by means of statistical control and a focus on subgroups. However, the next step required study of epidemiological samples that obviated the need to control for these third variables. An epidemiological study in London of children of normal IQ, all of whom had physical crippling, in which comparison was made between those with crippling due to brain disease or damage and those with crippling due to other causes (Seidel et al., 1975), provided the opportunity. The associations between organic brain dysfunction and psychiatric disorder in this sample were weaker but still substantial, indicating the likelihood of a causal relationship.

The third step required longitudinal data in connection with a "natural experiment" in which some children acquired a brain injury through some accident. A prospective study comparing children receiving a severe head injury and children receiving an orthopedic injury met that requirement (Rutter et al., 1983a). Again, a significant strong association was found between brain injury and psychiatric disorder. An additional test was provided by determining whether the psychiatric risk rose in conjunction with increasing severity of brain damage, i.e., a dose-response relationship. The data showed that to some extent it did. The causal hypothesis received support because epidemiological data had been able to provide quasi-experimental tests. Of course, the findings still leave open many questions on the processes by which brain damage creates a psychiatric risk and uncertainty remains on the degree of brain damage needed to give rise to a psychiatric vulnerability.

Lead Toxicity

The question of threshold for effects has been most discussed with respect to lead toxicity. It has been known for a long time that high blood lead levels lead to encephalopathy but there has been much uncertainty on whether lower levels of body lead of a degree that are common in the general population also carry psychological risks

(Rutter and Russell-Jones, 1983). The first systematic large scale epidemiological study to tackle that question was undertaken by Needleman et al. (1979) using dentine lead as a measure. It showed an association between raised lead levels and an IQ deficit of 4.5 points after controlling for a range of covariates (such as maternal IQ and socioeconomic status); also an association with hyperactivity and inattention. The problem faced in this and most other studies has been that raised lead levels are associated with psychosocial adversity and disadvantage. The inevitable question is whether the statistical adjustments provided an adequate control for these associated psychosocial risk factors. The dilemma is well posed by the findings from the well planned British epidemiological study by Smith et al. (1983), which incorporated improvements in the measurement of both dentine lead and of confounding variables, but it applies equally to other surveys (see Harvey, 1984; Harvey et al., 1988; Smith, 1985; Fulton, 1987). They found that an initial IQ deficit of some 5 points (associated with rather lower lead levels than those in the Needleman study) reduced to a nonsignificant difference of 2.7 points after correction for confounding variables. The investigators argued that the remaining deficit was likely to be due to unspecified and unmeasured confounding variables but equally it could be argued that the finding that nearly all studies fail to reduce the lead effect to zero suggests that the effect is real (whether it is statistically significant in any one study being heavily dependent on the sample size used). There is no epidemiological strategy that can resolve this dilemma at all decisively but the two New Zealand epidemiological/longitudinal studies have been helpful in two connections. The Dunedin study had the advantage that lead levels showed only a trivial association with social variables so that there was less opportunity for confounding effects (Silva et al., 1988). The results showed a nonsignificant effect of lead (as measured in blood) on IQ and scholastic attainment but a significant effect on behavior. The Christ church study (with a larger sample size—approximately 1,000 compared to about 600) was the first to use structural equation modelling to deal with error in the measurement of both predictor and outcome variables (an important advance) and found very small but significant lead effects on both scholastic and behavioral functioning (Fergusson, 1988; Fergusson et al., 1988a-c). The finding that consistent dose-response relationships (for IQ and attainment) remained after controlling for confounding variables supported the causal hypothesis. Inevitably, doubts remain but a small real effect of lead within ordinary population levels seems probable; however, clearly the effect must be very small and many of the published studies used samples too small to detect it at all reliably.

Family Discord

Numerous clinic and epidemiological studies have shown associations between serious chronic family discord and child psychiatric disorders (Emery, 1982); however, a variety of problems arise in the interpretation of this finding. First, there is the query as to whether the discord may have been caused by the child's behavioral disturbance, rather than the other way around. The prospective longitudinal data from Richman et al.'s (1982) epidemiological study showing, that family discord was associated with the *later* development of child psychiatric disorder, ruled out that possibility as a sufficient explanation. Second, there is the query as to whether the association could reflect a genetic, rather than environmental, effect. The finding that discord was strongly associated with child disorder in a sample all of whom had mentally ill parents made genetic mediation less likely (Rutter and Quinton, 1984), but the possibility has not as yet been subjected to a rigorous test. A third uncertainty is whether the risk arises from discord per se or rather from a broader pattern of psychosocial adversity of which discord is but one part. The need is to examine the effects of discord when it arises truly in isolation from other risk factors. This requires a focus on subgroups; the test for a main effect in the multivariate analysis does not serve the same purpose (Rutter, 1983). The few studies that have examined this question have suggested that most psychosocial risk factors have little effect when they really occur on their own (Rutter, 1979b; Kolvin et al., 1988), an unusual circumstance as most risk factors tend to come in multiples. A fourth query is whether the risk is family-wide (impinging somewhat similarly on all children) or whether it derives from a discordant parent-child relationship that is specific to the child in question. Curiously, this question has been subject to very little systematic investigation (in spite of the evidence suggesting the importance of differentiating between shared and non-shared environmental influences [Plomin and Daniels, 1987]). The need is to include both family-wide and child-specific variables and to make sib-sib comparisons. The study by Reitsma-Street et al. (1985) is one of the very few to have used the sib-comparison strategy, with findings suggesting that child-specific influences are likely to be of some importance. The issue is one that leads to the final query; namely, which specific mechanisms mediate the child psychiatric risk associated with family discord. Of all the questions, this is the one that has been least studied so far. Do the risks derive from the *lack* of a secure, consistent parent-child relationship or from the *stresses* associated with frequent arguing, quarrelling and hostility? The raised level of psychiatric disorder in children admitted to institutions in infancy suggests that the former may constitute part of the risk (Quinton and Rutter, 1988), but the data do not rule out the latter mechanism. Does the risk derive from an impaired relationship as such or rather from the fact that such relationships frequently go along with inadequate supervision and discipline or poor parenting more generally? These (and other) possibilities remain as matters for future epidemiological research agendas.

School Influences

Related issues arise in the interpretation of school effects. The London half of the London-Isle of Wight epidemiological comparison constituted the basis for a longitudinal study following the sample from entry to secondary school at age 11 to one year after school leaving some 6 to 8 years later (Rutter et al., 1979, Gray et al., 1980). Major differences between schools in rates of behavioral disturbance and in levels of scholastic attainment were found; these held up after controlling for differences in the intakes to the 12 schools studied. Moreover, the school variations were systematically associated with characteristics of the schools as social organizations. The finding implied causal effects associated with school experiences. However, two alternative explanations needed to be considered; first, that the school variations reflected influences from unmeasured aspects of the child's behavior or family background, and, secondly, that the child characteristics shaped the school rather than the reverse. Three more methodological steps have produced findings that have strengthened the causal inference. First, it was shown that the school features were more strongly associated with child characteristics at school exit than at school entry (Maughan et al., 1980)—a finding that rather runs against the notion that the qualities of the children shaped the school. Second, the opportunity was taken to examine effects on children's attendance and attainments of a change in school principal, in the absence of any change in the schools' catchment area (Ouston et al., 1985; Rutter, et al., 1986b). This natural experiment showed that in one of the three schools studied, the change in principal was followed by a marked improvement in children's levels of attendance and scholastic attainment; the second school showed somewhat similar but less dramatic improvements and the effects in the third school were quite modest. The combination of change over time associated with a quasi-experimental intervention strongly suggested a true school effect. The third advance, stemming from a longitudinal study of children's progress through elementary (primary) schools, involved improved statistical handling of the data together with the crucial distinction between school effects on *change* in scholastic attainment and those on final *level* of attainment (Mortimore et al., 1988). The results were striking in their demonstration that school effects predominated over family effects with respect to changes in reading skills following entry to junior school at age 7 years, but that family effects predominated for final level of attainment (as a consequence mainly of their effects on level at school entry). The implication is that family background had its main effect on the qualities that children brought with them at school entry but gains during the years that followed were more a function of the school attended. A somewhat similar distinction applied in Tizard et al.'s (1988) study of chilren's progress through infant schools (although the investigation was not primarily concerned with school influences). These studies were concerned with scholastic attainment rather than with psychiatric disorder, but the methodological implications apply equally to the effects of school experiences on children's behavior.

Area Influences

The Isle of Wight-London comparison showed that rates of child psychiatric disorder were twice as high in the metropolis (Rutter et al., 1975a); that this area difference was not a function of differential migration (Rutter and Quinton, 1977); and that it was largely explicable in terms of the greater frequency of family discord, disadvantage and disorganization in inner London (Rutter et al., 1975b). The suggestion was that there was something about living in the inner city that put families under stress and that, in turn, these family adversities led to a raised psychiatric risk for the children. However, the study was not able to delineate just what it was about city living that led to family stresses (Rutter, 1981b). Subsequent studies comparing metropolitan and rural areas have usually shown similar area differences (Lavik, 1977; Offord et al., 1987), although the higher psychiatric prevalence has not generally applied to nonmetropolitan urban areas (Kastrup, 1977). As already noted, the Chinese study by Shen et al. (1985) was unusual in showing that the psychiatric risk applied to isolated mountain communities rather than to the city but, again, the risk seemed to be associated with psychosocial adversity. Cederblad et al. (Rahim and Cederblad, 1984; Cederblad and Rahim, 1986) used the rather different research strategy of examining changes over time in psychiatric prevalence in an area undergoing urbanization; in spite of improved physical health, psychological disturbance increased. The epidemiological evidence points to area influences on family life and behavior, but further progress will depend on improved conceptualization and measurement of ecological variables.

Therapeutic Interventions

The last causal effect to be discussed concerns the consequences of therapeutic interventions. The main advantages of using epidemiological strategies for this purpose are that it is possible to examine possible benefits on a community-wide basis and that the interventions are those that operate in a real-life situation. However, there are the compensating disadvantages that it is much less easy to control the treatment qualities and that the families have not sought help for their children. The Rose and Marshall (1974) study of counseling and school social work in England, the Woodlawn (Kellam et al., 1975) evaluation of group therapy in the classroom and the Newcastle comparison of specific school-based methods of psychological treatment (Kolvin et al., 1981) were all pioneering in their use of epidemiological approaches for the evaluation of community-based treatment methods. Because of the complexity of the situations studied and of the data, it is not easy to draw succinct conclusions. The Woodlawn project provided inconclusive evidence of modest benefits, the Rose and Marshall findings on school counselling and social work were rather more positive and the Newcastle data indicated that group therapy and behavioral modification were of benefit, that parent counselling and teacher consultation were without much effect and compensatory "nurturing" of primary school children gave rise to intermediate effects. However, the findings were complicated and different outcome measures did not always agree with one another. The findings of the ambitious Newcastle project provide good evidence that psychological interventions can bring about worthwhile therapeutic gains, but it is less easy to derive clear messages on the specificity of effects or on the mechanisms involved in successful interventions.

METHODOLOGICAL ADVANCES

Why Use Epidemiology

As briefly reviewed in this paper, it is clear that epidemiological research in the field of child psychiatry has produced a wealth of useful findings over the last quarter of a century. Nevertheless, epidemiological studies are both difficult and expensive to undertake and it is necessary to ask whether clinic-based investigations might not be just as effective. There are several reasons why clinic studies involve serious limitations, but two main problems may be highlighted. First, clinic populations tend to be unrepresentative as a result of referral biases or other selective factors. Thus, they tend to include a misleadingly high proportion of subjects with multiple diagnoses just because referral will have been influenced by the occurrence of each separate condition (Berkson, 1946). Also, however, child patients who have been referred to clinics tend to differ systematically from those not referred, in ways that may distort findings on causal hypotheses. For example, Shepherd et al. (1971) in the Buckinghamshire study, found that referral was a function of family and parental characteristics as well as of child disorder.

Second, all the subjects attending clinics already manifest disorder so that, necessarily, the investigation of prior risk factors has to rely on retrospective recall, with the possible biases that this may entail. The prospective longitudinal study of other general population or high risk epidemiological samples avoids that problem. However, it is not just the avoidance of retrospective bias that is important. The use of longitudinal designs with samples of nonpatients exposed to risk factors has been crucial in showing the importance of "escape" from risk (Rutter, 1979b). Thus, although most adults who experience a serious breakdown in the parenting of their children have suffered serious adversities in their own upbringing, the converse does not apply (Quinton and Rutter, 1988). Many individuals who suffer gross deprivation develop into relatively well-functioning adults despite the hazards that they have faced. That observation has focused attention on the important phenomenon of psychological resilience (Anthony and Cohler, 1987; Masten and Garmezy, 1985; Rutter, 1985; Werner and Smith, 1982) and the possible operation of protective factors (Rutter, 1987a).

Longitudinal Designs

One of the major advances, therefore, has been the recognition of the increased power of epidemiological studies achieved by the inclusion of a longitudinal component (Rutter, 1988b,c). As noted, prospective designs are needed to investigate the reasons why so many individuals do *not* develop disorder after exposure to risk factors. They are also crucial for the testing of causal hypotheses because they allow the study of *change* over the period of risk exposure. As Farrington (1988) has argued persuasively, the demonstration of intraindividual change over time in relation to experience of hypothesized risk factor provides a powerful test of causal hypotheses. His own research (Farrington et al., 1986) and that of others (Warr, 1987) on the adverse effects of unemployment provides a good example of the use of this research strategy. Its value in relation to head injury (Rutter et al., 1983a), to maternal depression and family discord (Richman et al., 1982), to school influences (Mortimore et al., 1988) and to therapeutic interventions (Kellam et al., 1975; Kolvin et al., 1981) has already been noted.

It should be added that longitudinal data are also crucial in showing that some supposed consequences of risk factors actually antedated the hypothesized risk experience. For example, Block et al. (1986, 1988) noted that boys in families in which the parents subsequently divorced were already behaviorally distinctive before the divorce. Similarly, St. Claire and Osborne (1987), using data from the British 1970 birth cohort, showed that children who were later placed in foster care differed from other children prior to their fostering. The implication in both cases is that much of the risk stemmed from the family discord and disorganization that preceded the divorce or parenting breakdown rather than from the family break-up as an event.

An additional strength of longitudinal designs is that they allow a focus on chronic or persistent psychiatric disorders. This is potentially important because a high proportion of otherwise normal children exhibit transient disorders at some time during their development (Ghodsian et al., 1980). For many purposes there is an advantage in concentrating on those children who continue to show disorder over two or more time points (McGee et al., 1984a,b). Several studies have shown that psychosocial risk factors such as parental mental disorder (Rutter and Quinton, 1984) or living in a deprived inner city area (Rutter, 1979a) show a stronger association with persistent than with transient disorders.

Until recently, little has been made of adult outcome as a means of throwing light on child psychiatric disorders, but it has become evident that longitudinal studies to examine continuities and discontinuities between child and adult psychopathology provide a valuable research strategy (Robins and Rutter, in press). For example, Robins' several longitudinal investigations of males have shown consistent associations between conduct disturbance in childhood and antisocial personality disorder in adult life (Robins, 1978). Recent studies, using both the Epidemiologic Catchment Area study retrospective data (Robins, 1986) and prospective data from high risk groups (Quinton et al., in press) have shown a rather different picture in females. As in males, conduct disturbance constitutes a substantial risk factor for psychosocial functioning in adult life, but the outcome is much more varied, including personality disorders of other types together with affective disturbances. The findings raise questions about the classification of personality disorders and about the mechanisms involved in the risks for adult psychopathology associated with childhood conduct disturbance.

Sampling and Screening

Sometimes it is supposed that epidemiological studies must be of general population samples but this is not so. Indeed, the first convincing epidemiological elucidation of etiology in psychiatric disorders, Goldberger's demonstration that pellagra psychosis was due to nutritional deficiency, took place in mental hospitals. What is distinctive about epidemiological methods is the study of the distribution of disorders in a defined population, together with an examination of the factors that are associated with variations in that distribution (Weissman, 1987). Another advance in child psychiatric epidemiology has been the discriminating use of high risk samples to test particular causal hypotheses. As well as the several high risk studies already discussed, examples include the prospective study of infants shown to have chromosomal abnormalities on neonatal screening of large samples (Ratcliffe et al., in press; Walzer, 1985); the study of children involved in natural disasters (Earls et al., 1988; McFarlane et al., 1987), or exposed to nuclear risks (Cornely and Bromet, 1986), or subjected to a sniper attack in a school playground (Pynoos et al., 1987); and the study of children reared by mentally ill parents (reviewed by Rutter, 1987c). It is important that these investigations have been able to show when there is a lack of effect, as well as the impact, of different risk factors. For example, it was found that 3-year-old children living near the Three Mile Island nuclear reactor when there was an accident did not show any increase in psychological disturbance (Cornely and Bromet, 1986).

These high risk studies involved a focus on special groups who experienced a particular risk factor in order to test the hypotheses that there was a causal link between the risk factor and the later development of psychiatric disorder. In other cases, when it is necessary to study multiple risk factors or when it is important to assess the childrens' behavior *before* the risk experience (always an advantage when examining causal hypotheses), it is desirable to study the whole population longitudinally. This is because it is not possible to know in advance which individuals will experience the risk factors or who will develop disorder. The total population coverage strategy works well when dealing with relatively common risk factors and with relatively common psychological outcomes. However, for many purposes it constitutes a highly inefficient strategy because it requires that a large number of normal subjects must be assessed in order to identify a small number with disorder (Kraemer et al., 1987). It has been argued that a two stage design is a much more cost effective method (Shrout et al., 1986). In the first stage, a screening procedure is used on the total population to pick out individuals likely to have a disorder and in the second stage, a more definitive diagnostic procedure is used on this smaller selected subsample. For obvious reasons this two-stage approach is essential when studying disorders such as autism, anorexia nervosa, and obsessive compulsive disorders that have very low base rates. However, even with more common conditions, estimates of prevalence may often be obtained with greater accuracy and less cost using a two-stage design (Shrout et al., 1986).

Nevertheless, if such a design is to be employed successfully, a variety of methological issues need careful attention (Rutter, 1977). First, because of the modest levels of agreement between different data sources, it will usually be necessary to employ multiple screening measures (Achenbach et al., 1987a, b; Mattison et al., 1987). The Isle of Wight studies showed the importance of using both teacher and parent assessments and also indicated the need to involve child measures for some conditions. MacMillan et al. (1980) in the Newcastle study, went on to show that a multiple criterion screen was more efficient than any single screening instrument in 11- to 12-year-old children. Nicol et al. (1987) also developed a multiple criterion screen for toddlers, as has Place (1987) for adolescents. The second methodological issue concerns the need for screening measures that are both specific and sensitive for the psychiatric disorder of interest. Good broad band rating scales for completion by parents and by teachers are available (Barkley, 1988). However, there is a relative lack of well-tested parent or teacher questionnaires for more specific aspects of psychopathology such as anxiety, fears, depression, and social skills. There is an even greater lack of both broad and narrow band self-report questionnaires for completion by children and adolescents. During recent years most effort has gone into the development of scales to assess depression (Costello and Angold, 1988) and anorexic symptoms (Szmukler, 1985) and, within limits, screening for these disorders is possible, although more work is needed to test the instruments. Self-report measures for anxiety (Spielberger, 1973) and for fears (Miller et al., 1971; Ollendick, 1983) are available, and parent and child interviews for anxiety disorders (Silverman and Nelles, 1988) have recently been developed. These measures are likely to take on an increased importance in view of the evidence on the relatively high prevalence of anxiety disorders in childhood (see above). Also, a measure to assess social functioning, with parallel parent and child versions has been developed (John et al., 1987). (This usefully adds to the GAS measure of impaired general functioning [Shaffer et al., 1983].) There has been relatively little work on the qualities needed for a good screening questionnaire, but the issues have been well outlined by Burd et al. (1987), Murphy (1986), and by Costello and Angold (1988).

The third issue concerns the need in each epidemiological study to test the efficiency of screening through inclusion in the more intensive diagnostic stage of a random sample of individuals who were screen-negative, and to use the findings to calculate a corrected prevalence figure. If two samples are to be compared (as, for example, according to age or ethnic differences), this procedure must be carried out with each sample, as it cannot be assumed that there will be the same relationship among screening measures or between them and the diagnostic measures in each group. Thus, for example, using the Diagnostic Interview Schedule for Children (DISC), Edelbrock et al. (1985, 1986) found that the reliability of the child version and parent-child agreement were both greater in adolescents than in younger children. Also Breslau et al. (1988) found that the relationship between parent and child reports of psychopathology was different for depressed and nondepressed mothers.

In recent years most attention has been paid to the discrepancy between parent and child reports (with respect to both questionnaires and interviews), the usual finding being that parents report more conduct problems whereas children report more affective and other emotional difficulties (e.g., Angold et al., 1987; Edelbrock et al., 1986; Weissman et al., 1987b). The findings underline the importance of including child reports (at both the screening and diagnostic level) when studying affective and anxiety disorders in childhood and adolescence. However, although there has been useful study of possible reasons for the discrepancies (see also Breslau et al., 1988; Jensen et al., 1988a,b; Stavrakaki et al., 1987), and of rules for combining multiple sources of information (Reich and Earls, 1987), it cannot be said that the issue has been resolved. It seems plausible that children are likely to be more accurate informants on emotional symptomatology because the presence of phenomena such as anxiety or depression may not be readily observable by others. However, equally, it could be that young people tend to perceive feelings of negative affect as more serious than would adults and, hence, that the more severe depressive features perceived by others may be more valid indications of clinically significant psychopathology than those reported only by the children. Follow-up data would help decide between these alternatives. In the meanwhile, it is evident that it is desirable to include a child questionnaire in any screen for psychopathology disorders, especially so if there is a focus on affective or anxiety disorders.

Measures

The Isle of Wight studies, although innovative in using standardized interview methods, relied on measures that appear crude by present day standards. Several advances in measurement have taken place (see review chapters in Rutter et al., 1988b). Most strikingly, the development of structured interview schedules for adults (Endicott and Spitzer, 1978; Robins et al., 1981; Wing et al., 1967), together with the development of research diagnostic criteria (Feighner et al., 1972; Spitzer et al., 1978), led to similar advances in child psychiatry (see Edelbrock and Costello, 1988; Young et al., 1987, and rest of special section in the September 1987 issue of the *Journal*). As a consequence, there is now a range of standardized interview measures that are likely to give replicable diagnoses for most of the broader diagnostic categories. The newer instruments have clearly increased diagnostic discriminations and reliability—an important gain. Nevertheless, problems remain.

Two rather different interview approaches predominate. On the one hand there are the highly structured, questionnaire-style, respondent-based interviews in which there is complete standardization of the questions to be asked, with codings based almost entirely on the informant's affirmative or negative response to carefully designed closed questions that specify the behaviors of interest. These have the substantial advantage of obviating the need for interviewer judgment and therefore of removing one potential source of unreliability. However, there is the compensating disadvantage of reliance on the assumption that all subjects will interpret the questions in the same way and that their concepts will match those of the researcher. Also, necessarily, the information gained is restricted to that specifically covered by the questions, making it difficult to identify possible behaviors of interest outside the scope of the questions. On the other hand, there are the investigator-based interviews that seek to obtain detailed descriptions of behavior, which are then coded by the interviewer according to closely specified operationalized behavioral criteria. In these interviews, the structure lies in the concepts and coding rather than in the questions. The advantage is that it is easier to ensure that the codings match the concepts intended and to pick up unspecified behaviors of interest (because they will be evident in the descriptions). The compensating disadvantage is that, inevitably, there is greater reliance on interviewer skills and training, with an additional source of unreliability in interviewer judgments.

So far there has been relatively little direct comparison of the two forms of interview (but see Breslau, 1987; Carlson et al., 1987; Cohen et al., 1987). However, it seems that the two produce closely comparable information for many symptoms, but that the respondent-based interviews may tend to lead to an *over*estimate of psychopathology in the case of unusual behaviors (such as obsessions and psychotic phenomena) for which lay and clinical concepts may differ or in the case of some common behaviors (such as anxiety) where there is uncertainty on the cut off between the normal and the abnormal. However, the data are sparse and these conclusions must be regarded as very tentative. The matter warrants further study. Robins (1985) and Parker (1983) presented two rather different views on the validity of lay-administered questionnaire-style interviews for lifetime estimates of adult psychopathology; similar issues apply in the field of child measures.

Most epidemiological studies have relied on interview measures of one kind or another. But the Child Behavior Check List developed by Achenbach and Edelbrock (see Barkley, 1988) has been designed for survey use (as well as for other purposes) and has proved a useful measure of psychopathology in several large scale studies (see e.g., Achenbach et al., 1987a,b). It gives rise to behavioral syndromes that have some comparability with psychiatric diagnoses (see Achenbach, 1988) but it remains to be determined how satisfactory questionnaire scores are for individual diagnosis.

Most effort has been placed on the development of all-purpose interviews or questionnaires that tap a wide range of psychopathology. However, there has also been concern to develop interview and observational measures specifically to assess the behaviors associated with pervasive developmental disorders (e. g., Le Couteur et al., in press; Lord et al., in press; Rutter et al., 1988a; Schopler et al., 1985; Wing and Gould, 1978), as these conditions are not well dealt with in the wide range measures. However, apart from the observational approaches designed for PDD, and the general interview assessment developed by Kestenbaum and Bird (1978), there has been little development of standardized clinical observation methods in child psychiatry that might be applicable in epidemiological enquiries, although a range of detailed school and home observation schemes are available (see Reid et al., 1988). This would seem to be an aspect of diagnostic appraisal that requires additional work.

Because epidemiological research relies on the study of associations between psychiatric disorder and risk factors of various kinds, the development of measures of such risk variables has been equally important. An extensive range of family assessment methods is now available, many of which have been shown to have satisfactory reliability and validity (Jacob and Tennenbaum, 1988). Despite necessary concerns regarding possible bias in retrospective recall, it has also been possible to develop retrospective measures of the home environment that are reasonably robust (Holmes and Robins, 1987; Parker, 1983; Robins et al., 1985). Psychological testing has become increasingly discriminating and there have been important advances, too, in psychobiological measures, although substantial methodological problems remain (Ferguson and Bawden, 1988).

Combining Data Sources

Because diagnosis in child psychiatry often needs to be based on multiple sources of data, a key issue is *how* the various measures should be combined (Cohen et al., 1987). It is common clinical practice to accept any symptom as positive if any one informant reports it as definitely present. However, unless some measure of social impairment is also taken into account, this approach often leads to implausibly high prevalence estimates (Cohen et al., 1987). Moreover, it is also desirable to take into account possible sources of bias such as may arise if the parent-informant is depressed and thereby possibly likely to exaggerate the child's problem (Breslau et al., 1988; Ferguson and Horwood, 1987a,b), as well as variations in the reliability of the different instruments (Fergusson and Horwood, 1988). For some purposes relatively simple methods of combination may suffice, but in each study it is necessary to consider the nature of the latent variable that is represented by the diagnosis being investigated and the ways in which assessments of that latent variable may be distorted through unreliability and/or bias in the measuring instruments (Rutter and Pickles, in press). Structural equation modeling provides one effective way of dealing with the matter (see Fergusson and Horwood, 1987a,b).

Statistical Presentation of Epidemiological Data

Although epidemiologists have long been aware that estimates of prevalence, and of odd ratios for the increase in rates of psychiatric disorder associated with various psychosocial or organic risk factors, are much affected by random error, it is only relatively recently that it has become expected to provide confidence figures for the figures arrived at in any particular study. These are a great help in determining whether the estimates are likely to be stable across studies and should now be standard in the presentation of epidemiological data. However, as the recent controversy in the *American Journal of Public Health* makes clear, they are not a substitute for hypothesis testing and the use of levels of statistical significance (see e.g., Poole, 1987; Thompson, 1987).

CHALLENGES FOR THE FUTURE

It is evident that epidemiological research has accomplished a great deal in the last 25 years; equally, it is clear that many tasks remain. Inevitably, opinions are likely to differ on the priorities for future research, but certain challenges may be highlighted. It might be thought that the most basic need is to establish "true" prevalence figures for the complete range of child psychiatric disorders. Such data would be useful, but they would not be of much value on their own because of the following: (1) some diagnostic categories are of uncertain validity (Rutter, 1989); (2) clinical implications depend on social impairment as well as symptom patterns (a reason for ensuring separate measurement of the two); (3) there is no direct connection between prevalence and service needs (data on duration, response to treatment, and acceptability of intervention are also required [Rutter et al., 1970b]); (4) rates are likely to vary according to psychosocial (and other) circumstances; (5) preventive and therapeutic interventions need to be planned on the basis of knowledge on the factors that influence the onset and course of disorders; and (6) information on service utilization is also relevant (in that connection there is a paucity of studies on primary care [see Garralda and Bailey, 1986a,b]). Accordingly, it is highly desirable that epidemiological enquiries extend much more widely than previously in their aims. In doing so, certain needs stand out as requiring attention.

Developmental Perspectives

The crucial importance of adopting developmental perspectives has already been noted in several different connections. Thus, there are several conditions where it is necessary to investigate the reasons for major changes in prevalence with age, such as the rise in affective disorders and anorexia nervosa during adolescence. In order to do this, it will be crucial to use measures that are truly comparable across the age range to be studied (with empirical testing of their comparability) and to obtain data on the range of intrinsic and extrinsic factors that might account for the age trend. The investigation of age trends should include an evaluation of possible differences in the meaning of disorders arising at different ages (as shown, for example, by genetic loading, prognosis, or patterns of comorbidity). An additional aspect of developmental considerations is the need to determine the nature of continuities and discontinuities between the normal and the psychopathological. For example, which aspects of dysphoric mood show age trends parallel to those found for major depressive disorders or for bipolar affective conditions, which do not and, in each case, why? In which respects do the age trends in eating behavior and attitudes to body size and shape parallel those that apply to anorexia nervosa, and are the mechanisms similar?

A second developmental concern applies to the processes involved in continuities over time in psychopathology. The need to investigate this issue arises at both early and late age periods. For example, Richman et al. (1985) found that restlessness in boys at 3 years of age showed a strong association with psychiatric problems at 8 but that this did not apply in girls; why not? Also, both shyness and oppositional behavior show different patterns of correlates in boys and girls, with different parental responses (Maccoby and Jacklin, 1983; Radke-Yarrow et al., 1988; Simpson and Stevenson-Hinde, 1985; Stevenson-Hinde, 1988). What are the implications for the mechanisms underlying continuity and discontinuity? Similar issues arise with respect to the sex differences found for the adult sequelae of childhood conduct disturbance (Robins, 1986).

A third developmental question focuses on possible differences in the etiology and nature of disorders according to age on onset. Thus, the Isle of Wight study (Rutter, 1979a) highlighted the differences between disorders beginning for the first time in adolescence and those continuing into adolescence following an onset in earlier childhood; a difference also evident in the data from other studies (Robins and Hill, 1966; Werner and Smith, 1977) but little investigated up to now. A sequential over-lapping cohort epidemiological/longitudinal study extending from before adoles-cence to the late teens would seem to be indicated. Similarly, there is evidence from several studies that antisocial behavior of unusually early onset is particularly likely to result in persistently recidivist delinquency; an association with hyperactivity also predicts chronicity (Loeber and Le Blanc, in press; Farrington et al., in press; Rutter and Giller, 1983). A prospective epidemiological/longitudinal study starting in the preschool years and continuing into adolescence would be most helpful in delineat-ing the processes involved.

Comorbidity

In many respects the most striking finding to emerge from all epidemiological studies undertaken up to now has been the extremely high level of comorbidity (also found in clinic samples) (see e.g., McDermott, 1980; Anderson et al., 1987; Bird et al., 1988; Kashani et al., 1987). It is equally striking, however, that until very recently, research findings have not been analyzed in ways that take account of comorbidity. As a consequence, there is no means of knowing whether the features found to be associated with the same specified disorder under investi-gation in any particular study are truly related to that disorder or whether, instead, they stem from one or more of the unspecified and unanalyzed other disorders occurring in the same children. Several patterns of comorbidity stand out as likely to be particularly important, but there may well be others of equal consequence. First, there is a major overlap between conduct disorders and hyperkinetic/attention deficit syndromes (Rutter, 1988c; Shapiro and Garfinkel, 1986; Taylor, 1989; Taylor et al., 1988); second, between conduct disorders and drug abuse (Robins and McEvoy, in press); third, between depressive conditions and conduct disorders (Puig-Antich, 1982; Angold 1988a,b) or alcohol/drug abuse (Deykin et al., 1987); fourth, between depression and anxiety disorders (Strauss et al., 1988; Puig-Antich and Rabinovich, 1986; Bernstein and Garfinkel, 1986; Weissman et al., 1987a,b); fifth, between depression and anorexia/bulimia nervosa (Strober and Katz, in press); and sixth, between supposedly different types of anxiety disorder (Last et al., 1987). Various alternative hypotheses may be put forward to account for these comorbidity patterns. Thus, it could be that the impression of multiple disorders is misleading. Perhaps the reality is that many disorders typically have mixed patterns of symptomatology so that, for example, affective disorders characteristically involve an admixture of anxiety and depres-sive symptoms. Alternatively, it could be that the overlap stems from shared risk factors, such as temperamental adversity or family discord, that predispose to several otherwise different psychiatric disorders. For example, temperamental adversity could constitute the link between reading difficulties and conduct disorder. A variant of that suggestion is that the overlap between disorders derives from an overlap between risk factors. For example, in adult life depression and family discord are quite strongly associated. It could be that the discord predisposes to conduct disorders in the offspring and that parental depression leads to depressive disorders in the children, and, hence, that the comorbidity of conduct and depressive disorders is a consequence of the frequency with which family discord and adult depression are associated. A fourth possibility is that one disorder creates an increased risk for another condition; for example, in adult life, this seems to be the case for antisocial personality disorder in relation to depression (Cadoret et al., in press). Obviously, in any particular comorbidity pattern, this causal pathway needs to be considered in both directions. Fifth, it is possible that one disorder represents the early manifestations of the other as, for example, has been suggested for the link between oppositional disorder and conduct disorder. Sixth, it could reasonably be suggested that, at least in some instances, it is a mistake to conceptualize the disorders in categorical terms, rather the mixed pictures are an inevitable consequence of disorders deriving from risks associated with a range of dimensional variables (Achenbach, 1988). There is a great need to devise epidemiological/longitudinal studies designed to test and contrast these competing hypotheses.

Situation-Specificity

From Lapouse and Monk onwards, there has been the repeated observation that there is only modest agreement between teacher and parent reports of children's behavior. Clearly, to some extent this is a function of unreliability in measurement and differences in rates' perceptions (after all, teacher-teacher and mother-father agreement fall short of unity). However, there is reason to suppose that, in addition, there is a degree (sometimes a very marked degree) of situation-specificity with even quite severe handicapping disorders. The most obvious psychiatric example is provided by the syndrome of elective mutism in which children are completely mute in some circumstances, yet talk fluently in others (Kolvin and Fundudis, 1981; Kratochwill, 1981). To a lesser degree it applies to many other child psychiatric disorders. There is a substantial literature on situational determinants of delinquent behavior (Clarke, 1985), but it is only very recently that there has been any systematic attention to the psychological and psychiatric study of situational variations in psychiatric disturbance (Loeber and Dishion, 1984; Barkley and Edelbrock, 1987). This would appear to be an area warranting research investment; it requires attention both to the reliable valid assessment of disturbance in particular settings (using multiple measures) and a better conceptualization and measurement of situational qualities.

Etiology

Several examples have been given in this review of the use of epidemiological/ longitudinal research methods to tackle questions involving causal hypotheses. In spite of the difficulties of inferring causation from correlation, there are many ways in which epidemiology can be used to examine causal questions with respect to the onset, course, and remission of disorders (Rutter, 1981a). However, if this is to be done effectively it is necessary to go beyond cross-sectional correlations and associations. Whenever possible, it is desirable to seek for natural experiments that capitalize on changes over time (as with the effects on individuals of a head injury, a parental divorce, admission to an institution, a geographical move, or the experience of unemployment; or the effects on population groups of experiences such as the change in organization of a school, urbanization or industrialization, or a natural or man-made disaster—examples of all of which have been given above). Alternatively, the natural experiment may reside in the comparison of two groups that are initially similar but which undergo different experiences (as with between-schools comparisons, or rearing by mentally ill parents with different forms of psychiatric disorder, or comparisons between children born to severely disadvantaged parents who are brought up by them and children of the same parents who are adopted (see Schiff and Lewontin, 1986, for an example of the last situation). It is clear that the science and the art of this sort of epidemiology lies in the combination of strategic choice of suitably contrasting samples with the use of longitudinal data. As part of the study of etiological factors, it is clear that there would be much to be gained from the combination of epidemiological and genetic strategies. For example, in the adult field, the Camberwell Collaborative Depression Study has been informative in its combined study of the familiality of both adverse life events and depression (McGuffin et al., 1988). Similarly, both family genetic and twin strategies could be informative in examining age trends in affective disorder over the adolescent age period.

Links between Childhood and Adult Life

The last epidemiological focus to mention is the study of continuities and discontinuities between childhood and adult life (Rutter, 1989a). This is potentially important for several different reasons. First, data on the nature of linkages between child and adult psychiatric disorders should throw light on the nature of disorders at both age periods. Thus, as already noted, the different adult outcome in men and women of childhood conduct disturbances raises queries on the conceptualization of personality disorder (Hill et al., 1989; Robins, 1986; Rutter, 1987b). Similarly, the combination of the rather varied childhood antecedents of adult depressive disorder (Zeitlin, 1986) with prospective continuity when children with depressive disorders are followed into adult life (Harrington et al., unpublished; Kovacs and Gatsonis, in press; Kovacs et al., 1989b) raises questions about the possibility of different pathways with different forms of depressive disorder. Secondly, temporal linkages need to be investigated with respect to the range of mediating variables that have been postulated to account for the perpetuation of psychopathology risks associated with early adverse experiences (Maughan and Champion, in press; Rutter, 1989)—such as the shaping of one's own environment (Scarr and McCartney, 1983), the lack of planning and self-efficacy in dealing with life's challenges and changes (Quinton and Rutter, 1988), internal working models of relationships (Bretherton and waters, 1985), and low self-esteem or feelings of helplessness (Harris et al., 1987). For the reasons already discussed, epidemiological approaches using longitudinal data are needed in order that there can be an adequate assessment of "escape" from risk, of protective factors, and of the varied antecedents of adult outcomes. Continuities over time have to be examined both looking forwards and looking backwards (Rutter et al., 1983b).

CONCLUSION

Although necessarily brief in its coverage of individual topics, this review of child psychiatric epidemiology over the last 25 years has had to cover a wide territory. The time when epidemiology could be seen as the mere counting of heads of individuals with specified labels of disorder has long since passed. Instead, it has proved to be a highly flexible and effective means of answering a range of different questions that are important for therapy, policy, and practice. The advances stem from a combination of improved methods of measurement, diagnosis, and classification, and an enrichment of concepts and research strategies and tactics. Many difficult and challenging tasks remain, but we can move forward with confidence that the means are available, or can be devised, to tackle them.

REFERENCES

Abraham, S. F., Mira, M., Beumont, P. J. V., Sowerbutts, T. D. & Llewellyn-Jones, D. (1983), Eating behaviors among young women. *Med. J. Aust.*, 2:225–228.

Achenbach, T. M. (1988), Integrating Assessment and Taxonomy. In: *Assessment and Diagnosis in Child Psychopathology*, eds. M. Rutter, A. H. Tuma & I. S. Lann. New York: Guilford Press; London: David Fulton, pp. 300–343.

——Verhulst, F. C., Baron, G. D. & Akkerhuis, G. W. (1987a), Epidemiological comparisons of American and Dutch children: I. Behavioral/emotional problems and competencies reported by parents for ages 4 to 1–16. *J. Am. Acad. Child Adolesc. Psychiatry*, 26:317–325.

—— ——Edelbrock, C., Baron, G. D. & Akkerhuis, G. W. (1987b), Epidemiological comparisons of American and Dutch children. II. Behavioral/emotional problems reported by teachers for ages 6 to 11. *J. Am. Acad. Child Adolesc. Psychiatry,* 26:336–332.

American Psychiatric Association (1987), *Diagnostic and Statistical Manual of Mental Disorders (Third edition–Revised)—DSM-III-R.* Washington, DC: American Psychiatric Association.

Anderson, J. C., Williams, S., McGee, R. & Silva, P. A. (1987), DSM-III disorders in pre-adolescent children: prevalence in a large sample from the general population. *Arch. Gen. Psych.,* 44:69–76.

——Williams, S., McGee, R. & Silva, P. (in press), Cognitive and social correlates of DSM-III disorders in pre-adolescent children. *J. Am. Acad. Child Adolesc. Psychiatry.*

Angold, A. (1988a), Childhood and adolescent depression: I. Epidemiological and aetiological aspects. *Br. J. Psychiatry,* 152:501–507.

——(1988b), Childhood and adolescent depression. II. Research in clinical populations. *Br. J. Psychiatry,* 153:476–492.

——Weissman, M. M., John, K. et al. (1987), Parent and child reports of depressive symptoms in children at low and high risk of depression. *J. Child Psychol. Psychiatry,* 28:901–915.

Anthony, E. J. & Cohler, B. (1987), *The Invulnerable Child.* New York: Guilford Press.

Anthony, J. C., Folstein, M., Romanoski, A. J. et al. (1985), Comparison of the lay diagnostic interview schedule and a standardized psychiatric diagnosis: experience in Eastern Baltimore. *Arch. Gen. Psychiatry,* 42:667–675.

Apley, J. (1975), *The Child with Abdominal Pains (2nd Ed).* Oxford: Blackwell Scientific Publications.

Barkley, R. A. (1988), Child behavior rating scales and checklists. In: *Assessment and Diagnosis in Child Psychopathology,* eds. M. Rutter, A. H. Tuma & I. S. Lann. New York: Guilford Press; London: David Fulton, pp. 113–155.

——Edelbrock, C. (1987), Assessing situational variation in children's problem behaviors: the Home and School Situations Questionnaires. In: *Advances in Behavioral Assessment of Children and Families,* ed. R. Prinz. Greenwich, CT: JAI Press.

Beitchman, J. H., Peterson, M. & Clegg, M. (1987), Speech and language impairment and psychiatric disorder: the relevance of family demographic variables. *Child Psychiatry Hum. Dev.,* 18:191–207.

Beitchman, J. H., Nair, R., Clegg, M., Ferguson, B. & Patel, P. G. (1986), Prevalence of psychiatric disorders in children with speech and language disorders. *J. Am. Acad. Child Psychiatry,* 25:528–535.

Berg, C. Z., Whitaker, A., Davies, M., Flament, M. F. & Rapoport, J. L. (1988), The survey form of the Leyton obsessional inventory-child version: norms from an epidemiological study. *J. Am. Acad. Child Adolesc. Psychiatry,* 27:759–763.

Berger, M., Yule, W. & Rutter, M. (1975), Attainment and adjustment in two geographical areas: II. The prevalence of specific reading retardation. *Br. J. Psychiatry,* 126:510–519.

Berkson, J. (1946), Limitations of the application of four-fold table analysis to hospital data. *Biometrics,* 2:47–53.

Bernstein, G. A. & Garfinkel, B. D. (1986), School phobia: the overlap of affective and anxiety disorders. *J. Am. Acad. Child Psychiatry,* 25:235–241.

Bird, H. R., Canino, G., Rubio-Stipec, M. et al. (1988), Estimates of the prevalence of child-hood maladjustment in a community survey in Puerto Rico. *Arch. Gen. Psychiatry,* 45:1120–1126.

———Gould, M. S., Yager, T., Staghezza, B. & Canino, G. (in press), Risk factors for mal-adjustment in Puerto Rican children. *J. Am. Acad. Child Adolesc. Psychiatry.*

Block, J. H., Block, J. & Gjerde, P. F. (1986), The personality of children prior to divorce. *Child Dev.,* 57:827–840.

Block, J., Block, J. H., & Gjerde, P. F. (1988), Parental functioning and the home environment in families of divorce. *J. Am. Acad. Child Adolesc. Psychiatry,* 27:207–213.

Bohman, M., Bohman, I. L., Bjorck, P. O. & Sjoholm, E. (1983), Childhood psychosis in a northern Swedish county: some preliminary findings from an epidemiological survey. In: *Epidemiological Approaches in Child Psychiatry II,* ed. M. H. Schmidt & H. Remschmidt. Stuttgart/NY: Thieme Verlag/Thieme-Stratton, pp. 164–173.

Boudreault, M., Thivierge, J., Cote, R., Boutin, Y., Julien, Y. & Bergeron, S. (1988), Cognitive development and reading achievement in pervasive-ADD, situational-ADD and control children. *J. Child Psychol. Psychiatry,* 29:611–619.

Brask, B. H. (1967), The need for hospital beds for psychotic children: an analysis based on a prevalence investigation in the County of Arthus. *Ugeskr. Laeger,* 129:1559–1570.

Breslau, N. (1987), Inquiring about the bizarre: False positives in Diagnostic Interview Schedule for Children "DISC" ascertainment of obsessions, compulsions, and psychotic symptoms. *J. Am. Acad. Child Adolesc. Psychiatry,* 26:639–644.

———Davis, G. C. & Prabucki, K. (1988), Depressed mothers as informants in family history research—are they accurate? *Psychiatry Res.,* 24:345–359.

Bretherton, I. & Waters, E. eds. (1985), Growing points of attachment theory and research. *Monogr. Soc. Res. Child Dev.,* 50 (1-2, Serial No. 209).

Bryson, S. E., Clark, B. S. & Smith, I. M. (1988), First report of a Canadian epidemiological study of autistic syndromes. *J. Child Psychol. Psychiatry,* 29:433–445.

Burd, L., Fisher, W. & Kerbeshian, J. (1987), A prevalence study of pervasive developmental disorders in North Dakota. *J. Am. Acad. Child Adolesc. Psychiatry,* 26:700–703.

Button, E. J. & Whitehouse, A. (1981), Subclinical anorexia nervosa. *Psychol. Med.,* 11:509–516.

Cantwell, D. & Baker, L. (1987), *Developmental Speech and Language Disorders.* New York: Guilford Press.

Carlson, G. A., Kashani, J. H., Thomas, M. deF., Vaidya, A. & Daniel, A. E. (1987), Comparison of two structured interviews on a psychiatrically hospitalized population of children. *J. Am. Acad. Child Adolesc. Psychiatry,* 26:645–648.

Cadoret, R., Troughton, E., Moreno, L. & Whitters, A. (in press), Early life psychosocial events and adult affective symptoms. In: *Straight and Devious Pathways from Childhood to Adulthood,* ed. L. Robins & M. Rutter. Cambridge: Cambridge University Press.

Cederblad, M. & Rahim, S. I. A. (1986), Effects of rapid urbanization on child behaviour and health in a part of Khartoum, Sudan—I. Socio-economic changes 1965–1980. *Soc. Sci. Med.,* 22:713–721.

Clarke, R. V. G. (1985), Delinquency, environment and intervention. Second Jack Tizard Memorial Lectures. *J. Child Psychol. Psychiatry,* 26:505–523.

Cohen, P., Velez, N., Kohn M., Schwab-Stone, M. & Johnson, J. (1987), Child psychiatric diagnosis by computer algorithm: theoretical issues and empirical tests. *J. Am. Acad. Child Adolesc. Psychiatry,* 26:631–638.

Cooper, J. (1970), The Leyton Obsessional Inventory. *Psychol. Med.,* 1:48–64.

Cornely, P. & Bromet, E. (1986), Prevalence of behavior problems in three-year-old children living near Three Mile Island: a comparative analysis. *J. Child Psychol. Psychiatry,* 27:489–498.

Costello, E. J. & Angold, A. (1988), Scales to assess child and adolescent depression: checklists, screens, and nets. *J. Am. Acad. Child Adolesc. Psychiatry,* 27:726–737.

——Costello, A. J., Edelbrock, C. et al. (1988), Psychiatric disorders in pediatric primary care. *Arch. Gen. Psychiatry,* 45:1107–1116.

——(in press a), Developments in child psychiatric epidemiology, *J. Am. Acad. Child Adolesc. Psychiatry.*

——(in press b), Child psychiatric disorders and their correlates: a primary care pediatric sample. *J. Am. Acad. Child Adolesc. Psychiatry.*

Cox, A., Rutter, M., Yule, B. & Quinton, D. (1977), Bias resulting from missing information. *Br J. Prev. Soc. Med.,* 31:131–136.

Crisp, A. H., Palmer, R. L. & Kaluey, R. S. (1976), How common is anorexia nervosa? *Br. J. Psychiatry,* 128:549–554.

Deykin, E. Y., Levy, J. C. & Wells, V. (1987), Adolescent depression, alcohol and drug abuse. *Am. J. Public Health,* 77:178–182.

——MacMahon, B. (1979a), Viral exposure and autism. *Am. J Epidemiol.,* 109:628–638.

—— ——(1979b), The incidence of seizures among children with autistic symptoms. *Am. J. Psychiatry* 136:1310–1312.

Dowdney, L., Skuse, D., Heptinstall, E., Puckering, C. & Zur-Szpiro, S. (1987), Growth retardation and developmental delay amongst inner-city children. *J. Child Psychol. Psychiatry,* 28:529–541.

Douglas, J. W. B. (1973), Early disturbing events and later enuresis. In: *Bladder Control and Enuresis,* eds. I. Kolvin, R. MacKeith & S. R. Meadow. Clinics in Developmental Medicine, Nos. 48/49. London: Heinemann/SIMP, pp. 109–117.

Earls, F. (1980a), Epidemiological child psychiatry: an American perspective. In: *Psychopathology of Children and Youth: A Crosscultural Perspective,* ed. E. F. Purcell. New York: Macy Foundation.

——(1980b), Prevalence of behavior problems in 3-year-old children: a cross-national replication. *Arch. Gen. Psychiatry,* 37:1153–1157.

——(1982), Epidemiology and child psychiatry: future prospects. *Compr. Psychiatry,* 23:75–84.

——Jung, K. G. (1987), Temperament and home environment characteristics as causal factors in the early development of childhood psychopathology. *J. Am. Acad. Child Adolesc. Psychiatry,* 26:491–498.

——Smith, E., Reich, W. & Jung, K. G. (1988), Investigating psychopathological consequences of a disaster in children: a pilot study incorporating a structured diagnostic interview. *J. Am. Acad. Child Adolesc. Psychiatry,* 27:90–95.

Edelbrock, C. & Costello, A. J. (1988), Structured psychiatric interviews for children. In:

Assessment and Diagnosis in Child Psychopathology, ed. M. Rutter, A. H. Tuma & I. S. Lann. New York: Guilford Press, pp. 87–112.

——— ———Dulcan, M. K., Conover, N. C. & Kalas, R. (1986), Parent-child agreement on child psychiatric symptoms assessed via structured interview. *J. Child Psychol. Psychiatry,* 27:181–190.

——— ——— ———Kalas, R. & Conover, N. C. (1985), Age differences in the reliability of the psychiatric interview of the child. *Child Dev.,* 56:265–275.

Emery, R. E. (1982), Interparental conflict and the children of discord and divorce. *Psychol. Bull.,* 2:310–330.

Endicott, J. & Spitzer, R. L. (1978), A diagnostic interview: The Schedule for Affective Disorders and Schizophrenia. *Arch. Gen. Psychiatry,* 35:837–844.

Essen, J. & Peckham, C. (1976), Nocturnal enuresis in childhood. *Dev. Med. Child Neurol.,* 18:577–589.

Farrington, D. P. (1988), Studying changes within individuals: the causes of offending. In: *Studies of Psychosocial Risk: The Power of Longitudinal Data,* ed. M. Rutter. Cambridge: Cambridge University Press, pp. 158–183.

———Gallagher, B., Morley, L., St. Ledger, R. J. & West, D. J. (1986), Unemployment, school leaving, and crime. *British Journal of Criminology,* 26:335–356.

———Loeber, R. & van Kammen, W. B. (in press), Long-term criminal outcomes of hyperactivity-impulsivity-attention deficit and conduct problems in childhood. In: *Straight and Devious Pathways from Childhood to Adult Life,* ed. L. Robins & M. Rutter. New York: Cambridge University Press.

Faull, C. & Nicol, A. R. (1986), Abdominal pain in six-year olds: an epidemiological study in a new town. *J. Child Psychol. Psychiatry,* 27:251–260.

Feighner, J. P., Robins, E., Guze, S. B., Woodruff, R. A. & Winokur, G. (1972), Diagnostic criteria for use in psychiatric research. *Arch. Gen. Psychiatry,* 26:57–63.

Ferguson, H. B. & Bawden, H. N. (1988), Psychobiological measures. In: *Assessment and Diagnosis in Child Psychopathology,* ed. M. Rutter, A. H. Tuma & I. S. Lann. New York: Guilford Press, pp. 232–263.

Fergusson, D. M. (1988), A longitudinal study of dentine lead, cognitive ability and behaviour in a birth cohort of New Zealand children. PhD. Thesis, University of Otago, Dunedin.

———Horwood, L. J. (1987a), The trait and method components of ratings of conduct disorder. Part I. Maternal and teacher evaluations of conduct disorder in young children. *J. Child Psychol. Psychiatry,* 28:249–260.

——— ———(1987b), The trait and method components of ratings of conduct disorder. Part II. Factors related to the trait component of conduct disorder scores. *J. Child Psychol. Psychiatry,* 28:261–272.

——— ———(1988), Structural equation modelling of measurement processes in longitudinal data. In: *Studies of Psychosocial Risk: The power of longitudinal data,* ed. M. Rutter. Cambridge: Cambridge University Press, pp. 325–353.

Fergusson, J. E., Horwood, L. J. & Kinzett, N. G. (1988a), A longitudinal study of dentine lead levels, intelligence, school performance and behaviour. Part I. Dentine lead levels and exposure to environmental risk factors. *J. Child Psychol. Psychiatry,* 29:781–792.

———— ———— ———— ————(1988b), A longitudinal study of dentine lead levels, intelligence, school performance and behaviour. Part II. Dentine lead and cognitive ability. *J. Child Psychol. Psychiatry,* 29:793–809.

———— ———— ———— ————(1988c), A longitudinal study of dentine lead levels, intelligence, school performance and behaviour. Part III. Dentine lead levels and attention/activity. *J. Child Psychol. Psychiatry,* 29:811–824.

Flament, M. F., Whitaker, A., Rapoport, J. L., et al. (1988), Obsessive compulsive disorder in adolescence. *J. Am. Acad. Child Adolesc. Psychiatry,* 27:764–771.

Folstein, S. & Rutter, M. (1987), Autism; Familial aggregation and genetic implications. In: *Neurobiological Issues in Autism,* ed. E. Schopler & G. Mesibov. New York: Plenum, pp. 83–105.

Fredman, G. & Stevenson, J. (1988), Reading processes in specific reading retarded and reading backward 13-year-olds. *British Journal of Developmental Psychology,* 6:07–108.

Frith, U. (1985), The usefulness of the concept of unexpected reading failure. Comments on reading retardation revisited. *British Journal of Developmental Psychology,* 6:97–108.

Fulton, M., Thompson, G., Hunter, R., Raab, G., Laxen, D. & Hepburn, W. (1987), Influence of blood lead on the ability and attainment of children in Edinburgh. *Lancet,* 1:1221–1225.

Garner, D. M., Olmsted, M. P. & Garfinkel, P. E. (1983), Does anorexia nervosa occur on a continuum? Subgroups of weight-preoccupied women and their relationship to anorexia nervosa. *International Journal of Eating Disorders,* 2:11–20.

Garralda, M. E. & Bailey, D. (1986a), Psychological deviance in children attending general practice. *Psychol. Med.,* 16:423–429.

———— ————(1986b), Children with psychiatric disorders in primary care. *J. Child Psychol. Psychiatry,* 27:611–624.

Garrison, W. & Earls, F. (1985a), Change and continuity in behaviour problems from the pre-school period through school entry: an analysis of mothers' reports. In: *Recent Research in Developmental Psychopathology,* ed. J. E. Stevenson. Oxford: Pergamon, pp. 51–65.

———— ————(1985b), The social context of early human experience—preliminary findings from an epidemiological study of families with infants and preschool children. In: *Epidemiological Approaches in Child Psychiatry II,* ed. M. H. Schmidt & H. Remschmidt. Stuttgart/New York: Thieme Verlag/Thieme-Stratton, pp. 79–92.

Ghodsian, M., Fogelman, K., Lambert, L. & Tibbenham, A. (1980), Changes in behaviour ratings of a national sample of children. *Br. J. Soc. Clin. Psychol.,* 19:247–256.

Gillberg, C. (1984), Infantile autism and other childhood psychoses in a Swedish urban region. *J. Child Psychol. Psychiatry,* 25:35–43.

————Rasmussen, P., Carlstrom, G., Svenson, B. & Waldenstrom, E. (1982), Perceptual, motor and attentional deficits in six-year-old children. *J. Child Psychol. Psychiatry,* 23:131–144.

————Wahlstrom, J. (1985), Chromosome abnormalities in infantile autism and other childhood psychoses: a population study of 66 cases. *Dev. Med. Child Neurol.,* 27:293–304.

———— ————Forsman, A., Hellgren, L. & Gillberg, I. C. (1986), Teenage psychoses-epidemiology, classification and reduced optimality in the pre-, peri- and neonatal periods. *J. Child Psychol. Psychiatry,* 27:87–98.

Gollnitz, G., Teichmann, H., & Meyer-Probst, B. (1983). The interaction between biological and psychosocial risk factors in the epidemiology of brain function disturbances and the genesis of child-psychiatric disorders. In: *Epidemiological Approaches in Child Psychiatry II,* ed. M. H. Schmidt & H. Remschmidt. Stuttgart/New York: Thieme Verlag/Thieme-Stratton, pp. 108–120.

Gould, M. S., Wunsch-Hitzig, R. & Dohrenwend, B. P. (1980), Formulation of hypotheses about the prevalence, treatment and prognostic significance of psychiatric disorders in children in the United States. In: *Mental Illness in the United States: Epidemiological estimates,* eds. B. P. Dohrenwend, B. S. Dohrenwend, M. S. Gould, B. Link, R. Neugebauer & R. Wunsch-Hitzig. New York: Praeger.

Graham, P. J. ed. (1977), *Epidemiological Approaches in Child Psychiatry.* New York: Academic Press.

——(1979), Epidemiological studies. In: *Psychopathological Disorders of Childhood (2nd Ed),* ed. H. C. Quay & J. S. Werry. New York: Wiley.

——(1980), Epidemiological approaches to child mental health in developing countries. In: *Psychopathology of Children and Youth: A Cross-cultural Perspective,* ed. E. F. Purcell. New York: Macy Foundation.

——Rutter, M. & George, S. (1973), Temperamental characteristics as predictors of behavior disorders in children. *Am. J. Orthopsychiatry,* 43:328–339.

Gray, G., Smith, A. & Rutter, M. (1980), School attendance and the first year of employment. In: *Out of School: Modern Perspectives in Truancy and School Refusal.* Chichester: Wiley, pp. 343–370.

Haim, A. (1974), *Adolescent Suicide.* Translated by A. M. Sheridan Smith, London: Tavistock.

Harris, T., Brown, G. W. & Bifulco, A. (1987), Loss of parent in childhood and adult psychiatric disorder: the role of lack of adequate parental care. *Psychol. Med.,* 17:163–183.

Harvey, P. G. (1984), Lead and children's health—recent research and future questions. *J. Child Psychol. Psychiatry,* 25:517–522.

——Hamlin, M. W., Kumar, R., Morgan, G., Spurgeon, A. & Delves, H. T. (1988), Relationships between blood lead, behaviour, psychometric and neuropsychological test performance in young children. *Br. J. Dev. Psychol.,* 6:145–156.

Hawton, K. & Goldacre, M. (1982), Hospital admissions for adverse effects of medicinal agents (mainly self-poisoning) among adolescents in the Oxford region. *Br. J. Psychiatry,* 141:166–170.

Heptinstall, E., Puckering, C., Skuse, D., Start, K., Zur-Szpiro & Dowdney, L. (1987), Nutrition and mealtime behaviour in families of growth-retarded children. *Hum. Nutr. Appl. Nutr.,* 41A:390–402.

Hill, J., Harrington, R., Fudge, H., Rutter, M. & Pickles, A. (1989), The Adult Personality Functioning Assessment: development and reliability. *Br. J. Psychiatry,* 155:24–35.

Holmes, S. J. & Robins, L. N. (1987), The influence of childhood disciplinary experience on the development of alcoholism and depression. *J. Child Psychol. Psychiatry,* 28:399–415.

Howlin, P. & Rutter, M. (1987), The consequences of language delay for other aspects of development. In: *Language Development and Disorders,* ed. W. Yule & M. Rutter. Clinics in Developmental Medicine No. 101/102. London: MacKeith Press/Blackwell Scientific, pp. 271–294.

Jacob, T. & Tennenbaum, D. L. (1988), Family assessment methods. In: *Assessment and Diagnosis in Child Psychopathology,* ed. M. Rutter, A. H. Tuma & I. S. Lann. New York: Guilford Press, pp. 196–231.

Jensen, P. S., Taylor, J., Xenakis, S. N. & Davis, H. (1988a), Child psychopathology rating scales and interrater agreement: I. Parents' gender and psychiatric symptoms. *J. Am. Acad. Child Adolesc. Psychiatry,* 27:442–450.

——Xenakis, S. N., Davis, H. & Degroot, J. (1988b), Child psychopathology rating scales and interrater agreement. II. Child and family characteristics. *J. Am. Acad. Child Adolesc. Psychiatry,* 27:451–461.

John, K., Gammon, G. D., Prusoff, B. A. & Warner, V. (1987), The Social Adjustment Inventory for Children and Adolescents (SAICA): testing of a new semistructured interview. *J. Am. Acad. Child Adolesc. Psychiatry,* 26:898–911.

Johnson-Sabine, E., Wood, K., Patton, G., Mann, A. & Wakeling, A. (1988), Abnormal eating attitudes in London schoolgirls—a prospective epidemiological study: factors associated with abnormal response on screening questionnaires. *Psychol. Med.,* 18:615–622.

Jorm, A. F., Share, D. L., Maclean, R. & Matthews, R. (1986a), Cognitive factors at school entry predictive of specific reading retardation and general reading backwardiness. *J. Child Psychol. Psychiatry,* 27:45–54.

——Share, D. L., Matthews, R. & Maclean, R. (1986b), Behaviour problems in specific reading retarded and generl reading backward children. *J. Child Psychol. Psychiatry,* 27:33–43.

Kaffman, M. & Elizur, E. (1977), Infants who become enuretics. A longitudinal study of 161 kibbutz children. *Monogr. Soc. Res. Child Dev.,* 42(No. 2):170.

Karno, M., Golding, J. M., Sorenson, S. B. & Burnam, M. A. (1988), The epidemiology of obsessive-compulsive disorder in five US communities. *Arch. Gen. Psychiatry,* 45:1094–1099.

Kashani, J. H. & Orvaschel, H. (1988) Anxiety disorders in mid-adolescence. *Am. J. Psychiatry,* 145:960–964.

——Beck, M. C., Hoeper, E. W. et al. (1987), Psychiatric disorders in a community sample of adolescents. *Am. J. Psychiatry,* 144:584–589.

Kastrup, M. (1977), Urban-rural differences in 6 year olds. In: *Epidemiological Approaches in Child Psychiatry,* ed. P. J. Graham. London: Academic Press, pp. 181–194.

Kellam, S. G., Branch, J. D., Agrawal, K. C. & Ensminger, M. E. (1975), *Mental Health and Going to School: The Woodlawn Program of Assessment, Early Intervention and Evaluation.* Chicago: University of Chicago Press.

Kendell, R. E., Hall, D. J., Hailey, A. & Babigian, H. M. (1973), The epidemiology of anorexia nervosa. *Psychol. Med.,* 3:200–203.

Kestenbaum, C. J., & Bird, H. R. (1978), A reliability study of the Mental Health Assessment Form for school-age children. *J. Am. Acad. Child Psychiatry,* 17:338–347.

Kolvin, I. & Fundudis, T. (1981), Elective mute children: psychological development and background factors. *J. Child Psychol. Psychiatry,* 22:219–232.

———Garside, R. F., Nicol, A. R., Macmillan, A., Wolstenholme, F. & Leitch, I. M. (1981), *Help Starts Here: The Maladjusted Children in the Ordinary School.* London/New York: Tavistock.

———Miller, F. J. W., Fleeting, M. & Kolvin, P. A. K. (1988), Risk/protective factors for offending with particular reference to deprivation. In: *Studies of Psychosocial Risk: The Power of Longitudinal Data,* ed. M. Rutter. Cambridge: Cambridge University Press, pp. 77–95.

Kovacs, M. & Gatsonis, C. (in press), Stability and change in childhood-onset depressive disorders; longitudinal course as a diagnostic validator. In: *The Validation of Psychiatric Disorders,* ed. L. Robins & J. Barrett. New York: Raven.

———Paulauskas, S., Gatsonis, C. & Richards, C. (1989), Depressive disorders in childhood. III. A longitudinal study of comorbidity with and risk for conduct disorders. *J. Affective Disord.* 15:235–243.

Kraemer, H. C., Pruyn, J. P., Gibbons, R. D. et al. (1987), Methodology in psychiatric research. Report on the 1986 MacArthur Foundation Network I Methodology Institute. *Arch. Gen. Psychiatry,* 44:1100–1106.

Kratochwill, T. R. (1981), *Selective Mutism: Implications for Research and Treatment.* Hillsdale, NJ: Erlbaum.

Lapouse, R. (1965a), Who is sick? *Am. J. Orthopsychiatry,* 35:138–144.

———(1965b), The relationship of behavior to adjustment in a representative sample of children. *Am. J. Public Health,* 55:1130–41.

———Monk, M. A. (1958), An epidemiological study of behaviour characteristics in children. *Am. J. Public Health,* 48:1134–1144.

——— ———(1959), Fears and worries in a representative sample of children. *Am. J. Orthopsychiatry,* 29:803–818.

——— ———(1964), Behavior deviations in a representative sample of children: variation by sex, age, race, social class and family size. *Am. J. Orthopsychiatry,* 34:436–446.

Last, C. G., Hersen, M., Kazdin, A. E., Finkelstein, R. & Strauss, C. C. (1987), Comparison of DSM-III separation anxiety and over-anxious disorders: demographic characteristics and patterns of comorbidity. *J. Am. Acad. Child Adolesc. Psychiatry,* 26:527–531.

Lavik, N. (1977), Urban-rural differences in rates of disorder. In: *Epidemiological Approaches in Child Psychiatry,* ed. P. J. Graham. London: Academic Press, pp. 223–274.

Le Couteur, A., Rutter, M., Lord, C. et al. (in press), Autism Diagnostic Interview: a standardized investigator-based instrument. *J. Autism Dev. Disord.*

Links, P. S. (1983), Community surveys of the prevalence of childhood psychiatric disorders. *Child Dev.,* 54:531–548.

Loeber, R. & Dishion, T. J. (1984), Boys who fight at home and school: family conditions influencing cross-setting consistency. *J. Consult. Clin. Psychol.,* 52:759–768.

———LeBlanc, M. (in press), Toward a developmental criminology. In: *Crime and Justice, an Annual Review,* ed. M. Tonry & N. Morris. Chicago: University of Chicago Press.

Lord, C., Rutter, M., Goode, S. et al. (in press), Autism Diagnostic Observation Schedule: a standardized observation of communicative and social behavior. *J. Autism Dev. Disord.*

Lotter, V. (1966), Epidemiology of autistic conditions in young children. I: Prevalence. *Soc. Psychiatry,* 1:124–137.

Maccoby, E. E. & Jacklin, C. N. (1983), The 'person' characteristics of children and the family as environment. In: *Human Development: An Interactional Perspective,* ed. D. Magnusson & V. L. Allen. New York: Academic Press, pp. 76–91.

Macmillan, A., Kolvin, I., Garside, R. F., Nicol, A. R. & Leitch, I. M. (1980), A multiple criterion screen for identifying secondary school children with psychiatric disorder: characteristics and efficiency of screen. *Psychol. Med.,* 10:265–276.

McCarthy, P., Fitzgerald, M. & Smith, M. A. (1984), Prevalence of childhood autism in Ireland. *Ir. Med. J.,* 77:129–130.

McDermott, P. A. (1980), Prevalence and constituency of behavioural disturbance taxonomies in the regular school population. *J. Abnorm. Child Psychol.,* 4:523–536.

McFarlane, A. C., Plicansky, S. K. & Irwin, C. (1987), A longitudinal study of the psychological morbidity in children due to a natural disaster. *Psychol. Med.,* 17:727–738.

McGee, R. & Share, D. (1988), Attention-deficit disorder-hyperactivity and academic failure: which comes first and what should be treated? *J. Am. Acad. Child Adolesc. Psychiatry,* 27:318–325.

——Silva, P. A. & Williams, S. (1984a), Behaviour problems in a population of seven-year-old children: prevalence, stability and types of disorder—a research report. *J. Child Psychol. Psychiatry,* 25:251–259.

—— —— ——(1984b), Perinantal neurological, environmental and developmental characteristics of seven-year-old children with stable behaviour problems. *J. Child Psychol. Psychiatry,* 25:573–586.

——Williams, S., Share, D. L. Anderson, J. & Silva, P. A. (1986), The relationship between specific reading retardation, general reading backwardness and behavioural problems in a large sample of Dunedin boys: a longitudinal study from five to eleven years. *J. Child Psychol. Psychiatry,* 27:597–610.

McGuffin, P., Katz, R. & Bebbington, P. (1988), The Camberwell Collaborative Depression Study: III. Depression and adversity in the relatives of depressed probands. *Br. J. Psychiatry,* 152:775–782.

Magnusson, D. (1988), *Paths through Life: A Longitudinal Research Program.* Hillsdale, NJ: Erlbaum.

——Bergman, L. R. (in press), Pattern approach to the study of pathways from childhood to adulthood. In: *Straight and Devious Pathways from Childhood to Adulthood,* eds. L. Robins & M. Rutter. New York: Cambridge University Press.

Masten, A. S. (in press), Toward a developmental psychopathology of early adolescence. In: *Early Adolescent Transitions,* ed. M. D. Levine & E. R. McAnarney. Lexington, MA: Health.

——Garmezy, N. (1985), Risk, vulnerability,and protective factors in developmental psychopathology. In: *Advances in Clinical Child Psychology, Vol. 8,* ed. B. B. Lahey & A. E. Kazdin. New York: Plenum Press.

Mattison, R. E., Bagnato, S. & Strickler, E. (1987), Diagnostic importance of combined parent and teacher ratings on the Revised Behavior Problem Checklist. *J. Abnorm. Child Psychol.*, 15:617–662.

Maughan, B. & Champion, L. (in press), Risk and protective factors in the transition to adult life. In: *Successful Aging: Perspectives from the Behavioral and Social Sciences*, ed. P. Baltes & M. Baltes. New York: Cambridge University Press.

———Gray, G. & Rutter, M. (1985), Reading retardation and antisocial behaviour: a follow-up into employment. *J. Child Psychol. Psychiatry*, 26:741–758.

———Mortimore, P., Ouston, J. & Rutter, M. (1980), Fifteen Thousand Hours: a reply to Heath and Clifford. *Oxford Reviews of Education*, 6:289–303.

Maziade, M., Caperaa, P., Laplante, B. et al. (1985), Value of difficult temperament among 7 year olds in a general population for predicting psychiatric diagnosis at age 12. *Am. J. Psychiatry*, 142:943–946.

Miller, F. J. W., Court, S. D. M., Walton, W. S. & Knox, E. G. (1960), *Growing Up in Newcastle-upon-Tyne*. London: Oxford University Press.

Miller, L. C., Barrett, C. L., Hampe, E. & Noble, H. (1971), Factor structure of childhood fears. *J. Consult. Clin. Psychol.*, 39:264–268.

Minde, K. & Minde, R. (1977), Behavioural screening of pre-school children—A new approach to mental health? In: *Epidemiological Approaches in Child Psychiatry*, ed. P. J. Graham. London: Academic Press, pp. 139–164.

Monck, E. & Graham, P. (1988, Dec.), *Suicidal ideation in a total population of 15–19 year old girls*. Paper presented at Multi-Disciplinary Workshop on "Suicidal Behaviour of Adolescents," Paris.

Moreau, D. L. & Weissman, M. M. (in press), Anxiety symptoms across childhood and adolescence in nonpsychiatrically referred youngsters. In: *Anxiety Across the Life Span: A Developmental Perspective on Anxiety and Anxiety Disorders*, ed. C. Last. New York: Springer Publications.

Mortimore, P., Sammons, P., Stoll, L., Lewis, D. & Ecob, R. (1988), *School Matters: The Junior Years*. Wells, Somerset: Open Books.

Murphy, J. M. (1986), Diagnosis, Screening, and "Demoralization": epidemiological implications. *Psychiatr. Dev.*, 2:101–133.

Needleman, H. L., Gunnoe, C., Leviton, A. et al. (1979), Deficits in psychologic and classroom performance of children with elevated dentine lead levels. *N. Engl. J. Med.* 300:689–695.

Nichols, P. L. & Chen, T. C. (1981), *Minimal Brain Dysfunction—A Prospective Study*. Hillsdale, NJ: Lawrence Erlbaum.

Nicol, A. R., Stretch, D. D., Fundudis, T., Smith, I. & Davison, I. (1987), The nature of mother and toddler problems—I. Development of a multiple criterion screen. *J. Child Psychol. Psychiatry*, 28:739–754.

Offord, D. R. & Boyle, M. H. (1986), Problems in setting up and executing large-scale psychiatric epidemiological studies. *Psychiatr. Dev.*, 3:257–272.

——— ———(in press), Ontario child health study: correlates of disorder. *J. Am. Acad. Child Adolesc. Psychiatry*.

——— ———Szatmari, P. et al. (1987), Ontario Child Health Study. II. Six-month prevalence of disorder and rates of service utilization. *Arch. Gen. Psychiatry*, 44:832–836.

Ollendick, T. H. (1983), Reliability and validity of the revised fear survey schedule for children (FSSC-R). *Behav. Res. Ther.,* 21:685–692.

Oppel, W. C., Harper, P. A. & Rider, R. V. (1968), Social, psychological and neurological factors associated with enuresis. *Pediatrics,* 42:627–641.

Orvaschel, H. & Weissman, M. M. (1986), Epidemiology of anxiety disorders in children: a review. In: *Anxiety Disorders of Childhood,* ed. R. Gittleman, New York: Wiley, pp. 58–72.

Ouston, J., Maughan, B. & Rutter, M. (1985), *Change and innovation in secondary schools.* Final report to the Department of Education and Science.

Parker, G. (1983), *Parental Overprotection: A Risk Factor in Psychosocial Development.* New York: Grune & Stratton.

Petersen, A. C. (1988), Adolescent development. *Annu. Rev. Psychol.,* 39:583–607.

Place, M. (1987), The relative value of screening instruments in adolescence. *J. Adolesc.,* 10:227–240.

Platt, S., Hawton, K., Kreitman, N., Fagg, J. & Foster, J. (1988), Recent clinical and epidemiological trends in parasuicide in Edinburgh and Oxford: a tale of two cities. *Psychol. Med.,* 18:405–418.

Plomin, R. & Daniels, D. (1987), Why are children in the same family so different from one another? *Behavioral Brain Science,* 10:1–15.

Poole, C. (1987), Beyond the confidence interval. *Am. J. Public Health,* 77:195–199.

Puig-Antich, J. (1982), Major depression and conduct disorder in prepuberty. *J. Am. Acad. Child Psychiatry,* 21:118–128.

——Rabinovich, H. (1986), Relationship between affective and anxiety disorders in childhood. In: *Anxiety Disorders of Childhood,* ed. R. Gittelman. Chichester/New York: Wiley, pp. 136–156.

Pynoos, R. S., Frederick, C., Nader, K. et al. (1987), Life threat and post traumatic stress in school-age children. *Arch. Gen. Psychiatry,* 44:1057–1063.

Quinton, D. & Rutter, M. (1988), *Parental Breakdown: The Making and Breaking of Intergenerational Links.* Aldershot: Gower.

—— ——& Gulliver, L. (in press), Continuities in psychiatric disorder in the children of psychiatric patients. In: *Straight and Devious Pathways from Childhood to Adulthood,* ed. L. Robins & M. Rutter. Cambridge: Cambridge University Press.

Radke-Yarrow, M., Richters, J. & Wilson, W. E. (1988), Child development in a network of relationships. In: *Relationships within Families: Mutual Influecnes,* ed. R. A. Hinde & J. Stevenson-Hinde. Oxford: Clarendon Press, pp. 48–67.

Rahim, S. I. A. & Cederblad, M. (1984), Effects of rapid urbanization on child behaviour and health in a part of Khartoum, Sudan. *J. Child Psychol. Psychiatry,* 25:629–641.

Ratcliffe, S. G., Jenkins, J. & Teague, P. (in press), Cognitive and behavioural development of the 47,XYY child. In: *Cognitive and Psychosocial Dysfunctions Associated with Sex Chromosome Abnormalities,* ed. D. Berch & B. Bender. Washington, DC: American Association for the Advancement of Science.

Reich, W. & Earls, F. (1987), Rules for making psychiatric diagnoses in children on the basis of multiple sources of information. *J. Abnorm. Child Psychol.,* 15:601–616.

Reid, J. B., Baldwin, D. V., Patterson, G. R. & Dishion, T. J. (1988), Observations in the assessment of childhood disorders. In: *Assessment and Diagnosis in Child Psychopathology,* ed. M. Rutter, A. H. Tuma & I. S. Lann. New York: Guilford Press; London: Fulton, pp. 156–195.

Reitsma-Street, M., Offord, D. R. & Finch, T. (1985), Pairs of same-sexed siblings discordant for antisocial behaviour. *Br. J. Psychiatry,* 146:415–423.

Richman, N., Stevenson, J. & Graham, P. J. (1982), *Pre-school to School: A Behavioral Study.* London: Academic Press.

———— ———— ————(1985), Sex difference in outcome of pre-school behaviour problems. In: *Longitudinal Studies in Child Psychology and Psychiatry: Practical Lessons from Research Experience,* ed. A. R. Nicol. Chichester: Wiley, pp. 75–89.

Robins, L. (1978), Sturdy childhood predictors of adult antisocial behaviour: replications from longitudinal studies. *Psychol. Med.,* 8:611–622.

————(1985), Epidemiology: reflections on testing the validity of psychiatric interviews. *Arch. Gen. Psychiatry,* 42:918–924.

————(1986), The consequence of conduct disorder in girls. In: *Development of Antisocial and Prosocial Behavior: Research Theories and Issues,* ed. D. Olweus, J. Block & M. Radke-Yarrow. New York: Academic Press, pp. 385–414.

————Helzer, J. E., Croughan, J. & Ratcliff, K. S. (1981), National Institute of Mental Health Diagnostic Interview Schedule: its history, characteristics, and validity. *Arch. Gen. Psychiatry,* 38:381–389.

————Hill, S. Y. (1966), Assessing the contributions of family structure, class and peer groups to juvenile delinquency. *Journal of Criminal Law, Criminology Police Science,* 57:325–334.

————McEvoy, L. (in press), Conduct problems as predictors of substance abuse. In: *Straight and Devious Pathways from Childhood to Adulthood,* ed. L. Robins & M. Rutter. Cambridge: Cambridge University Press.

————, Rutter, M. eds. (in press), *Straight and Devious Pathways from Childhood to Adulthood.* Cambridge: Cambridge University Press.

————Schoenberg, S. P., Holmes, S. J., Radcliff, K., Benham, A. & Works, J. (1985), Early home environment and retrospective recall: a test for confordance between siblings with and without psychiatric disorders. *Am. J. Orthopsychiatry,* 55:27–41.

Rodgers, B. (1983), The identification and prevalence of specific reading retardation. *Br. J. Educ. Psychol.,* 53:369–373.

Rose, G. & Marshall, T. F. (1974), *Counseling and School Social Work: An Experimental Study.* London: Wiley.

Rutter, M. (1977), Surveys to answer questions. In: *Epidemiological Approaches in Child Psychiatry,* ed. P. J. Graham. London: Academic Press, pp. 1–30.

————(1978), Family, area and school influences in the genesis of conduct disorders. In: *Aggression and Antisocial Behaviour in Childhood and Adolescence,* ed. L. Hersov, M. Berger & D. Shaffer. *(Journal of Child Psychology and Psychiatry* Book Series No. 1). Oxford: Pergamon.

————(1979a), *Changing Youth in a Changing Society: Patterns of Adolescent Development and Disorder.* London: Nuffield Provincial Hospitals Trust (1980, Cambridge, MA: Harvard University Press).

____(1979b), Protective factors in children's responses to stress and disadvantage. In: *Primary Prevention of Psychopathology: Vol. 3: Social Competence in Children,* ed. M. W. Kent & J. E. Rolf. Hanover, NH: University Press of New England, pp. 49–74.

____(1981a), Epidemiological/longitudinal strategies and causal research in child psychiatry. *J. Am. Acad. Child Psychiatry,* 20:513–544.

____(1981b), The city and the child. *Am. J. Orthopsychiatry,* 51:610–625.

____(1983), Statistical and personal interactions: Facets and perspectives. In: *Human Development: An Interactional Perspective,* ed. D. Magnusson & V. Allen. New York: Academic Press, pp. 295–319.

____(1985), Resilience in the face of adversity: protective factors and resistance to psychiatric disorder. *Br. J. Psychiatry,* 147:598–611.

____(1987a), Psychosocial resilience and protective mechanisms. *Am. J. Orthopsychiatry,* 57:316–331.

____(1987b), Temperament, personality and personality disorder. *Br. J. Psychiatry,* 150:443–458.

____(1987c), Parental mental disorder as a psychiatric risk factor. In: *American Psychiatric Association's Annual review, Vol. 6,* ed. R. E. Hales & A. J. Frances. Washington, DC: American Psychiatric Association Inc., pp. 647–663.

____(1988a, May), *Age changes in depressive disorders: some developmental considerations.* Paper presented at the Society for Research in Child Development Workshop on "The Development of Affect Regulation and Dysregulation," Vanderbilt University.

____(1988b), *Studies of Psychosocial Risk: The Power of Longitudinal Data.* Cambridge: Cambridge University Press.

____(1988c), Epidemiological approaches to developmental psychopathology. *Arch. Gen. Psychiatry,* 45:486–500.

____(1989a), Pathways from childhood to adult life. Sixth Jack Tizard Memorial Lecture. *J. Child Psychol. Psychiatry,* 30:23–51.

____(1989b), Age as an ambiguous variable in developmental research. *International Journal of Behavioral Development,* 12:1–34.

____(1989c), Attention deficit disorder, hyperkinetic syndrome: conceptual and research issues regarding diagnosis and classification. In: *Attention Deficit Disorder and Hyperkinetic Syndrome,* ed. T. Sagvolden & T. Archer. Hillsdale, NJ: Erlbaum, pp. 1–24.

____Chadwick, O. & Shaffer, D. (1983a), Head injury. In: *Developmental Neuropsychiatry,* ed. M. Rutter. New York: Guilford Press, pp. 83–111.

____Cox, A., Tupling, C., Berger, M. & Yule, W. (1975a), Attainment and adjustment in two geographical areas. I. The prevalence of psychiatric disorder. *Br. J. Psychiatry,* 175:493–509.

____Giller, H. (1983), *Juvenile Delinquency: Trends and Perspectives.* Harmondsworth, Middx: Penguin (1984, New York: Guilford Press).

____Graham, P., Chadwick, O. F. D. & Yule, W. (1976a), Adolescent turmoil: fact or fiction? *J. Child Psychol. Psychiatry,* 17:35–56.

____ ____Yule, W. (1970a), *A Neuropsychiatric Study in Childhood.* London: Heinemann/SIMP.

_____Izard, C. & Read, P. eds. (1986a), *Depression in Young People: Developmental and Clinical Perspectives.* New York: Guilford Press.

_____Le Couteur, A., Lord, C., Macdonald, H., Rios, P. & Folstein, S. (1988a), Diagnosis and subclassification of autism: Concepts and instrument development. In: *Diagnosis and Assessment in Autism,* ed. E. Schopler & G. Mesibov. New York: Plenum, pp. 239–259.

_____Maughan, B., Mortimore, P. & Ouston, J., with Smith, A. (1979), *Fifteen Thousand Hours: Secondary Schools and Their Effects on Children.* London: Open Books; Cambridge, MA: Harvard University Press.

_____ _____Ouston, J. (1986b), The study of school effectiveness. In: *School Drop Outs: After the Storm Comes . . . .?,* ed. J. C. van der Wolf & J. J. Hox. Lisse: Swets and Zeitlinger, pp. 32–43.

_____Pickles, A. (in press), Improving the quality of psychiatric data. In: *Methodological Issues in Longitudinal Research,* ed. D. Magnusson & L. Bergman. Cambridge: Cambridge University Press.

_____Quinton, D. (1977), Psychiatric disorder: ecological factors and concepts of causation. In: *Ecological Factors in Human Development,* ed. H. McGurk. Amsterdam: North-Holland.

_____ _____(1984), Parental psychiatric disorder: effects on children. *Psychol. Med.,* 14:853–880.

_____ _____Liddle, C. (1983b), Parenting in two generations: looking backwards and looking forwards. In: *Families at Risk,* ed. N. Madge. London: Heinemann Educational, pp. 60–98.

_____Russell Jones, R. eds. (1983), *Lead Versus Health: Sources and Effects of Low Level Lead Exposure.* Chichester: Wiley.

_____Sandberg, S. (1985), Epidemiology of child psychiatric disorder: methodological issues and some substantive findings. *Child Psychiatry Hum. Dev.,* 15:209–233.

_____Tizard, J. & Whitmore, K. eds. (1979b), *Education, Health and Behaviour.* London: Longmans (Reprinted 1981, Melbourne, FA: Krieger).

_____ _____Yule, W., Graham, P. & Whitmore, K. (1976b), Research Report: Isle of Wight Studies 1964–1974. *Psychol. Med.,* 6:313–332.

_____Tuma, A. H. & Lann, I. S. eds. (1988b), *Assessment and Diagnosis in Child Psychopathology.* New York: Guilford Press.

_____Yule, B., Quinton, D., Rowlands, O., Yule, W. & Berger, M. (1975b), Attainment and adjustment in two geographical areas. III. Some factors accounting for area differences. *Br. J. Psychiatry,* 126:520–533.

_____Yule, W. (1975), The concept of specific reading retardation. *J. Child Psychol. Psychiatry,* 6:181–197.

_____ _____Graham, P. (1973), Enuresis and behavioural deviance: Some epidemiological considerations. In: *Bladder Control and Enuresis,* ed. I. Kolvin, R. MacKeith & S. R. Meadow. Clinics in Developmental Medicine Nos. 48/49. London: Heinemann/SIMP.

St. Claire, L. & Osborne, A. F. (1987), The ability and behaviour of children who have been "in-care" or separated from their parents. *Early Child Development and Care,* 28(No. 3, Special Issue).

Scarr, S. & McCartney, K. (1983), How people make their own environments: a theory of genotype → environmental effects. *Child Dev.,* 54:424–435.

Schachar, R., Rutter, M. & Smith, A. (1981), The characteristics of situationally and pervasively hyperactive children: implications for syndrome definition. *J. Child Psychol. Psychiatry,* 22:375–392.

Schiff, M. & Lewontin, R. (1986), *Education and Class: The Irrelevance of IQ Genetic Studies.* Clarendon Press: Oxford.

Schmidt, M. H., Esser, G., Allehoff, W. et al. (1983), Prevalence and meaning of cerebral dysfunction in eight-year-old children in Mannheim. In: *Epidemiological Approaches in Child Psychiatry II,* ed. M. H. Schmidt & H. Remschmidt. Stuttgart/New York: Thieme Verlag/Thieme-Stratton, pp. 121–137.

———— ——— ———Geisel, B., Laught, M. & Woerner, W. (1987), Evaluating the significance of minimal brain dysfunction—results of an epidemiological study. *J. Child Psychol. Psychiatry,* 25:803–821.

———Remschmidt, H., eds. (1983), *Epidemiological Approaches in Child Psychiatry II.* Stuttgart/New York: Thieme Verlag/Thieme-Stratton.

Schopler, E., Reichler, R. J. & Renner, B. R. (1985), *Childhood Autism Rating Scale (CARS).* New York: Irvington Publishers.

Seidel, U. P., Chadwick, O. F. D. & Rutter, M. (1975), Psychological disorders in crippled children: a comparative study of children with and without brain damage. *Dev. Med. Child Neurol.,* 17:563–573.

Shaffer, D. (1986), Developmental factors in child and adolescent suicide. In: *Depression in Young People: Developmental and Clinical Perspectives,* ed. M. Rutter, C. E. Izard and P. B. Read. New York: Guilford Press, pp. 383–396.

———Garland, A., Gould, M., Fisher, P. & Trautman, P. (1988), Preventing teenage suicide. *J. Am. Acad. Child Adolesc. Psychiatry,* 27:675–687.

———Gould, M. S., Brasic, J., et al. (1983), A children's global assessment scale (CGAS). *Arch. Gen. Psychiatry,* 40:1228–1231.

Shapiro, S. K. & Garfinkel, B. D. (1986), The occurrence of behavior disorders in children: the interdependence of attention deficit disorder and conduct disorder. *J. Am. Acad. Child Psychiatry,* 25:809–819.

Share, D. L., McGee, R., McKenzie, D., Williams, S. & Silva, P. A. (1987), Further evidence relating to the distinction between specific reading retardation and general reading backwardness. *British Journal of Developmental Psychology,* 5:35–44.

Shen, Y-C., Wang, Y-F. & Yang, X-L. (1985), An epidemiological investigation of minimal brain dysfunction in six elementary schools in Beijing. *J. Child Psychol. Psychiatry,* 26:777–787.

Shepherd, M., Oppenheim, B. & Mitchell, S. (1971), *Childhood Behaviour and Mental Health.* London: University of London Press.

Shrout, P. E., Skodel, A. E. & Dohrenwend, B. P. (1986), A multi-method approach for case identification: first stage instruments. In: *Mental Disorders in the Community: Progress and Challenge,* ed. J. E. Barrett. New York: Guilford Press.

Silva, P. A. (1987), Epidemiology, longitudinal course, and some associated factors. In: *Language Development and Disorders,* ed. W. Yule & M. Rutter. Clinics in

Developmental Medicine No. 101/102. Oxford: Mac Keith Press/Blackwell Scientific Publications, pp. 1–15.

_____Hughes, P., Williams, S. & Faed, J. M. (1988), Blood lead, intelligence, reading attainment, and behaviour in eleven year old children in Dunedin, New Zealand. *J. Child Psychol. Psychiatry,* 29:43–52.

_____McGee, R. & Williams, S. (1985), Some characteristics of nine year old boys with general reading backwardness and specific reading retardation. *J. Child Psychol. Psychiatry,* 26:407–421.

Silverman, W. K. & Nelles, W. B. (1988), The Anxiety Disorders Interview Schedule for children. *J. Am. Acad. Child Adolesc. Psychiatry,* 27:772–778.

Simpson, A. E. & Stevenson-Hinde, J. (1985), Temperamental characteristics of three- to four-year-old boys and girls and child-family interactions. *J. Child Psychol. Psychiatry,* 26:43–53.

Smith, M. (1985), Recent work on low level lead exposure and its impact on behavior, intelligence, and learning. *J. Am. Acad. Child Psychiatry,* 24:24–32.

_____Delves, T., Lansdown, R., Clayton, B. & Graham, P. (1983), The effects of lead exposure on urban children: the Institute of Child Health/Southampton study. *Dev. Med. Child Neurol,* 25:Suppl. 47.

Speilberger, C. D. (1973), *Manual for the State-Trait Anxiety Inventory for Children.* Palo Alto, CA: Consulting Psychologists Press.

Spitzer, R. L., Endicott, J. & Robins, E. (1978), Research diagnostic criteria. *Arch. Gen. Psychiatry,* 35:773–782.

Stavrakaki, C., Vargo, B., Roberts, N. & Boodoosing, L. (1987), Concordance among sources of information for ratings of anxiety and depression in children. *J. Am. Acad. Child Adolesc. Psychiatry,* 26:733–737.

Steffenburg, S. & Gillberg, C. (1986), Autism and autistic-like conditions in Swedish rural and urban areas: a population study. *Br. J. Psychiatry,* 149:81–87.

Stein, Z. A., Susser, M. W. & Wilson, A. E. (1965), Families of enuretic children. I. Family type and age. II. Family culture, structure and organisation. *Dev. Med. Child Neurol.,* 7:658–676.

Steinhausen, H-C., Gobel, D., Breinlinger, M. & Wohlleben, B. (1986), A community survey of infantile autism. *J. Am. Acad. Child Psychiatry,* 25:186–189.

Stevenson, J. (1984), Predictive value of speech and language screening. *Dev. Med. Child Neurol.,* 26:528–538.

_____(1988), Which aspects of reading ability show a 'hump' in their distribution? *Applied Cognitive Psychology,* 2:77–85.

_____Richman, N. & Graham, P. (1985), Behaviour problems and language abilities at 3 years and behavioural deviance at 8 years. *J. Child Psychol. Psychiatry,* 26:215–230.

Stevenson-Hine, J. (1988), Individuals in relationships. In: *Relationships within families: Mutual Influences,* ed. R. A. Hinde & J. Stevenson-Hine. Oxford: Clarendon Press. pp. 68–80.

Strauss, C. C., Last, C. G., Hersen, M. & Kazdin, A. E. (1988), Association between anxiety and depression in children and adolescents with anxiety disorders. *J. Abnorm. Child Psychol.,* 16:57–68.

Strober, M. & Katz, J. (in press), Depression in the eating disorders: a review and analysis of descriptive, family and biological findings. In: *Diagnostic Issues in Anorexia Nervosa and Bulimia Nervosa,* ed. D. M. Garner & P. E. Garfinkel. New York: Brunner/Mazel.

Szmuckler, G. I. (1985), Review: the epidemiology of anorexia nervosa and bulimia. *J. Psychiatr. Res.,* 19:143–153.

Taylor, E. (1989), On the epidemiology of hyperactivity. In: *Attention Deficit Disorder and Hyperkinetic Syndrome,* ed. T. Sagvolden & T. Archer. Hillsdale, NJ: Erlbaum, pp. 31–52.

————Sandberg, S. & Rutter, M. (1988), *An epidemiological study of childhood hyperactivity.* Report to the Medical Research Council, London.

Thompson, W. D. (1987), Statistical criteria in the interpretation of epidemiological data. *Am. J. Public Health,* 77:191–194.

Thorndike, R. L. (1963), *The Concepts of Over- and Underachievement.* New York: Teachers College, Columbia University.

Tizard, B., Blatchford, P., Burke, J., Farquhar, C. & Plewis, I. (1988), *Young Children at School in the Inner City.* Hillsdale, NJ/Hove & London, UK: Erlbaum.

Van der Wissel, A. & Zegers, F. E. (1985), Reading retardation revisited. *British Journal of Developmental Psychology,* 3:3–9.

Velez, C. N. & Cohen, P. (1988), Suicidal behavior and ideation in a community sample of children: maternal and youth reports. *J. Am. Acad. Child Adolesc. Psychiatry,* 27:349–356.

————Johnson, J. & Cohen, P. (in press), The children in the community project: a longitudinal analysis of selected risk factors for childhood psychopathology. *J. Am. Acad. Child Adolesc. Psychiatry.*

Verhulst, F. C. & Althaus, G. W. (1988), Persistence and change in behavioral/emotional problems reported by parents of children aged 4–14: an epidemiological study. *Acta Psychiatr. Scand. [Suppl.* 339] 77.

————Van Der Lee, J. H., Althaus, G. W., Sanders-Woudstra, J. A. R., Timmer, F. C. & Donkhorst, I. D. (1985), The prevalence of nocturnal enuresis: do DSM criteria need to be changed? *J. Child Psychol. Psychiatry,* 26:989–993.

Vikan, A. (1985), Psychiatric epidemiology in a sample of 1510 ten-year-old children. I. Prevalence. *J. Child Psychol. Psychiatry,* 26:55–75.

Walzer, S. (1985), X chromosome abnormalities and cognitive development: implications for understanding normal human development. *J. Child Psychol. Psychiatry,* 26:177–184.

Warr, P. (1987), *Work, Unemployment and Mental Health.* London: Clarendon Press.

Weissman, M. M. (1987), Foreword to Section V, Psychiatric Epidemiology. In: *American Psychiatric Association Annual Review, Vol. 6,* ed. R. E. Hales & A. J. Frances. Washington, DC: American Psychiatric Press, pp. 572–588.

————Gammon, G. D., John, K. et al. (1987a), Children of depressed parents: increased psychopathology and early onset of major depression. *Arch. Gen. Psychiatry,* 44:847–853.

————Wickramaratne, P., Warner, V. et al. (1987b), Assessing psychiatric disorders in children: discrepancies between mothers' and children's reports. *Arch. Gen. Psychiatry,* 44:747–753.

Werner, E. E. & Smith, R. S. (1977), *Kauai's Children Come of Age*. Honolulu: University Press of Hawaii.

———— ————(1982), *Vulnerable but Invincible: A Study of Resilient Children*. New York: McGraw Hill.

Wing, J. K., Birley, J. L. T., Cooper, J. E., Graham, P. & Isaacs, A. D. (1967), Reliability of a procedure for measuring and classifying 'present psychiatric state.' *Br. J. Psychiatry,* 113:499–515.

Wing, L. & Gould, J. (1978), Systematic recording of behaviors and skills of retarded and psychotic children. *Journal of Autism and Childhood Schizophrenia,* 8:79–97.

———— ————(1979), Severe impairments of social interaction and associated abnormalities in children. *J. Autism Dev. Disord.,* 9:11–30.

Wolkind, S. (1985), The first years: pre-school children and their families in the inner city. In: *Recent Research in Developmental Psychopathology,* ed. J. E. Stevenson. Oxford: Pergamon Press, pp. 203–212.

————Kruk, S. (1985), From child to parent: early separation and the adaptation to motherhood. In: *Longitudinal Studies in Child Psychology and Psychiatry: Practical Lessons from Research Experience,* ed. A. R. Nicol. Chichester: Wiley, pp. 53–74.

World Health Organization (in press), *ICD-10: 1988 Draft of Chapter V, Categories F00-F99, Mental, Behavioural and Developmental Disorders, Clinical Descriptions and Diagnostic Guidelines.* Geneva: WHO.

Young, J. G., O'Brien, J. D., Gutterman, E. M. & Cohen, P. (1987), Research on the clinical interview. *J. Am. Acad. Child Adolesc. Psychiatry,* 26:613–620.

Yule, W. (1973), Differential prognosis of reading backwardness and specific reading retardation. *Br. J. Educ. Psychol.,* 43:244–248.

————(1981), The epidemiology of child psychopathology. In: *Advances in Clinical Child Psychology, Vol. 4,* ed. B. B. Lahey & A. E. Kazdin. New York: Plenum.

Zeitlin, H. (1986), *The Natural History of Psychiatric Disorders in Children* (Institute of Psychiatry Maudsley monograph no. 29). Oxford: Oxford University Press.

Zuckerman, B., Stevenson, J. & Bailey, V. (1987), Stomachaches and headaches in a community sample of preschool children. *Pediatrics,* 79:677–682.

8

High-Risk Children in Young Adulthood: A Longitudinal Study from Birth to 32 Years

Emmy E. Werner
University of California, Davis

The developmental courses of high-risk and resilient children were analyzed in a follow-up study of members of a 1955 birth cohort on the island of Kauai, Hawaii. Relative impact of risk and protective factors changed at various life phases, with males displaying greater vulnerability than females in their first decade and less during their second; another shift appears under way at the beginning of their fourth decade. Certain protective factors seem to have a more general effect on adaptation than do specific risk factors.

Even in the most discordant and impoverished homes, and beset by physical handicaps, some children appear to develop stable and healthy personalities, and display a remarkable degree of resilience in the face of life's adversities. Such youngsters have recently become the focus of attention of a handful of researchers who have asked what the protective factors are in these children and in their caregiving environment that ameliorate, or buffer, their responses to stressful life events. But, in contrast to the well-established track record of mental health studies of individuals who develop serious disorders, research on protective factors and individual resilience is still in its infancy, "a new scientific region to explore" (Anthony, 1978, p. 3).

Based on a paper presented at the 1988 annual meeting of the American Orthopsychiatric Association in San Francisco.

KAUAI LONGITUDINAL STUDY

One of the largest interdisciplinary investigations of the roots of resiliency in vulnerable children is a prospective longitudinal study of a multiracial cohort of 698 infants born in 1955 on the island of Kauai, Hawaii. Beginning in the prenatal period, the Kauai Longitudinal Study has monitored the impact on development of a variety of biological and psychosocial risk factors, stressful life events, and protective factors in early and middle childhood, late adolescence, and, now, young adulthood (Werner, 1986; Werner, Bierman, & French, 1971; Werner & Smith, 1977, 1982). The principal goals of the Kauai Longitudinal Study were *a)* to document, in naturalistic fashion, the course of all pregnancies and their outcomes in an entire community from the prenatal period until the offspring reached adulthood, and *b)* to assess the long-term consequences of perinatal complications and adverse early rearing conditions on the individuals' physical, cognitive, and psychosocial development.

Along the way, we learned that *both* vulnerability (susceptibility to negative developmental outcomes under high risk conditions) and resiliency (successful adaption following exposure to stressful life events) are relativistic concepts that do not preclude change over time.

From its inception, this has been a multidisciplinary study. Public health nurses recorded the reproductive histories of the women, and interviewed them in each trimester of pregnancy, noting any exposure to physical or emotional trauma. Physicians monitored any complications that occurred during the prenatal, labor, delivery, and neonatal periods. Nurses and social workers interviewed the mothers in the postpartum period and when the children were one and ten years old. They also observed the interaction of parents and offspring in the home. Pediatricians and psychologists independently examined the children at ages two and ten. They assessed their physical, intellectual, and social development, and noted any physical handicaps, and learning or behavior problems.

From the beginning of the study we also recorded information on the material, intellectual, and emotional aspects of the family environment, including stressful life events that brought discord or disruption to the family unit.

When the children reached school age, their teachers evaluated their academic progress and classroom behavior. In addition, the children were given a wide range of aptitude, achievement, and personality tests in the elementary grades and in high school. We also, with permission of the parents, had access to the records of the public health, educational, and social service agencies in the community, and to the files of the local police and family court. Last, but not least, we gained the individual perspectives of the members of the birth cohort when we interviewed them at ages 18 and at ages 30–32.

High-Risk Children

It should be emphasized that most of the infants in this cohort were born without complications after uneventful pregnancies, and grew up in supportive home environments. But one third of the infants could be considered "at risk" because they had experienced moderate to severe degrees of perinatal stress, were born into poverty, were reared by mothers with little formal education, and lived in a family environment troubled by discord, desertion, or divorce, or marred by parental alcoholism or mental illness. Two out of three of these at-risk children, all of whom encountered four or more such cumulative risk factors before the age of two, developed serious learning or behavior problems by the age of ten, or had delinquency records, mental health problems, or teenage pregnancies by the age of 18. Surprisingly, however, one out of every three of them (30 males, 42 females)—some 10% of the total cohort—developed instead into competent, confident, and caring young adults.

Looking back over the lives of these 72 resilient individuals, we contrasted their behavioral characteristics and caregiving environment with those of the high-risk youth of the same age and sex who had developed serious coping problems at ages ten or 18. We found a number of characteristics within the individuals, within their families, and outside the family circle that contributed to their resilience.

Even as infants, the temperamental characteristics of the resilient subjects elicited positive attention from family members as well as from strangers. By the age of one, both boys and girls were more frequently described by their caregivers as "very active;" the girls as "affectionate" and "cuddly," the boys as "good-natured" and "easy to deal with." The resilient infants had fewer eating and sleeping habits that distressed their parents than did the high-risk infants who later developed serious learning or behavior problems.

As toddlers, the resilient boys and girls already tended to meet the world on their own terms. The pediatricians and psychologists who examined them at age 20 months noted their alertness and autonomy, their tendency to seek out novel experiences, and their positive social orientation, especially among the girls. They were more advanced in communication, locomotion, and self-help skills than the children who later developed serious learning and behavior problems.

In elementary school, teachers reported that the resilient children got along well with their classmates. They had better reasoning and reading skills than high-risk children who developed problems, especially the girls. Though not especially gifted, these children used whatever skills they had effectively. Both parents and teachers noted that they had many interests and engaged in activities and hobbies that were not narrowly sex-typed. Such activities provided solace in adversity and a reason for pride.

By the time they graduated from high school, the resilient youth had developed a positive self-concept and an internal locus of control. On the California

Psychological Inventory (CPI), they displayed a more nurturant, responsible, and achievement-oriented attitude toward life than their high-risk peers who developed coping problems. The resilient girls were also more assertive, achievement-oriented, and independent.

The resilient boys and girls tended to grow up in families with four or fewer children, with a space of two years or more between themselves and their next sibling. Few had experienced prolonged separations from their primary caretaker during the first year of life. All had the opportunity to establish a close bond with at least one caregiver from whom they received plenty of positive attention when they were infants.

Some of this nurturing came from substitute parents, such as grandparents or older siblings, or from the ranks of neighbors and regular baby-sitters. Such substitute parents played an important role as positive models of identification. Maternal employment and the need to take care of younger siblings contributed to the pronounced autonomy and sense of responsibility noted among the resilient girls, especially in households where the father was absent.

Resilient boys were often first-born sons who did not have to share their parents' attention with many additional children. There were some males in the family who could serve as a role model (if not the father, then a grandfather, older cousin, or uncle). Structure, rules, and assigned chores were part of their daily routine in adolescence.

The resilient boys and girls also found emotional support outside their own families. They tended to have at least one, and usually several, close friends, especially the girls. They relied on an informal network of kin and neighbors, peers and elders, for counsel and support in times of crisis. Some had a favorite teacher who became a role model, friend, and confidant for them.

Participation in extracurricular activities played an important part in the lives of the resilient youth, especially activities that were cooperative enterprises. For still others, emotional support came from a youth leader, or from a minister or church group. With their help the resilient children acquired a faith that their lives had meaning and that they had control over their fate.

We noted in our analyses that as disadvantage and the number of stressful life events accumulated, more such protective factors were needed as counterbalance in the lives of these high-risk individuals, to ensure a positive developmental outcome.

THE 30-YEAR FOLLOW-UP

When we had last interviewed the members of the 1955 birth cohort, at age 18, we were aware that the maximum period for mental breakdown was still ahead of the high-risk youth (Werner & Smith, 1982). We did not yet know how well they would adapt to the demands of the adult world of work, marriage, and parenthood.

Since 1985, we have been involved in a follow-up of these resilient youth and of comparison groups of high-risk subjects from the 1955 birth cohort who had previously developed problems. Our follow-up has had two general objectives: *1)* to trace the long-term effects of stressful life events in childhood and adolescence on the adult adaptation of men and women who were exposed to poverty, perinatal stress, and parental psychopathology; and *2)* to examine the long-term effects of protective factors (personal competencies, sources of support) in childhood and adolescence on their adult coping.

The present follow-up finds our cohort at a stage which provides an opportunity to reappraise and modify the initial mode of adult living established in the previous decade. The transition period at age 30 is biologically the peak of adulthood, a time of great energy, but also among the most stressful points in the adult life cycle (Levinson, 1986). We believe, as did Lowenthal and her colleagues (1977), that such a transitional life stage *a)* maximizes individuals' awareness of their life circumstances, *b)* yields insights into the ways in which individuals adapt to stressful life situations, and *c)* increases their readiness to discuss these matters.

METHOD

During 1985–86, we located some 80% ($N = 545$) of the survivors of the 1955 birth cohort. The majority still live on Kauai and among them are most of the former "problem" children. Some 10% have moved to other Hawaiian islands (Oahu, Maui, and Hawaii), most to Honolulu. Another 10% live on the U.S. mainland, some 2% live abroad. Among those who moved away from Kauai are many of the resilient individuals.

The instruments administered in individual sessions with the subjects are: a checklist of stressful life events, Rotter's Locus of Control scale, the EAS Temperament Survey for Adults (Buss & Plomin, 1984), and a structured interview. The interview assesses the subjects' perception of major stressors and support in their adult lives: in school, at work, and in their relationships with their spouses or mates, their children, parents, in-laws, siblings, and friends. It concludes with an assessment of the individual's state of health, satisfaction, and well-being at the present stage of life.

In addition, we have access to the records of the District and Circuit courts in Kauai, in Honolulu, and on the other outer islands. They contain civil, criminal, and family court files which are open to the public and cover the period since our last follow-up at age 18. These files contain not only records of major violations of the law, but also information on such domestic problems as desertion, divorce, delinquent child support payments, and spouse and child abuse.

We also have access to the state-wide mental health registry which records diagnoses and treatment outcomes for all members of the 1955 birth cohort (and their parents) who have received in-or out-patient mental health services since the last follow-up, and to the records of the State Department of Health which registers marriage licenses, and birth and death certificates.

So far, we have follow-up data in adulthood on every member of the 1955 cohort who has been a defendant in a criminal or civil law suit, or whose marriage ended in divorce by age 30. We also have follow-up data on 86% of the resilient subjects, 90% of the teenage parents, 75% of the offspring of alcoholics, 75% of the delinquents, and 80% of the individuals who had developed mental health problems by the age of 18.

RESULTS

Stressful Life Events

More than half of the stressful life events that significantly increased the likelihood of having a criminal record or an "irrevocably broken marriage" by age 30 for members of this cohort took place in infancy and early childhood. Among the events with negative effects on the quality of adult coping for both men and women were: *1)* the closely spaced birth of a younger sibling in infancy (less than two years after birth of the index child); *2)* being raised by a mother who was not married at the time of the child's birth; *3)* having a father who was permanently absent during infancy or early childhood; *4)* prolonged disruptions of the family life and separations from the mother during the first year of life (these included unemployment of the major breadwinner, illness of the parent, and major moves); and *5)* having a mother who worked outside the home without stable substitute child care during the first year of the child's life.

A significantly higher proportion of males with a criminal record (including promotion of harmful drugs, theft and burglary, assault and battery, rape, and attempted murder) experienced such disruptions of their family unit in their early years, as did the men and women whose marriages had ended in divorce by age 30.*

For the females, teenage pregnancies, teenage marriages, marital conflict, problems in their relationships with their fathers, and financial problems in their teens also significantly increased the likelihood of divorce by age 30; for the males, it was the absence of the father, as well as the death of the mother, or of a grandparent or close friend before age 10. Such events occurred in significantly greater frequency among children in this birth cohort who had been born and raised in chronic poverty.

---

* Tables and figure summarizing these and other findings in this section may be obtained directly from the author.

Resilient Individuals

Now let us examine some of the competencies and sources of support that characterized those members of the cohort who had been resilient children. So far, we have follow-up data in adulthood on 62 (26 males, 36 females), of whom one third are of Japanese descent, one third Philippino, and one third part-Hawaiian mixtures. All had grown up in poverty and had previously coped successfully with the effects of perinatal stress, parental psychopathology, or discord and disruption in their family units. They had graduated from high school during the height of the energy crisis and joined the workforce during the worst recession since the Great Depression. In spite of these economic constraints, these young men and women are coping well with the demands of one of the most stressful periods in the adult life cycle.

Education and vocation. Both men and women in this group are highly achievement-oriented. With few exceptions, they have pursued education beyond high school (three out of four have some college education) and are satisfied with their performance in school. With the exception of one male and three females, they are currently in full-time employment; the women predominantly in semiprofessional and managerial positions, the men in the professions or in skilled trades and technical jobs. Three out of four are satisfied with their current work. In terms of both educational and vocational accomplishments, these high-risk individuals from economically poor backgrounds have fared as well or better than low-risk comparison groups of the same sex and age. The majority of the resilient men and women list career or job success as their primary objective at this stage of life, followed by self-fulfillment; fewer choose such traditional objectives as a happy marriage or children.

Marriage. The resilient women have made more transitions into multiple life trajectories than the resilient men. Eighty-five percent are married and work, among them the 75% who have young children. In contrast, only 40% of the resilient men are currently married, and only 35% have children.

The significant gender difference in life trajectories observed in this group may be, in part, a consequence of the recent women's liberation movement, but it may also represent realistic adaptations to economic circumstances, similar to those reported by Elder (1974) for the *Children of the Great Depression.* Whatever the reasons, there seems to be a greater reluctance among the resilient males than among the resilient females to make commitments to marriage, or to remarry if their first marriage ends in divorce.

A significantly higher proportion of males than females in this group report that the break-up of a long-term relationship between the ages of 18 and 30 has been a source of great stress to them (53% males vs 31% females). The expectations from such a long-term relationship also differ significantly by gender. The majority of both males and females want permanency and security from marriage, but a significantly higher proportion of females expect intimacy and sharing from such a relationship (69.2% female vs 38.5% male).

Children. For those among the resilient adults who are parents, the primary goal for their children is acquisition of personal competencies and skills. A significantly higher proportion of resilient women than men expects high achievement from their offspring, and stress early independence in their sons and daughters. In contrast, a significantly higher proportion of resilient men than women considers the "opportunity to care for others" as the most positive aspect of being a parent (71.4% males vs 20.8% females), and tolerates dependence in their young children (71.4% vs 19.0%). These are the same individuals who were rated as more "androgynous" in their interests and activities by their parents and teachers in childhood and adolescence.

Sources of worry. The greatest source of worry among the resilient men and women at this stage in their lives appears to be problems of family members, especially the health of parents or in-laws, or divorces among parents or siblings. Work conditions are reported as major worries by a higher proportion of men; a significantly higher proportion of women tend to worry about their children.

At age 30, the proportion of self-reported health problems is significantly higher among these high-risk resilient individuals than among low-risk comparison groups (46% vs 15%). Some 55.6% of the resilient men report health problems that appear related to stress, such as back problems, dizziness and fainting spells, problems with overweight, and ulcers. Most of the health problems reported by 40% of the resilient women are related to pregnancy and childbirth (emergency D & C, miscarriages, C-sections, toxemia of pregnancy, and premenstrual migraine headaches).

Sources of support. The overwhelming majority of the resilient men and women at age 30 consider personal competence and determination to be their most effective resources in coping with stressful life events. On Rotter's Locus of Control Scale, both sexes scored significantly (more than 2 *SD*) below the standardization group in the *internal* direction (as they did on the Fear subscale on the EAS Adult Temperament Scale).

Both sexes also value the support of a spouse or mate, and faith and prayer. In fact, faith and prayer were significantly more often reported as sources of support by resilient high-risk individuals than by their low-risk peers of the same age (33% vs 15%). But the resilient women draw on a significantly larger number of sources of support (including friends, older relatives, siblings, co-workers, mental health professionals, and self-help groups) than do the resilient men. In contrast, the resilient males seem to rely more exclusively on their own resources, with some additional support from spouses or parents. They less frequently derive emotional support from friends and co-workers.

Life satisfaction. Despite some continuing financial worries and the stress of multiple transitions into work, marriage, and parenthood, three out of four among the resilient men and women in their early thirties consider themselves "happy" or "satisfied" with their current status in life. Indeed, a significantly higher proportion of the high-risk resilient individuals than their low-risk peers rate themselves as "happy" and "delighted" with their current life circumstances (44% vs 10%).

It appears from this preliminary analysis of our 30-year interview data that most resilient individuals who had coped successfully with adversity in childhood and adolescence are also competent in coping with their adult responsibilities. But, as at age 18, more resilient women tend to weather stressful life events with less impairment to their health; they also rely on more sources of support than do resilient men.

A relatively high proportion of the men in this group appears to be reluctant to commit themselves to sustained intimate relationships. Success in these individuals may have been attained at the cost of spontaneous enjoyment of life (see Cohler, 1987, p. 406). One such individual, recently divorced, summed up his attitude when queried about the most important thing that happened in his life so far:

> The realization of how harsh life really is—how relationships can leave deep, within, hurts that don't seem to go away. With understanding and care, much can be accomplished—with sincere motivation and determination. Believe in yourself, and accomplish the best you can do, and know it is your own achievement that brings you along. Enjoy life and respect it.

Cohler (1987), in an excellent review chapter, pointed out that there are still relatively few studies of the manner in which people use reflection upon their own past experiences as a resource to promote later resilience. Looking back at their lives, many of the resilient men and women in our study commented, with some surprise, on their own strength and accomplishments:

F1: I feel good about myself—actually going through a lot of hurdles and having survived it, I know now I can make it on my own . . .

F2: I like myself . . . I surprise myself a lot with the knowledge I gained from all the jobs and the people I've met in the jobs. Lots of opportunities came my way . . .

M1: The struggle to succeed strengthened me—gave me confidence.

Others look forward to the challenges ahead in their lives:

M2: I've accomplished a lot—some of my goals I wanted to reach, but I am always setting new goals.

M3: I thank God that he gave me the power and strength to be where I am. I just think I am 30 years young—I have so much more to do in my life—I cannot believe I've gone through 30 years. I can't possibly do all I want to do in 60–70 years . . .

F3: I feel good—I feel that things are really rolling, moving along. It's neat to be married, to get to know a person better, to build a relationship . . . I feel young to be 30 . . .

A few sense a time clock ticking away, and feel that they have fallen short of the mark, in spite of considerable attainment:

F4: 30? I feel that every day of my life I am starting from new. 30 scares me—I am not young anymore. Well—I do feel 30. I look in the mirror and see the first white hair.

M4: Ten years go by in a snap, sitting in my living room, on my easy chair—and now I am 30 . . . I am still trying to figure out what I am supposed to accomplish, I haven't done the best I could. I can do more.

Thus, not all of the resilient individuals are happy and satisfied with their life situation in their early thirties. One male and two females rated themselves as either "unhappy" or "mostly dissatisfied." While no one in the resilient group has had periods of sustained unemployment or run afoul of the law, 20% of the resilient men and women who married were divorced by the time they reached age 30. Two of the resilient women (one the daughter of a mentally ill mother) have had to seek help from mental health professionals since graduating from high school. Two males and one female had problems with substance abuse in their early twenties, but are now rehabilitated.

Positive Change

By the same token, we may ask if positive changes have taken place among the high-risk children who had developed problems during their teens. Have protective factors operated in their lives to turn the balance toward resiliency? Preliminary follow-up data suggest some answers for two high-risk groups: *1)* teenage mothers whose status *a)* deteriorated or *b)* improved in the third decade of life; *2)* delinquents *a)* with and *b)* without a criminal record by age 30.

Teenage mothers. So far we have obtained follow-up information in adulthood on 24 of the 28 teenage mothers in this birth cohort (one had died of cancer). Ten had established stable relationships with a spouse or mate by the time they reached their late twenties, and had also improved their financial lot. The others were either divorced or separated, and had serious financial worries. They either lived in chronic poverty or were supported by welfare agencies.

Teenage mothers whose lot improved had less anxious, insecure relationships with their caregivers as infants, and a stronger feeling of security as part of their family in adolescence than teenage mothers whose lot deteriorated. A higher proportion of "successful" teenage mothers modeled themselves after mothers who had held a steady job when the teenagers were children, and a smaller proportion had problems in their relationship with their fathers in adolescence.

A sociable disposition, an internal locus of control, and more nurturant, responsible and flexible attitudes characterized the teenage mothers whose lot improved in their twenties and early thirties. The unimproved group tended to consist of women who were more anxious, dependent, and inhibited and believed that events happened to them as a result of factors beyond their control.

A significant proportion of improved teenage mothers had sought additional education beyond high school and prepared themselves for skilled, semiprofessional or managerial positions. While they went to school, their sources of child-care differed from those of the teenage mothers who did not seek further education and who are now found mostly in unskilled positions as adults. A higher proportion of improved teenage mothers relied on help by siblings, friends, or in-laws; among the unimproved, care was mostly extended by the young women's parents, possibly increasing their dependency.

Those who improved in status reported the following balance of protective factors: their own determination, high social support, and a moderate amount of stressful life events. Our numbers are small, but we note that our findings are similar to those reported by Furstenberg and his associates in his follow-up of black teenage mothers in the Baltimore area (Furstenberg, Brooks-Gunn, & Morgan, 1987).

Delinquent youth. Thirty-one individuals (26 males, 5 females) from the 1955 birth cohort had a criminal record by age 30. While most had been delinquents in adolescence (involved in burglary, car theft, and larceny), it must be kept in mind that they constituted a minority of all delinquents—about one third ($N = 27/89$). Identifying prospective criminals at an early age is of greater practical importance than identifying potential juvenile delinquents, most of whom turn out to be only temporary nuisances (Werner, 1987).

As in the Cambridge Study in Delinquent Development, conducted among London working youth (Farrington, Gallagher, Morley, St. Ledger, & West, 1988; West, 1982), we found among the "crime resistant" delinquents a much smaller proportion considered to be troublesome by their classroom teachers and their parents during middle childhood. Among those who entered an adult criminal career, a significantly higher proportion had been considered dishonest by both teachers and parents, and had exhibited temper tantrums, uncontrolled emotions, and extreme irritability, aggression, and bullying behavior in the classrooms at age ten.

Delinquents who did not commit any adult crimes also had significantly higher scores in early childhood on developmental examinations that assessed their sensory-motor and social competence. In addition, they were less frequently considered to be in need of mental health services by age ten than those who went on to commit adult crimes.

Last, but not least, the presence of an intact family unit in childhood, and especially in adolescence, was a major protective factor in the lives of delinquent youth who turned out to be only temporary or minor offenders. Five out of six of the delinquents with an adult criminal record came from families where either the mother or the father was absent during their adolescence because of separation or divorce. Only one out of four among the delinquents without an adult crime record grew up in a home where either the mother or the father was permanently absent in their teens. Delinquents without a later crime record also had a lower divorce rate by age 30 than did those with a criminal record.

DISCUSSION

Three types of protective factors emerge from our analyses of the developmental course of high-risk children from infancy to adulthood: *1)* dispositional attributes of the individual, such as activity level and sociability, at least average intelligence, competence in communication skills (language, reading), and an internal locus of control; *2)* affectional ties within the family that provide emotional support in times of stress, whether from a parent, sibling, spouse, or mate; and *3)* external support systems, whether in school, at work, or church, that reward the individual's competencies and determination, and provide a belief system by which to live.

The preliminary findings reviewed here also suggest that such protective factors may have a more generalized effect on adaption in childhood, adolescence, or adulthood than do specific risk factors or stressful life events such as poverty, perinatal stress, parental alcoholism or psychopathology, and teenage pregnancy.

The qualities that define individual resilience have been demonstrated in children from different ethnic groups, different socioeconomic strata, and different cultural contexts; among the multiracial children of Kauai, as well as among black children on the U.S. mainland, and Caucasian children in the U.S. and in Europe (Garmezy, 1985; Rutter, 1985; Werner, in press). Rutter has summed them up succinctly:

Resilience . . . seems to involve several related elements. Firstly, a sense of self-esteem and self-confidence; secondly, a belief in one's own self-efficacy and ability to deal with change and adaptation; and thirdly, a repertoire of social problem solving approaches. (Rutter, 1985, p. 607)

The influence of protective factors that enhance resilience in high-risk children appears to operate both directly and indirectly as chain reactions over time. A major challenge ahead of us is the examination of each of the individual links in such longitudinal chains.

Our longitudinal data indicate that the relative impact of risk and protective factors changed from infancy through early and middle childhood to late adolescence and young adulthood. At each developmental stage there was a shifting balance between stressful life events that heightened individual vulnerability, and protective factors that enhanced resilience. This balance changed not only with the stages of the life cycle, but also with the gender of the individual.

Both our own and other American and European studies have shown repeatedly that boys are more vulnerable than girls when exposed to biological insults and caregiving deficits in the first decade of life, but that this trend is reversed when females become more vulnerable in late adolescence, especially with the onset of early childbearing. Judging from our follow-up data, by the age of 30 the balance appears to be shifting back in favor of the women.

An individual is able to cope so long as the balance among risks, stressful life events, and protective factors is manageable. But when risk factors and stressful life events outweigh the protective factors, even the most resilient individual can develop problems. They may be serious coping problems, or of the less visible type whose symptoms are internalized, as with the stress-related health problems we noted among some of the resilient males in their early thirties, and their difficulties in establishing intimate, committed relationships.

For the clinician, intervention may be conceived as an attempt to shift the balance for the client from vulnerability to resilience, either by decreasing exposure to stress-related health risks or life events (such as the impact of parental alcoholism, psychopathology, or divorce), or by increasing the number of protective factors (communication and problem-solving skills, or sources of emotional support) available. For the researcher, the challenge of the future is to discover how the chain of direct and indirect linkages between protective factors is established over time so as to foster escape from adversity for vulnerable children.

REFERENCES

Anthony, E. J. (1978). A new scientific region to explore. In E. J. Anthony, C. Koupernik, & C. Chiland (Eds.), *The child and his family: Vol. 4, Vulnerable children*, New York: Wiley.

Buss, A. H., & Plomin, R. (1984). *Temperament: Early developing personality traits.* Hillsdale, NJ: Erlbaum.

Cohler, B. J. (1987). Adversity, resilience and the study of lives. In E. J. Anthony & B. J. Cohler (Eds.), *The invulnerable child.* New York: Guilford.

Elder, G. H. (1974). *Children of the Great Depression: Social change in life experience.* Chicago: University of Chicago Press.

Farrington, D. P., Gallagher, B., Morley, L., St. Ledger, R. J., & West, D. (1988). Are there any successful men from criminogenic backgrounds? *Psychiatry, 51,* 116–130.

Furstenberg, F., Brooks-Gunn, J., & Morgan, S. P. (1987). *Adolescent mothers in later life.* New York: Cambridge University Press.

Garmezy, N. (1985). Stress-resistant children: The search for protective factors. In *Recent research in developmental psychopathology* (Journal of Child Psychology and Psychiatry, Book Suppl. vol. 4). Oxford: Pergamon Press.

Levinson, D. J. (1986). A conception of adult development. *American Psychologist, 41,* 3–13.

Lowenthal, M., Thurnher, M., & Chiriboga, D. (1977). *Four stages of life.* San Francisco: Jossey-Bass.

Rutter, M. (1985). Resilience in the face of adversity: Protective factors and resistance to psychiatric disorder. *British Journal of Psychiatry, 147,* 598–611.

Werner, E.E. (1986). Resilient offspring of alcoholics: A longitudinal study for birth to age 18. *Journal of Studies on Alcohol, 47,* 34–40.

Werner, E.E. (1987). Vulnerability and resiliency in children at risk for delinquency: A longitudinal study from birth to young adulthood. In J.D. Burchard & S.N. Burchard (Eds.), *The prevention of delinquent behavior.* Beverly Hills: Sage.

Werner, E.E. (in press). Protective factors and individual resilience. In S.J. Meisels & J.P. Shonkoff (Eds.), *Handbook of early intervention: Theory, practice and analysis.* Cambridge, England: Cambridge University Press.

Werner, E.E., Bierman, J., & French, F. (1971). *The children of Kauai.* Honolulu: University of Hawaii Press.

Werner, E.E., & Smith, R.S. (1977). *Kauai's children come of age.* Honolulu: University of Hawaii Press.

Werner, E.E., & Smith, R.S. (1982). *Vulnerable but invincible: A longitudinal study of resilient children and youth.* New York: McGraw-Hill.

West, D.J. (1982). *Delinquency: Its roots, careers and prospects.* London: Heinemann.

9

Ontario Child Health Study:
Correlates of Disorder

David R. Offord, Michael H. Boyle, and Yvonne Racine

McMaster University, Ontario, Canada

Data from the Ontario Child Health Study were used to examine the prevalence and selected correlates of conduct disorder, hyperactivity, emotional disorder, and somatization in children 4 to 16 years of age by informant (parent and teacher for children 4 to 11, and parent and youth for children 12 to 16). The results indicate that the prevalence and pattern of correlates of the individual disorders differ in important ways by informant. This suggests that we need to understand the factors that influence assessments provided by informants from different contexts (e.g., parents and teachers) before combining information from them to arrive at singular classifications. Key Words: childhood behavior disorders, risk factors, correlates, surveys.

The Ontario Child Health Study (OCHS) was an interview survey of 1,869 families, including 3,294 children. The primary objective of the OCHS was to estimate the prevalence of psychiatric disorders among Ontario children, 4 to 16 years of age. Data were also gathered on correlates of disorders. The OCHS was carried out in the Province of Ontario, a large and varied geographic area of 412,582 square miles, with a population of over 8.5 million persons, almost 1.7 million of these being children between the ages of 4 and 16 in 1983. The OCHS was commissioned by the Ministry of Community and Social Services of the Province of Ontario, which is responsible for the delivery of children's mental health services in the Province. Key ministry officials recognized that sound epidemiological data would facilitate plan-

Reprinted with permission from *Journal of American Academy of Child and Adolescent Psychiatry,* 1989, Vol. 28, No. 6, 856–860. Copyright © 1989 by the American Academy of Child and Adolescent Psychiatry.

This study was supported by the Ministry of Community and Social Services, Ontario, and was carried out by the Child Epidemiology Unit, Department of Psychiatry, McMaster University, and the Child and Family Centre, Chedoke Division, Chedoke-McMaster Hospitals, Hamilton, Ontario.

ning for more effective, comprehensive services for children delivered in an equitable manner across the various regions of Ontario.

METHOD

Sampling

The sampling design and measurement of disorder of the OCHS have been covered in detail elsewhere (Boyle et al., 1987) and will be summarized here. The target population included all children born between January 1, 1966, and January 1, 1979, whose usual place of residence was a household dwelling in Ontario. The survey excluded three groups of children representing 3.3% (55,100 of 1,687,200) of the population of children 4 to 16 years of age: those children living on Indian reserves (13,800); those in collective dwellings such as institutions (4,830), and those living in dwellings constructed after June 1, 1981 (Census Day) (36,500). The sampling unit consisted of all household dwellings listed in the 1981 Census of Canada. The sample frame (source of subjects) was the 1981 census. Selection was done by stratified, clustered, random sampling from the census file of household dwellings (Statistics Canada, 1982).

Interviewers collected information from the female head of the household (parents), teachers, and youth 12 to 16. With the exception of the school information, all the data were collected during a home visit. The survey work was carried out during January and February of 1983 by Statistics Canada, which is the federal government agency responsible for producing the census and other governmental reports. The participation rate among eligible households was high (91.1%) and the refusal rate was low (3.9%).

Measures

The survey investigated four childhood psychiatric disorders: conduct disorder, hyperactivity, and emotional disorder (neurosis) in children 4 to 11, and these three plus somatization disorder in adolescents 12 to 16 years of age. To measure each of the four disorders, scales were composed of problem behaviors (items) summed to form a score. *DSM-III* criteria guided the selection of items for each scale. The item content for the emotional disorder scale was chosen to reflect elements of the *DSM-III* categories of overanxious disorder, affective disorder, and obsessive compulsive disorder. The Child Behavior Checklist (CBCL) (Achenbach and Edelbrock, 1981) furnished the basic pool of items for the scales. When items from the CBCL did not adequately describe a particular criterion, additional items were generated. The resulting checklist was termed the Survey Diagnostic Instrument (SDI). Similar checklists were used for the three types of informants: parents, teachers, and adolescents, 12 to 16. Checklist items applicable to a particular disorder were grouped to form a scale. Each item could be scored 0, 1, or 2, indicating responses of "never or not true," "sometimes or somewhat true," and "often or very true," respectively.

Checklist scale scores were converted to binary ratings of disorder based on their ability to discriminate best the presence or absence of a diagnosis made by a child psychiatrist. Separate thresholds were established for each data source for the two age groups. The completion rate on the teacher form in the older age group was too low for use in measuring disorder and was not used. Thus, a 4- to 11-year-old child could have a disorder on the basis of parent or teacher, or both parent *and* teacher. Similarly, a 12- to 16-year-old adolescent could have a disorder on the basis of parent or adolescent or both parent and adolescent. Children and adolescents had to score below the thresholds for both sources to be considered nondisordered in each category. In addition, children and adolescents were excluded from analyses if data from one or both informants were incomplete.

Definition of Correlates

The nine correlates of psychiatric disorders examined included two in the sociodemographic domain (low income and urban/rural), three in the parental-family area (family dysfunction, parent treated for nerves, and parent arrested), and four pertaining to the child (age, sex, repeated a grade, and chronic medical illness). The definitions for variables that are not self-explanatory include the following:

Low income: Total family income in preceding year (1982) was <$10,000.

Urban/rural: Urban areas are those with a population of >25,000. Rural areas include both small urban areas (population 3,000 to 25,000) and rural areas (population <3,000).

Family dysfunction: A score above 26, on a range of 12 to 48, on the 12-item General Functioning subscale derived from the McMaster Family Functioning Assessment Device (Byles et al., 1988).

Parent treated for nerves: Parent reports that self or partner was treated at some time for nerves or a nervous condition.

Parent arrested: Parent reports that self or partner was at some time arrested or charged with an offense other than a traffic violation.

Age: 4 to 11 or 12 to 16.

Failed a grade: Parent reports that child failed or repeated a grade at some time during his or her school career.

Chronic medical illness: Parent reports that child has one or more illnesses or conditions which are usually chronic in duration (>6 months).

RESULTS

Table 1 presents the 6-month prevalence of psychiatric disorders by age and informant (parent and teacher for children 4 to 11, and parent and youth for children 12 to 16). Other data on the distribution of these disorders in the population are presented elsewhere (Offord et al., 1987). Weighting of the data to reflect the household probability of selection, its size, and the age and sex distribution of children, had minimal effects on prevalence estimates (Offord et al., 1987), so only unweighted (actual responses) are presented here and used in subsequent analyses.

In the 4- to 11-year-old age group, conduct disorder and hyperactivity are more common in boys than in girls regardless of informant (parent or teacher). The prevalence rates of teacher-identified cases are higher than those of parent-identified cases for these two disorders for both boys and girls. In contrast, parent-identified cases of emotional disorder are more common in girls than in boys, while the reverse is true for teacher-identified cases. For boys, parents and

TABLE 1
Six-Month Prevalence (per 100) of Psychiatric Disorders by Age
and by Informant

| | Informant | | | |
| | Parent | | Teacher/Youth | |
Group	Boys	Girls	Boys	Girls
Age 4 to 11	($N = 710$)	($N = 718$)	($N = 710$)	($N = 718$)
Conduct disorder	1.4	0.4	4.9	1.8
Hyperactivity	2.1	0.8	7.3	2.5
Emotional disor-				
der	5.8	7.1	5.8	4.2
One or more dis-				
orders (95%				
confidence in-	7.2	7.8	13.4	6.4
terval)	(±2.7)	(±2.8)	(±3.6)	(±2.6)
Age 12 to 16	($N = 607$)	($N = 624$)	($N = 607$)	($N = 624$)
Conduct disorder	4.0	1.9	7.2	2.9
Hyperactivity	3.1	1.4	4.0	1.8
Emotional disor-				
der	2.3	4.0	2.6	9.8
Somatization	2.0	3.8	3.0	8.7
One or more dis-				
order (95% con-	8.1	7.7	12.4	17.1
fidence interval)	(±3.4)	(±3.0)	(±3.8)	(±4.3)

teachers identify the same percentage of children with emotional disorder, while for girls, parents identify more cases than do teachers. For one or more of the three disorders, the rates of parent-identified cases are almost the same for boys and girls, but the rate of teacher-identified cases in boys is over twice the rate for girls. Between informants, the prevalence of one or more disorders for boys is almost twice as high among teachers as parents; for girls, however, parents identify a slightly higher percentage as having one or more disorders compared to teachers. It should be noted that in the validity substudy which involved clinical workups by child psychiatrists (Boyle et al., 1987), the prevalence of diagnosed cases of somatization in the 4-to-11 age group was too low to act as a standard for setting scale thresholds.

In 12- to 16-year-olds, the prevalence rates of youth-identified cases are substantially higher than those of parent-identified cases for conduct disorder in boys and emotional disorder and somatization in girls. As with the younger age group, conduct disorder and hyperactivity are more common in boys than in girls, regardless of informant. Emotional disorder and somatization, on the other hand, are more common in girls than in boys for both parents and youth. In the case of one or more disorders, parent-identified cases are slightly more common in boys than in girls, while youth-identified cases are noticeably more common in girls than in boys.

The agreement between informants (not shown) is low. For example, in 4- to 11-year-old boys, parents identify 51 children with one or more disorders and teachers identify 95 children. Both sources agree on the presence of one or more disorders in only 9.6% (14 of 146) of the boys. The corresponding percentage for girls in this age group is 3.9%. In the 12- to 16-year-old age group, these percentages for boys and girls are 16.1% and 16.8%, respectively.

Correlates of Disorder

Table 2 displays the results of the logistic regression analyses of the strength of the association (odds ratio: OR) between selected correlates and individual psychiatric disorders based on parental data, for children 4 to 16. It should be noted that the identical comparison group was used in each of these analyses, that is, children without any parent-identified disorders. The logistic regression analyses permit the determination of the independent contribution of a correlate to the prediction of a disorder. In the model tested for each disorder, all nine correlates were forced in and testing was done for the following interactions: age by each of the correlates, and sex by each of the correlates. Only significant interactions ($p < 0.05$) appear in the table.

In the case of conduct disorder, family dysfunction has a strong, independent relationship to this disorder (OR = 7.2). Other main effects include parent arrested and age 12 to 16. There is one significant interaction involving sex of the child and parent treated for nerves. The relative strength of the association of boys compared to girls to conduct disorder is significantly higher in families where the parents have been treated for nerves than in families where this is not so (ORs = 6.1 and 1.0, respectively). For hyperactivity, there are two significant main effects, family dysfunction and failed a grade. The one significant interaction indicates that the relationship between chronic medical illness in the child and hyperactivity is significantly higher in the younger (OR = 8.1) than the older children (OR = 1.4).

In emotional disorder, there are three significant main effects: family dysfunction, parent treated for nerves, and chronic medical illness in the child. A significant interaction between age and income level was observed. The relationship between

TABLE 2
Relative Odds in Logistic Regression Analyses Between Selected Correlates and Individual Psychiatric Disorders, By Parent Informant, for Children Aged 4 to 16

	Disorder			
Correlate	Conduct	Hyper-activity	Emotional	Somatiza-tion[a]
Low income	2.2	1.7	[e]	1.5
Urban residence	0.8	1.8	1.2	1.4
Family dysfunc-tion	7.2[b]	4.5[b]	4.0[b]	6.5[b]
Parent treated for nerves	[c]	1.3	2.6[b]	[f]
Parent arrested	3.2[b]	0.7	1.5	1.6
Age 12–16	2.6[b]	[d]	[e]	–
Male	[c]	1.6	0.9	[f]
Failed a grade	1.6	2.4[b]	0.9	0.6
Chronic medical illness	3.2[b]	[d]	2.7[b]	3.9[b]

[a] 12 to 16-year-olds only.

[b] $p < 0.05$.

[c] Parent treated; male vs. female, 6.1. Parent not treated; male vs. female, 1.0. Interaction significant at $p < 0.05$.

[d] Age 12–16; illness vs. not, 1.4. Age 4–11; illness vs. not, 8.1. Interaction significant at $p < 0.05$.

[e] Age 12–16; low income vs. not, 0.5. Age 4–11; low income vs. not, 4.4. Interaction significant at $p < 0.05$.

[f] Males; parent treated vs. not, 5.5. Females; parent treated vs. not, 0.8. Interaction significant at $p < 0.05$.

low income and emotional disorder is higher in younger (OR = 4.4) than in older children (OR = 0.5). Lastly, in the case of somatization, family dysfunction and chronic medical illness have significant main effects. The one significant interaction involves sex and parent treated for nerves and somatization is higher for boys (OR = 5.5) than for girls (OR = 0.8).

Table 3 presents the results of the logistic regression analyses of the strength of the association between the selected correlates and individual psychiatric disorders identified either by teachers (for children aged 4 to 11) or by the youths themselves (for the 12- to 16-year-old age group). The analyses and the format for presenting the data are identical to those used in Table 2.

For conduct disorder, three correlates have significant independent effects in pre-

TABLE 3

Relative Odds in Logistic Regression Analyses Between Selected
Correlates and Individual Psychiatric Disorders by Teacher/Youth
Informant, for Children Aged 4 to 16

	Disorder			
Correlate	Conduct	Hyper-activity	Emotional	Somatiza-tion[a]
Low income	[c]	3.5^b	1.9	2.2
Urban residence	1.1	1.4	2.0^b	1.6
Family dysfunc-tion	2.9^b	2.3^b	2.6^b	3.2^b
Parent treated for nerves	1.3	1.3	1.6	[f]
Parent arrested	1.2	0.7	1.5	[g]
Age 12–16	[c]	0.6^b	[d]	–
Male	1.9^b	2.2^b	[d, e]	[f, g]
Failed a grade	1.9^b	1.4	[e]	1.2
Chronic medical illness	1.7	2.3^b	1.7	1.5

[a] 12–16-year-olds only.

[b] $p < 0.05$.

[c] Age 12–16; low income vs. not, 1.9. Age 4–11; low income vs. not, 9.9. Interaction significant at $p < 0.05$.

[d] Age 12–16; male vs. female, 0.3. Age 4–11; male vs. female, 1.5. Interaction significant at $p < 0.05$.

[e] Males; failed vs. not, 2.9. Females; failed vs. not, 0.6. Interaction significant at $p < 0.05$.

[f] Males; parent treated vs. not, 0.2. Females; parent treated vs. not, 1.6. Interaction significant at $p < 0.05$.

[g] Males; parent arrested vs. not, 10.1. Females; parent arrested vs. not 0.6. Interaction significant at $p < 0.05$.

dicting disorders: family dysfunction, male sex, and failed a grade. The one significant interaction indicates that the relationship between low income and teacher/ youth-identified conduct disorder is higher in younger compared to older children (ORs = 9.9 and 1.9, respectively).

In the case of hyperactivity, five correlates have an independent positive association with this disorder: low income, family dysfunction, male sex, and chronic medical illness. One other main effect has an independent association with disorder, namely, age 12 to 16 (OR = 0.6). No significant interactions are present. Two correlates, urban residence and family dysfunction, are related to emotional disorder. There are two significant interactions. The relationship between being male and emotional disorder varies by child age (OR = 1.5 at age 4 to 11 and OR = 0.3 at age 12 to 16). Also, the relationship between failed a grade and emotional disorder varies by child sex (OR = 2.9 among males and OR = 0.6 among females). Finally, in somatization, there is one main effect, family dysfunction. Again, there are two significant interactions. The relationship between parent treated for nerves and somatization varies by child sex (OR = 0.2 among boys and OR = 1.6 among girls). In addition, the association between parent arrested and somatization is higher among males (OR = 10.1) than it is among females (OR = 0.6).

Table 4 examines, using a logistic regression analysis, the strength of relationship between selected correlates and conduct disorder versus emotional disorder. Two correlates, urban/rural residence and chronic medical illness, were dropped because there was no indication from the literature that they would be differentially related to conduct disorder and emotional disorder. Further, the disorders used in this analysis were pure disorders, that is, when they occurred in a child, there was never any co-existing psychiatric disorder of the ones measured in the OCHS. This strat-

TABLE 4

Relative Odds in Logistic Regression Analyses Between Selected
Correlates and Conduct Disorder (Pure) versus Emotional Disorder
(Pure), for Children Aged 4 to 16

Correlate	Relative Odds
Low income	0.7
Family dysfunction	0.6
Parent treated for nerves	0.3[a]
Parent arrested	1.0
Age 12 to 16	[b]
Male	[b]
Failed a grade	2.9

[a] $p < 0.05$.

[b] Age 12–16; males vs. females, 33.5. Age 4–11; males vs. females, 3.5. Interaction significant at $p < 0.05$.

egy ensured that any differences found between the two disorders could not be due to one or more co-existing disorders. The results show that the only variable with a significant main effect in differentiating the two disorders is parent treated for nerves. The presence of this variable is associated with a reduced prevalence of conduct disorder compared to emotional disorder. There is one significant interaction involving age and sex. In the older age group, being a male is a stronger predictor of conduct disorder (compared to emotional disorder) than it is in the younger age group (ORs = 33.5 and 3.5, respectively).

DISCUSSION

A major finding is that the prevalence and correlates of disorder are different in important ways as a function of informant. For instance, the prevalences of teacher-identified conduct disorder and hyperactivity, in boys and girls, far exceed the rates of the parent-identified disorders in the 4- to 11-year-old age group. In emotional disorder, in this age group, however, the prevalence in girls is greater for parent-identified compared to teacher-identified cases; in boys, the prevalence rates are identical.

The patterns of correlates also show differences as a function of informant. For instance, while parent arrested is a significant correlate of parent-identified conduct disorder, it is not for the other (teacher or youth)-identified condition. In contrast, low income is strongly related to teacher-identified conduct disorder (4- to 11-age group) but not to parent-identified conduct disorder (across both age groups). It should be pointed out, however, that when age is involved in an interaction, as occurs with teacher- or youth-identified conduct disorder, the effects of age and informant are confounded. In the case in point, the relationship between low income and conduct disorder is reported to vary significantly as a function of age. To what extent this finding is due to age differences or informant differences is impossible to know from this study.

Another complicating factor is that in the case of parent-identified disorder, the informant for disorder is the same as the informant for the correlate identification. Thus, these two variables might be expected to be positively correlated because they both are describing negative aspects of the child and the family, and share the same informant. The fact that family dysfunction continues to have a significant relationship to individual disorders when the disorders are identified by other than the parent provides some evidence that unifying characteristics may exist among assessments provided by different informants. However, tempering this inference is the observation that the magnitude of the association between family dysfunction and disorder is much higher for those with parent-identified disorder than for those with disorder identified by other informants. Also, family dysfunction appears to be somewhat indiscriminate in its relationship with disorder. The ORs between family dysfunction and the different types of disorder are not much different in magnitude within informants.

The finding that, apart from symptomatology, there are few distinguishing characteristics in the correlate realm between conduct disorder and hyperactivity is in agreement with the literature (Werry et al., 1987). Werry and his colleagues found that anxiety disorder in children tended to have a specific relationship with parental anxiety. The finding in this study that the only variable showing a significant, independent, and specific relationship to emotional disorder compared to conduct disorder was parent treated for nerves provides support for this finding.

In summary, the analyses done here illustrate that case ascertainment depends heavily on who provides information for assessment. The lack of agreement between informants on the individuals who exhibit clinically important symptomatology is strong evidence that the identification of childhood disorder is much influenced by the perception of informants and the contexts in which assessments are done. This finding is in full agreement with a recent meta-analysis of child/adolescent behavioral and emotional problem ratings provided by different informants (Achenbach et al., 1987).

In addition to disagreements between informants on cases, the analyses here suggest that child features associated with disorder may also vary by informant. For example, low income, parent treated for nerves, parent arrested, and chronic medical illness show evidence of having a different relationship with disorder, depending on informant. If differences such as these stand up on further investigation, it would provide additional evidence that childhood disorder should be treated and studied as a contextual phenomenon and not a unitary attribute that is an essential component of the child's personality.

These findings have two important consequences for the way childhood psychiatric disorder is measured and studied. First, combining information from different informants to measure childhood disorder may be ill advised. If child features associated with disorder vary by informant, there is a risk of attenuating or masking these associations when informant assessments are combined. This would occur, for example, if economic disadvantage was associated strongly with teacher assessments of childhood externalizing problems and weakly associated with parent assessments of childhood externalizing problems, as in this study. In such instances, the method used to combine information from different informants could have important effects on inferences made about associated features of disorder. Invariably, these inferences would be biased to a greater or lesser extent by the rules developed for combining information. Second, the usefulness of information provided by informants in different contexts should be evaluated. The factors that influence respondent judgements about emotional and behavioral problems of children are poorly understood. It is known, for example, that parents and teachers identify different children as cases. The present data suggest, in addition, that there may be differences in the child characteristics that give rise to problem ratings given by different informants. However, the extent to which ratings provided by different informants are valid or useful against the usual criteria of etiology, prognosis and response to treatment is not known. Seeking to evaluate the usefulness of informant-identified childhood disorder may prove to be a more profitable line of inquiry than continuing to study childhood disorder without due attention to the informants and contexts from which assessment data arise.

REFERENCES

Achenbach, T. M. & Edelbrock, C. S. (1981), Behavioral problems and competencies reported by parents of normal and disturbed children aged four through sixteen. *Monogr. Soc. Res. Child Dev.*, 46(1) (Serial No. 188):1–78.

Achenbach, T. M., McConaughy, S. H., & Howell, C. T. (1987), Child/adolescent behavioral and emotional problems: implications of cross-informant correlations for situational specificity. *Psychol. Bull.*, 101:213–232.

Boyle, M. H., Offord, D. R., Hofmann, H. G., et al. (1987), Ontario Child Health Study: I. Methodology. *Arch. Gen. Psychiatry*, 44:826–831.

Byles, J., Byrne, C., Boyle, M. H., & Offord, D. R. (1988), Ontario Child Health Study: reliability and validity of the General Functioning subscale of the McMaster Family Assessment Device. *Fam. Process*, 27:97–104.

Offord, D. R., Boyle, M. H., Szatmari, P., et al. (1987), Ontario Child Health Study: II. Six-month prevalence of disorder and rates of service utilization. *Arch. Gen. Psychiatry*, 44:832–836.

Statistic Canada (1982), *Census Directory*, Ottawa, Canada: Minister of Supply and Services.

Werry, J. S., Reeves, J. C. & Elkind, G. S. (1987), Attention deficit, conduct, oppositional, and anxiety disorders in children: I. A review of research on differentiating characteristics. *J. Am. Acad. Child Adolesc. Psychiatry*, 26:133–143.

10

The UCLA-University of Utah Epidemiologic Survey of Autism: Recurrence Risk Estimates and Genetic Counseling

Edward R. Ritvo

UCLA School of Medicine, Los Angeles

Lynn B. Jorde

University of Utah, Salt Lake City

Anne Mason-Brothers and B.J. Freeman

UCLA School of Medicine, Los Angeles

Carmen Pingree

University of Utah, Salt Lake City

Marshall B. Jones

University of Pennsylvania, Hershey Medical School

William M. McMahon, P. Brent Petersen, and William R. Jenson

University of Utah, Salt Lake City

Amy Mo

UCLA School of Medicine, Los Angeles

The authors recently reported, in this journal, an epidemiological survey of autism in Utah. Twenty (9.7%) of the 207 families ascertained had more than one autistic child. Analyses of these data revealed that autism is 215 times more frequent among the siblings of autistic patients

Reprinted with permission from *American Journal of Psychiatry,* 1989, Vol. 146, No. 8, 1032–1036. Copyright © 1989 by the American Psychiatric Association.

Supported by the Dresher, Bennin, Kunin, Miano, and Gergans family funds at UCLA; and by the George S. and Dolores Doré Eccles Foundation, the Herbert I. and Elsa B. Michael Foundation, the Marriner S. Eccles Foundation, and the Castle Foundation in Salt Lake City, Utah.

than in the general population. The overall recurrence risk estimate (the chance that each sibling born after an autistic child will develop autism) is 8.6%. If the first autistic child is a male the recurrence risk estimate is 7%, and if a female 14.5%. These new recurrence risk estimates should be made available to all individuals who have autistic children and are interested in family planning.

A consensus has been reached over the past two decades by investigators throughout the world concerning autism (1, 2). It is now recognized as a specific behaviorally defined syndrome that produces irregularities in development and characteristic disturbances in relatedness, language, and responses to sensory stimuli (3). Symptoms are usually manifested before 30 months of age and are expressive of CNS dysfunction rather than psychological trauma, as was formerly thought. Most likely, more than one etiological factor and pathological process will be found that can produce the syndrome. In two-thirds of the patients, brain dysfunction is so extensive that they score in the mentally retarded ranges on standard IQ scales (4). The vast majority of patients require lifelong supervision and social support. However, mild cases occur, and some of these patients can live independently, marry, and become parents (5).

While no specific pathognomonic signs or CNS pathology is known, biomedical findings have been reported that characterize subgroups of patients. These findings include hyperserotonemia (6); decreased b-wave amplitude in the electroretinogram (7); decreased post-rotatory nystagmus (8); decreased cerebellar Purkinje cells at autopsy (9); nonspecific abnormal EEGs, MRIs, CT scans, pneumoencephalograms, and autopsy findings (3, 10); and possible cerebellar abnormalities as seen on MRI (11, 12). Autism is also known to occur in association with other diseases (2, 3).

Prior epidemiologic surveys estimated the prevalence of autism to be between 2 and 21 per 10,000 in the general population and the sibling risk to be 2% (10). Although these surveys were based on relatively small populations and used different ascertainment techniques, diagnostic criteria, and methods, the latter figure is widely quoted and cited in *DSM-III*. It indicates that siblings of autistic children have a 50-fold higher risk of autism than the general population. While risks are most often based on the total number of siblings of an affected individual, it is also useful to estimate the recurrence risk, which is based only on the siblings born after the first affected individual in each sibship. This compensates for those couples who limit reproduction after the birth of an affected child (13) (a phenomenon called stoppage). For comparability with previous studies, we report a sibling risk that is based on the total number of siblings of autistic subjects. In addition, we report recurrence risks that are based on the siblings born after the first autistic subject in each sibship. To our knowledge, recurrence risks estimated in the latter fashion have not previously been reported for autism. In only one survey to date have the siblings of autistic probands been given psychiatric examinations. Baird and August (14) diagnosed as autistic three (5.9%) of 51 siblings of 29 probands; they did not evaluate the parents.

In order to provide a more accurate and comprehensive database to explore these and related issues, we conducted an epidemiologic survey of autism in the state of Utah. On the basis of the survey, the best estimate for the prevalence of autism is 4 per 10,000 in the general population, and the sex ratio is 4 males to 1 female (15).

In this report we present the data on multiple-incidence families from the survey and recurrence risk estimates. These findings provide new guidelines for genetic counseling of families with autistic children. The overall recurrence risk for autism is 8.6%, and it varies with the sex of the firstborn autistic child—7.0% if a male and 14.5% if a female. The sibling risk for autism is 4.5%.

METHOD

Our recent epidemiologic survey of autism in the state of Utah (15) employed a four-level ascertainment system, *DSM-III* criteria, and a team of highly experienced clinicians who conducted blind diagnostic evaluations throughout the state. A total of 489 possibly autistic individuals born between 1960 and 1984 and living in Utah during the survey (1984–1988) were ascertained, and 241 were diagnosed as autistic. They came from 187 single-incidence families and 20 multiple-incidence families. The latter contained a total of 46 autistic siblings. Genetic research shows no excess of inbreeding or consanguinity in Utah, and the gene pool is fully representative of North American and European Caucasian populations (16, 17).

For the purposes of this study we defined sibling risk as the number of autistic siblings of the firstborn autistic child divided by the total number of siblings of the firstborn autistic child or, stated differently, the percentage of all the firstborn autistic child's siblings who are themselves autistic. Recurrence risk was determined by the later sibling method (13). This is the number of autistic siblings born after the first autistic child divided by the total number of siblings born after the first autistic child. In multiple-incidence families it is the number of autistic siblings born after the second autistic sibling divided by all siblings born after the second autistic sibling.

RESULTS

Figure 1 shows the birth order and IQ scores of first-degree relatives in the 20 multiple-incidence families identified in the survey.

Because 70% of the population of Utah identify themselves as practicing the Mormon religion, separate analyses were conducted to determine if this factor influ-

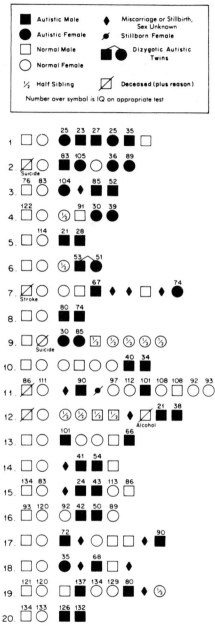

Figure 1. Birth Order and IQs of Autistic Probands and Their Siblings in 20 Families With Multiple Incidences of Autism in Utah Survey. The first two symbols on the left of each family represent the parents.

enced the distribution and prevalence of autism. No influence was found except for larger family size, which is common for members of this religion (18). Table 1 shows family sizes and sex ratios among Mormons and non-Mormons. The mean number of siblings per family was greatest when both parents were Mormon (4.31 siblings), less when only one parents was (3.0 siblings), and smallest when neither parent was (2.51 siblings). The male to female sex ratio of nonautistic siblings was approximately equal in Mormon (0.96) and non-Mormon (0.91) families. The autistic male to female sex ratio was lower in Mormon (3.18, 23.9% female) than non-Mormon (4.33, 18.8% female) families, but this difference was not significant ($\chi^2 = 0.55$, df = 1, p>0.10).

Table 2 shows the distribution of family sizes, sex ratios, and IQ scores in the single-incidence and multiple-incidence groups. The mean number of siblings was approximately equal in both single-incidence and multiple-incidence families (3.79 versus 3.90 siblings). The sex ratio of the nonautistic siblings was also approximately equal in both groups (0.96 for single-incidence and 0.88 for multiple-incidence families). The sex ratio of autistic siblings was lower in the multiple-incidence group than in the single-incidence group (2.54, 28.3% female versus 4.19, 19.3% female). Unfortunately, there were too few females (N = 13) in

TABLE 1
Family Sizes and Sex Ratios in Mormon and Non-Mormon
Families in Utah Survey

Item	All Families	Both Parents Mormons	One Parent Mormon	Non-Mormons
Family factors				
Siblings	787	620	54	113
Nonautistic	554	453	36	65
Autistic	233	167	18	48
Families	207	144	18	45
Siblings per family	3.80	4.31	3.00	2.51
Sex of siblings				
Nonautistic siblings				
Male	271	222	18	31
Female	283	231	18	34
Sex ratio	0.96	0.96	1.0	0.91
Autistic siblings				
Male	184	127	18	39
Female	49	40	0	9
Sex ratio	3.76	3.18	—	4.33

the multiple-incidence group to permit clinically meaningful statistical analyses of these data. However, the intergroup difference in sex ratio of autistic siblings warrants further study when larger populations are available.

The birth order of autistic children was determined separately for sibships of size 2 and for sibships of size 3 or more (see Table 3). In sibships of size 2 there was a significant tendency for autistic children to be first-born in Mormon families, non-Mormon families, and in all the families combined. In informative sibships of size 3 or larger there was a nonsignificant tendency in the non-Mormon families for autistic children to be born later but no such tendency in the Mormon families.

Table 4 shows the proportion of multiple-incidence families and recurrence risk

TABLE 2
Family Sizes, Sex Ratios, and IQs in Families With Single and
Multiple Incidences of Autism in Utah Survey

Item	All Families	Single-Incidence Families	Multiple-Incidence Families
Family factors			
Siblings	787	709	78
Nonautistic	554	522	32
Autistic	233	187	46
Families	207	187	20
Siblings per family	3.80	3.79	3.90
Sex of siblings			
Nonautistic siblings			
Male	271	256	15
Female	283	266	17
Sex ratio	0.96	0.96	0.88
Autistic siblings			
Male	184	151	33
Female	49	36	13
Sex ratio	3.76	4.19	2.54
IQ and sex of siblings			
>70			
Male	67	54	13
Female	10	5	5
Sex ratio	6.70	10.80	2.60
50–69			
Male	46	39	7
Female	12	11	1
Sex ratio	3.83	3.55	7.0
<50			
Male	69	56	13
Female	26	19	7
Sex ratio	2.65	2.95	1.86

TABLE 3
Birth Order of Autistic Children in Informative Sibships of Size 2 and
Size 3 or More in Utah Survey

Item	All Families				Mormon Families				Non-Mormon Families				Families With One Mormon Parent			
	N	%	p	Z	N	%	p	Z	N	%	p	Z	N	%	p	Z
Two-child sibships	28	—	—	—	15	—	—	—	8	—	—	—	5	—	—	—
Firstborn	22	79	<0.001[a]	—	11	73	0.06[a]	—	7	88	0.04[a]	—	4	80	0.19[a]	—
Secondborn	6	21	—	—	4	27	—	—	1	12	—	—	1	20	—	—
Sibships of three or more	153	—	>0.27[b]	0.60	121	—	>0.49[b]	0.01	22	—	>0.18[b]	0.88	10	—	>0.18[b]	0.89

[a]Binomial probability test.
[b]One-tailed, partial Mann-Whitney U test.

TABLE 4

Recurrence Risk Estimates[a] of Autism in Families in Utah Survey (Later Sibling Method)

Family Category	Total Families	Proportion of Multiple-Incidence Families			Recurrence Risk			
		Multiple-Incidence Families		95% Confidence Limits	All Siblings Born After Proband	Autistic Siblings Born After Proband	Recurrence Risk Estimate	95% Confidence Limits
		N	%					
All	207	20	9.7	6.0–14.5	302	26	8.6	5.8–12.2
With male firstborn autistic child	166	15	9.0	5.2–14.4	236.5[b]	16.5	7.0	4.3–11.2
With female firstborn autistic child	41	5	12.2	2.2–22.2	65.5[b]	9.5	14.5	6.7–24.7
Multiple-incidence families	—	—	—	—	17[c]	6	35.3	12.6–58.0

[a]Estimates based on 241 diagnosed autistic children less eight (two with fragile X chromosome, five adopted, and one with no family information), yielding 233 autistic children from 207 families; 233 total autistic children less 46 from multiple-incidence families yields 187 autistic probands from single-incidence families, plus 20 multiple-incidence families yields a total of 207 families.
[b]Includes firstborn concordant twin autistic child, who is counted as one-half.
[c]Seventeen siblings born after the second autistic child.

estimates. The overall recurrence risk was 8.6%; it indicates that siblings born after one autistic child were 215 times more likely to have autism than siblings of nonautistic children (the rate in the general population is 4 per 10,000). The sibling risk was 4.5% (95% confidence limits = 2.8%–6.2%). The 95% confidence limits for recurrence risk and sibling risk indicate that the two do not differ significantly.

The recurrence risk in the informative multiple-incidence families was 35.3%, which indicates that siblings born after two autistic children are 883 times more likely to have autism than are siblings of nonautistic children. This is an approximate figure, since it is based on only eight informative families in which 17 siblings were born after the second autistic child (Figure 1, families 1–3, 11, 14–16, 18). Furthermore, it could be higher because it is possible that six fathers (Figure 1, families 1, 3, 7, 11, 13, 19) may be autistic adults (5).

Recurrence risks were also determined for families in which the firstborn autistic child was a male and in which it was a female. This was done to assess the hypothesis that families with firstborn autistic females are more likely to have a proposed familial form of autism, an assumption we have previously discussed and employed to divide data for analyses, e.g., a threshold polygenic model in which the female threshold is higher than that of the males (19–21). The results indicate that families in which the firstborn is an autistic female have a nonsignificant higher recurrence risk (14.5% versus 7.0%, $\chi^2 = 2.8$, df = 1, p>0.10).

DISCUSSION

The overall recurrence risk of 8.6% indicates that autism is 215 times more frequent among siblings born after an autistic child than in the general population and has great clinical significance and implications for genetic counseling. It is consistent with data from our prior studies of twins (20) and multiple-incidence families (21) which indicate that there may be a subtype of autism that is genetically influenced. In addition, we found by assessing parents as well as siblings of probands in our Utah population that autism does not aggregate in families with cognitive processing pathology (22). This lends support to the corollary hypothesis that there may be genetic influences unique to autism, rather than to the notion that autism is on the extreme end of a continuum of inherited cognitive processing pathology, as has been suggested by Bartak et al. (23).

The findings on birth order show a significant trend in sibships of size 2 for the autistic child to be firstborn but no such relationship in larger sibships. This is consistent with a recently published reanalysis by one of us (M.B.J.) (13) of our earlier data derived from a nationally solicited survey of multiple-incidence families (21). That reanalysis demonstrated that families with autism tend to stop having children after the birth of an affected child, providing that child is not the firstborn. This phenomenon, referred to as stoppage, must be accounted for when determining recurrence risks and when testing models of inheritance, as we have previously discussed (20, 21).

Comparing our results to those of prior studies reveals interesting differences. While the sibling risk cited in *DSM-III* is 2%, we found it to be 4.5%. This difference may reflect our having conducted the most extensive survey to date and our having selected a large population ideally suited for epidemiological research. The recurrence risk of 8.6% is larger still. The later sibling method factors out possible effects of stoppage, which, although slight in our study, have been shown to operate in families of autistic children (13).

At this time the combined evidence for a genetically influenced type or types of autism does not precisely fit a specific mode of Mendelian inheritance. Data from previous studies (20, 21) (see references 2, 3, and 10 for review) suggest that autosomal inheritance is a possibility for one subtype. Even granting this assumption, however, we are still left with the question of what proportion of autistic patients has the proposed genetic type. As with any disease, patients with autism too mild to be diagnosed or too severe to survive or to be diagnosed cannot be identified, thus making estimates for determining possible genetic modes of transmission from clinical data alone quite imprecise. Only when the autistic phenotype or genotype can be specified with biomedical markers will we be better able to determine prevalence, recurrence risks, and modes of genetic transmission (24).

On the basis of the data presented in this report, we are counseling parents of our autistic patients that if they have another child, there is an overall 8.6% chance of having another autistic child (7% if they already have an autistic boy, 14.5% if they already have an autistic girl, and 35% if they already have two autistic children). We present this information as being preliminary and take pains to carefully explain the limited data upon which our estimates are based.

REFERENCES

1. Volkmar FR, Cohen DJ: Neurobiologic aspects of autism (editorial). N Engl J Med 1988; 318:1390–1392
2. Ritvo ER, Freeman BJ: A medical model of autism: etiology, pathology and treatment. Pediatr Ann 1984; 13:298–305
3. Coleman M, Gillberg C: The Biology of the Autistic Syndromes. New York, Praeger, 1985
4. Freeman BJ, Ritvo ER, Needleman R, et al: The stability of cognitive and linguistic parameters in autism: a five-year prospective study. J Am Acad Child Psychiatry 1985; 24:459–464
5. Ritvo ER, Brothers AM, Freeman BJ, et al: Eleven possibly autistic parents (letter). J Autism Dev Disord 1988; 18:139–143

6. Yuwiler A, Geller E, Ritvo E: Biochemical studies on autism, in Handbook for Neurobiochemistry, vol 10. Edited by Lajtha A. New York, Plenum, 1985

7. Ritvo ER, Creel D, Realmuto G, et al: Electroretinograms in autism: a pilot study of b-wave amplitudes. Am J Psychiatry 1988; 145:229–232

8. Ritvo ER, Ornitz EM, Eviatar A, et al: Decreased postrotatory nystagmus in early infantile autism. Neurology 1969; 19:653–658

9. Ritvo ER, Freeman BJ, Scheibel AB, et al: Lower Purkinje cell counts in the cerebella of four autistic subjects: initial findings of the UCLA-NSAC autopsy research report. Am J Psychiatry 1986; 143:862–866

10. Ornitz EM: Autism, in Handbook of Child Psychiatric Diagnosis. Edited by Last CG, Hersen M. New York, John Wiley & Sons (in press)

11. Courchesne E, Yeung-Courchesne R, Press GA, et al: Hypoplasia of cerebellar vermal lobules VI and VII in autism. N Engl J Med 1988; 318:1349–1354

12. Ritvo ER, Garber HJ: Cerebellar hypoplasia and autism (letter). N Engl J Med 1988; 319:1152

13. Jones MB, Szatmari P: Stoppage rules and genetic studies of autism. J Autism Dev Disord 1988; 18:31–41

14. Baird TD, August GJ: Familial heterogeneity in infantile autism. J Autism Dev Disord 1985; 15:315–321

15. Ritvo ER, Freeman BJ, Pingree C, et al: The UCLA-University of Utah epidemiologic survey of autism: prevalence. Am J Psychiatry 1989; 146:194–199

16. Woolf CM, Stephens FE, Mulaik DD, et al: An investigation of the frequency of consanguineous marriages among the Mormons and their relatives in the United States. Am J Hum Genet 1956; 8:236–252

17. McLellan T, Jorde LB, Skolnick MH: Genetic distances between the Utah Mormons and related populations. Am J Hum Genet 1984; 36:836–857

18. Martin TK, Heaton TB, Bahr SJ (eds): Utah in Demographic Perspective. Salt Lake City, Signature Books, 1986

19. Carter CO: Genetics of common single malformations. Br Med Bull 1976; 32:21–26

20. Ritvo ER, Freeman BJ, Mason-Brothers A, et al: Concordance for the syndrome of autism in 40 pairs of afflicted twins. Am J Psychiatry 1985; 142:74–77

21. Ritvo ER, Spence MA, Freeman BJ, et al: Evidence for autosomal recessive inheritance in 46 families with multiple incidences of autism. Am J Psychiatry 1985; 142:187–192

22. Freeman BJ, Ritvo ER, Mason-Brothers A, et al: Psychometric assessment of first-degree relatives of 62 autistic probands in Utah. Am J Psychiatry 1989; 146:361–364

23. Bartak L, Rutter M, Cox A: A comparative study of infantile autism and specific developmental language disorders, I: the children. Br J Psychiatry 1975; 126:127–145

24. Ritvo ER, Mason-Brothers A, Menkes JH, et al: Association of autism, retinoblastoma, and reduced esterase D activity (letter). Arch Gen Psychiatry 1988; 45:600

Part III

FAMILY ISSUES

The impact on families and children is what links the issues addressed by the papers in this section: divorce, sibling relationships, working mothers, physical handicap, and incest. In the first paper, Hetherington provides an overview of a longitudional study of the effects of divorce and remarriage on children's adjustment, which she and her collegues have conducted over the past seven years. The great strength of this investigation lies in its methodology.

Recognizing that the assessment of the long-term effects of divorce is made difficult by the fact that there are significant variables involved—the ages of children at the time of initial separation and the sequences of family reorganizations and family experiences following divorce—Hetherington selected a research strategy designed to curtail confounding by these variables by means of careful sample selection. The study was composed of 144 middle-class white parents and their children; half of the children were from divorced, mother-custody families and the other half from nondivorced families. Boys and girls were equally represented in each group. A target child who was four years of age at the beginning of the study and his or her parents were studied at two months, one year, two years and six years following divorce. At the time of the six-year follow-up, the groups were expanded to include 30 sons and 30 daughters in each of three groups—a remarried mother/stepfather group; a nonremarried mother/stepfather group; and a nondivorced group. Although the generalizability of the findings to other ages and other patterns of family reorganization is limited within these carefully defined parameters, the findings are clear and unequivocal.

Individual characteristics, such as children's temperament, family relations, and extrafamilial factors, played an important role in exacerbating or buffering children from negative consequences associated with their parent's marital transitions. Although boys in divorced families and children of both sexes in remarried families showed more problems in adjustment than did children in nondivorced families, some also showed remarkable resiliency. Hetherington answers the question of the enduring effects of divorce and remarriage on children by indicating that she has revised her original view of divorce as inevitably pathogenic. Rather, depending upon the characteristics of the child, available resources, subsequent life experiences, and especially interpersonal relationships, children may be "survivors, losers, or winners of their parents' divorce or remarriage."

The second paper in this section addresses a relatively neglected research area. Although differences among characteristics of siblings relationships are familiar, the

217

correlates of these differences have been less well studied. Stocker, Dunn, and Plomin address this gap in an investigation of the extent to which maternal behavior, children's temperament, age, and family structure are associated with dimensions of sibling relationships in a sample of 96 intact Caucasian families with younger siblings aged three to six years and older siblings aged five to 10 years. During home visits, mothers were interviewed and observed interacting with their children in both structured and unstructured settings. Sibling relationships were rated along dimensions of conflict, cooperation, control, and competition, whereas mothers' behavior was conceptualized as reflecting control-intrusiveness, affection, attention, and responsiveness. The pattern of findings is rich and complex. Both maternal behavior, differences in mothers' behavior to their two children, and child temperament, as well as the age of the younger sibling, added independently to the prediction of sibling relationships.

Although the authors caution against generalizing the results to relationships among siblings of different ages living in other types of families, the findings highlight the importance of taking into account children's individual characteristics when assessing their dyadic relationships, as well as the nature of their relationships with other family members.

In the third paper in this section, the focus of inquiry shifts to that of working mothers and their families. The paper by Scarr, Phillips, and McCartney reviews the literature on the effects of mothers' employment on marital relations, on the development of their children, and on mothers themselves. It can be seen as a reprise of the section on maternal employment outside the home, which appeared in the 1985 Annual Progress. In introducing that section, we characterized the idea that the mother who works outside the home is necessarily doing harm to her youngsters even if they are provided with adequate substitute care as a "sacred cow" continuing to persist, despite overwhelming research evidence to the contrary. Much the same conclusion is reached by Scarr and her collegues five years later.

During this interval no new evidence has appeared to show that maternal employment per se is a major issue in either marital relations or child development. Rather, the circumstance of the family, the attitudes and expectations of fathers and mothers, and the distribution of time available have significant impact. Fears about child care are not based on scientifically demonstrated facts but instead on socially determined theories about mothers' roles and obligations to their families. Working mothers are here to stay. More and more women are entering the work force when their children are very young. In discussing the needs of working parents and their families, Scarr et al. point out that the combined responsibilities of motherhood and paid employment are an enormous burden that needs to be shared more equitably by fathers and by society as a whole, and they present a set of recommendations directed toward accomplishing this end.

The next study in this section is a report of an investigation that extends the search for risk and protective factors contributing to adaptation into the area of physical handicap. Varni, Rubenfeld, Talbot, and Setoguchi examine the contribution of both family function and temperament to the psychologic adjustment of children with visible physical deformities. The results indicate that better psychologic and social adjustment is associated with both less family conflict and less emotional temperaments. Moreover, the interaction between temperamental emotionality and family cohesion significantly predicts both internalizing and externalizing behavior problems. The findings are consistent with those of other investigations that have sought to identify factors contributing to successful coping in the face of a wide range of stressors. However, as the authors point out, family and temperamental factors accounted for less that half the variance in psychologic and social adjustment. Although the findings of this study can provide guidance for interventions designed to attempt to enhance the psychologic and social adaptation of children with limb deformaties, the search for additional risk and protective factors needs to continue.

The final report in this section by Everson, Hunter, Runyon, and Edelsohn on maternal support following disclosure of incest adds to the growing body of literature on the sexual abuse of children. Specifically, these workers have sought to identify factors contributing to the degree of support offered by mothers to their sexually abused children. A limited data base has been maximally exploited through the application of sophisticated statistical techniques. The findings parallel the results of other studies in identifying substantial variability in how mothers respond to reports of incest within their families. Less than one-half of 84 mothers were classified as consistently supportive of their children, and one quarter consistently sided with their male partners.

A very thoughtful discussion examines the consequences of lack of maternal support for victims of incest, including increased likelihood of being required to testify in court and being placed in foster care. The authors suggest that professional bias in the form of holding a victim's mother as responsible as the perpetrator-father may contribute to the mother's increased alienation from her child. A disclosure of incest is a crisis for child and family. However, child protective service workers and mental health, legal, and medical professionals exercise some control over subsequent events. The authors urge less emphasis on the mother's contribution to the occurrence of incest and more emphasis on her contribution to her child's recovery.

11

Coping with Family Transitions: Winners, Losers, and Survivors

E. Mavis Hetherington
University of Virginia, Charlottesville

This article presents the results of a longitudinal study of the effects of divorce and remarriage on children's adjustment. It was found that individual characteristics, such as children's temperament, family relations, and extrafamilial factors, played an important role in exacerbating or buffering children from negative consequences associated with their parents' marital transitions. Although boys in divorced families and children in remarried families showed more problems in adjustment than did children in nondivorced families, some also showed remarkable resiliency in the face of multiple life stressors.

One of the things that is notable in studies of family transitions is the great diversity in the response of parents and children to divorce and remarriage. Most family members undergo an initial period of emotional distress and disrupted functioning following divorce but recover within a 2–3-year period if the divorce is not compounded by continued stress and adversity. Some parents and children show intense and enduring deleterious outcomes. Others show delayed effects, appearing to adapt well in the early stages of family reorganization but having problems or developmental disruptions that emerge at a later time. Finally, a substantial minority of adults and children are able to cope constructively with the challenges of divorce and remarriage and emerge as psychologically enhanced and exceptionally competent and fulfilled individuals. In this article I will examine some of the long-term outcomes of divorce and remarriage as well as the factors that contribute to children being survivors, winners, or losers following these family transitions.

This paper was presented as the Presidential Address at the Meetings of the Society for Research in Child Development, April 1987, in Baltimore.

One difficulty in attempting to assess the long-term effects of divorce on parents and children and the factors that may mediate these outcomes is that sequences of family reorganizations and family experiences following divorce vary widely, and the timing of these events may be critical in predicting the long-term adjustment of family members. For most parents and children, divorce is only one in a series of family transitions that follow separation. Life in a single-parent household following divorce is usually a temporary condition since 80% of men and 75% of women will remarry. About 25% of children will spend some time in a stepparent family before they are young adults. Moreover, since the divorce rate is higher in subsequent marriages than in first marriages, some parents and children encounter a series of divorces, periods in a one-parent household, and remarriages.

VULNERABILITY AND PROTECTIVE FACTORS

Garmezy (1983) and Rutter (1983) have underscored the importance of vulnerability and protective factors that modulate responses to stress. Rutter (1983) has advanced a chemical analogy, saying that these factors are largely inert on their own but serve as catalysts in combination with stressful events. When such variables increase the effect of stressors they may be viewed as vulnerability factors; when they diminish the effects of stressors they an be seen as protective factors. After reviewing the literature on the stressors of childhood, Garmezy (1983) concluded that a triad of protective factors repeatedly emerges. The first of these are positive personality dispositions, the second a supportive family milieu, and the third external societal agencies that function as support systems for reinforcing and strengthening children's coping efforts. The effects of this triad of protective factors are not automatic, for as Rutter (1987) has emphasized, protection does not lie in the availability of potentially supportive resources but in the use made of them. As we will see, some children are less able or willing than others to seek out or use available resources when coping with the marital transitions of their parents.

Different protective or vulnerability factors may shape the adaptation of individuals to different family transitions at different times. In addition, adaptation to family transitions may depend on the experiences that have preceded these changes. For example, it should be kept in mind that, in remarriage, the challenge for the child is coping with changes trigged by the addition rather than the loss of a family member as it was in divorce. Moreover, remarriage follows a period of time in a one-parent household. The response to divorce will be influenced by predivorce family relationships, and adjustment and roles and relations in the one-parent household will shape the child's subsequent response to the addition of a stepparent. It seems reasonable to assume that as the salient vulnerability and protective factors shift in different phases following a marital transition, some discontinuities in the coping and adjustment of individuals in response to these family reorganizations will occur.

THE VIRGINIA LONGITUDINAL STUDY OF DIVORCE AND REMARRIAGE

In order to examine vulnerability and protective factors that contribute to children's long-term adjustment to divorce and remarriage, I am going to discuss a 6-year follow-up of a longitudinal study of divorce and remarriage that I began in collaboration with Martha and Roger Cox (Hetherington, Cox, & Cox, 1982). The sample in the original study was composed of 144 well-educated, middle-class white parents and their children. Half of the children were from divorced, mother-custody families, and the other half were from nondivorced families. Within each group, half were boys and half were girls. A target child who was 4 years of age at the beginning of the study and his or her parents were studied at 2 months, 1 year, 2 years, and 6 years following divorce.

In the 6-year follow-up, the subjects were residential parents and their children in 124 of the original 144 families who were available and willing to continue to participate in the study. A new group of families matched on demographic characteristics with the original sample was added in order to expand the size of the groups to 30 sons and 30 daughters in each of three groups—a remarried mother/stepfather group; a nonremarried, mother-custody group; and a nondivorced group—a total of 180 families. For some analyses, the remarried group was broken down into those who were remarried less than 2 years and those remarried longer than 2 years. The cross-sectional analyses of families 6 years after divorce for the most part were based on the expanded sample, the longitudinal analyses on the original sample.

ADJUSTMENT IN THE 2 YEARS FOLLOWING DIVORCE

During the first 2 years following divorce, most children and many parents experienced emotional distress; psychological, health, and behavior problems; disruptions in family functioning; and problems in adjusting to new roles, relationships, and life changes associated with the altered family situation. However, as is reported in other studies, by 2 years following divorce, the majority of parents and children were adapting reasonably well and certainly were showing great improvement since the time of the divorce. Some continuing problems were found in the adjustment of boys and in relationships between divorced custodial mothers and their sons. Boys from divorced families, in comparison to boys in nondivorced families, showed more antisocial, acting-out, coercive, noncompliant behaviors in the home and in the school and exhibited difficulties in peer relationships and school achievement. In contrast, girls from divorced families in which remarriages had not occurred were functioning well and had positive relationships with their custodial mothers.

In considering these results, two things must be kept in mind. First, this study involves only mother-custody families, and there is evidence that children adjust better in the custody of a parent of the same sex (Camara & Resnick, 1988; Santrock &

Warshak, 1986; Zill, 1988). Second, age of the child may be an important factor in sex differences in children's responses to divorce and remarriage. The children were 4 years of age at the beginning of this study, on the average, 6 at the 2-year assessment, and 10 at the time of the 6-year assessment. Reports of more severe and long-lasting disruption of behavior in boys than girls following their parents' divorce have tended to come from studies of preadolescent children. Our children however, were just entering adolescence at the time of the 6-year follow-up, and this is a time when behavior problems in girls and conflicts in the interactions between daughters and mothers in divorced mother-custody families may emerge (Hetherington, 1972; Wallerstein, Corbin, & Lewis, 1988).

The 6-year follow-up had not been planned as part of the original study. We initiated the 6-year follow-up because we were concerned that at 2 years after divorce we had not followed these families long enough to see a restabilizing in the mother-son relationship and a final readjustment of the sons. Moreover, it was apparent that the effects of divorce alone could not be considered in appraising the long-term adjustment of the children since remarriages were presenting new adaptive challenges to many of our parents and children. Let us turn now to the triad of individual, familial, and extrafamilial factors that protect the child or that put the child at risk for long-term adverse consequences following marital transitions.[1]

TEMPERAMENT AND PERSONALITY

Although many individual characteristics protected children or made them vulnerable to long-term adverse effects following their parents' marital transitions, I will focus only on the child's temperament. Temperament will be used to illustrate the complexity of interactions of such individual characteristics with risk and protective factors in determining long-term adjustment. However, it should be noted that other individual characteristics, such as intelligence, age, and sex, were important, with more intelligent children being more resilient, older children being more affected than younger children by extrafamilial factors, and younger children coping more readily than late preadolescent or early adolescent children with their parent's remarriage. Finally, marked sex differences were found in response to divorce and remarriage: boys were more adversely affected than girls by divorce and life in a mother-custody one-parent household, and girls had more long-term difficulty than boys in adjusting to the introduction of a stepfather (Hetherington, Cox, & Cox, 1985).

Temperamentally difficult children have been found to be less adaptable to change and more vulnerable to adversity than are temperamentally easy children. However,

---

[1]For more details and data on individual differences and family relationships in this 6-year follow-up study, see Hetherington, 1987, 1988, in press.

the research literature on the relation between early temperament and later adjustment is confused and inconsistent, and the discussion about to ensue is a good example of the complexities involved.

One of the problems in this area is that much of the work on infant temperament relies on parents' reports—often retrospective ones. In this study, retrospective parental ratings of children's temperament as infants and current parent and observer ratings of temperament were available at each of four times. However, in assessing the role of children's temperament in their adaptation to divorce, it seemed desirable to obtain a measure of temperament before the divorce had occurred and one that might be less biased than parental ratings. We were fortunate in being able to have temperament ratings made by nurses based on pediatric records of well-baby visits during the first 2 years of life on a large subset of our sample. These included ratings of irritability, soothability, fearfulness, activity, sociability, and irregularity or difficulty in basic biological functions such as sleep, feeding, and elimination. The nurses' ratings of infant temperament better predicted later child behaviors than did mothers' ratings of infant temperament, and the mothers' ratings of infant temperament better predicted their own later behavior toward the child, although they also were significantly but modestly correlated with the child's behavior. Nurses' ratings of infant temperament in the first 6 months of life did not predict later behavior; therefore, only ratings in the 6-month to 2-year period were included. Fathers' ratings of early infant temperament did not seem to be related to anything.

Although individual differences in temperament may be biologically based, Rutter (1987) has noted that the increased risk of the temperamentally difficult child is, in part, attributable to transactions with the parent. He proposes that the difficult child is more likely to be both the elicitor and the target of aversive responses by the parent, while in times of stress the temperamentally easy child is not only less likely to be the recipient of criticism and displaced anger and anxiety but also is more able to cope with adversity when it hits. We found some support for this position in our 6-year follow-up data, but these interactions were modified by the personality problems of the parent (a composite index of depression, irritability, and anxiety), parental stress (a composite index of negative stressful life events occurring in the last year and daily hassles recorded six times in the past month), and parental support systems. Under conditions of a stable maternal personality and low stress there were no differences in the conditional probabilities of mothers responding more negatively to difficult, as compared with easy children, although difficult children emitted more aversive behavior. Thus, unless temperamental difficulty was compounded by other risk factors, there was no difference in the conditional probability of aversive maternal responses. However, the presence of either personality problems in the mother or high levels of stress increased the probability of negative behaviors in mothers. Furthermore the co-occurrence of these risk factors significantly increased maternal aversive responses over the level found with either stress or personality problems alone. These effects occurred more often with temperamentally difficult children, with sons, and with divorced nonremarried mothers.

These effects were moderated in a somewhat unexpected way by the availability of social supports. Under conditions of low stress and few maternal personality problems, the availability of supports had no effect on the aversive behaviors of mothers in dealing with either easy or difficult children. Surprisingly, the availability of supports also had no effects in situations involving a combination of maternal personality problems, high stress, and a difficult child. Apparently, then, there were not enough deleterious factors under low stress conditions to need support. Under high stress conditions, however, the compounding of deleterious factors was so great that it overwhelmed the effects of these resources. Furthermore, the data suggest that, even when supports were available, multiply stressed mothers did not use them effectively. Supportive resources had their greatest effect in moderating maternal responses toward difficult children when only maternal personality problems or only life stresses were present.

The effects of personality problems and/or stress in the responses of fathers and stepfathers to difficult and easy children were similar to the pattern found in mothers. However, fathers who had been remarried longer than 2 years, in contrast to those remarried for a shorter time and to nondivorced fathers, were more likely to target girls than boys with aversive responses. Fathers were also not able to use extrafamilial supports to moderate their aversive responses when they were under duress. This inability of fathers in contrast to mothers to solicit or utilize emotional support from friends and family was frequently found. For many men their wives were the only persons to whom they would disclose their feelings or turn for solace. When there was an alienated or discordant marriage, or a divorce, their one source of support was gone. Mothers, on the other hand, sought emotional support and confided in a wide network of friends and family. We found similar sex differences in the ability to self-disclose and to obtain emotional support in boys and girls, and these differences increased with age.

Overall, the data are consistent with Rutter's proposal that temperamentally difficult children are likely to be the target of their parents' aversive responses; moreover, we have identified some of the conditions under which this occurs. Let us turn now to his second proposal, that is, that temperamentally difficult children are less able than temperamentally easy children to cope with this abusive behavior from parents when it occurs. To do this, we examined the relation between temperament, an index of family stress, a composite index of support available to the child, and an index of the child's adaptability at age 10.

No differences in the adaptive ability of easy and difficult children were observed under conditions of low stress and high support. Under conditions in which supports were not readily available, increased frequency of family stressors led to less adaptive behavior among both easy and difficult children, although easy children were more adaptable than difficult ones. Under conditions of high availability of protective factors, however, a very different pattern emerged. For difficult children, a linear relation between stress and adaptive behavior was obtained. Increased stress was associated with less adaptability. For the temperamentally easy children, a curvilinear relation emerged: under supportive conditions, these children actually developed more adaptive skills when stress levels were moderate than when either extremely low or high. For temperamentally easy children, then, some practice in solving stressful problems under supportive conditions enhanced their later abilities to delay gratification, to persist on difficult tasks, and to be flexible and adaptive on problem-solving tasks and in social relations. In addition, if stresses did not occur simultaneously but were distributed across time, these children could cope with them more easily. The simultaneous occurrence of multiple stressors or a series of unresolved stresses with no available protective resources had the most deleterious outcomes for children's long-term adjustment. As Rutter has stated, "Inoculation against stress may be best provided by controlled exposure to stress in circumstances favorable to successful coping or adaptation" (Rutter, 1987, p. 326). However, when stressful life events outweigh available protective factors, even the most resilient child can develop problems (Werner, 1988). These differences were more marked in children from divorced and remarried families than in children from nondivorced families, and the effects of temperament and family type were greater for boys than for girls.

Our analysis is relatively gross, grouping together diverse family stressors and diverse protective factors. As will be seen, different stressors and resources are salient for children in different families. Familial factors are especially potent for young children, and extrafamilial experiences, stresses, and resources in the school and the peer group become increasingly important as children grow older. In addition, goodness of fit between stressors and protective factors is critical. For example, a close relationship with one parent is the best protection against the adverse consequences of rejection or emotional disturbance in the other parent; and, among older children, good peer relationships or a close relationship with one good friend can buffer against acrimonious relations with a sibling. Let us turn now to family relationships that make children vulnerable or protect them from long-term adverse consequences following divorce and remarriage.

FAMILY RELATIONSHIPS

How do family relationships buffer or exacerbate children's long-term adjustment to divorce and remarriage? Remember that our divorced-mother-custody families are what we might call "stabilized" divorced families since they have been divorced for an average of 6 years and are well beyond the initial crisis. We separated our stepfamilies into those remarried more or less than 2 years, making the tenuous assumption that the crisis period and the period needed for stabilization following remarriage would be about the same as that in divorce. Family interactions in our different types of families will be described first, and then the association of these interactions with the long-term adjustment of the children will be discussed.

The findings indicate that mother-son relationships in the divorced nonremarried families and parent-child relationships in newly remarried families, particularly with stepdaughters, were problematic. Divorced nonremarried mothers continued to exhibit many of the behaviors with their sons 6 years after divorce that were seen 2 years after divorce. More differences in punishment and control than in warmth and affection distinguished divorced mothers from mothers in the other family types. Divorced mothers were ineffectual in their control attempts and gave many instructions with little follow-through. They tended to nag, natter, and complain and were often involved in angry, escalating coercive cycles with their sons. Spontaneous negative "start-ups," that is, negative behavior initiated following neutral or positive behavior by the other person, were twice as likely to occur between mothers and sons in divorced families as in nondivorced families. Moreover, once these negative interchanges between divorced mothers and sons occurred, they were likely to continue longer than in any other dyad in any family type. The probability of continuance of a negative response was higher in the divorced mother-son dyads than in any other parent-child dyad, with the exception of daughter and stepfathers in the early stages of remarriage. In spite of these conflicts, however, it might be best to view the relationship of custodial mothers and their early adolescent sons as intense and ambivalent rather than as purely hostile and rejecting since warm feelings were also expressed in many of these dyads.

Both sons and daughters in divorced families were allowed more responsibility, independence, and power in decision making than were children in nondivorced families. In the words of Robert Weiss (1979), "these children grow up faster." They successfully interrupted their divorced mothers, and their mothers yielded to their demands more often than in other families. In some cases this greater power and independence resulted in an egalitarian, mutually supportive relationship. In other cases, especially when the emotional demands or responsibilities required by the mother were inappropriate, were beyond the child's capabilities, or interfered with the child's normal activities, resentment, rebellion, or behavior problems often followed.

Finally, divorced mothers monitored their children less closely than did mothers in nondivorced families. They knew less about where their children were, who they were with and what they were doing than did mothers in two-parent households. In addition, children in one-parent households were less likely than those in the two-parent households to have adult supervision in parental absence. Both Weiss (1979) and Wallerstein and Kelly (1980) report that one way children cope with their parents' divorce is by becoming disengaged from the family. We found, too, that boys from divorced families were spending significantly less time in the home with their parents or other adults and more time alone or with peers than were any of the other children. Stepsons were also significantly more disengaged than were sons in non-divorced families.

In contrast to the situation with divorced mothers and sons, few differences were observed in the relationship between divorced mothers and their daughters and those of mothers and daughters in nondivorced families. In fact, mothers and daughters in mother-headed families express considerable satisfaction with their relationship 6 years after divorce. One exception to this happy picture, however, is found among divorced mothers with early-maturing daughters. Family conflict was higher in all three family situations for early-maturing girls versus late-maturing girls, but it was most marked between mothers and daughters in single-parent households. Early maturity in girls was associated with premature weakening of the mother-child bond, increased parent-child conflict, and greater involvement with older peers. Past research suggests that divorced mothers and daughters may experience problems as daughters become pubescent and involved in heterosexual activities (Hetherington, 1972). Thus, the difficulties in interactions between these early-maturing girls and their divorced mothers may be precursors of more intense problems yet to come.

It is important to distinguish between those stepfamilies in the early stages of remarriage, when they are still adapting to their new situation, and those in later stages, when family roles and relationships should have been worked through and established. The early stage of remarriage may be a honeymoon period when the parents, if not the children, want to make the family relationship successful. Neither mothers nor stepfathers were successful in controlling and monitoring their children's behavior in stepfamilies, although controls were more successful in mothers who had been remarried for more than 2 years. In the first 2 years following remarriage, conflict between mothers and daughters was high. These daughters also exhibited more demandingness, hostility, coercion, and less warmth toward both parents than did girls in divorced or nondivorced families. Their behavior improved over the course of remarriage, but, even 2 years after remarriage, these girls were still more antagonistic and disruptive with their parents than were girls in the other two family types.

The behavior of stepsons with their mothers and stepfathers was very different than that of stepdaughters. Although mothers and stepfathers initially viewed sons as extremely difficult, the son's behavior improved over time. Boys whose mothers had been remarried for over 2 years were showing no more aggressive, noncompliant behavior in the home or in the school than were boys in nondivorced families (Hetherington et al., 1985). It should be noted that this improvement may be found only when the remarriage has occurred before adolescence. In another study (Hetherington & Clingempeel, 1988), we found that even 2 years following their mother's remarriage, both early adolescent boys and girls were exhibiting many behavior problems. In this study, although stepfathers continued to view stepchildren, especially stepdaughters, as having more problems than nondivorced fathers saw in their children, they reported greater improvement among stepsons and greater warmth and involvement with them than with stepdaughters. In fact, stepsons in longer remarried families frequently reported being close to their stepfathers, enjoying their company, and seeking their advice and support.

What might explain these differences in responses to their mother's remarriage by sons and daughters? Some answers are found in the different patterns of correlations between marital satisfaction and children's responses in nondivorced and remarried families. Among nondivorced couples, closeness of the marital relationship and support by the spouse for participation in child rearing were positively related to parental warmth and involvement with the child and negatively to parent-child conflict. Among the stepfamilies, however, there occurred what might appear to be an anomalous finding. As in other studies (Brand, Clingempeel, & Bowen-Woodward, 1988; Bray, 1987), among remarried families, closeness in the marital relationship and active involvement in parenting by the stepfather were associated with high levels of conflict between the child and both the mother and the stepfather. These conditions were also associated with high rates of behavior problems, especially when the stepchild was a girl. For sons, these relations were significant in the early but not the later stages of remarriage.

How can we explain these unexpected results? It seems likely that, in the early stages of remarriage, new stepfathers are viewed as intruders or competitors for the mother's affection. Since boys in divorced families often have been involved in coercive or ambivalent relationships with their mothers, in the long run, they may have little to lose and something to gain from the remarriage. In contrast, daughters in one-parent families have played more responsible, powerful roles than girls in nondivorced families and have had more positive relationships with their divorced mothers than have sons. They may see both their independence and their relationship with the mother as threatened by a new stepfather, and therefore resent the mother for remarrying. This was reflected in sulky, resistant, ignoring, critical behavior by daughters toward their remarried mothers and stepfathers. Furthermore, it is notable that positive behavior of stepfathers toward stepdaughters did not correlate with the girls' acceptance of their stepfathers in the early stages of remarriage. No matter how hard stepfathers tried, their stepdaughters rejected them.

Early adolescence may be a particularly difficult age in which to gain acceptance of stepparents by stepchildren. The adolescent's increased striving for independence from the family and their concerns about their awakening sexuality may make them especially resistant to the introduction of a stepfather. Most adolescents do not like to think of their parents as sexual objects, and it is difficult, when parents remarry, not to recognize them as such. Stepchildren often distort reasonable displays of affection by the newly married couple into something inappropriate or unacceptable.

Moreover, the lack of biological relatedness between the stepfather and the pubescent daughter may heighten concerns about what constitutes appropriate forms of affection between them. As it turns out, early adolescent children (i.e., from approximately 9 to 15 years of age) are more resistant to the introduction of a stepparent than are either older or younger children (Hetherington & Anderson, 1987). Most younger children in supportive homes with "normal" levels of conflict eventually accept a warm and involved stepfather. Older adolescents are future oriented and are anticipating leaving the home. For them, the presence of a stepfather to some extent relieves their own responsibilities for the economic and emotional well-being of the mother.

It has been said that there is considerable ambiguity in the role of a stepparent (Cherlin, 1981). How does the stepfather deal with this ambiguity, particularly in the face of ambivalence or active antagonism from his stepchildren? In the first 2 years following remarriage, stepfathers reported themselves to be relatively low in felt affection for their stepchildren, but they reported spending time with them attempting to establish relationships. In fact, although they expressed less strong positive affect during this period, they also showed fewer negative, critical responses than did the nondivorced fathers: they resembled polite strangers. Biological fathers, on the other hand, were freer in expressing affection and in criticizing their children for poor personal grooming, for not doing their homework, not cleaning up their rooms, and for fighting with their siblings. However, they also were more involved and interested in the activities of their children. Stepfathers were far less supportive initially of their stepsons than their stepdaughters, managing to remain relatively pleasant in spite of the aversive behavior they encountered from their stepdaughters. Two years after remarriage, however, they were more impatient than earlier, and intensely hostile exchanges sometimes ensued between stepfathers and stepdaughters, especially concerning parental authority and respect for the mother.

Although stepfamilies change over time, stepfathers remained much less authoritative and much more disengaged than were fathers in nondivorced families (Hetherington, 1987). Many stepfathers wanted to minimize the amount of time, effort, and interference with their own needs and their marital relationships that child rearing entailed. A frequently heard complaint was "I married her, not her kids," or on confronting disruptive behavior on the part of stepchildren, "That's their mother's problem not mine." Indeed, a sequence analysis of observed family interactions in our study indicated that a pattern of "mother command/child noncomply/father intervene" was found significantly less in the remarried than in the nondivorced families. Although the number of authoritative stepfathers increased modestly over time for boys, authoritative behavior by stepfathers with daughters decreased; disengagement doubled as the remarriage went on. In addition, even for boys after 2 years of remarriage, disengagement remained the predominant parenting style of stepfathers. Even in longer remarriages, many stepfathers and stepchildren did not mention each other when asked to identify the members of their families.

How does parental behavior protect the child or put the child at risk for developing problem behaviors? As Diana Baumrind (1973) has been telling us for many years, authoritarian, disengaged, and permissive parenting styles are more likely than authoritative parenting to be associated with the development of behavior problems and low social and cognitive competence in children. Generally, we found the same thing, although the effects varied somewhat with sex of the child and sex of the parent.

Authoritative parenting was associated with high social competence and low rates of behavior problems, especially with low externalizing problems, and especially among boys. Authoritative parenting involving warmth and firm but responsive control was particularly important in divorced and remarried custodial parents in protecting children from the adverse effects of marital transitions. Thus, in coping with stressful life events, a supportive, structured, predictable parent-child relationship plays a critical protective role.

An exception to this positive relation between authoritative parenting and child outcomes was found, however, among stepfathers and stepchildren. Both authoritative and authoritarian parenting in stepfathers were related to high rates of behavior problems in both stepdaughters and in stepsons in the first 2 years of remarriage. These two parenting styles both involve high levels of control, although the former involves warm, responsive control while the latter is punitive, coercive, and rigid. Apparently, any kind of active control by the stepfather is initially aversive to the stepchild. After 2 years, though, authoritative parenting by stepfathers was related to fewer behavior problems and greater acceptance of the stepfather by stepsons than before, but was not, even at this time, significantly related to stepdaughter's behavior. The best strategy of the stepfather in gaining acceptance of the stepchildren thus seems to be one where there is no active attempt initially to take over, shape, and control the child's behavior. Instead, a period of time is needed, first to work at establishing a relationship and to support the mother in her parenting, followed, later, by more active authoritative parenting. Such a strategy leads to constructive long-term outcomes, at least for boys.

By the time these children were 10, maternal behaviors had more impact on the anti-social and prosocial behavior as well as the self-esteem of girls than of boys in all family types. In contrast, biological fathers in nondivorced families had more impact on such behaviors in boys. In families remarried for over 2 years, stepfathers also played a significant role in modifying prosocial and problem behaviors in stepsons. Moreover, although only one-quarter of our noncustodial fathers were seeing their children once a week or more, those who were warm, involved, and reasonably competent played a positive role in their son's development when there was also low conflict between the divorced spouses. Over all, the salience of the same-sexed parent increased markedly from the preschool years to age 10.

SIBLING RELATIONSHIPS

Although considerable research has been done on parent-child relationships in divorced and remarried families, there is little work on the role siblings may play in exacerbating or buffering the effects of marital transitions (Hetherington & Clingempeel, 1988; Wallerstein et al., 1988). Two alternative hypotheses might be offered about siblings and the marital transitions of their parents. One would be that siblings become increasingly rivalrous and hostile as they compete for scarce resources of parental love and attention following their parents' divorce or remarriage. Alternatively, siblings in families that have gone through marital transitions may view relationships with adults as unstable, untrustworthy, and painful and turn to each other for solace, support, and alliance.

Four main findings were apparent in our data. First, siblings in stepfamilies and boys in divorced families had more problematic relationships than siblings in nondivorced families or girls in divorced families. They were more aggressive, avoidant, and rivalrous and were less warm and involved than other siblings. Negative start-ups, reciprocated aggression, and long chains of aggressive, coercive behaviors with siblings were more common among stepchildren than among children in nondivorced families but were most frequently found among sons in divorced families. These behaviors were more frequent if the target child was interacting with a male sibling. Second, sibling relationships in stepfamilies improved over time but remained more disturbed than those in nondivorced or divorced families. Disengagement and avoidance of female children toward their siblings remained more common in stepfamilies than other families, even 2 years after remarriage. Third, any sibling dyad involving a boy was more troubled than those involving only girls. Not only were boys seen as exhibiting more aversive behaviors than girls, but girls behaved in a less congenial fashion when interacting with brothers than sisters. Both sons and daughters in stepfamilies and daughters in divorced families were less likely to initiate conversations or activities and more likely to refuse or ignore overtures on the part of a male than a female sibling. Brothers were not getting much support from their female siblings in these families. Fourth, older girls in divorced families often played a supportive, nurturing role in relationships with younger female siblings. Daughters in divorced families were more involved in teaching, play, and caretaking activities with their younger sisters than were other children. Usually this was associated with positive outcomes (e.g., higher rates of prosocial behavior, lower externalizing, and better peer relationships) in both the female sibling caregiver and the recipient of the care. Sometimes the close relationship found between female siblings became too enmeshed, however, and was associated with adverse outcomes.

We used cluster analysis to identify four styles of sibling relationships (Hetherington, 1988). One of these was a small cluster that included less than 10% of our children and that was characterized by very high warmth, involvement, and communication, along with very low rivalry and aggression. These children spent little time playing with other children, most of their time with each other, were dependent on one another, and fiercely protective of each other. Although they were nurturant and empathetic with each other, they showed little sensitivity or concern with the feelings of adults or peers. They scored moderately high on internalizing, sometimes got into problems with parents and teachers, and were usually neglected rather than rejected on peer nominations. These relationships seemed to be pathologically intense, enmeshed, symbiotic, and restrictive. These siblings were most likely to be girls and to be found in divorced or remarried families and in families where the child had no regular contact or involvement with an affectionate, involved adult. This enmeshment, then, tends to occur under stressful life conditions without available adult support.

To our initial question, whether marital transitions promote productive alliances or competition between siblings, the answer is clear in our study: Ambivalent or hostile, alienated relationships were more common in siblings in remarried families and in boys in divorced families than among siblings in nondivorced families. Companionate, caring relationships, on the other hand, were more common in nondivorced families and in female siblings in divorced families. Furthermore, sibling rivalry, aggression, and disengagement played a more important role in increasing externalizing, antisocial behavior and in decreasing prosocial behavior in divorced and remarried families than did warmth, support, and involvement in protecting siblings from adverse developmental consequences. Positive sibling relationships, however, played a more important buffering role among older than among younger children and in the advanced rather than the earlier stages of marital transitions. In the early stages of divorce and remarriage the effects of parent-child relationships were so powerful that sibling relationships could do little to moderate them.

GRANDPARENTS

Grandparents offer support not only to their divorced and remarried children but also to their grandchildren. Studies of black families have found that children in homes in which there is a mother and grandmother are better adjusted than those in which the mother is alone (Kellam, Adams, Brown, & Ensminger, 1982; Kellam, Ensminger, & Turner, 1977). At 6 years following divorce, about half of our grandparents and stepgrandparents lived within 100 miles of their divorced children; only a few mothers who were unemployed or had not remarried were living with their parents. In our white, middle-class families, the divorced custodial mothers appreciated the emotional, economic, and child-care support offered by grandparents, but, when they were economically independent, they preferred to live alone and have grandparents accessible. When divorced women lived with their parents, they often reported feeling infantilized and not treated as adults by their parents. Loss of independence, shared control over their children, conflicts about discipline, and the divorced mother's social life were frequent areas of disagreement. Relationships between divorced mothers and residential grandmothers were frequently ambivalent, although this ambivalence was not as frequently found with residential grandfathers.

For both parents of the custodial and the noncustodial parent, frequency of contact with grandchildren was related to proximity. In our divorced families, amount of contact by children with the parents of the noncustodial parent was directly related to the amount of contact maintained by the noncustodial parent (see also Furstenberg, 1988). Since for most children contact with the noncustodial father decreased over time—especially if he remarried—so did contact with those grandparents. However, 6 years after divorce, half of our parents of noncustodial fathers reported that they had as much or more contact with their grandchildren as before the divorce.

When divorced parents remarried, the complexity of the child's social network increased dramatically. Involvement of stepgrandparents with stepchildren was related to age of the child at the time of remarriage and whether the stepfather had children from a previous marriage. When there were no biological grandchildren and when stepgrandchildren were young at the time of the remarriage, stepgrandparents became more actively involved.

But contact is one thing, influence another. What role do grandparents play in increasing or buffering risks for children in divorced and remarried families? Our findings are congruent with those of Cherlin and Furstenberg (1986). In most cases, there was little evidence that grandparents play a potent role in the social, emotional, and cognitive development of their grandchildren unless they live in the home. In fact, there was a low positive correlation between the number of behavior problems in grandchildren and the amount of contact with grandparents. The more problems, the more contact. Grandparents were called in to help with difficult children, especially in families headed by a divorced nonremarried mother. Grandparents are thus the parent's reserves when things go wrong. Cherlin and Furstenberg (1986, p. 183) have said, "Grandparents in America are like volunteer firefighters: they are required to be on the scene when needed but otherwise keep their assistance in reserve." Even so, one exception should be noted to the finding that grandparents have a negligible influence on the adjustment of their grandchildren. Involved grandfathers may have salutary effects on the social behavior and achievement of boys in divorced-mother-custody families, and increased conflict between divorced mothers and residential grandmothers increases externalizing behavior in boys. In general, however, the relationship with nonresidential grandparents had little direct influence on the long-term adjustment of grandchildren. The effects of support by the grandparents were mediated by changed maternal behavior in response to such support.

SCHOOLS AND PEERS

As the children became older, schools and peers played an increasingly salient role in their adjustment to divorce and remarriage. We had found earlier that, even in the preschool period, the social and cognitive development of young children from divorced families was enhanced if children were in schools with explicitly defined schedules, rules, and regulations and with consistent, warm discipline and expectations for mature behavior. Just as authoritative parents played a protective function for children going through family transitions, authoritative schools play a buffering role for children undergoing stress. Under stress, children gained security in a structured, safe, predictable environment. I had earlier predicted that this effect might be most marked in young children under high stress since they may not be able to exert internal control and may require more external controls than either less stressed or more mature children. Even at age 10, though, we found that authoritative teachers and school environments attenuated adverse outcomes for children in divorced and remarried families and in nondivorced families with high conflict. This protective effect of authoritative schools is most marked for boys, for children with difficult temperaments, and for children exposed to multiple stressful life events.

Attainments in school also modified adverse or salutary outcomes for children from divorced and remarried families. Academic achievement and, for boys only, athletic achievement were associated with fewer behavior problems than those found in their less academically successful peers among children in divorced and remarried families.

Peer relationships did not play roles as protective or vulnerability factors in preschool children but became more influential with age. Children who were actively rejected by their peer group or who did not have one close friend showed increased long-term problems in adjustment. Moreover, it did not take a high level of general popularity to enhance development. A supportive relationship with a single friend could moderate the adverse consequences of marital transitions and could modify the effects of rejection by other children.

About one-third of adolescent children become disengaged from the family following divorce and remarriage. They become involved in school activities and the peer group or, if they are fortunate, they attach themselves to a responsive adult or to the family of a friend. Whether these are desirable coping mechanisms depends on the child's family situation and on the particular activities and type of associates with which the child becomes involved. If they are socially constructive activities and the child's associates are well adjusted, this move can be advantageous.

Undesirable activities and an antisocial or delinquent peer group, on the other hand, usually have disastrous consequences. When disengagement from the family occurs, however, contact with an interested, supportive adult plays a particularly important role in buffering the child against the development of behavior problems.

WINNERS, LOSERS, AND SURVIVORS

Which children are the winners, losers, and survivors 6 years after divorce? Cluster analyses of observational, interview, and standardized tests were done on the measures of current adjustment for all children in our sample, and for boys and girls separately. These analyses included the children in all family groups, that is, with nondivorced parents, with divorced nonremarried custodial mothers, and with remarried mothers. The clusters were fairly similar for boys and girls, although some sex differences will be noted. Although five clusters of children emerged, children from divorced or remarried families were overrepresented in only three; these are discussed in this article. The first cluster was clearly maladaptive, and the last two involved more successful coping.

One cluster involved *aggressive, insecure* children. These children manifested multiple problems in multiple settings. They were noncompliant, impulsive, and aggressive in the home, with their parents and siblings, in the school, and in the peer group. These children were prone both to impulsive, irritable outbursts and to sullen, brooding periods of withdrawal. They were unpopular with peers; in fact, 70% of the children in this group did not have a close friend. Moreover, they had difficulties in school: placement in special classes, poor grades, referrals for disciplinary problems, and retention in grade were more common in this group than in any other group of children. These children had few or no areas of satisfaction and attainment, and this was reflected in their exceptionally low levels of self-esteem. In short, these were lonely, unhappy, angry, anxious, insecure children.

What kinds of attributes, experiences, and family relationships were associated with this pattern of adjustment? First, there were three times as many boys as girls in this group, although girls from remarried families and boys with divorced, nonremarried mothers and recently remarried mothers were overrepresented. The homes of these children were characterized by high levels of negative affect, conflict, and unsatisfactory conflict-resolution styles in parents involving verbal or physical attacks, power assertion, or withdrawal rather than compromise. Authoritative parenting was rarely found with these children. They were more likely to be exposed to disengaged, neglecting, or ineffectually authoritarian parenting styles. Boys in this group had been temperamentally difficult children early in life, and their behavior problems seem to have been exacerbated by family conflict or divorce. In these late preadolescent or early adolescent children, the relationship with the same-sexed parent was especially significant for the development of behavior problems or competence. Boys in this aggressive, insecure cluster tended to have no close relationship with an adult male. Many of these boys had unavailable fathers or fathers or stepfathers who actively rejected them. However, the behavior of divorced custodial mothers was also important for sons. Boys in this cluster with divorced mothers also had conflicted or alienated relations with their mothers. Their mothers also tended to work full time. In this study, full-time maternal employment in divorced mothers was associated with adverse outcomes for boys but positive outcomes for girls. In contrast to parental relationships with boys, girls in this cluster in all types of families had poor relationships with their mothers and were unaffected by their relationships with their fathers.

Children in two other clusters can be labeled *opportunistic-competent* and *caring-competent* children; individuals in both clusters appeared to be adapting exceptionally well. Children in both clusters were high in self-esteem, popular with their peers and teachers, and low in behavior problems. In addition, they were performing at an average or above average level academically. Both groups of children were described by others as curious, energetic, assertive, self-sufficient, and as having wide-ranging interests and skills in interpersonal relations. In addition, children in both groups were unusually competent, flexible, and persistent in dealing with demanding or stressful situations. A manipulative, opportunistic quality was apparent, however, among the opportunistic-competent children and not among the caring-competent children. Nearly equal numbers of girls and boys were in the opportunistic-competent group, and they were more frequently found in divorced and remarried families and in nondivorced families with high conflict than in nondivorced families with low conflict. The family-conflict level in these families was higher for girls than for boys. Parents reported that these children, even when they were young, had attempted to use disagreements and conflicts between parents for their own gains. They often played parents off against one another, thereby exacerbating the parents' acrimony. Although these children had close, supportive relationships with at least one parent—usually a parent of the same sex—they often had one parent who rejected or neglected them and/or who had problems in personal adjustment.

The egocentric, manipulative quality in these opportunistic-competent children was frequently remarked by interviewers and observers. These children were oriented toward people in power, such as parents and teachers and even peers with high status or resources. Their attempts to ingratiate themselves with such powerful people were often done with considerable grace, charm, and humor and were usually successful. The friendships of these children, however, were often short-lived. Children in this group seldom had the same best friends from one testing session to another. Finally, almost all of the girls in this group had working mothers and had been encouraged by their mothers to be autonomous and independent. These maternal characteristics were found in this cluster for girls but not for boys.

Children in the caring-competent cluster were similar to those in the opportunistic cluster in many ways. In social relations, however, they were less manipulative. They got along well with adults and peers, but they were less concerned about prestige and power in their relationships. Although they were cooperative, there was less striving to gain the attention and approbation of adults. Friendships were more stable and less likely to be focused on high-status peers. In fact, caring-competent children often befriended children who were neglected or even rejected by the peer group. There was a notable difference, however, in prosocial behavior: the children in this group were higher in helping and sharing than children in any other group.

Can we identify differences in the experiential factors that might differentiate between the opportunistic-competent and caring-competent children? The most striking factor is that the caring-competent cluster is comprised almost totally of girls. Only five of the 23 children in this cluster were boys, and none of these boys had divorced, nonremarried mothers. In contrast, over half of the girls in this cluster were daughters of divorced, nonremarried mothers with whom they had a close relationship. Experiences in a one-parent, mother-headed family seemed to have a positive effect for these girls. Like the girls in the opportunistic-competent cluster, these girls had working mothers who encouraged their children in mature independent behavior. They had mothers who usually were warm and supportive but not always available. A salient characteristic in the backgrounds of both the opportunistic-competent and caring-competent children was contact with a caring adult, whether a parent, other relative, teacher, or neighbor. However, the most notable experience in the background of caring-competent girls, but not the opportunistic-competent children, was that they had assumed responsibility for the care of others even at this young age. This usually involved the care and nurturance of younger siblings; in seven cases, however, it involved supporting a physically ill, lonely, alcoholic, or depressed mother, and in three cases it involved helping to care for an aged or physically feeble grandparent. This early required helpfulness was the most powerful factor in predicting later membership in the caring-competent cluster. These responsibilities, clearly associated with what Weiss (1979) has called "growing up faster" in divorced one-parent households, seem to have enhancing effects for girls but not for boys. The adverse experiences, for boys, of living in a one-parent, mother-headed household seem to counteract any possible salutary effects of early caretaking responsibilities.

CONCLUSION

What can be said in response to the frequent query, What enduring effects do divorce and remarriage have on children? When I began to study children in divorced families, I had a pathogenic model of divorce. However, after more than 2 decades of research on marital transitions, I would have to respond: depending on the characteristics of the child, particularly the age and gender of the child, available resources, subsequent life experiences, and especially interpersonal relationships, children in the long run may be survivors, losers, or winners of their parents' divorce or remarriage.

REFERENCES

Baumrind, D. (1973). The development of instrumental competence through socialization. In A. D. Pick (Ed.), *Minnesota symposia on child psychology.* Vol. 7. Minneapolis: University of Minnesota Press, 1973.

Brand, E., Clingempeel, W. E., & Bowen-Woodward, K. (1988). Family relationships and children's psychological adjustment in stepmother and stepfather families: Findings and conclusions from the Philadelphia Stepfamily Research Project. In E. M. Hetherington & J. D. Arasteh (Eds.), *Impact on divorce, single parenting, stepparenting on children* (pp. 299–324). Hillsdale, NJ: Erlbaum.

Bray, J. H. (1987, August). *Becoming a stepfamily.* Symposium presented at the meeting of the American Psychological Association, New York.

Camara, K. A., & Resnick, G. (1988). Interparental conflict and cooperation: Factors moderating children's post-divorce adjustment. In E. M. Hetherington & J. Arasteh (Eds.), *Impact of divorce, single parenting, and stepparenting on children* (pp. 169–195). Hillsdale, NJ: Erlbaum.

Cherlin, A. (1981). *Marriage, divorce, remarriage: Changing patterns in the postwar United States.* Cambridge, MA: Harvard University Press.

Cherlin, A., & Furstenberg, F. F., Jr. (1986). *The new American grandparent: A place in the family, a life apart.* New York: Basic.

Furstenberg, F. F. (1988). Child care after divorce and remarriage. In E. M. Hetherington & J. D. Arasteh (Eds.), *Impact on divorce, single-parenting, and stepparenting on children* (pp. 245–261). Hillsdale, NJ: Erlbaum.

Garmezy, N. (1983). Stressors of childhood. In N. Garmezy & M. Rutter (Eds.), *Stress, coping, and development in children* (pp. 43–84). New York: McGraw-Hill.

Hetherington, E. M. (1972). Effects of fathers' absence on personality development in adolescent daughters. *Developmental Psychology, 7,* 313–326.

Hetherington, E. M. (1987). Family relations six years after divorce. In K. Pasley & M. Ihinger-Tollman (Eds.), *Remarriage and stepparenting today: Current research and theory* (pp. 185–205). New York: Guilford.

Hetherington, E. M. (in press). The role of individual differences and family relations in coping with divorce and remarriage. In P. Cowan & E. M. Hetherington (Eds.), *Advances in family research: Vol. 2. Family transitions.* Hillsdale, NJ: Erlbaum.

Hetherington, E. M. (1988). Parents, children and siblings six years after divorce. In R. Hinde & J. Stevenson-Hinde (Eds.), *Relationships within families.* Cambridge: Cambridge University Press.

Hetherington, E. M., & Anderson, E. R. (1987). The effects of divorce and remarriage on early adolescents and their families. In M. D. Levine & E. R. McArney (Eds.), *Early adolescent transitions* (pp. 49–67). Lexington, MA: Heath.

Hetherington, E. M., & Clingempeel, W. G. (1988, March). *Coping with remarriage: The first two years.* Symposium presented at the Southeastern Conference on Human Development, Charleston, SC.

Hetherington, E. M., Cox, M., & Cox, R. (1982). Effects of divorce on parents and children. In M. Lamb (Ed.), *Nontraditional families* (pp. 233–288). Hillsdale, NJ: Erlbaum.

Hetherington, E. M., Cox, M., & Cox, R. (1985). Long-term effects of divorce and remarriage on the adjustment of children. *Journal of American Academy of Psychiatry,* **24**, 518–830.

Kellam, S. G., Adams, R. G., Brown, C. H., & Ensminger, M. A. (1982). The long-term evolution of the family structure of teenage and older mothers. *Journal of Marriage and the Family,* **4**, 539–554.

Kellam, S. G., Ensminger, M. E., & Turner, R. J. (1977). Family structure and the mental health of children: Concurrent and longitudinal community-wide studies. *Archives of General Psychiatry,* **34**, 1012–1022.

Rutter, M. (1983). Stress, coping, and development: Some issues and some questions. In N. Garmezy & M. Rutter (Eds.), *Stress, coping, and development in children* (pp. 1–42). New York: McGraw-Hill.

Rutter, M. (1987). Psychosocial resilience and protective mechanisms. *American Journal of Orthopsychiatry,* **57**, 316–331.

Santrock, J. W., & Warshak, R. A. (1986). Development of father custody relationships and legal/clinical considerations in father-custody families. In M. E. Lamb (Ed.), *The father's role: Applied perspectives* (pp. 135–166). New York: Wiley.

Wallerstein, J. S., Corbin, S. B., & Lewis, J. M. (1988). Children of divorce: A ten-year study. In E. M. Hetherington & J. Arasteh (Eds.), *Impact of divorce, single-parenting and step-parenting on children* (pp. 198–214). Hillsdale, NJ: Erlbaum.

Wallerstein, J. S., & Kelly, J. B. (1980). *Surviving the breakup: How children and parents cope with divorce.* New York: Basic.

Weiss, R. S. (1979). Growing up a little faster: The experience of growing up in a single-parent household. *Journal of Social Issues,* **35**, 97–111.

Werner, E. E. (1988). Individual differences, universal needs: A 30-year study of resilient high risk infants. *Zero to Three Bulletin of National Center for Clinical Infant Programs,* **8**, 1–5.

Zill, N. (1988). Behavior, achievement, and health problems among children in stepfamilies: Findings from a national survey of child health. In E. M. Hetherington & J. D. Arasteh (Eds.), *Impact of divorce, single-parenting and stepparenting on children* (pp. 325–368). Hillsdale, NJ: Erlbaum.

12

Sibling Relationships: Links with Child Temperament, Maternal Behavior, and Family Structure

Clare Stocker, Judy Dunn, and Robert Plomin
The Pennsylvania State University

The extent to which maternal behavior, children's temperament, age, and family structure variables—jointly and independently—are associated with dimensions of sibling relationships is investigated in a sample of 96 families with younger siblings aged 3–6 years and older siblings aged 5–10 years. During home visits, mothers were interviewed and observed with their children in structured and unstructured settings. Together the 4 sets of predictor variables accounted for 22%–40% of the variance in measures of the sibling relationship. Maternal behavior, particularly differences in mothers' behavior to their 2 children, child temperament, and younger siblings' age added independently to the prediction of sibling relationships. Family structure variables were less important in accounting for variance in sibling relationships than were the other groups of predictors. The implications of these findings for understanding differences in siblings' relationships in early and middle childhood are discussed.

Marked differences between characteristics of siblings' relationships have been noted in most studies of siblings, yet there is little information about the correlates of these differences. The issue is an important one for both psychologists and parents. Differences in the ways that siblings behave toward one another may be associated

Reprinted with permission from *Child Development,* 1989, Vol. 60, 715–727. Copyright © 1989 by the Society for Research in Child Development, Inc.

This investigation was funded by a grant from the National Science Foundation (BNS 8643938). We would like to thank the families in the Colorado Adoption Project for their willing participation in our study. We are grateful to Robin DeWitt, Anastasia Galanopoulos, Kathy Purfield, and Betty Rhea for their help in rating videotapes and collecting data.

with their adjustment and personality and with diverse aspects of sociocognitive development (Daniels, Dunn, Furstenberg, & Plomin, 1985; Dunn, 1983, 1988; Dunn & Munn, 1985, 1986a, 1986b; McHale & Gamble, 1987). Parents frequently express anxiety about what role their own behavior plays in the development of their children's sibling relationships (Clifford, 1959; Newson & Newson, 1970).

Most attempts to understand differences in sibling relationships have examined the influence of family structure variables, such as birth order and the age difference between siblings (Abramovitch, Pepler, & Corter, 1982; Brody, Stoneman, & MacKinnon, 1982; Cicirelli, 1972; Furman & Buhrmester, 1985; Koch, 1960; Minnett, Vandell, & Santrock, 1983). Results from these studies are inconsistent and have yielded few insights into the processes through which characteristics of the sibling relationship develop.

Investigations of the links between parental behavior and sibling relationships have been more illuminating. Several studies report associations between maternal behavior and the sibling relationship. For example, maternal behavior toward first-born children has been shown to correlate with the quality of the relationship that develops between the first- and second-born children (Dunn & Kendrick, 1982; Howe, 1986; Stewart, Mobley, Van Tuyl, & Salvador, 1987). It appears likely that *differential* maternal treatment of the siblings within a family may be important in addition to traditional between-mother measures. More conflictual and less friendly sibling relationships have been reported in families in which mothers were differentially affectionate, responsive, or controlling toward their children (Brody, Stoneman, & Burke, 1987; Bryant & Crockenberg, 1980; Daniels et al., 1985; Hetherington, 1988; McHale & Gamble, 1987).

In addition to the mother-child relationship, the temperamental or personality characteristics of each sibling are likely to be related to the relationship that develops between them. Surprisingly little research has examined the associations between children's temperament and their sibling relationships. However, in a study of 40 same-sex sibling pairs 4–10 years of age, Brody and his colleagues found that children who were highly active, emotionally intense, and low in persistence directed more agonistic behavior toward their siblings during an observational session than children who were rated low on these dimensions (Brody et al., 1987; see also Dunn & Munn, 1988).

Although much research has explored the influence of children's birth order on their sibling relationships, relatively few studies have examined the impact of the age of first- and second-born children independent of birth order. Yet children's rapid social and cognitive development during early childhood suggests that age may be an important predictor of characteristics of sibling relationships (Beardsall, 1987).

The goal of the present study was to examine the extent to which variance in the sibling relationship could be accounted for—jointly and independently—by mothers' behavior, by siblings' temperament, by siblings' age, and by family structure variables (age spacing, gender combination, and adoptive status). We predicted that more conflictual and less friendly sibling relationships would be found in families where maternal differential behavior was marked. On the basis of Brody et al.'s study (1987), we hypothesized that child temperament would also be associated with the quality of sibling relationships. These issues are addressed with data from a longitudinal study of 96 families in which mothers and siblings were studied in their homes when the younger siblings were 3–6 years and the older siblings were 5–10 years.

METHOD

Subjects

Subjects were 96 mother-sibling-sibling triads. Younger siblings ranged in age from 37 to 79 months ($M = 56.1$, SD $= 8.56$), and older siblings were 56–129 months old ($M = 91.9$, SD $= 14.20$). The average age gap between siblings was 35.6 months. Forty-four of the sibling dyads were same-gender (25 brother-brother, 19 sister-sister) and 52 were mixed-gender (25 older brother–younger sister, 27 older sister–younger brother). Sixty-four of the families had two children, 27 had three children, and five families had four children. The sample included 41 adoptive families, in which both siblings were adopted and were biologically unrelated, and 55 nonadoptive families. The subjects are a subsample of the Colorado Adoption Project (CAP), a longitudinal prospective study of environmental and genetic influences on behavioral development (Plomin, DeFries, & Fulker, 1988). All CAP families with a younger sibling between the ages of 3 and 6 were asked to participate in the study. There was a 95% acceptance rate. In the total sample, no significant differences have been found between adoptive and nonadoptive families, in a variety of environmental features, in parental characteristics, or in children's scores on a wide range of developmental measures (Plomin et al., 1988).

Procedure

Each family was visited in their home for approximately 2 hours. Mothers and siblings were videotaped for 30 min while they participated in six play settings. The settings were designed to draw out particular features of the sibling relationship and varied in the amount of structure they imposed on the children. In the first setting, siblings built a tower together and mothers counted the number of blocks in the tower (six 15-sec trials; adapted from Graziano, French, Brownell, & Hartup, 1976). In the second game (marble-pull, cooperation; based on Madsen & Kagan, 1973) the children worked together to make a marble drop into a hole in a wooden board (four 30-sec trials). In the third setting (marble-pull, competition), the children played the same game but competed with each other in order to get the marble into the hole on their side of the board (four 15-sec trials). Mothers participated in both marble-pull games by dropping the marble onto the board to start the game. In the fourth setting, siblings and mothers played together with a set of farm toys for 5 min; the children continued to play with the farm set for an additional 5 min with the mother absent for the fifth setting. In the last setting, the siblings were given a can of Playdoh, and one cookie cutter and one rolling pin was provided between them. They played for 5 min with the mother absent.

The siblings were next observed during a 30-min unstructured session. Siblings were asked to stay in the same room but were told they could play together or separately. The observer did not provide any play materials and the children played with their own toys. Mothers were instructed to continue their normal routine as much as possible. Mothers were present on average for a third of the unstructured period, a proportion similar to that found in other studies of siblings in middle childhood (Beardsall, 1987). The session was audiotaped, and the children's verbal interaction was coded later. Finally, mothers participated in a 45-min, open-ended interview that included questions in three areas: their differential behavior to the two children, the nature of the children's sibling relationship, and the children's temperamental characteristics.

Measures

Maternal behavior. Mothers' behavior to each sibling during each videotaped setting was rated on four 5-point scales, similar to those employed in a previous study (Dunn & Plomin, 1986): Control-intrusiveness, Affection, Attention, and Responsiveness. The Control scale ranged from (1) no intruding or directive remarks, does not handle game pieces or take on child's role, to (5) many directive comments, controls child physically, takes child's part in game, organizes child's play. The scale for Affection ranged from (1) negative or discouraging remarks, no positive remarks, no physical affection, to (5) many positive comments, many smiles, positive physical contact. The Attention scale ranged from (1) not watching child for most of the session, no comments to child, to (5) many comments to the child throughout the session. The Responsiveness scale ranged from (1) mother does not share child's excitement or disappointment, ignores many of the child's requests or comments, to (5) immediately responds to child's comments and questions, expands on child's comments, shares child's excitement or disappointment, responds to child's subtle gestures. Total scores on each of these scales were created by adding maternal scores for each scale from each setting.

In addition to examining the relation of these direct measures of maternal behavior to each child, the differences in how a mother behaved to her two children were also examined. Maternal differential scores were derived by calculating the absolute difference of the rating of maternal behavior to one sibling from the rating of her behavior to the other sibling. Measures of relative maternal differential behavior were derived by subtracting the mother's score to the younger sibling from her score to the older sibling. Since, in general, mothers directed more affection, control, attention, and responsiveness to younger siblings than to older siblings, the results from analyses using both types of differential measures were very similar. We therefore report below only results from analyses of the absolute-difference scores.

Sibling relationship. Measures of the sibling relationship are from three sources: the videotaped settings, the unstructured observation, and the maternal interview. Although there were moderate positive intercorrelations between measures from the different sources (Dunn, Stocker, & Plomin, 1988), the information from the three sources highlights different features of the siblings' relationship, and we therefore chose to analyze the measures from these sources separately.

1. Videotaped settings. Coders who had not rated maternal behavior rated each child's behavior to his or her sibling from the videotapes. Four 5-point scales were used: Conflict, Cooperation, Control, and Competition. For Conflict, the scale ranged from (1) no physical aggression or teasing, no verbal hostility, no protests or disputes, to (5) intense aggression, physical aggression, frequent criticism of other's actions. The scale for Cooperation ranged from (1) no attempts to cooperate, refusal to cooperate or follow suggestions, to (5) frequent attempts to cooperate with sibling, responds promptly to suggestions or questions, frequent sustained conversation, innovatory suggestions for cooperative play. The Control scale ranged from (1) no controlling, bossy, or directive statements, no physical acts of interference with other's actions, to (5) frequent bossy, directive, or controlling comments, physical interference with sibling's play, takes over sibling's play. For Competition, the scale ranged from (1) no signs of rivalry or competitiveness, no competitive statements, no complaints about turns, no disruption of mother-sibling interaction, to (5) frequent signs of above, aggression in winning, disparaging remarks about sibling to mother.

The means and standard deviations for children's scores on each scale in each setting revealed acceptable distributions of scores in 22 of the 24 scales. The exceptions were in the competitive marble-pull game, where more than 90% of the scores on Conflict and Cooperation fell on one point of the scales. Thus, we omitted Conflict and Cooperation scores from this setting. Because the focus for this analysis was on the dyad's relationship rather than each child's behavior toward the other, *pair* scores were calculated by adding together younger siblings' and older siblings' ratings on these measures (see Dunn et al., 1988). The average correlations across the six settings for Conflict, Competition, Cooperation, and Control were .50, .35, .29, and .34, respectively. Given these significant correlations, and in order to obtain more global sibling relationship measures, total scores were created by adding the pair's ratings from each of the six settings. The Conflict and Competition scales were significantly correlated ($r = .59$) and had similar patterns of relations with the other measures used in the study. Therefore, in order to reduce the number of dependent variables, we decided not to include Conflict in further analyses.

2. Unstructured observations. During the 30-min unstructured session, the observer coded the following behaviors exhibited by each sibling on a 10-sec time base: invite joint interaction, cooperate, show/give, help, imitate, smile/laugh, caretake, intense positive affect, intense negative affect, positive physical affection, interfere, protest/prohibit, tease, hit, fuss/cry. The following dyadic behaviors were also coded: joint play/activity, pretend play, conflict, and parallel play. The audiotape of the unstructured observation was coded per speaker tone on the following verbal items that each child addressed to the sibling: complains about sibling, disparages, directs, compares self positively with sibling, compares self negatively with sibling, joint "we" statements (see Gottman, 1983), questions, negotiates, disconfirms, and justifies/explains own behavior. After preliminary analysis, infrequently occurring items were combined: cooperate with help, tease with hit, and positive physical affection with smile/laugh.

In order to represent the dyad's interaction for these analyses we included *dyadic* scores (behaviors coded for the dyad such as conflict, joint play) and *pair* scores (combined scores of the two children on behaviors originally coded for each child individually) in a principal components analysis with orthogonal rotation. Two factors with eigenvalues greater than 1.0 were retained for rotation; these accounted for 40.1% of the variance. The first factor represented negative behavior and included pair scores on protest/prohibit, disconfirm, and tease/hit, which loaded .83, .80, and .43, respectively; this factor accounted for 32.7% of the rotated variance. The second factor was characterized by positive behavior and included pair scores on cooperate/help, positive physical/smile, and joint "we" statements, and the dyadic measure pretend play, which loaded .67, .63, .56, and .59, respectively. The second factor accounted for 62.3% of the rotated variance. A positive and a negative scale were created using standardized Z scores of these items.

3. Maternal interview. Mothers were asked 17 questions about dimensions of the siblings' relationship and about each child's behavior toward the sibling. The questions were open ended and the interviewer rated mothers' responses on 6-point scales ranging from 0 (almost never/rarely) to 5 (regularly/just about every day).[1] Mothers' responses were included in a principal components analysis with orthogonal rotation. Two factors with eigenvalues greater than 1 were retained for rotation. They accounted for 34.4% of the variance. The first factor represented positive behavior and included the measures joint play, desire to be with sibling, and affection to sibling, which loaded .90, .89, and .36, respectively. This factor accounted

---

[1]A copy of the interview is available from the first author at Department of Individual and Family Studies, S-110 Henderson Building, The Pennsylvania State University, University Park, PA 16802.

for 53.2% of the rotated variance. Negative behaviors loaded on the second factor and included jealousy of the sibling with the father, jealousy of the sibling with the mother, physical aggression, competition, and frequency of fights, which loaded .78, .76, .36, .35, and .38, respectively, and accounted for 46.8% of the rotated variance. Based on these loadings, a positive and a negative scale were created using standardized Z scores. In summary, eight measures of the sibling relationship were originally used: Conflict, Competition, Control, and Cooperation from the video settings, the positive and negative scales from the unstructured observation, and the positive and negative scales from the maternal interview.

Children's temperamental characteristics. A semistructured interview with the mother assessed dimensions of each child's temperament based on Buss and Plomin's (1984) system of temperament: activity, fear, anger, sociability, and shyness. In addition, because of the likelihood that emotionality plays a role in sibling relationships, three items were added to assess frequency and intensity of emotional upset and ease of recovery from emotional upset. The interviewer continued to use standard probes to expand mothers' descriptions of each temperament dimension until the interviewer was satisfied that an adequate rating could be made on a 1–5 low-high scale.

Family structure variables. Family structure variables consisted of adoptive status, age spacing, and gender composition of the sibling pair. Adoptive status was coded as 1 for adoptive families and 2 for nonadoptive families. Age spacing between the siblings was assessed as the difference in months between the older sibling's and younger sibling's ages. Preliminary analyses indicated that there were no mean differences or differences in the patterns of correlations between the measures used in this study for boy-boy versus girl-girl pairs, or for older brother–younger sister versus older sister–younger brother pairs. Therefore, same-gender pairs (coded as 1) were compared to mixed-gender pairs (coded as 2) in these analyses.

Intercoder Agreement

Two coders independently rated maternal behavior on 10 videotapes. The interrater correlations for maternal Control, Affection, Attention, and Responsiveness were .80, .83, .72, and .84 for older siblings and .96, .93, .93, and .91 for younger siblings. A second pair of coders independently rated the siblings' behavior on 10 different videotapes. The correlations between the raters on Conflict, Cooperation, Control, and Competition were .95, .91, .86, and .98, respectively. Interrater correlations for behaviors coded during the unstructured observation ranged from .65 to 1.00 ($M = .86$). These correlations were based on two coders' independent codings of 10 videotapes and two home visits to pilot families.

Test-Retest Reliabilities

Test-retest reliabilities for all measures were computed on a separate sample of 30 families. The families were visited twice at a 2-week interval and participated in identical procedures during both sessions. The test-retest reliabilities for the maternal behavior measures from the videotaped settings were: to the older sibling—Control .83, Affection .65, Attention .80, and Responsiveness .69; to the younger sibling—Control .80, Affection .72, Attention .75, and Responsiveness .67. The correlations for the sibling relationship measures from the videotaped settings were: .58 for Control, .48 for Cooperation, .38 for Competition, and .42 for Conflict. In the unstructured observation, the test-retest correlation for the positive scale was .48, while for the negative scale it was .00. In the unstructured situation, positive behaviors occurred three times more often than negative behaviors. Negative behaviors may have occurred too infrequently to provide a reliable sample in only a 30-min observation. Therefore the negative scale was dropped from further analyses. The positive and negative scales from the maternal interview had high test-retest correlations: .64 and .79, respectively. Test-retest correlations for the eight temperament measures averaged .42 for the older sibling and .44 for the younger. These correlations are lower than in studies of paper-and-pencil parental ratings of temperament (Buss & Plomin, 1984). Nonetheless, as indicated in the following section, the temperament measures were associated with sibling relationship variables from the videotaped observations, maternal interviews, and unstructured situation.

RESULTS

Correlations are first reported between the six indices of the sibling relationship (Competition, Cooperation, and Control from the video settings, the positive and negative scales from the maternal interview, and the positive scale from the unstructured observation) and (1) maternal behavior measures, (2) child temperament measures, (3) siblings' age, and (4) family structure variables. Following these univariate analyses, multivariate analyses are presented that *(a)* describe the joint prediction of sibling relationships by these four categories of correlates, and that *(b)* compare their independent contribution to the prediction of sibling relationships.

Correlations between Maternal Behavior and the Sibling Relationship Measures

Table 1 presents the Pearson product-moment correlations between the sibling relationship and differential maternal behavior, maternal behavior (direct) to

TABLE 1

Correlations Between Maternal Behavior and Sibling Relationship Measures

MEASURES OF THE SIBLING RELATIONSHIP

	Video Settings			Maternal Interview		Unstructured
	Competition	Cooperation	Control	Positive	Negative	Positive
Differential maternal behavior:						
Differential control	.22*	-.21	.12	-.16	.12	-.02
Differential affection	.18	.10	.22*	-.02	.12	.12
Differential attention	.34*	-.20	.19	-.14	.14	-.10
Differential responsiveness	.24*	-.02	.34*	-.24*	-.11	.07
Maternal behavior direct to older sibling:						
Control	.30*	-.04	.27*	.17	-.07	.08
Affection	.08	-.05	-.03	.12	.13	-.01
Attention	.18	.03	.06	.16	.08	.03
Responsiveness	-.00	.04	-.13	.11	.12	-.03
Maternal behavior direct to younger sibling:						
Control	.39*	-.20	.30*	.06	-.01	.04
Affection	.14	.00	.03	.08	.13	-.01
Attention	.44*	-.17	.29*	.05	.09	-.07
Responsiveness	.08	.02	-.05	.07	.10	-.04

* $p < .05$.

TABLE 2
Correlations Between Children's Temperament and Sibling Relationship Measures

MEASURES OF THE SIBLING RELATIONSHIP

	Video Settings			Maternal Interview		Unstructured
	Competition	Cooperation	Control	Positive	Negative	Positive
Older sibling:						
Activity	.02	−.02	.02	−.12	.05	−.07
Shyness	−.29*	.08	−.23*	.03	.06	.05
Sociability	.00	.06	.02	−.07	−.08	−.02
Frequency of upset ...	.11	−.10	−.01	.02	.24*	−.27*
Intensity of upset	.13	−.12	−.02	−.13	.17	−.12
Recovery from upset ..	.17	−.13	.12	.11	.31*	−.04
Anger	−.03	.03	−.20	.07	.14	−.04
Fear	.10	−.12	.04	.17	.27*	−.08
Younger sibling:						
Activity	.21*	−.19	.12	.15	.22*	.06
Shyness	−.10	.07	−.11	.18	.17	−.07
Sociability	.14	−.23*	.10	−.02	.15	.21*
Frequency of upset ...	.02	−.14	−.02	.00	.13	−.27*
Intensity of upset	.22*	−.18	.21*	−.15	.08	−.08
Recovery from upset ..	−.15	.12	−.21*	.03	−.08	−.06
Anger	.28*	−.19	.11	.17	.18	−.05
Fear	−.01	.07	.06	−.01	.12	.04

* $p < .05$.

older sibling, and maternal behavior (direct) to younger sibling. The results indicate that maternal behavior correlated with the dimensions of the sibling relationship, primarily as assessed in the videotaped settings. Interestingly, differential maternal behavior yielded a different pattern of associations with sibling relationships than did maternal behavior directed toward each child. As predicted, maternal differential behavior was associated with more conflictual sibling relationships. Maternal differential responsiveness was positively correlated with the sibling dyad's competition and control in the videotaped settings and negatively correlated with the positive scale from the maternal interview. Differential maternal control and differential attention were positively associated with the dyad's competition and differential maternal affection with the siblings' control in the videotaped situation. Affection and responsiveness as direct rather than differential measures of maternal behavior were not related to the sibling measures. However, maternal control to both the older and younger sibling and maternal attention to the younger sibling were significantly positively related to the dyad's control and competition in the video settings.

Correlations between Siblings' Temperamental Characteristics and the Sibling Relationship Measures

The Pearson product-moment correlations between children's temperamental characteristics and the sibling relationship measures are presented in Table 2. Temperament was also associated with the quality of the sibling relationship, although the associations differed for the older and younger siblings. Older siblings' shyness was correlated with less controlling and competitive sibling relationships as assessed in the video setting. Younger siblings' sociability was associated with less cooperation in the video settings but with a more positive relationship as observed in the unstructured situation. Younger siblings' anger and intensity of emotion were associated with more competitive sibling relationships in the video settings. Younger siblings' intensity of emotional upset was positively correlated, and their speed of recovery from upset was negatively correlated, with control in the video settings. Their activity was associated with a more competitive relationship in the video settings and a more negative relationship as described by the mother. For older siblings, frequency of emotional upset was associated with a more negative relationship as described by the mother, and for both older and younger siblings it was negatively correlated with the positive scale from the unstructured observation. Finally, older siblings' speed of recovery from emotional upset and fear were positively associated with the negative scale from the maternal interview. The pattern of correlations between temperament and the sibling relationship measures differed slightly for boys and girls, but these differences were not above a chance level of occurrence.

TABLE 3

Correlations Between Siblings' Age, Family Structure Variables, and Sibling Relationship Measures

MEASURES OF THE SIBLING RELATIONSHIP

	Video Settings			Maternal Interview		Unstructured
	Competition	Cooperation	Control	Positive	Negative	Positive
Sibling age:						
Older sibling	−.32*	.17	−.19	−.24*	−.18	.28*
Younger sibling	−.39*	.39*	−.27*	.01	−.35*	.09
Family structure:						
Adoptive status	−.00	−.02	.05	.13	−.14	.03
Gender composition	−.21*	−.04	−.23*	.24*	.04	.06
Age difference	−.10	−.04	−.02	−.26*	.01	.25*

* p < .05.

Correlations between Siblings' Age and the Sibling Relationship Measures

The correlations presented in Table 3 show that, in general, older, second-born children had more positive and less negative sibling relationships than second-born children who were younger. Younger siblings' age was negatively correlated with the sibling pair's competition and control and positively correlated with their cooperation in the videotaped settings. Mothers rated younger second-borns' sibling relationships more negatively than older second-borns'. In addition, older siblings' age was positively correlated with the positive scale from the unstructured observation and negatively related to both competition in the videotaped settings and the positive maternal interview scale.

Correlations between Family Structure Variables and the Sibling Relationship Measures

Table 3 also shows that there were no significant relations between adoptive status and any of the sibling relationship measures. Same-gender pairs were less controlling and competitive in the video settings and were described by their mothers as having a more positive relationship than mixed-gender pairs. Siblings with larger age spacing had less positive relationships as assessed by the maternal interview but were observed to be more positive than pairs with small age spacing in the unstructured situation.

Multivariate Analyses of the Correlates of Sibling Relationships

Because the interpretation of these univariate associations is complicated by overlap among the predictor variables, two types of multiple regression analyses were conducted. The first type examined the variance in sibling relationships that could be explained *jointly* by maternal behavior, child temperament, siblings' age, and family structure variables. The second type examined the unique variance in the sibling relationship measures accounted for by each of the four sets of predictors (see Cohen & Cohen, 1975).

Variance in the sibling relationship measures explained jointly by maternal behavior, child temperament, sibling age, and family structure variables. Preliminary multiple regression analyses were conducted to select variables from the maternal behavior and child temperament domains that independently added to the prediction of the sibling relationship variables. For example, the 12 maternal variables were entered into stepwise multiple regression analyses to predict each of the six sibling relationship measures. With this procedure, three maternal variables were retained for further analysis of Competition, four for Control, and three for Cooperation. The

TABLE 4
Variance in Sibling Relationship Measures Explained by Maternal Behavior, Child Temperament, Age, and Family Structure Variables

MEASURES OF THE SIB RELATIONSHIP	R^2	F	df	Maternal Behavior	Change in R^2	Child Temperament	Change in R^2	Child Age	Change in R^2	Family Structure[a]	Change in R^2
Video setting:											
Competition ..	.40*	10.72	5,82	Differential responsiveness (+) Control to older sib (+)	13*	Older sib shyness (−) Younger sib recovery from upset (−)	.09*	Younger sib age (−)	.10*		
Cooperation ..	.22*	6.02	4,83	Differential affection (−)	.01	Younger sib sociability (−) Younger sib intensity of upset (−)	.06*	Younger sib age (+)	.12*		
Control	.39*	7.29	7,79	Differential responsiveness (+) Control to older sib (+)	.14*	Younger sib recovery from upset (−) Older sib anger (−) Older sib shyness (−)	.12*	Younger sib age (−)	.02	Gender composition (−)	.03
Maternal interview:											
Positive	.22*	3.84	6,82	Differential responsiveness (−)	.07*	Younger sib anger (+) Younger sib intensity of upset (−) Older sib fear (+)	.05	Older sib age (−)	.05*	Gender composition (+)	.03
Negative	.30*	6.65	5,79	Differential responsiveness (−) Differential affection (+)	.09*	Older sib recovery from upset (+)	.09*	Younger sib age (−)	.08*	Adoptive status (−)	.04
Unstructured positive	.27*	5.98	5,82	Differential affection (+) Differential attention (−)	.04	Older sib frequency of upset (−) Younger sib frequency of upset (−)	.15*			Age spacing (+)	.07*

[a] Adoptive status, gender composition, age spacing.
* $p < .05$.

same procedure was used to select temperament variables; between three and five were retained for analyses of the sibling relationship measures.

Next, the selected child temperament and maternal behavior variables were included in a multiple regression together with older siblings' age, younger siblings' age, and the family structure variables of adoptive status, age spacing, and gender composition. Table 4 indicates which variables in combination most parsimoniously predicted the sibling relationship measures as well as the amount of variance that they explained. For example, the first entry in Table 4 indicates that from the three maternal behavior variables, four temperament variables, two sibling age variables, and three family structure variables entered, 40% of the variance in siblings' competition was explained by a combination of two maternal behavior variables, two child temperament variables, and younger siblings' age. The positive or negative sign for each predictor indicates the direction of its relation with the sibling relationship measures.

Table 4 shows that between 22% and 40% of the variance in the different measures of the sibling relationship was explained by combinations of temperament, maternal behavior, children's age, and family structure variables; the variables were effective in accounting for the variance in measures of the relationship from each of the three sources—videotaped settings, maternal interview, and unstructured observation.

Maternal behavior, especially differential responsiveness and affection and control direct to the older sibling, predicted more negative and less positive sibling relationships. Both siblings' frequency of upset and younger siblings' intensity of upset were associated with less positive and more conflictual sibling relationships. Older siblings' shyness and younger siblings' speed of recovery from upset predicted less conflictual sibling relationships in the video settings. Younger siblings' age predicted less conflictual and more cooperative relationships in the videotaped settings and more positive maternal interview ratings.

Variance in the sibling relationship explained uniquely by mother behavior, child temperament, sibling age, and family structure variables. We next compared the independent contribution of the four sets of predictors. In four separate hierarchical multiple regression analyses, each set of predictors was added after the other three in order to determine the unique variance it contributed to the prediction of sibling relationships.

The results in Table 4 show that both maternal behavior and child temperament added unique variance to the prediction of most sibling relationship measures. On average, child temperament explained an additional 9% of the variance after maternal behavior, siblings' age, and family structure were entered into the hierarchical multiple regression. Maternal behavior independently added 8% to the prediction of sibling relationship measures on average. Younger siblings' age also added independently to the variance in the sibling dyad's Competition and Cooperation in the video setting and in maternal reports of negative interaction. Older siblings' age added uniquely to the variance of only one measure, the positive scale from the maternal interview. Family structure variables also were significant for one sibling relationship measure. Sibling pairs with a large age gap were more positive in the unstructured observation than those with a small age gap.

DISCUSSION

Differences in sibling relationships can, to a significant extent, be accounted for by maternal behavior, children's temperamental characteristics, their age, and family structure variables. Our results confirmed the findings of previous studies showing connections between differential parental behavior and conflictual sibling relationships (Brody et al., 1987; Bryant & Crockenberg, 1980; Daniels et al., 1985; Hetherington, 1988; McHale & Gamble, 1987). As in Bryant and Crockenberg's and Brody et al.'s studies, most mothers directed more affection, attention, control, and responsiveness to the younger sibling than to the older sibling. Therefore, it should not be assumed that in families in which mothers direct more behavior to the older sibling, sibling relationships are also more conflictual. The evidence that maternal differential behavior is a powerful predictor of sibling relationships provides important support for the significance of nonshared environment for children's development (Plomin & Daniels, 1987). However, the causal direction of the connections remains unclear. Maternal behavior may be a consequence of the negative relationship between the siblings rather than a cause. Longitudinal analyses are under way that will help to clarify the direction of effects.

Evidence that children's temperamental characteristics accounted for a significant percent of the unique variance in sibling relationships measures highlights the importance of taking account of children's individual characteristics when assessing their dyadic relationships (Stevenson-Hinde & Hinde, 1986). Different dimensions of temperament in older and younger siblings were associated with the relationship measures.

Younger siblings' age added notably to the prediction of the siblings' relationship in the videotaped structured settings. Sibling dyads that included an older second-born were more cooperative and less conflictual than those with a younger second-born, perhaps because some younger second-born children had difficulty participating in the marble-pull games and were likely to become upset. While these age effects may partly reflect the constraints of the structured settings, mothers also rated sibling relationships with an older second-born as less negative than those with a younger second-born, suggesting that the behavior is not limited to these specific settings.

In the structured and unstructured observations, older firstborns were less competitive and more positive than younger firstborns despite mothers' reports to the contrary. A similar discrepancy was found for age spacing. These results may be spurious, or mothers may have higher expectations for older children and judge their behavior more harshly than younger firstborns' behavior. It is also possible that older firstborns were particularly aware of the observer's presence and behaved more kindly than usual to their sibling during the observation.

There was no evidence that adoptive status affected the quality of siblings' relationships in families in which both siblings were adopted. This is important information for adoptive parents who may fear that their children might be less close than siblings in nonadoptive families. However, future research should explore the possibility of interaction effects between adoptive status and other family structure variables.

In conclusion, then, the study suggests that to understand siblings' relationships we need to focus both on characteristics of the children within the relationship and on children's relationships with other family members. Caution must be exercised in generalizing the results: our sample was limited to intact Caucasian families, and thus may not speak to the correlates of sibling relationships in other types of families. Future research should investigate links between children's relationships with their siblings and both their mothers and fathers to consider, for instance, whether differential paternal and maternal behavior have similar effects or complement or confound each other. It will be important, too, to examine whether the correlates of siblings' relationships found in early and middle childhood remain stable as children grow toward adolescence. More research is clearly needed; nevertheless, the results provide an encouraging first step toward understanding a relationship that is for most individuals the longest lasting in their lives.

REFERENCES

Abramovitch, R., Pepler, D., & Corter, C. (1982). Patterns of sibling interaction among preschool-age children. In M. E. Lamb & B. Sutton-Smith (Eds.), *Sibling relationships: Their nature and significance across the lifespan* (pp. 61–86). Hillsdale, NJ: Erlbaum.

Beardsall, L. (1987). *Sibling conflict in middle childhood.* Unpublished doctoral dissertation, University of Cambridge, Cambridge.

Brody, G., Stoneman, Z., & Burke, M. (1987). Child temperaments, maternal differential behavior, and sibling relationships. *Developmental Psychology, 23*, 354–362.

Brody, G., Stoneman, Z., & MacKinnon, C. (1982). Role asymmetries in interactions among school-aged children, their younger siblings and their friends. *Child Development, 53*, 1364–1370.

Bryant, B., & Crockenberg, S. (1980). Correlations and dimensions of prosocial behavior: A study of female siblings and their mothers. *Child Development, 51*, 354–362.

Buss, A., & Plomin, R. (1984). *Temperament: Early developing personality traits.* Hillsdale, NJ: Erlbaum.

Cicirelli, V. (1972). The effect of the sibling relationship on concept learning of young children taught by child teachers. *Child Development, 43*, 282–287.

Clifford, E. (1959). Discipline in the home: A controlled study of parental practices. *Journal of Genetic Psychology,* **95**, 45–82.

Cohen, J., & Cohen, P. (1975). *Applied multiple regression/correlation analysis for the behavioral sciences.* Hillsdale, NJ: Erlbaum.

Daniels, D., Dunn, J., Furstenberg, F., & Plomin, R. (1985). Environmental differences within the family and adjustment differences within pairs of adolescent siblings. *Child Development,* **56**, 764–774.

Dunn, J. (1983). Sibling relationships in early childhood. *Child Development,* **54**, 787–811.

Dunn, J. (1988). *The beginnings of social understanding.* Cambridge, MA: Harvard University Press.

Dunn, J., & Kendrick, C. (1982). *Siblings: Love, envy and understanding.* Cambridge, MA: Harvard University Press.

Dunn, J., & Munn, P. (1985). Becoming a family member: Family conflict and the development of social understanding in the second year. *Child Development,* **56**, 480–492.

Dunn, J., & Munn, P. (1986a). Sibling quarrels and maternal intervention: Individual differences in understanding and aggression. *Journal of Child Psychology and Psychiatry,* **27**, 583–595.

Dunn, J., & Munn, P. (1986b). Siblings and the development of prosocial behavior. *International Journal of Behavioral Development,* **9**, 265–284.

Dunn, J., & Munn, P. (1988). *Temperament and the developing relationship between young siblings.* Manuscript submitted for publication.

Dunn, J., & Plomin, R. (1986). Determinants of maternal behavior toward three-year-old siblings. *British Journal of Developmental Psychology,* **4**, 127–137.

Dunn, J., Stocker, C., & Plomin, R. (1988). *Assessing the relationship between young siblings.* Manuscript submitted for publication.

Furman, W., & Buhrmester, D. (1985). Children's perception of the qualities of sibling relationships. *Child Development,* **56**, 448–461.

Gottman, J. M. (1983). How children become friends. *Monographs of the Society for Research in Child Development,* **48**(3, Serial No. 201).

Graziano, W., French, D., Brownell, C., & Hartup, W. W. (1976). Peer interaction in same- and mixed-aged triads in relation to chronological age and incentive condition. *Child Development,* **47**, 707–714.

Hetherington, E. M. (1988). Parents, children and siblings six years after divorce. In R. A. Hinde & J. Stevenson-Hinde (Eds.), *Relations among relationships* (pp. 311–331). Oxford: Oxford University Press.

Howe, N. (1986). *Socialization, social cognitive factors and the development of the sibling relationship.* Unpublished doctoral dissertation, University of Waterloo, Waterloo, Canada.

Koch, H. L. (1960). The relation of certain formal attributes of siblings to their attitudes held towards each other and towards their parents. *Monographs of the Society for Research in Child Development,* **24**(4, Serial No. 78).

Madsen, W. C., & Kagan, S. (1973). Mother-directed achievement of children in two cultures. *Journal of Cross-cultural Psychology,* **4**, 221–228.

McHale, S. M., & Gamble, W. C. (1987). Sibling relationships and adjustment of children with disabled brothers and sisters. *Journal of Children in Contemporary Society,* **19**, 131–158.

Minnett, A., Vandell, D., & Santrock, J. (1983). Effects of sibling status on sibling interaction. *Child Development,* **54**, 1064–1072.

Newson, J., & Newson, E. (1970). *Four years old in an urban community.* Harmondsworth: Penguin.

Plomin, R., & Daniels, D. (1987). Why are children in the same family so different from one another? *Behavioral and Brain Sciences,* **10**, 1–16.

Plomin, R., DeFries, J. C., & Fulker, D. W. (1988). *Nature and nurture in infancy and early childhood.* New York: Cambridge University Press.

Stevenson-Hinde, J., & Hinde, R. A. (1986). Changes in associations between characteristics and interactions. In R. Plomin & J. Dunn (Eds.), *The study of temperament: Changes, continuities and challenges* (pp. 115–129). Hillsdale, NJ: Erlbaum.

Stewart, R. B., Mobley, L. A., Van Tuyl, S. S., & Salvador, M. A. (1987). The firstborn's adjustment to the birth of a sibling: A longitudinal assessment. *Child Development,* **58**, 341–355.

13

Working Mothers and Their Families

Sandra Scarr and Deborah Phillips
University of Virginia
Kathleen McCartney
University of New Hampshire

The topic of maternal employment and its effects on the family is receiving considerable attention as more and more mothers enter the work force when their children are very young. This article reviews the effects of mothers' employment on marital relations, on the development of their children, and on mothers themselves. Research shows that maternal employment per se is not the major issue in either marital relations or child development. Rather, the circumstances of the family, the attitudes and expectations of fathers and mothers, and the distribution of time available have important effects. The needs of working mothers for social supports, such as parental leave, spouse support, child care, and better wages are considered.

"A woman's work is never done," or so goes the old adage about women's responsibilities to the home. Women who are mothers of babies and young children spend even more hours on their family roles than do non-mothers or mothers with older children. If one adds to home care and motherhood full-time employment in the labor force, a mother's job requires 50% more hours than that of working fathers and single people without children (Nock & Kingston, in press; Rexroat & Shehan, 1987).

Women all over the world work longer hours than men (Tavris & Wade, 1984). Mothers work longer hours than anyone else because their family responsibilities to household and children are not equally shared by fathers—anywhere. In industrialized countries, whether in the Western or Eastern worlds, mothers do the majority of the shopping, house cleaning, cooking, laundry and child care, in addition to their paid employment. Whereas fathers in these societies work an average of

Reprinted with permission from *American Psychologist*, 1989, Vol. 44, No. 11, 1402–1409. Copyright © 1989 by the American Psychological Association, Inc.

50 hours per week in combined employment and household work, mothers work an average of 80 hours per week at the same tasks (Cowan, 1983).

The degree to which most fathers do not share the family work with their wives is vividly demonstrated by Rexroat and Shehan (1987) in a study of 1,618 White couples from the 1976 wave of the Panel Study of Income Dynamics. Whereas in the case of childless working couples and empty nesters, wives worked an average of 5 to 9 hours more per week than their husbands in combined employment and housework, in families with infants and preschool children, mothers worked 16 to 24 hours more per week than did fathers. The actual total hours per week worked by employed mothers of children under age three was 90!

Despite the enormous number of hours worked by most mothers in the world, the self-reports of mothers who are also employees demonstrate that their multiple roles are often not experienced as more stressful than the lives experienced by women with fewer roles and obligations (Crosby, 1987). These seemingly contradictory observations of actual workload and self-perceptions of well-being need to be resolved (Coleman, Antonucci, & Adelmann, 1987; Gove & Zeiss, 1987). Either the Puritans were right that hard work is good for the soul, or there is some self-selection of healthy women into complicated and demanding roles (Epstein, 1987; Reppetti, Matthews & Waldron, pp. 1394–1401).

In this article, we consider the implications of parental, particularly maternal, employment for family relationships and family well-being. Other articles in this Public Forum section take up the effects of women's employment on the physical and mental health of both mothers and non-mothers.

WHY DO MOTHERS WORK?

Most women in the labor force work primarily because the family needs the money and secondarily for their own personal self-actualization. Because of the decline in real family income from 1973 to 1988 (Congressional Budget Office, 1988), most families find it essential for both parents to work to support them at a level that used to be achieved by one wage-earner, and in many families two earners are required to keep the family out of poverty. Most divorced, single, and widowed mothers must work to avoid poverty.

However, most would not leave their paid employment, even if the family did not need the money (DeChick, 1988). Indeed, 56% of full-time homemakers say that they would choose to have a career if they had it to do all over again, and only 21% of working mothers would leave their current jobs to stay at home with the children (DeChick, 1988). Professional career women are a small but vocal minority of women who value the social and political equality of women's employment, and their endorsement of mothers' employment is consistent with their position. Surveys of working class mothers, with jobs as waitresses, factory workers, and domestics, show that these women are quite committed to their jobs (Hiller & Dyehouse, 1987), satisfied with their diverse roles, and would not leave the labor force even if they did not need the money. The social psychology of the workplace, with its social support, adult companionship, and contacts with the larger world, may explain the phenomenon (Repetti, Matthews, & Waldron, this issue). Like most men, most women want to participate in the larger society.

Several recent studies of mothers of newborns and infants show that returning to work soon after a birth is primarily a function of previously high involvement in the labor force and positive attitudes about mothers' employment, even among families who are economically marginal (Avioli, 1985; Greenstein, 1986; Pistrang, 1984). Mothers who are not employed during their child's infancy are less likely to have been employed prior to the birth and are more likely to have negative attitudes about maternal employment, regardless of the economic situation of the family. For more affluent mothers, attitudes carried more weight than any other factor (Greenstein, 1986). Thus, economic necessity may propel most women into the labor force, but other factors entice them to reenter after having a baby and to stay employed.

Regardless of the reasons, working mothers are here to stay. The Department of Labor projects that by 1995 roughly two thirds of all new labor force entrants will be women (Johnston, 1987), and 80% of those in their childbearing years are expected to have children during their work life. Yet, we as a nation are still ambivalent about mothers who work and whose children's care is delegated to others, and about their diminished time for responsibilities to husbands whose careers are generally presumed to be preeminent.

The major issues discussed in this article are the impact of mothers' employment on their marital relationships and on their children.

WORKING MOTHERS' MARITAL RELATIONSHIPS

Like other adults, mothers vary in their career ambitions, their sex-role expectations, and the degree to which they receive spousal support for their employment. Many reviews of research on mothers' employment show that such mediating factors are crucial to interpreting any effects of maternal employment on family relationships (Anderson-Kulman & Paludi, 1986; Locksley, 1980; Simpson & England, 1982; Smith, 1985). For women, spousal support is a key to the success of dual-career families; it is not maternal employment per se that affects marital satisfaction, but "the law of husband cooperation" (Bernard, 1974, p. 162). Husband cooperation includes positive attitudes toward maternal employment and cooperation with household and child care tasks (Bernardo, Shehan, & Leslie, 1987; Gilbert, 1985, 1988). Mothers who receive little or no spouse support, in either attitudes toward their employment or in participation in child care and household tasks, are indeed stressed by their multiple roles (Anderson-Kulman & Paludi, 1986; Pleck, 1985).

Mothers who receive a great deal of positive spouse support feel positive about their spouses and their lives. For mothers, the quality of their roles matters more than how many or how seemingly stressful they are (Baruch & Barnett, 1987).

Husbands' appreciation for and enjoyment of their wives' employment depended both on their degree of participation in family affairs and on their own perceptions of work and family life (Pleck, 1985; Simpson & England, 1982). Gilbert (1985) found that men with children in dual-career families can be classified as traditional, participant, and role-sharing, depending on the degree to which they share household and child-care responsibilities.[1] Men who participate more in the family claim to be content with, even proud of, their wives employment (Wortman, 1987), but outside pressures also affect their support of their wives' careers.

> The responses from men in the study indicate that for men who do experience role conflict, the tension often centers around wanting to support their spouses' career aspirations and to be involved in parenting and household roles while at the same time wanting to have their own career aspirations put first. Being highly competitive, experiencing high work demands, and working in an environment hostile to men's involvement in family roles . . . all contribute to the tension. (Gilbert, 1985, p. 104)

For dual-career parents, their satisfactions as couples often depend on their socialization experiences and current attitudes about male and female roles (Aldous, 1982; Pepitone-Rockwell, 1980). Role-sharing and participatory men are more likely to see maternal employment as opportunities for the wife to have greater independent identity, more social interaction, and greater intellectual companionship, opportunities that are less often cited by traditional men. Because of their more egalitarian beliefs about gender roles and women's rights, such fathers appreciate and applaud their wives' careers, even though they also perceive family costs.

Costs of maternal employment more often cited by nontraditional men include decreased leisure time, increased time spent on household tasks, and decreased sexual activity due to fatigue and lack of time (Gilbert, 1985; Voyandoff & Kelly, 1984). Traditional arrangements in which the father is less involved with child care and household responsibilities have some perceived advantages for fathers, but even traditional men acknowledge the contribution of maternal employment to increased family income. That they do not share family responsibilities has a negative effect on wives' perceptions of the marital relationship, but not evidently on theirs (Bernardo et al., 1987; Gilbert, 1988; Pleck, 1985).

---

[1]Traditional husbands do little to support their wives' employment by participating in family affairs. Participatory fathers take some responsibility for child care but do not do household chores. Role-sharing husbands take more responsibility for both children and home, but few (even in the university community studied) were found to share equally with the wife.

The costs and benefits of maternal employment have a positive balance for both husbands and wives in most working families (see Crosby, 1987; Gilbert, 1985; Wortman, 1987). Satisfactions and dissatisfactions of marital partners depend on attitudes toward gender roles and the degree to which they can manage time and effort (Voyandoff & Kelly, 1984). For mothers, satisfactions also depend on spouse support for their household and maternal roles and on their work commitment prior to becoming mothers; mothers with previously high work commitments who stay home for five or more months after a birth report greater irritability, greater depression, decreased marital intimacy, and lower self-esteem than mothers with previously low work commitments (Pistrang, 1984). For men, satisfactions depend primarily on the degree to which they are inconvenienced by maternal employment in exchange for larger family income (Gilbert, 1985, 1988).

MATERNAL EMPLOYMENT AND CHILD DEVELOPMENT

National concerns about the possible plight of children of working mothers prompted a large review of research in 1982 by the National Academy of Sciences (Kamerman & Hayes, 1982). A distinguished panel of social scientists reviewed all of the evidence and concluded that there were no consistent effects of maternal employment on child development. Rather, they said, maternal employment cannot have a single set of consistent effects on children because mothers work for various reasons and begin or interrupt work when their children are at various ages; furthermore, their employment is in contexts of various families and communities that support or do not support mothers' multiple roles.

Lois Hoffman (1984) reviewed 50 years of research on maternal employment, most of it predicated on the assumption that maternal employment should have negative effects on child development. Indeed, some of the investigators found that young sons were slightly disadvantaged by the loss of maternal attention in the early years. Of course, they were presumably in some form of day care, which may not have been of high quality.

Her reexamination of the data showed that daughters of employed mothers were often reported to be more self-confident, to achieve better grades in school, and to more frequently pursue careers themselves than were the daughters of nonemployed mothers. Whereas most sons had role models of competent, employed fathers, daughters of employed mothers also had such a model of achievement. Hoffman also noted that few investigators asked how maternal employment could benefit children by higher family income, higher self-esteem for mothers, a less sharp distinction between male and female roles, and a more positive role model for both sons and daughters for later in their own lives (Gottfried & Gottfried, 1987; Weinraub, Jaeger, & Hoffman, 1988).

When both parents in families with preschool children are employed, the fathers *do not* spend significantly more time on child care or household chores than do fathers in single-earner families (Bernardo et al., 1987; Nock & Kingston, in press). In fact, employed mothers also reduce their household work hours, primarily in categories of homemaking chores, rather than in child care activities (Nock & Kingston, in press). Thus, when both parents of preschool children are employed, both fathers and mothers spend about the same total amount of time in direct interaction with their children as do parents in families in which only fathers are employed. The biggest differences between the two-earner and one-earner families with preschool children are the distribution of time spent with children on weekdays versus weekends and in time spent on non-child care chores (Nock & Kingston, in press). Both parents in one-earner families have more leisure time for themselves.

Differences between one-earner and two-earner families with school-age children and adolescents are less pronounced but also involve a decrease in the amount of time spent on homemaking chores, for both employed fathers and mothers (Nock & Kingston, in press).

All in all, the question of what effects (if any) maternal employment has on children is not a productive one because it ignores the many contextual features of family life that moderate the effects of maternal employment (Grossman, Pollack, & Golding, 1988). We do know that

> the straightforward results of bad emotional, social, and intellectual outcomes for children of working mothers were not found, but no research can rule out yet unstudied subtleties. All we know is that the school achievement, IQ test scores, and emotional and social development of working mothers' children are every bit as good as that of children whose mothers do not work. (Scarr, 1984, p. 25)

WORKING FAMILIES AND CHILD CARE

Child care is *not* a women's issue; it is a family issue. However, the lack of high-quality, affordable child care has more impact on working mothers than on any others. Not only is there a critical shortage of high-quality child care in this country, but there also is such ambivalence about providing child care that we have a shameful national dilemma: More than 50% of American mothers of infants and preschool children are now in the labor force and require child care services, but there is no coherent national policy on parental leaves or on child care services for working parents.

With the exception of federal child care provided during the Great Depression and World War II, public provision of child care has been reserved for nonmainstream, generally poor families (Phillips & Zigler, 1987; Steinfels, 1973). Day care began in settlement houses in the 1850s for poor mothers who had to work because their husbands were inadequate providers or because they were not married. Early education, on the other hand, was begun by middle and upper class mothers who sponsored nursery schools and kindergartens to give their advantaged children good social and intellectual experiences (Scarr & Weinberg, 1986).

Today, the historical split between early education and day care is no longer tenable. Middle and upper class women have the same needs for work-related, full-day child care as do minority, poor, and single mothers. As of 1986, 51% of married mothers and 49% of single mothers were working (Kahn & Kamerman, 1987). Similarly, by 1985, 62% of both Black and White young children had working mothers. As a consequence, high rates of employment are now common to mothers of all races and marital statuses.

In sum, working mothers have become an everyday part of children's lives, of family life, and of our economic structure (Scarr, Phillips, & McCartney, 1988). Prior distinctions in the degree of child care use by children of different ages and in patterns of use by women with different demographic characteristics have merged into a universal pattern of extensive use. However, even this extensive, mainstream reliance on child care has not ensured that the child care needs of working families are adequately addressed (Hewlett, 1986; McCartney & Phillips, 1989). Kahn and Kamerman (1987) estimated that direct federal funding for child care programs actually decreased by 18% in real dollars between 1980 and 1986.

HOW DOES THE UNITED STATES COMPARE?

The U.S. policies on child care and maternal leaves are an anomaly among industrialized countries. The United States, among 100 countries, is the sole exception to the rule of providing paid, job-protected maternal leaves as national policy (Kamerman, 1986, 1989). Only five states require employers to provide temporary disability insurance, and federal law requires that pregnant women be eligible for these disability benefits. Even among private businesses that provide maternity benefits, this generally means an unpaid leave with no guarantee of reinstatement.

All other industrialized countries have some maternal leave policy. Sweden has one of the most extensive policies: Mothers and fathers have the right to a leave following childbirth that is paid at 90% of one parent's wages for 9 months, followed by a fixed minimum benefit for 3 additional months. Swedish parents may also take an unpaid, but job-protected, leave until their child is 18 months old and may work a six-hour day until their child is eight years old. In Italy, women are entitled to a 6-month job-protected leave, paid at a flat rate equal to the average wage for women workers. At the conclusion of this period, an unpaid, job-protected leave is also available for one year. In France, a job-protected maternity leave of 6 weeks before childbirth and 10 weeks after is provided.

Other countries also have much more systematic child care policies in conjunction with parental leave policies. As of 1986, Sweden had placed 38% of preschoolers with working mothers in subsidized child care programs (Leijon, 1986). France, Italy, Spain, and all of the Eastern European countries have more than half of their infants, toddlers, and preschool children in subsidized child care because their mothers are in the labor force. France, for example, maintains a system of preschools, open to all children two to six years old, and partially subsidized care is available for children under age two. Comparable figures concerning children in subsidized child care in the United States are not available, itself a sign of inattention.

WHY THE POLICY GAP?

Cherished beliefs about maternal care have led us historically as a nation to favor marginal support for mothers to stay home with their babies, through paternal employment and through Aid to Families with Dependent Children (AFDC), rather than support for women's attainment of economic independence. Until the last few years, when employment and training opportunities for women on AFDC were begun as an experiment in several states, poor women with young children had no option but to accept the degradation of poverty-on-the-dole. Now poor mothers are captives of a system that is moving from AFDC to Workfare, which, even in the best of circumstances, does not sustain support for child care for more than one year after these mothers achieve the minimum-wage jobs for which they are being trained.

Working parents need options. One option currently under congressional consideration is an *unpaid* parental (read that as 95% maternal)[2] leave. Many mothers cannot afford to take months off from their jobs, especially without pay; unpaid leaves for divorced and single mothers and for women married to men who earn the minimum wage are not very useful.

Even among mothers who can afford the unpaid leaves, not all *want* to be away from their careers for more than a few months after the birth of a child. Upon serious and honest reflection, they consider themselves to be better parents when they work and mother, rather than attempt only one role, or their careers are such that there are professional costs for taking four to six months out of the office. These women do not want extended maternal leaves; they want high-quality child care, and some want fulfilling, well-compensated, part-time work opportunities.

Policies that create strong incentives for mothers to stay at home for extended periods or that require them to go to work soon after a birth are based on conflicting assumptions about the nature of women's participation in the society and assumptions about infants' needs. There are many reasons that most women would prefer to remain in close contact with their newborns. For one, many women need a rest period after a birth, especially if the pregnancy or the birth was difficult. For

---

[2]Sweden pays parents 90% of their salaries for one parent to take off nine months with a new infant. In practice, 95% of the leave is taken by mothers, even though there is an additional incentive for the parents to share the leave time with the baby.

another, many new mothers need two or more months to establish reliable breast-feeding and to allow their babies to settle into a reasonably predictable routine. How long should a maternal leave be for either the mother's or the infant's benefit? Neither a mandatory child care nor a mandatory maternal leave policy suits all families. What we need are equally attractive options so that families can choose how best either to take advantage of quality child care while parents work or to arrange an extended leave for parents, usually the mother, to care for the baby. Still, many families (and policymakers) suffer great guilt and anxiety about mothers' return to work and placing infants and toddlers in child care. Psychological research has addressed their fears.

EFFECTS OF CHILD CARE ON CHILDREN

In psychological research, child care is often treated as a uniform arrangement that can be objectively characterized as "nonmaternal care" by investigators who in fact rarely study child care settings. By the same illogic, "home care" is treated uniformly as though all families were alike and is assumed to be preferred to other child care arrangements. Child care settings vary from babysitters in one's own home, to family day care in another's home, to centers that care for more than 100 infants and young children. The quality of these settings varies enormously in terms of their abilities to promote children's development and to provide support for working parents. Families also vary from abusive and neglectful of children's needs to supportive and loving systems that promote optimal development. So it is with other child care settings.

Recent reviews of the child care literature by psychologists of different theoretical persuasions agree that high-quality child care has no detrimental effects on intellectual or language development (Belsky, 1986; Clarke-Stewart, 1989; Scarr et al., 1988). In fact, high-quality day care settings have been shown to compensate for poor family environments (Ramey, Bryant, & Suarez, 1985) and to promote better intellectual and social development than children would have experienced in their own homes. The media and parents are most concerned about the possible effects of child care on attachments of infants to their mothers and on children's possible social deviance. The earliest research questioned whether child caregivers replaced mothers as children's primary attachment figure. Concerns that daily separations from mother might weaken the mother–child bond were a direct heritage of the work on children in orphanages (e.g., Spitz, 1945). Early evidence provided no suggestion that nonmaternal child care constitutes a milder form of full-time institutionalization. Attachment was not adversely affected by enrollment in the university-based child care centers that provided the early child care samples. Bonds formed between children and their caregivers did not replace the mother–child attachment relationship (Belsky & Steinberg, 1978; Etaugh, 1980; Kagan, Kearsley, & Zelazo, 1978).

Now that infant day care is the modal middle-class experience, a new debate about infant day care and attachment has arisen. The critics question whether full-time nonmaternal care in the first year of life increases the probability of insecure attachments between mothers and infants (Belsky & Rovine, 1988). Although the new literature has many limitations (Clarke-Stewart, 1989; Clarke-Stewart & Fein, 1983; McCartney & Galanopoulos, 1988; Phillips, McCartney, Scarr, & Howes, 1987; Scarr et al., 1988), there is near consensus among developmental psychologists and early childhood experts that child care per se does not constitute a risk factor in children's lives; rather, poor quality care and poor family environments can conspire to produce poor developmental outcomes (Alliance for Better Child Care, 1988; Howes, Rodning, Galluzzo, & Myers, 1988).

Research on the effects of child care on children's social development has yielded contradictory findings. Although some studies report no differences in social behavior between children with and without child care experience (Golden et al., 1978; Kagan et al., 1978), others show that children who had nonmaternal child care are more socially competent (Clarke-Stewart, 1984; Gunnarsson, 1978; Howes & Olenick, 1986; Howes & Stewart, 1987; Phillips, McCartney, & Scarr, 1987; Ruopp, Travers, Glantz, & Coelen, 1979), and others suggest lower levels of social competence (Haskins, 1985; Rubenstein, Howes, & Boyle, 1981). Positive outcomes include teacher and parent ratings of considerateness and sociability (Phillips et al., 1987), observations of compliance and self-regulation (Howes & Olenick, 1986), and observations of involvement and positive interactions with teachers (McCartney, 1984; Ruopp et al., 1979; Vandell & Powers, 1983). Haskins's (1985) study of a high-quality child care program for disadvantaged infants and preschool children found that, at kindergarten, teachers rated these children higher on scales of aggression than children with community-based child care or no nonmaternal care experience. (Behavior management training of caregivers in the day care center decreased aggression by 80% for later cohorts of children in this program; Finkelstein, 1982). However, children who spent comparable amounts of time in community-based child care programs were the least aggressive children in the study, so that the relationship of aggression to day care experience was not established.

WHAT IS QUALITY CHILD CARE?

Working parents are necessarily concerned about "what is quality?" in child care. Researchers have found that child care quality, operationalized by a number of policy-relevant variables, is important to young children's development. The most important of these factors are small child-caregiver ratio, small group size, caregiver training in child development, and stability of the child's care experience (see Bruner, 1980; Phillips, 1987; Ruopp et al., 1979; Scarr et al., 1988). These variables, in turn, appear to exert their influence by facilitating constructive and sensitive interactions among caregivers and children, which, in turn, promote positive social and cognitive development.

CONCLUDING COMMENTS

In our opinion, many of the fears about child care are not based on scientifically demonstrated facts but socially determined theories about mothers' roles and obligations to their families (Scarr et al., 1988). Of course, it is important for parents to arrange competent care for their children while they work, but it is not clear that mothers have to provide this care on a continuous basis during the entire first year, either for infants' well-being or for their own.

Critics of child care sometimes write as though working parents do not function as parents at all. For example, the term, "maternal absence," was used to describe employed mothers in the title of a recent article in the prestigious journal *Child Development* (Barglow, Vaughn, & Molitor, 1987). The terms "maternal absence" and "maternal deprivation" seem uncomfortably close to and conjure up the specter of neglected, institutionalized infants.[3] Some seem to forget that employed mothers are typically with their babies in the mornings, evenings, weekends, and holidays, which for most fully employed workers constitutes about half of the child's waking time.[4] Furthermore, when the child is ill, mothers are more likely than other family members to stay at home with the child (Hughes & Galinsky, in press).

The quality of maternal care, just like other child care arrangements, depends on many aspects of the home situation and mothers' mental health. The fantasy that mothers at home with young children provide the best possible care neglects the observation that some women at home full time are lonely, depressed, and not functioning well (see Crosby, 1987; Pistrang, 1984). Home care does not promise quality child care.

---

[3]Research on maternal deprivation reached an emotional climax in the 1950s, when Spitz (1945), Bowlby (1951), and others claimed that institutionalized infants wasted away for want of maternal care. Reanalyses of the evidence (Ernst, 1988; Yarrow, 1961) found that lack of sensory and affective stimulation in typical institutions of the day caused infants to languish both intellectually and emotionally. Longitudinal studies of institutionalized children showed that their later adjustment problems owed more to their continued deprivation throughout childhood than to deprived infant care (Ernst, 1988).

[4]Consider five working days/week for 49 weeks of the year: 1.5 hours in the morning and 3 hours of the child's waking time in the late afternoon and evening, for a sum of 4.5 of the approximately 14 hours of the child's daily waking time. The caregiver accounts for approximately 9 hours, 2 hours of which the child typically spends in a nap. (A half hour is allocated for transportation.) The sum of work week hours of parents employed full time is 1,102; for caregivers, 1,715.

To the parental sum, add weekends (2 days/work week) for 49 weeks, a sum of 1,274. To that, add three weeks of vacation time and 10 days of personal and sick leave (for self and child) during the work weeks, a sum of 455.

By these calculations, the typical, fully employed parents spend 2,831 hours with the child; caregivers spend approximately 1,715.

WORKING FAMILIES OF THE FUTURE

For the children of working families, the most pressing issue for the future is quality of care—care that will encourage and support all aspects of child development. In most cases, families will provide quality care themselves and try to buy it for their children while they work. Unfortunately, quality care costs more than inadequate care, and many parents today cannot afford good care without employer or public support.

For working parents, the most pressing family issues are shared family responsibilities, spousal support, and the affordability and availability of consistent, dependable child care. Working parents, especially mothers on whom most of the household and child care burdens fall, are constantly threatened psychologically by makeshift child care arrangements that fail unexpectedly and by the high cost of quality child care. Reluctance, even among high-income families, to hire household help means that mothers work more hours than they would need to if some income was invested in household help, rather than in consumer goods (Cowan, 1983; Scarr, 1984).

For policymakers at federal and state levels, the most pressing issues are how to fund a system of quality child care, regulate those aspects of quality that can be legislated and enforced, and coordinate efforts with the private sector and at all levels of government. If one could point to one "magic bullet" to improve the child care system in the United States, it would have to be money—more funding for every aspect of the child care system. Until the United States recognizes the rights of women to participate fully in the life of the society, through motherhood, employment, and political life, we will continue to fail to make appropriate provisions for the care of children of working families.

If statistical projections are correct, nearly 70% of mothers with infants and young children will be employed, most full-time, by the mid-1990s (Hofferth & Phillips, 1987). Such women will be devoted to their families, as they are now, but they will continue to be overworked and harassed by inadequate family supports, especially child care. One hopes that through concerted advocacy for women's rights and child care, there will be some improvements in their lives and in those of their families. Here are our suggestions:

1. Fathers should assume more personal responsibility for planning and implementing family life. At present, many fathers are willing to "fill in" or "help out" with family chores that they and the society consider the mother's responsibility. Indeed, such men are often heard to congratulate themselves on their efforts to aid their wife in her chores (Gilbert, 1985; Wortman, 1987). Fathers today "babysit" their children. Have you ever heard a mother say that she is "babysitting" her children? Even the U.S. Bureau of Census counts father-care as a form of child care alongside nonrelative care and child care centers. Attitudes must change to make the

lives of working mothers more tolerable. One would not be likely to see an article on the effects of paternal employment on marital relations and child development, unless the father were unemployed.

2. Children have traditionally been the individual responsibility of families in this society, regardless of inequities in their life chances. Children's fates have been tied exclusively to the fates of their parents, unless there were legal infractions of neglect and abuse statutes, in which case society has stepped in tentatively and temporarily. Can we not as a society recognize that children are also a community responsibility? They are the next generation for all of us, regardless of who their parents are. Many countries have family allowances that compensate parents for the extraordinary financial costs of rearing children. Child care costs can be subsidized by the society, just as public educational costs are shared by all. Few citizens today object to public support of education for children from ages 5 to 18. Why should they object to child care and early education for children from age 1 to 5?

3. We must recognize changes in American families that make sole support for children more difficult than it has been in the past. Changes in the earning capacity of service workers, who cannot support a family on a full-time job, means that most families will require more than one worker. Increasing diversity in family composition means that children will be cared for in a variety of settings that may or may not include their biological parents. Single parents, mostly mothers who have been divorced or never married, are poor and cannot pay the full costs of child care while they work. They must be subsidized for child care, or they will have to live on welfare.

4. We can encourage employers to take more responsibility for the necessary balance of family and work life of their employees. Recently, in both Britain and the United States, some companies have recognized the shrinking labor pool projected for the 1990s and proposed measures to assist working families, and thereby they have become more attractive employers (Gardner, 1988a, 1988b). Proposals include now-familiar assistance with finding child care, provision of subsidies or on-site child care, and novel approaches (for these countries) such as paid and job-guaranteed maternal leaves for extended periods. Given the opposition of the National Chamber of Commerce to even an unpaid maternal leave for only 12 weeks, these changes may not come in the foreseeable future. Federal legislation will be required for paid, extended parental or maternal leaves to become a reality for most workers.

5. In Europe, North America, and most other parts of the world, mothers are economically disadvantaged compared with men and with non-mothers, especially if they are single parents. In the United States, more than 50% of single mothers and their young children are poor; in Australia, 65% of single mothers and their children are poor. These figures compare to poverty rates for single mothers of 35% to 39% for most of Europe and only 8.6% in Sweden (Smeedling & Torrey, 1988). Poverty

rates for all families with children vary from a low of 5.1% in Sweden to a high of 17.1% in the United States (with Australia next to the bottom at 16.9%).

Employed women in the United States earn about 70% of men's wages. Even in Sweden, where women's earnings per hour are more than 90% of men's earnings, women work an average of 10 hours less per week than men and fill virtually all the part-time jobs (Leijon, 1986). Moreover, Swedish women are found in a much narrower band of occupations than are men, primarily concerned with "nursing, care, and services" (Leijon, 1986). It appears that, even when helpful options of parental leaves and subsidized child care are available, many mothers are economically disadvantaged, unless supported by a male worker. Rather than pursuing demanding, well-paid careers, they have part-time, lower status jobs. The combined responsibilities of motherhood and paid employment are an enormous burden that needs to be shared more equitably by fathers and by society as a whole.

REFERENCES

Aldous, J. (1982). *Two paychecks: Life in dual-earner families.* Beverly Hills, CA: Sage.

Alliance for Better Child Care. (1988, March). *Statement in support of the ABC Child Care Bill.* Washington, DC: Author.

Anderson-Kulman, R.E., & Paludi, M.A. (1986). Working mothers and the family context: Predicting positive coping. *Journal of Vocational Behavior, 28,* 241–253.

Avioli, P. S. (1985). The labor-force participation of married mothers of infants. *Journal of Marriage and the Family, 47,* 739–745.

Barglow, P., Vaughn, B.E., & Molitor, N. (1987). Effects of maternal absence due to employment on the quality of infant–mother attachment in a low-risk sample. *Child Development, 58,* 945–954.

Baruch, G.K., & Barnett, R.C. (1987). Role quality and psychological well-being. In F.J. Crosby (Ed.), *Spouse, parent, worker: On gender and multiple roles* (pp. 91–108). New Haven, CT: Yale University Press.

Belsky, J. (1986). Infant day care: A cause for concern? *Zero to Three, 6*(5), 1–9.

Belsky, J., & Rovine, M.J. (1988). Nonmaternal care in the first year of life and the security of infant–parent attachment. *Child Development, 59,* 157–176.

Belsky, J., & Steinberg, L.D. (1978). The effects of daycare: A critical review. *Child Development, 49,* 929–949.

Bernard, J. (1974). *The future of motherhood.* New York: Dial Press.

Bernardo, D.H., Shehan, C.L., & Leslie, G.R. (1987). A residue of tradition: Jobs, careers, and spouses' time in housework. *Journal of Marriage and the Family, 49,* 381–390.

Bowlby, J. (1951). *Maternal care and mental health.* Geneva, Switzerland: World Health Organization.

Bruner, J. (1980). *Under five in Britain.* London: Oxford University Press.

Clarke-Stewart, A. (1984). Day care: A new context for research and development. In M. Perlmutter (Ed.), *The Minnesota Symposia on Child Psychology: Vol. 17. Parent–child interaction and parent–child relations in child development* (pp. 61–100). Hillsdale, NJ: Erlbaum.

Clarke-Stewart, A. (1989). Infant day care: Malignant or maligned? *American Psychologist, 44*, 266–273.

Clarke-Stewart, A., & Fein, G. (1983). Early childhood programs. In M. Haith & J. Campos (Eds.), *Handbook of child psychology: Vol. 2. Infancy and developmental psychobiology* (pp. 917–1000). New York: Wiley.

Coleman, L.M., Antonucci, T.C., & Adelmann, P.K. (1987). Role involvement, gender, and well-being. In F.J. Crosby (Ed.), *Spouse, parent, worker: On gender and multiple roles* (pp. 138–153). New Haven, CT: Yale University Press.

Congressional Budget Office. (March 1988). *New report on family income.* Washington, DC: Author.

Cowan, R.S. (1983). *More work for mother: The ironies of household technology from the open hearth to the microwave.* New York: Basic Books.

Crosby, F.J. (Ed.). (1987). *Spouse, parent, worker: On gender and multiple roles.* New Haven, CT: Yale University Press.

DeChick, J. (1988, July 19). Most mothers want a job, too. *USA Today,* p. D1.

Epstein, C.F. (1987). Multiple demands and multiple roles: The conditions of successful management. In F.J. Crosby (Ed.), *Spouse, worker, parent: On gender and multiple roles* (pp. 23–25). New Haven, CT: Yale University Press.

Ernst, C. (1988). Are early childhood experiences overrated? A reassessment of maternal deprivation. *European Archives of Psychiatry and Neurological Sciences, 237,* 80–90.

Etaugh, C. (1980). Effects of nonmaternal care on children: Research evidence and popular views. *American Psychologist, 35,* 309–319.

Finkelstein, N. (1982). Aggression: Is it stimulated by daycare? *Young Children, 37,* 3–9.

Gardner, M. (1988a, June 9). Home with the kids—job break without penalty. *Christian Science Monitor,* p. 23.

Gardner, M. (1988b, June 30). Family-friendly corporations. *Christian Science Monitor,* p. 32.

Gilbert, L.A. (1985). *Men in dual-career families: Current realities and future prospects.* Hillsdale, NJ: Erlbaum.

Gilbert, L.A. (1988). *Sharing it all: The rewards and struggles of two-career families.* New York: Plenum Press.

Golden, M., Rosenbluth, L., Grossi, M.T., Policare, H.J., Freeman, H., Jr., & Brownlee, E.M. (1978). *The New York City Infant Day Care Study.* New York: Medical and Health Research Association of New York City.

Gottfried, A., & Gottfried, A. (Eds.). (1987). *Maternal employment and children's development: Longitudinal research.* New York: Plenum.

Gove, W.R., & Zeiss, C. (1987). Multiple roles and happiness. In F.J. Crosby (Ed.), *Spouse, parent, worker: On gender and multiple roles* (pp. 125–137). New Haven, CT: Yale University Press.

Greenstein, T.N. (1986). Social–psychological factors in perinatal labor force participation. *Journal of Marriage and the Family, 48,* 565–571.

Grossman, F.K., Pollack, W.S., & Golding, E. (1988). Fathers and children: Predicting the quality and quantity of fathering. *Developmental Psychology, 24,* 82–91.

Gunnarsson, L. (1978). *Children in day care and family care in Sweden* (Research Bulletin No. 21). Gothenburg, Sweden: University of Gothenburg.

Haskins, R. (1985). Public aggression among children with varying day care experience. *Child Development, 57,* 689–703.

Hewlett, S. (1986). *A lesser life.* New York: Morrow.

Hiller, D.V., & Dyehouse, J. (1987). A case for banishing "dual-career marriages" from the research literature. *Journal of Marriage and the Family, 49,* 787–795.

Hofferth, S.L., & Phillips, D.A. (1987). Child care in the United States, 1970 to 1995. *Journal of Marriage and the Family, 49,* 559–571.

Hoffman, L.W. (1984). Work, family, and the socialization of the child. In R. D. Parke (Ed.), *Review of child development research* (Vol. 7, pp. 223–281). Chicago: University of Chicago Press.

Howes, C., & Olenick, M. (1986). Family and child care influences on toddlers' compliance. *Child Development, 57,* 202–216.

Howes, C., Rodning, C., Galluzzo, D., & Myers, L. (1988). Attachment and child care: Relationships with mother and caregiver. *Early Childhood Research Quarterly, 3,* 403–416.

Howes, C., & Stewart, P. (1987). Child's play with adults, toys, and peers: An examination of family and child-care influences. *Developmental Psychology, 23,* 423–430.

Hughes, D., & Galinsky, E. (in press). Relationships between job characteristics, work/family interference, and marital outcomes. *Early Childhood Research Quarterly.*

Johnston, W.B. (1987). *Workforce 2000: Work and workers for the 21st century.* Indianapolis, IN: Hudson Institute.

Kagan, J., Kearsley, R.B., & Zelazo, P.R. (1978). *Infancy: Its place in human development.* Cambridge, MA: Harvard University Press.

Kahn, A.J., & Kamerman, S.B. (1987). *Child care: Facing the hard choices.* Dover, MA: Auburn House.

Kamerman, S. (1986). Maternity, paternity, and parenting policies: How does the United States compare. In S.A. Hewlett, A.S. Ilchman, & J.J. Sweeney (Eds.), *Family and work: Bridging the gap* (pp. 53–66). Cambridge, MA: Ballinger.

Kamerman, S. (1989). Child care, women, work and the family: An international overview of child care services and related policies. In J. Lande, S. Scarr, & N. Gunzenhauser (Eds.), *The future of child care in the United States* (pp. 93–110). Hillsdale, NJ: Erlbaum.

Kamerman, S., & Hayes, C.D. (Eds.). (1982). *Families that work: Children in a changing world.* Washington, DC: National Academy Press.

Leijon, A. (1986). The origins, progress, and future of Swedish family policy. In S.A. Hewlett, A.S. Illchman, & J.J. Sweeney (Eds.), *Family and work: Bridging the gap* (pp. 31–38). Cambridge, MA: Ballinger.

Locksley, A. (1980). On the effects of wives' employment on marital adjustment and companionship. *Journal of Marriage and the Family, 42,* 337–346.

McCartney, K. (1984). The effects of quality of day care environment upon children's language development. *Developmental Psychology, 20,* 244–260.

McCartney, K., & Galanopoulos, A. (1988). Child care and attachment: A new frontier the second time around. *American Journal of Orthopsychiatry, 58,* 16–24.

McCartney, K., & Phillips, D. (1989). Motherhood and child care. In B. Birns & D. Haye (Eds.), *Different faces of motherhood* (pp. 157–183). New York: Plenum.

Nock, S.L., & Kingston, P.W. (in press). Time with children: The impact of couples' worktime commitments. *Social Forces.*

Pepitone-Rockwell, F. (1980). *Dual-career couples.* Beverly Hills, CA: Sage.

Phillips, D. (Ed.). (1987). *Quality in child care: What does research tell us?* Washington, DC: National Association for the Education of Young Children.

Phillips, D., McCartney, K., & Scarr, S. (1987). Child care quality and children's social development. *Developmental Psychology, 23,* 537–543.

Phillips, D., McCartney, K., Scarr, S., & Howes, C. (1987). Selective review of infant day care research: A cause for concern! *Zero to Three,7*(1), 18–21.

Phillips, D., & Zigler, E. (1987). The checkered history of federal child care regulations. In E. Rothkops (Ed.), *Review of research in education* (pp. 3–41). Washington, DC: American Educational Research Association.

Pistrang, N. (1984). Women's work involvement and experience of new motherhood. *Journal of Marriage and the Family, 46,* 433–447.

Pleck, J.H. (1985). *Working wives/working husbands.* Beverly Hills, CA: Sage.

Ramey, C.T., Bryant, D.M., & Suarez, T.M. (1985). Preschool compensatory education and the modifiability of intelligence: A critical review. In D. Detterman (Ed.), *Current topics in human intelligence (pp. 247–296).* Norwood, NJ: Ablex.

Repetti, R.L., Matthews, K.A., & Waldron, I. (1989). Effects of paid employment on women's mental and physical health. *American Psychologist, 44,* 1394–1401.

Rexroat, C, & Shehan, C. (1987) The family life cycle and spouses' time in housework. *Journal of Marriage and the Family, 49,* 737–750.

Rubenstein, J., Howes, C., & Boyle, P. (1981). A two year follow-up of infants in community based day care. *Journal of Child Psychology and Psychiatry, 22,* 209–218.

Ruopp, R., Travers, J., Glantz, F., & Coelen, C. (1979). *Children at the center: Final results of the National Day Care Study.* Boston, MA: Abt Associates.

Scarr, S. (1984). *Mother care/other care.* New York: Basic Books.

Scarr, S., Phillips, D., & McCartney, K. (1988). *Facts, fantasies and the future of child care in America.* Unpublished manuscript.

Scarr, S., & Weinberg, R.A. (1986). The early childhood enterprise: Care and education of the young. *American Psychologist, 41,* 1140–1146.

Simpson, I.H., & England, P. (1982). Conjugal work roles and marital solidarity. In J. Aldous (Ed.), *Two paychecks: Life in dual-earner families.* Beverly Hills, CA: Sage.

Smeedling, T.M., & Torrey, B.B. (1988). Poor children in rich countries. *Science, 242,* 873–877.

Smith, D.S. (1985). Wife employment and marital adjustment: A cumulation of results. *Family Relations, 34,* 483–490.

Spitz, R. (1945). Hospitalism: An inquiry into the genesis of psychiatric conditions in early childhood. *Psychoanalytic Studies of the Child, 1,* 53–74.

Steinfels, M. (1973). *Who's minding the children: The history and politics of day care in America.* New York: Simon & Schuster.

Tavris, C., & Wade, C. (1984). *The longest war: Sex differences in perspective.* New York: Harcourt Brace Jovanovich.

Vandell, D.L., & Powers, C.P. (1983). Day care quality and children's free play activities. *American Journal of Orthopsychiatry, 53,* 493–500.

Voyandoff, P. & Kelly, R.F. (1984). *Journal of Marriage and the Family, 46,* 881–892.

Weinraub, M., Jaeger, E., & Hoffman, L. (1988). Predicting infant outcome in families of employed and non-employed mothers. *Early Childhood Research Quarterly, 3,* 361–378.

Wortman, C. (1987, October). Coping with role overload among professionals with young children. In K.P. Matthews (Chair), *Workshop on Women, Work and Health.* Workshop conducted at the meeting of the MacArthur Foundation, Hilton Head, SC.

Yarrow, L. (1961). Maternal deprivation: Toward an empirical and conceptual evaluation. *Psychological Bulletin, 58,* 459–490.

14

Family Functioning, Temperament, and Psychologic Adaptation in Children With Congenital or Acquired Limb Deficiencies

James W. Varni, Lori Ann Rubenfeld, Darlene Talbot, and Yoshio Setoguchi

University of California, Los Angeles

Family functioning and child temperament variables were investigated as predictors of psychologic and social adaptation in 42 children with congenital or acquired limb deficiencies. Higher psychologic and social adaptation were seen when there was more family cohesion and moral-religious emphasis and organization, in combination with less family conflict. With regard to child temperament, more emotionality predicted greater internalizing and externalizing behavior problems and less social competence. In addition to the main effects of the family functioning and child temperament predictor variables, the interaction between family cohesion and child emotionality significantly predicted both internalizing and externalizing behavior problems. The findings are discussed in terms of the risk and protective effects of family functioning domains and temperament on the psychologic and social adaptation of children with visible physical handicaps. Abbreviations: UCLA, University of California, Los Angeles; EAS, Emotionality, Activity, Sociability/Shyness Scales.

Limb deficiencies in children are the result of trauma, disease, and congenital causes.[1] Much of the literature on children and adolescents with limb deficiencies has focused on the problems of the amputee, whether traumatic or disease-related

Reprinted with permission from *Pediatrics,* 1989, Vol. 84, No. 2, 323–330. Copyright © 1989 by the American Academy of Pediatrics.

This research was supported by grants from the Shriners Hospitals for Crippled Children research fund and the Milo B. Brooks Foundation for Limb Difficient Children.

(e.g., osteosarcoma). Clinical observations have described children and adolescents who have suffered an amputation as a result of disease or trauma as manifesting depression, anxiety, and loss of self-esteem.[2-5] Recent research studies[6,7] have begun the empirical process of identifying the potentially modifiable predictors of the psychologic and social functioning of children with congenital or acquired limb deficiencies.

As a group, children with chronic physical handicaps have been found to be at risk for psychologic adjustment problems.[8,9] There is considerable variability in the adaptation of individual children to their physical handicap, however, with some children functioning well psychologically, whereas other children exhibit psychologic maladjustment.[8] This variance in psychologic adaptation has resulted in a search for the factors that might potentially mediate the relationship between pediatric chronic disorders and psychologic functioning.[10]

Two factors that have received increasing empirical attention as potential mediators of psychologic adaptation to pediatric chronic disorders are family functioning[11] and child temperament.[12] The family has been hypothesized as a critical determinant of the child's earliest and continuing adaptation to chronic illness and physical handicaps.[13,14] Although a rapidly growing empirical literature has generally supported the hypothesized relationship between various dimensions of family functioning and child adaptation to chronic illness and handicapping conditions, few empirical investigations exist in the published literature concerning the relationship between temperament and the psychologic adaptation of chronically ill and handicapped children.

Theoretically, a generally accepted precise definition of the temperament construct continues to elude investigators.[15] Certain common characteristics do appear to emerge from the diverse viewpoints of the major theories, however.[16] For the purposes of our study, we decided that the theoretical perspective and measurement methodology of Buss and Plomin[17] was most appropriate in testing our hypothesis. Essentially, Buss and Plomin define temperament as a set of inherited personality traits that appear early in life. They propose two defining characteristics of their temperament construct: (1) the personality traits are genetic in origin, like other psychologic and cognitive dispositions that they theorize are inherited (e.g., intelligence), and (2) the personality traits appear in infancy, more specifically, during the first year of life, which they theorize distinguishes temperament from other groups of personality traits, both inherited and acquired. Thus, Buss and Plomin have selected personality traits that they theorize appear in infancy, provide a foundation for later personality development, and exclude transient individual differences. They include inheritance as part of their definition of temperament and exclude personality traits that originate solely as a result of environmental influences.

In investigating the hypothesized relationship between temperament and child psychologic adaptation, it is essential to select an assessment instrument that measures the temperament construct while minimizing confounding with measures of psychologic adjustment.[18] Garrison and Earls[18] have concluded that, in more recent temperament questionnaires, there has been an attempt to minimize confounding by carefully wording instrument items to reflect more global behavioral patterns rather than specific psychologic or social problems. Buss and Plomin's temperament model reflects their theoretical and methodologic approach of selecting global characteristics that are theoretically inheritable and relatively stable across time. These hypothesized constitutionally based personality traits are operationally defined to measure the global behavioral patterns of emotionality, activity, and sociability/shyness. Thus, as concluded by Garrison and Earls,[18] the type of temperament assessment instrument developed by Buss and Plomin might best be used to minimize potential overlap with measures of psychologic adjustment. Therefore, from both theoretical and methodologic perspectives, the Buss and Plomin temperament model appears well suited for the purposes of predicting psychologic adaptation.

Chess and Thomas[19] have postulated that temperament characteristics must be considered within the context of the environment to predict psychologic adjustment. They emphasize that environmental/temperament interaction is critical in understanding the psychologic adaptation of physically handicapped children. Within this interactionist model, temperament characteristics may predispose children to certain patterns of behavioral adjustment or maladjustment, but the manifestation of adaptational or dysfunctional functioning is significantly influenced by the interplay between child temperament and environmental demands. In other words, child temperament characteristics that maximally "fit" or "match" the demands imposed by the child's social environment are expected to result in more favorable adaptation compared with those that represent a relatively "poor fit." Although this Goodness-of-Fit theoretical model is intuitively appealing, there has been relatively little research to investigate its validity, particularly in terms of children with chronic illness or physical handicaps.

Consequently, the objective of the present study was to investigate both the potential direct effects of family functioning and child temperament on the psychologic and social adaptation of children with congenital or acquired limb deficiencies, as well as to empirically test the hypothesized interaction effects of family functioning and child temperament in predicting child psychologic and social adaptation to chronic physical handicap.

METHOD

Subjects

Subjects were selected from the population of families having children with congenital or acquired limb deficiencies who were receiving treatment at the Child Amputee Prosthetics Project at the University of California, Los Angeles (UCLA)

Rehabilitation Center. The subjects for the present study were participants in a large ongoing research project (Child and Adolescent Needs Project) designed to assess the psychologic and social needs of children and adolescents with limb deficiencies and their families. Candidates for study participation had to be English speaking and between the ages of 6 to 13 years. Through systematic review of the weekly clinic schedules of the Child Amputee Prosthetics Project, 45 children were identified for the research project. Three families chose not to participate. The number of children participating in the study was 42 (27 boys and 15 girls), typically, as part of their routine annual evaluations. The mean age of the children was 8.4 years, with a range of 6 to 13 years (SD = 2.3). In this sample, 36 children had congenital limb loss, and 6 children had acquired limb loss. The mean family socioeconomic status based on the Hollingshead[20] four-factor index was 43.5 (SD = 11.8), indicating an average middle-class family socioeconomic status.

Predictor Variables

Family Functioning. The construct of family functioning was measured by the Family Environment Scale.[21] The Family Environment Scale is a 90-item true or false questionnaire comprised of ten 9-item subscales that measure the social environmental characteristics of the family. In the 10 subscales, three underlying domains, or sets of dimensions are assessed: the relationship dimensions, the personal growth dimensions, and the system maintenance dimensions. The relationship dimensions are measured by the cohesion, expressiveness, and conflict subscales, in which are assessed the degree of commitment, help, and support family members provide for one another; the extent to which family members are encouraged to act openly and to express their feelings directly; and the amount of openly expressed anger, aggression, and conflict among family members. The personal growth or goal orientation dimensions are measured by the independence, achievement orientation, intellectual-cultural orientation, active-recreational orientation, and moral-religious emphasis subscales. In these subscales the following are assessed: the extent to which family members are assertive, self-sufficient, and make their own decisions; the extent to which activities (such as school and work) are cast into an achievement-oriented or competitive framework; the degree of interest in political, social, intellectual, and cultural activities; the extent of participation in social and recreational activities; and the degree of emphasis on ethical and religious issues and values. The system maintenance dimensions are measured by the organization and control subscales, which assess the degree of importance of clear organization and structure in planning family activities and responsibilities; and the extent to which set rules and procedures are used to run family life. Cronbach α internal consistency reliabilities for the 10 subscales range from .61 to .78. Two-month test-retest reliabilities range from .68 to .86. The Family Environment Scale is currently one of the most widely used measures of family functioning, with considerable content, face, and construct validity.[21] This instrument was completed by the parents of each child (typically, the child's mother).

Child temperament. The construct of child temperament was measured by the EAS Temperament Survey,[17] an acronym for the Emotionality, Activity, and Sociability/ Shyness scales of the Colorado Childhood Temperament Inventory.[22] That inventory represents a factor-analyzed merger between the nine temperament dimensions of Chess and Thomas[19] and the items of the original EASI (Emotionality, Activity, Sociability, Impulsivity).[23] The 20-item EAS Temperament Survey for Children: Parent Ratings was completed by the children's parents on a rating scale from 1 (not characteristic or typical of your child) to 5 (extremely characteristic or typical of your child) to 5 (extremely characteristic or typical of your child). Examples of the EAS items include: (1) Emotionality, e.g., "Child gets upset easily," "Child reacts intensely when upset"; (2) Activity, e.g., "Child is always on the go," "Child prefers quiet, inactive games to more active ones" (reversed scored); (3) Shyness, e.g., "Child makes friends easily" (reversed scored); (4) Sociability, e.g., "Child prefers playing with others rather than alone," "Child finds people more stimulating than anything else." The internal consistencies of the scales average .83, and have content, face, and construct validity.[17] Test-retest reliabilities at 1 month range from .71 to .78.[24]

Degree of limb loss. As part of the overall Child and Adolescent Needs Project at the UCLA Child Amputee Prosthetics Project, we developed the Degree of Limb Loss Scale. Upper body limb loss was scored as follows: Forequarter, 8; shoulder disarticulation, 7; above elbow, 6; elbow disarticulation, 5; below elbow, 4; wrist disarticulation, 3; transcarpal/metacarpal, 2; partial hand, 1. Lower body limb loss was scored as: hemicorporectomy, 9; hemipelvectomy, 8; hip disarticulation, 7; above knee, 6; knee disarticulation, 5; below knee, 4; ankle disarticulation, 3; transtarsal, 2; partial foot, 1. Complete/partial phocomelia and proximal femoral focal deficiency were scored using this scale according to the length of the limb. Total limb loss was calculated as the sum of the upper and lower limb loss ratings.

Criterion Variable

Child psychologic and social adaptation. The construct of child psychologic and social adaptation was measured by the Child Behavior Checklist-Parent Report form.[25] The Child Behavior Checklist consists of 118 behavior problem items and 20 social competence items. Standardized scores for internalizing (e.g., depression, anxiety, withdrawal) and externalizing (e.g., acting out, aggression) dimensions of behavior problems, and social competence (interpersonal relationships, school performance, activities involvement) are provided. Cutoff points on the distributions of total behavior problem and social competence scores have yielded good separation between children referred to mental health clinics and community nonreferred samples.[25] In the Child Behavior Checklist standardization sample, intraclass correlations were in the .90s for interparent agreement, one-week test-retest reliability, and interinterviewer reliability.[25] Across all demographic groups, referral status (mental health clinic-referred children vs randomly selected community nonreferred children) accounted for more variance in total behavior problems and social competence scores than any other factor.[25] Normative data, stratified for three age groups (4 to 5 years, 6 to 11 years, 12 to 16 years) and sex, are available for 1300 community nonclinic-referred and 2300 mental health clinic-referred children between the ages of 4 and 16 years. Extensive analyses have yielded principal component solutions for the 118 behavior problem items that are different for the two sexes and three age groups. However, the two second-order principal components of Internalizing Behavior Problems and Externalizing Behavior Problems exist for all sexes and age groups and can serve as summary scales of behavior problems. The same holds true for the 20 items of the Social Competence summary scale. Thus, the analyses of psychologic and social adjustment are based on the three summary scales across all ages and sex. With standard procedures and available norms,[25] scores in all scales were computed as normalized T scores.

Procedure

The mothers of the children identified as possible study participants were informed of the study when they were scheduling a regular clinic appointment. Subsequently, they were mailed a packet containing more information about the study, an informed consent form, and half of the larger study questionnaires to be completed by the mother, her child, and, when appropriate, the child's father. Two days before the scheduled clinic appointment, the mothers were phoned and reminded to bring the questionnaires with them to the appointment. At the time of the scheduled clinic appointment, both the child and mother were met by a research team member and the signed consent form was obtained as well as verbal assent from the child. Consent from both the parent and the child was necessary for study participation. They were subsequently given more information about the study as well as the opportunity to ask questions, and they then were asked to complete the remaining questionnaires. The research team member was available at all times to answer any questions regarding the administered instruments. This research protocol was approved by the Institutional Review Board at UCLA.

Statistical Analysis for Interaction Model

Plomin and Daniels[26] emphasized the need for statistical approaches that take into account the relationship between temperament characteristics and environmental context, requiring analytic procedures that evaluate the independent contributions of temperament and environment separately in the prediction of psychologic adaptation (main or direct effects), as well as incremental prediction when the temperament/ environment relationships are considered (interaction effects). Support for a Goodness-of-Fit model is dependent on results indicating that statistically significant additional variance is accounted for by the temperament × environment interaction term in predicting psychologic adaptation after partialling out the main effects of temperament and environment through the use of hierarchical multiple regression analysis.[27] As pointed out by Plomin and Daniels,[26] a major advantage of the hierarchical multiple aggression approach is the ability to analyze continuous variation. Because child temperament, family psychosocial environment, and psychologic and social adaptation are continuous variables in the present study, then hierarchical multiple regression analysis was deemed the appropriate statistical procedure for testing the main and interaction effects of the independent (predictor) variables on the dependent (criterion) variable.[27]

RESULTS

Demographic Variables

Sex was significantly correlated with internalizing behavior problems ($r = -.33$, $P < .02$), but not with externalizing behavior problems ($r = -.19$, not significant) or social competence ($r = .06$, not significant). Age and socioeconomic status were not significantly correlated with internalizing/externalizing behavior problems or with social competence. Notably, degree of limb loss was not significantly correlated with internalizing behavior problems ($r = 00$, not significant), externalizing behavior problems ($r = -.04$, not significant), or social competence ($r = -.02$, not significant).

Family Functioning

In Table 1, the means, standard deviations, and the zero-order correlations between family functioning and internalizing/externalizing behavior problems and social competence are shown. To control for the number of correlations, we set the significant level at $P < .01$. More family cohesion was associated with fewer internalizing behavior problems ($r = -.45$, $P < .001$), fewer externalizing behavior problems ($r = -.44$, $P < .005$), and more social competence ($r = .36$, $P < .01$). A similar pattern is evident for family organization and moral-religious emphasis. In contrast, more family conflict was associated with more of both internalizing ($r = .43$, $P < .005$) and externalizing ($r = .53$, $P < .001$) behavior problems. Intellectual-cultural orientation was significantly positively associated with social competence, but not with internalizing/ externalizing behavior problems.

Next, three separate multiple regression analyses[27] were conducted to statistically predict the three criterion (dependent) variables of internalizing/externalizing behavior problems and social competence by the family predictor (independent) variables. Only those family functioning variables that were significantly associated with each criterion variable for the zero-order correlations were entered into the three separate multiple regression analyses. For each regression analysis, age and sex were entered initially to control for these demographic variables. Then, the zero-order significant family functioning variables were entered as a group on one step in each of the separate regression analyses. The R^2, F, and P values described for each group of family functioning variables represents the increment in R^2 accounted for after we controlled for age and sex.

Family cohesion, conflict, moral-religious emphasis, and organization accounted for 39% of the variance in internalizing behavior problems ($R^2 = .392, F = 6.94, P < .0003$). These same four family functioning variables accounted for 42% of the variance in externalizing behavior problems ($R^2 = .417, F = 7.15, P < .0003$). Family cohesion, intellectual-cultural orientation, and moral-religious emphasis accounted for 25% of the variance in social competence ($R^2 = .249, F = 4.11, P < .01$).

TABLE 1
Family Functioning and Psychologic and Social Adaptation

Family Functioning Predictor Variables	Intercorrelations			T Scores	
	Internalizing Behavior Problems	Externalizing Behavior Problems	Social Competence	Means*	SD
Cohesion	−.45§	−.44‡	.36†	60.4	11.50
Expressiveness	−.07	−.13	.04	57.8	11.00
Conflict	.43‡	.53§	−.23	45.5	9.43
Independence	.12	.07	−.03	52.2	10.01
Achievement orientation	−.06	.10	.18	48.7	9.05
Intellectual-cultural orientation	−.25	−.23	.36†	52.1	13.84
Active-recreational orientation	−.01	−.09	.22	50.4	13.51
Moral-religious emphasis	−.57§	−.49§	.41‡	56.0	11.91
Organization	−.48§	−.45†	.13	56.4	10.84
Control	−.19	−.07	.04	52.8	10.94

* T scores. Internalizing Behavior Problems· mean = 52.71, SD = 8.95; Externalizing Behavior Problems: mean = 53.19, SD = 10.4ʻ: Social Competence: mean = 51.14, SD = 8.55.
†$P < .01$.
‡ $P < .005$.
§ $P < .001$.

Child Temperament

In Table 2, the means, standard deviations, and the zero-order correlations between child temperament and internalizing/externalizing behavior problems and social competence are shown. The significance level was again set at $P < .01$. More emotionality was associated with more internalizing behavior problems ($r = .48$, $P < .001$), more externalizing behavior problems ($r = .58$, $P < .001$), and less social competence ($r = -.55$, $P < .001$). Sociability, shyness, and activity temperament characteristics were not significantly associated with the dependent variables.

Next, three separate multiple regression analyses[27] were conducted to statistically predict the three criterion variables. Only those child temperament variables that were significantly associated with each criterion variable for the zero-order correlations were entered into the three separate multiple regression analyses. For each regression analysis, age and sex were entered initially to control for these demographic variables. Then, the zero-order significant child temperament variables were entered as a group on one step in each of the separate regression analyses. The R^2, F, and P values for each group of child temperament variables represents the increment in R^2 accounted for after we controlled for age and sex.

Child emotionality accounted for 23% of the variance in internalizing behavior problems ($R^2 = .234$, $F = 13.59$, $P < .0007$). Child emotionality accounted for 39% of the variance in externalizing behavior problems ($R^2 = .391$, $F = 13.52$, $P < .0001$). For social competence, child emotionality accounted for 28% of the variance ($R^2 = .284$, $F = 15.65$, $P < .0003$).

Family Functioning/Child Temperament Interactions

To reduce the probability of obtaining chance findings as a function of the large number of possible interaction terms, only those family functioning and child temperament variables that were significant zero-order predictors of the criterion variables were retained for the computation of the interaction terms.

TABLE 2
Temperament and Psychologic and Social Adaptation

Temperament Predictor Variables	Intercorrelations			Means	SD
	Internalizing Behavior Problems	Externalizing Behavior Problems	Social Competence		
Emotionality	.48*	.58*	-.55*	2.50	0.98
Activity	-.20	-.05	-.09	4.00	0.65
Shyness	-.09	-.12	-.07	2.12	0.83
Sociability	.16	.30	-.10	3.72	0.67

* $P < .001$.

Separate hierarchical multiple regression analyses[27] were conducted for each criterion variable, initially entering into the regression analysis age, sex, and the significant family functioning and child temperament predictor variables for each criterion variable. The interaction term was then entered as the last step in the equation. Because of the small subject to variable ratio, these analyses should be interpreted with caution. The family cohesion × child emotionality interaction term was a significant predictor of internalizing behavior problems ($R^2 = .08$, $F = 5.06$, $p < .03$) and externalizing behavior problems ($R^2 = .06$, $F = 4.27$, $P < .05$) after we controlled for age, sex, and the family functioning and child temperament main effects. None of the other interaction terms was a significant predictor of psychologic and social adaptation.

To determine the Goodness-of-Fit relationship of the family cohesion × child emotionality interaction term, we divided the family cohesion data at the mean and calculated the correlation between child emotionality and internalizing and externalizing behavior problems when there is greater or lesser family cohesion. When family cohesion is greater, child emotionality did not significantly predict internalizing ($r = .28$, $P > .05$) or externalizing ($r = .35$, $P > .05$) behavior problems. In contrast, when family cohesion is less, child emotionality significantly predicted both internalizing ($r = .43$, $P < .02$) and externalizing ($r = .53$, $P < .003$) behavior problems.

DISCUSSION

The results of the present study of the hypothesized predictors of psychologic and social adaptation in children with congenital or acquired limb deficiencies indicate that demographic variables (age, sex, socioeconomic status, degree of limb loss) are generally not significant predictors of adaptation, but rather potentially modifiable dynamic social environment variables (family functioning domains) and child personality traits (temperament characteristics) do explain a significant amount of the variance in adaptation. The differential findings of the various family functioning predictors on the adaptation of the children to limb deficiency suggests the need to measure multiple domains of family functioning for their potential differential influence on psychologic and social adjustment rather than simply recording only a global index of family functioning that may obscure important and unique family functioning-child temperament/adaptation relationships.

The pattern of results suggests that aspects of the child's temperament and family psychosocial environment are statistically significant predictors of psychologic and social adaptation in children with congenital or acquired limb deficiency. In general, more family cohesion, moral-religious emphasis and organization, in combination with less family conflict, predicted better psychologic and social adaptation. With regard to child temperament, greater emotionality predicted greater internalizing/

externalizing behavior problems and lesser social competence. In addition to the main effects of the family functioning and child temperament predictor variables, the interaction between family cohesion and child emotionality significantly predicted both internalizing and externalizing behavior problems.

The findings of the significant direct effects of various aspects of the family psychosocial environment are consistent with the recent empirical literature in which the predictive relationship between family functioning and child psychologic and social adaptation in chronically ill and handicapped children is examined.[11,28] The significant direct effects of components of child temperament on psychologic and social adaptation are also consistent with the recent empirical literature on the predictive relationship of child temperament on adaptation in physically handicapped children.[12]

The finding of only two statistically significant interaction terms in predicting psychologic and social adaptation is consistent with the extant empirical literature. As emphasized by Plomin and Daniels, "It is considerably easier to talk about temperament interactions than it is to find them."[26] The statistically significant prediction of both internalizing and externalizing behavior problems by the family cohesion/child emotionality interaction, although statistically consistent with the longitudinal analyses from the New York Longitudinal Study of Thomas and Chess[29] and more recent research by Lerner and associates,[30,31] are of a magnitude that does not provide empirical evidence for the clinical significance of the Goodness-of-Fit theoretical model. Rather, from the perspective of clinical significance, the findings might be more parsimoniously interpreted as providing evidence for the positive direct benefits of family cohesion on child psychologic and social adjustment along the full spectrum of the child emotionality temperament dimension. These findings of the positive direct effects of family cohesion on child psychologic and social adjustment are consistent with other recent studies with chronically ill and handicapped children using the same assessment instruments.[11,28]

Finally, the results have implications for primary and secondary prevention efforts. A major focus of this study was to attempt to identify potentially modifiable risk and protective factors that might enhance the psychologic and social adaptation of children with congenital or acquired limb deficiencies through intervention. The findings suggest several paths in this regard. For instance, family therapy might facilitate a reduction in family conflict and an increase in family cohesion and organization. Specifically increasing family cohesion might function as a protective factor for those children at risk for psychologic adjustment problems. It should be pointed out that a considerable amount of the observed variability in child psychologic and social adjustment was not accounted for by the predictor variables. Additional predictors recently investigated include daily stress and social support from friends, classmates, parents, and teachers.[6] By also delineating family functioning and child temperament as risk and protective factors, this study may serve to provide empirical guidance for future intervention studies in which there is an attempt to enhance the psychologic and social adaptation of children with congenital or acquired limb deficiencies and other visible physical handicaps who are at increased risk for psychologic and social adjustment problems.[32]

REFERENCES

1. Setoguchi Y, Rosenfelder R. *The Limb Deficient Child*. Springfield, IL: Charles C Thomas; 1982

2. Boren HA. Adolescent adjustment to amputation necessitated by bone cancer. *Orthop Nurs.* 1985;4:30–32

3. Henker FO. Body-image conflict following trauma and surgery. *Psychosomatics.* 1979;20:812–820

4. Kashani JH, Frank RG, Kashani SR, Wonderlich SA, Reid JC. depression among amputees. *J Clin Psychiatry.* 1983;44:256–258

5. Shukla GD, Sahu SC, Tripathi RP, Gupta DK. A psychiatric study of amputees. *Br J Psychiatry.* 1982;141:50–53

6. Varni JW, Rubenfeld LA, Talbot D, Setoguchi Y. Stress, social support, and depressive symptomatology in children with congenital/acquired limb deficiencies. *J Pediatr Psychol.* In press

7. Varni JW, Rubenfeld LA, Talbot D, Setoguchi Y. Determinants of self-esteem in children with congenital/acquired limb deficiencies. *J Dev Behav Pediatr.* 1989;10:13–16

8. Wallander JL, Varni JW, Babani L, Banis HT, Wilcox KT. Children with chronic physical disorders: Maternal reports of their psychological adjustment. *J Pediatr Psychol.* 1988;13:197–212

9. Cadman D, Boyle M, Szatmari P, Offord DR. Chronic illness, disability, and mental health and social well-being: findings of the Ontario Child Health Study. *Pediatrics.* 1987;79:805–813

10. Varni JW. Stress, moderator variables, and adaptation in pediatric chronic disorders. Presented at the annual meeting of the American Psychological Association; August 1987; New York, NY

11. Varni JW, Wilcox KT, Hanson V. Mediating effects of family social support on child psychological adjustment in juvenile rheumatoid arthritis. *Health Psychol.* 1988;7:421–431

12. Wallander JL, Hubert NC, Varni JW. Child and maternal temperament characteristics, goodness of fit, and adjustment in physically handicapped children. *J Clin Child Psychol.* 1988;17:336–344

13. Varni JW. *Clinical Behavioral Pediatrics: An Interdisciplinary Biobehavioral Approach.* New York, NY: Pergamon; 1983

14. Johnson SB. The family and the child with chronic illness. In DC Turk, RD Kerns, eds. *Health, Illness, and Families: A Life-Span Perspective.* New York, NY: John Wiley & Sons, 1985:220–254

15. Hubert NC, Wachs TD, Peters-Martin P, Gandour MJ. The study of early temperament: measurement and conceptual issues. *Child Dev.* 1982;53:571–600

16. Goldsmith HH, Buss AH, Plomin R, et al. Roundtable: what is temperament? Four approaches. *Child Dev.* 1987;58:505–529

17. Buss AH, Plomin R. *Temperament: Early Developing Personality Traits.* Hillsdale, NJ: Erlbaum; 1984

18. Garrison WT, Earls FJ. *Temperament and Child Psychopathology.* Newbury Park, CA: Sage; 1987

19. Chess S, Thomas A. *Temperament in Clinical Practice.* New York, NY: Guilford; 1986

20. Hollingshead AB. *Four-Factor Index of Social Status.* New Haven, CT: Yale University, 1975

21. Moos RH, Moos BS. *Family Environment Scale Manual.* 2nd ed. Palo Alto, CA: Consulting Psychologists Press; 1986

22. Rowe DC, Plomin R. Temperament in early childhood. *J Pers Assess.* 1977;41:150–156

23. Buss AH, Plomin R. *A Temperament Theory of Personality Development.* New York, NY: John Wiley & Sons; 1975

24. Gibbs MV, Reeves D, Cunningham CC. The application of temperament questionnaires to a British sample: issues of reliability and validity. *J Child Psychol Psychiatry.* 1987;28:61–77

25. Achenbach TM, Edelbrock CS. *Manual for the Child Behavior Checklist and Revised Child Behavior Profile.* Burlington, VT: University of Vermont; 1983

26. Plomin R, Daniels D. The interaction between temperament and environment: methodological considerations. *Merrill-Palmer Q.* 1984;30:149–162

27. Cohen J, Cohen P. *Applied Multiple Regression/Correlation Analysis for the Behavioral Sciences.* Hillsdale, NJ: Erlbaum; 1983

28. Varni JW, Babani L, Wallander JL, Roe TF, Frasier SD. Social support and self-esteem effects on psychological adjustment in children and adolescents with insulin-dependent diabetes mellitus. *Child Family Behav Ther.* 1989;11:1–17

29. Thomas A, Chess S. Genesis and evolution of behavioral disorders: From infancy to early adult life. *Am J Psychiatry.* 1984;141:1–9

30. Lerner JV. The import of temperament for psychosocial functioning: tests of a goodness of fit model. *Merrill-Palmer Q.* 1984;30:177–188

31. Lerner JV, Lerner RM, Zabski S. Temperament and elementary school children's actual and rated academic performance: a test of a "goodness-of-fit" model. *J Child Psychol Psychiatry.* 1985;26:125–136

32. Varni JW, Wallander JL. Pediatric chronic disabilities: Hemophilia and spina bifida as examples. In: DK Routh, ed. *Handbook of Pediatric Psychology.* New York, NY: Guilford; 1988:190–221

15

Maternal Support Following Disclosure of Incest

Mark D. Everson, Wanda M. Hunter, and Desmond K. Runyon
University of North Carolina, Chapel Hill
Gail A. Edelsohn
Johns Hopkins University, Baltimore
Martha L. Coulter
University of South Florida, Tampa

The level of maternal support to incest victims following disclosure was found to be more closely related to perpetrator than to child character- istics. Lack of maternal support was significantly associated with foster placement and higher psychopathology scores in a clinical interview. Evidence is presented challenging the validity of maternal behavioral reports in assessments of incest victims.

Sexually abused children are psychologically vulnerable for short-term (Friedrich, Urquiza, & Beilke, 1986; Gomes-Schwartz, Horowitz, & Sauzier, 1985; Mannarino & Cohen, 1986; White, Halpin, Strom, & Santilli, 1986) and long-term (Bagley & Ramsay, 1985–86; Briere & Runtz, 1985) mental health problems. Especially at risk are children who have been victimized by their fathers or father-figures because issues of betrayal and concern about family well-being compound the trauma of sexual vic- timization (Adams-Tucker, 1982; Burgess & Holmstrom, 1978; Herman, Russell, & Trocki, 1986). Consequently, the disclosure of incest precipitates a crisis for child and family (Simrel, Berg, & Thomas, 1979; Summit, 1983). Such a crisis fits Rutter's description (1987) of a "key turning point" in the child's life, a time "when a risk tra- jectory may be redirected onto a more adaptive path."

What distinguishes children who negotiate this "key turning point" in an adaptive

Reprinted with permission from *American Journal of Orthopsychiatry,* 1989, Vol. 59, No. 2, 197–207. Copyright © 1989 by the American Orthopsychiatric Association, Inc.
Research was supported by NCCAN grant 90CA0421, with additional support from NIJ grant 85-IJ-CX-0066.

fashion from children who develop emotional problems? A growing body of literature points to social support as an effective mediator of life stress for adults (Cobb, 1976; Dean & Lin, 1977). Similarly, longitudinal studies of vulnerable children (Block & Block, 1980; Freud & Burlingham, 1943; Rutter, 1979; Werner & Smith, 1982) find that affective support, especially from the child's parents, serves as an important protective mechanism. A second protective factor related to a child's successful coping is high self-esteem (Garmezy, 1985) which in turn is enhanced by positive and secure love attachments (Bretherton, 1985; Main, Kaplan, & Cassidy, 1985). Bowlby's observation (1973), that attachment behavior (even in adolescents and adults) grows stronger during times of trouble or crisis, supports the finding that parents, especially mothers as primary attachment figures, are important to their children's ability to cope.

Yet, at the time of disclosure, when the child needs acceptance, protection, and reassurance, some mothers respond with disbelief, rejection, or blame (Herman, 1981; Summit, 1983). The disclosure of incest differs from other family crises in that the mother is asked to believe something she may not want to believe, to interpret something that is at best difficult for her to comprehend, and to resolve the conflict between her roles as central support figure to both her child and her male partner at a time when her own social, emotional, and economic supports may be at risk.

In recent years, a few researchers have attempted to categorize the degree of maternal support offered to sexually abused children in clinical samples. Estimates of the percentage of supportive mothers in these samples have ranged from 27% to 56% (Adams-Tucker, 1982; Meyer, 1985; Lyon & Kouloumpos-Lenares, 1987). Among intrafamilial cases of abuse, maternal support of the child has been found to vary in predictable ways according to the intensity of the mother's relationship with the perpetrator, mothers being most supportive when they are no longer married to the perpetrator (Faller, 1984).

An even smaller number of studies have attempted systematically to relate maternal support to child outcomes following disclosure. Adams-Tucker reported that the children in her sample who were not supported by the adults on whom they depended were diagnosed with far more emotional disturbance than their supported counterparts. The Tufts New England Medical Center report (1984) indicated that while the presence of maternal support did not relate to improved outcomes for sexual abuse victims, lack of support was associated with the child's removal from home and increased behavioral disturbances.

The theoretical and clinical literatures are consistent in suggesting that while maternal support is crucial for ameliorating the harmful effects of father-perpetrated incest, it is frequently diminished because of the mother's role conflict. As part of a longitudinal investigation of the effects of social and institutional response on child victims of intrafamilial sexual abuse (Runyan, Everson, Edelsohn, Hunter, & Coulter, 1988), a cross-sectional analysis of our study population was conducted with the following objectives: *1)* to determine whether degree of maternal support is associated with child or case characteristics, *2)* to determine whether social or institutional response is related to maternal support, and *3)* to investigate further the relationship between maternal support and child mental health functioning.

METHOD

Subjects

The sample, ranging in age from 6 to 17 years, was recruited from 11 county social service agencies in North Carolina over a 28-month period. In exchange for their referral of substantiated victims of intrafamilial sexual abuse, these agencies were provided with written summaries of the child mental health assessments conducted as a part of the study.

Out of a total of 124 referrals, 14 families refused to participate. Ten children were evaluated but were subsequently determined to be ineligible because they were too young, not substantiated as sexually abused, or found not to reside in one of the study counties. From the resulting sample of 100 children, 88 children were selected for the current study. These included all 84 children who were living with their biological mothers at the time of disclosure. For several analyses, four additional children with no discernible source of support were included to contrast the absence of maternal support with both ambivalent support and active nonsupport. The remaining 12 children were in the care of stepmothers, grandmothers, foster mothers, or aunts. These children were excluded from this study because the duration and intensity of these relationships varied so widely.

The sample was 84% female with an average age of 11.9 years. Sixty percent of the children were white and 40% black. Level of maternal education was somewhat skewed; 36% of the mothers had less than a high school degree and only 4% held college degrees.

Fathers or father-figures predominated as perpetrators: 30% were biological fathers, 41% were stepfathers, 17% were the mother's "boyfriends" and 12% were a mixed group comprised of brothers, uncles, and cousins. Seventy percent of the children had experienced penetration or oral-genital contact. Length of abuse ranged from one recent incident (7 cases) to 12 years of chronic abuse (2 cases), with a mean of 23 months.

Procedure and Instruments

Children were evaluated within the first two weeks following disclosure in all but a few cases. The evaluation included the Child Assessment Schedule (Hodges, 1987; Hodges & Cools, in press; Hodges, Kline, Stern, Cytryn, & McKnew, 1982) and a semistructured interview about the history of abuse, disclosure, and family (especially maternal) reaction to the allegation of abuse. In addition, the child's mother was asked to complete the Child Behavior Checklist (Achenbach & Edelbrock, 1981, 1983). Lastly, the child's protective services worker was asked to provide additional information on the abuse allegations, family background, and familial response to the sexual abuse report.

The *Child Assessment Schedule* (CAS) is a structured psychiatric interview developed for clinical assessment of school-aged children in clinical or research settings. Interrater reliability is good (coefficients ranging from .84 to .92) and a variety of groups of "problem children" have been found to differ significantly on this measure, further attesting to its reliability and validity (Garbarino, Guttman, & Seeley, 1986). Abnormal responses were summed across the 226 items for a general psychopathology score and within subscales to generate assessments of depression, anxiety and fears, self-image, conduct disorders, and somatic complaints.

The *Child Behavior Checklist, Parent form,* (CBCL) is an extensively-used instrument, with established validity and reliability, designed to assess social competence and behavior problems among children from preschool age through adolescence (Achenbach & Edelbrock, 1983). For our analyses, we used T scores for Total Behavior Problems and the Internalizing Behavior and Externalizing Behavior scales.

We developed the *Parental Reaction to Incest Disclosure Scale* (PRIDS) (Table 1) to provide a structured measure of a parent's reaction and support following disclosure of sexual abuse. The total score is derived by adding clinical ratings of parental support in three areas, Emotional Support, Belief of Child, and Action

TABLE 1
Parental Reaction to Incest Disclosure Scale (PRIDS)

DEFINITION	WEIGHT
Emotional Support	
Is committed to child and provides meaningful support.	2
Is somewhat committed and supportive.	1
Vacillates in ability and/or desire to support child.	0
Unsupportive, yet not hostile or abandoning.	−1
Is threatening or hostile; has abandoned child psychologically.	−2
Belief of Child	
Makes clear, public statement of belief.	2
Makes weak statements of belief.	1
Wavers in belief of child or is undecided.	0
Makes weak statements of disbelief.	−1
Totally denies abuse occurred.	−2
Action Toward Perpetrator	
Actively demonstrates disapproval of perpetrator's abusive behavior	
(e.g. seeks separation, forces treatment, cooperates with criminal prosecution).	1
Remains passive; refuses to take sides.	0
Chooses perpetrator over child at child's expense.	−1

Toward Perpetrator, with a possible range of $+5$ (most supportive) to -5 (least supportive). The intercorrelations of these three clinical ratings ranged from the mid-.60s to the high .70s.

In this study, the PRIDS was used to measure the reaction and support of the biological mother. For most children, the examiner completed the PRIDS on the basis of the interview with the child, discussion with the referring child protective services worker, and an interview with the child's mother when she was available. Thirty-eight children either had already entered our larger longitudinal study (Runyan et al., 1988) before this instrument was developed or were scored initially for a parent-figure other than the biological mother. In these cases, the PRIDS was determined by review of the interview record. The reliability of assigning the support score by record review was evaluated by comparing both interrater reliability from the record review ($r = .96$), and by comparing ratings from blinded record reviews with the ratings assigned by the original interviewers ($r = .95$). It appears that record review and assignment by the interviewer were equally reliable methods of scoring.

Statistical Analysis

The relationships among child, family, and perpetrator characteristics; child disposition and decisions about prosecution; and maternal support were analyzed using Student's t-test and analysis of variance. Because the PRIDS does not generate scores that can be assumed to be truly ratio in nature, we also analyzed these data using the Kruskal-Wallis and Wilcoxon Rank Sum tests. Since both the parametric and nonparametric forms of analysis identified the same significant relationships, we have chosen to present only the more familiar parametric analysis. Comparisons between the children, grouped by the level of maternal support, and psychological status were analyzed with analysis of variance using Scheffe's technique to identify specific subgroup relationships. Fisher's r to Z transformations were used in this study to compare correlations between maternal support groups.

RESULTS

Maternal Support Classifications

Mothers were classified as "supportive" of their children if their scores on the PRIDS were $+3$ or above, "ambivalent" if their scores fell in the $+2$ to -2 range, and "unsupportive" if their ratings fell at or below -3. In our sample 44% of the 84 mothers were categorized as providing consistent support during the period following disclosure of sexual abuse, 32% were classified as ambivalent or providing inconsistent support, and the remaining 24% were unsupportive or rejecting of their children. In describing results from statistical analyses of the data, we refer to supportive mothers as the High Support group, unsupportive mothers as the Low Support group, and the children who have no mother-figure as the Mother Absent group.

Family Characteristics

As shown in Table 2, maternal support was not significantly related to the child's gender, age, or race, nor to the mother's educational level. However, the data suggested that children in the 16- to 18-year-old group received somewhat higher levels of maternal support than those in other age groups ($p = .07$). The level of maternal support was found to be highly related to the offender's relationship to the mother; mothers were significantly more supportive of their children if the offender were an ex-spouse than if he were someone with whom the women had a current relationship. In addition, a significant Spearman correlation of .45 ($p<.0001$) between PRIDS scores and rankings of the offender-mother relationship (i.e. ex-spouses, biological father and wife, stepfather and wife, unmmaried sexual partners) indicated

TABLE 2
Mean Maternal Support Score by Family Characteristics

| CHARACTERISTIC | N | \multicolumn{3}{c}{MATERNAL SUPPORT} | | |
		M	(SD)	STATISTIC
Child's Gender				
Male	14	2.4	(2.6)	$t = 1.65$, NS
Female	70	.7	(3.5)	
Child's Age				
6–9 yrs	24	1.3	(3.1)	$F(3,80) = 2.42$, $p = .07$
10–12 yrs	23	1.4	(3.2)	
13–15 yrs	27	− .3	(3.5)	
16–18 yrs	10	2.7	(3.1)	
Race				
Black	34	1.0	(3.6)	$t = .03$, NS
White	50	1.0	(3.3)	
Mother's Education[a]				
< HS grad	20	1.8	(2.9)	$t = − 1.37$, NS
≥ HS grad	43	.5	(3.6)	
Mother/Child Relationship to Offender[b]				
Ex-wife/biol. father	14	3.9	(0.92)	$F(3,71) = 5.98$, $p = .001$[c]
Wife/biol. father	19	1.0	(3.3)	
Wife/stepfather	28	.4	(3.7)	
Girlfriend	14	− .6	(2.7)	

Mother's education level unknown for 11 subjects.
Remaining 9 subjects had diverse family relationships with offender, therefore not easily categorized.
Scheffe's tests of pairwise comparisons revealed significant difference ($p<.05$) between ex-wife and all other groups.

an inverse relationship between level of maternal support and the recency and intensity of the offender-mother relationship. Specifically, mothers were most supportive and protective of their children when the offender was an ex-spouse and least supportive when the perpetrator was a current boyfriend. Maternal support ratings fell into an intermediate range in cases in which the mother was currently married to the perpetrator, whether he was the child's biological father or stepfather.

Table 3 presents maternal support as a function of the perpetrator's admission or denial of guilt. Not surprisingly, women were much more likely to be supportive of their children if the perpetrator confirmed the sexual involvement. It is noteworthy that none of the 14 perpetrators identified as the mother's boyfriends admitted guilt while over one-third of the accused biological fathers did so.

We also evaluated the relationship of maternal support to three aspects of case management: out-of-home placement, juvenile court testimony by the child, and criminal prosecution. The results are summarized in Table 3. Children who were removed from home and placed in foster or institutional care after the report of sexual abuse had mothers who were dramatically lower in the support they provided the child than mothers whose children were not removed. In fact, of the 15 children placed in foster or institutional care, 12 had mothers classified as unsupportive of the child. Only 2 of 45 mothers whose children were not removed were so classified (Fisher's exact test, $p<.0001$). Twenty-four children were removed from their homes and placed with relatives. Their maternal support ratings fell into an intermediate range.

To determine whether legal interventions were contingent on the level of support provided by the incest victim's mother, we tracked each case for a period of five

TABLE 3
Mean Maternal Support Score by Postdisclosure Circumstances

CIRCUMSTANCE	N	M	(SD)	STATISTIC
		\multicolumn{2}{c}{MATERNAL SUPPORT}	
Offender Response[a]				
Admit	19	3.4	(1.3)	$t=6.06, p<.0001$
Deny	52	−.1	(3.5)	
Child Placement				
Remains home	45	2.7	(2.3)	$F=30.2, p<.0001$[b]
Extended family	24	.5	(3.2)	
Foster/institutional	15	−3.2	(2.2)	
Child Testimony[c]				
Yes	11	−1.0	(3.2)	$t=2.12, p<.04$
No	69	1.3	(4.0)	
Criminal Prosecution[c]				
Yes (or pending)	49	1.2	(3.4)	$t=1.91$, NS
No	32	.9	(3.5)	

[a] In 13 cases, responses were ambivalent or not available to data collection.
[b] Scheffe's tests of pairwise comparisons revealed differences between all pairs ($p<.05$).
[c] Follow-up data not available for all cases.

months. Most of the cases in the current study resulted in juvenile court hearings, but only 11 of the children were required to testify at the hearings. Children who were asked to testify had mothers who were significantly less supportive than children who were not required to testify at the juvenile court hearing. In contrast, there was no evidence that maternal belief in the child's account of abuse and emotional support systematically influenced the decision to criminally prosecute the offender. By the end of the five-month tracking period, 49 of the 81 cases for which there were reliable data were either being actively prosecuted or were pending prosecution. Mean levels of maternal support within the "prosecution pending" and the "no prosecution" subgroups did not differ significantly.

Child Psychological Functioning

A major focus of the study was the degree to which maternal support might affect the child's mental health functioning during the period of time immediately after disclosure. To explore this issue, we compared the CAS scores and the CBCL scores of the support subgroups using analysis of variance. Because the Mother Absent group consisted of only four children, it was combined with the Low Support group to form a None/Low Support group.

As shown in Table 4, the three resulting groups were significantly different from one another on overall psychological functioning as measured by the CAS Total Psychopathology score. A comparison of the group means suggests that the High Support and Ambivalent Support groups were essentially equivalent in the degree of psychological distress exhibited soon after disclosure. In contrast, children in the

TABLE 4

Means and Anovas for Measures of Psychological Status as a Function of Maternal Support

MEASURE	MATERNAL SUPPORT GROUP		
	NONE/LOW	AMBIVALENT	HIGH
CAS			
Total psychopathology[a]	53.1	38.8	41.4
Depression[b]	13.3	8.1	9.7
Self-image[c]	4.4	3.2	3.2
Somatic complaints	5.1	3.6	3.9
Acting out	6.8	6.0	5.9
Anxiety/fears	10.8	8.5	9.2
CBCL			
Total problems	67.3	65.3	63.2
Internalization	64.5	62.7	61.4
Externalization	64.2	63.3	60.0

None/Low, Ambivalent, and High groups are composed of 24, 26, and 37 cases respectively with CAS scores, and 10, 25, and 30 cases respectively with CBCL scores.
[a] $F(2,84) = 4.93$, $p = .009$.
[b] $F(2,84) = 4.55$, $p = .01$.
[c] $F(2,84) = 3.08$, $p = .05$.

None/Low Support group displayed significantly higher levels of psychopathology than children in either the High or Ambivalent groups ($p < .05$).

There were also significant group effects for the Depression and Self-Image subscales of the CAS. In both cases, the means for the None/Low Support subgroup were inflated relative to their peers in the other two groups. However, Scheffe's tests revealed only the None/Low vs Ambivalent comparison to be statistically significant ($p < .05$) for Depression while none of the pairwise comparisons for Self-Image was significant.

We were also interested in the question of how children in the Mother Absent group fared relative to children in the Low Support group with mothers, albeit unsupportive or rejecting ones. Mother Absent children had higher mean scores for Total CAS Psychopathology (61.4 vs 51.4) and for three of the five CAS subscales. However, because of the small sample sizes, only the Somatic Complaints subscale reached statistical significance, with Mother Absent children reporting more psychosomatic problems than Low Support children (means of 7.7 vs 4.6 respectively; $t = 2.07, 22, p = .05$). Children in the Low Support group displayed more psychological disturbance on two of the CAS subscales, with the Self Image subscale reaching statistical significance (means of 4.8 vs 2.0 respectively; $t = 2.45, 22, p = .02$).

Maternal Report and Clinical Interview

While total psychopathology scores varied significantly by maternal support group, mothers' reports of behavior problems on the CBCL did not (see ANOVA comparisons, Table 4). In an effort to understand this inconsistency better, we correlated the CBCL ratings of the three support groups (Low, Ambivalent, and High) with the CAS psychopathology scores of their children. As shown in Table 5, the correlation between CBCL and CAS scores for the sample collapsed across support

TABLE 5

Comparison of Correlations between CAS Total Psychopathology Score and CBCL Scores by Maternal Support Group

		MATERNAL SUPPORT GROUP		
CORRELATIONS	TOTAL SAMPLE ($N = 63$)	LOW ($N = 10$)	AMBIVALENT ($N = 23$)	HIGH ($N = 30$)
CAS × CBCL Total[a]	.36*	− .32	.20	.63**
CAS × CBCL Internalizing[b]	.27*	− .42	.08	.56**
CAS × CBCL Externalizing[c]	.34*	− .29	.28	.54*

[a] Pairwise differences: Low-Ambivalent ($Z = − 1.78, p = .08$), Ambivalent-High ($Z = − 1.83, p = .06$), and Low-High ($Z = − 2.53, p = .02$).
[b] Pairwise differences: Low-Ambivalent ($Z = − 1.76, p = .08$), Ambivalent-High ($Z = 1.87, p = .06$), and Low-High ($Z = − 2.54, p = .02$).
[c] Pairwise differences: Low-Ambivalent ($Z = − 1.95, p = .05$), Ambivalent-High ($Z = − 1.07$, NS), and Low-High ($Z = − 2.13, p = .03$).
* $p < .01$, ** $p < .001$.

groups was a modest .36. However, when the correlations were computed separately for each support group a clear pattern emerged. The correlations for the Low Support and Ambivalent Support groups were—.32 and .20; while neither is significantly different from a correlation of zero, the comparison between them approaches significance ($p = .08$). In contrast, the correlation between supportive mothers' reports of their children's functioning on the CBCL and the responses of their children to the CAS was .63. This correlation of supportive mothers' reports with child interview data was significantly different from the correlation coefficient for nonsupportive mothers ($p = .02$) and nearly so when compared to ambivalent mothers ($p = .06$). These findings suggest that among the Low and Ambivalent Support groups, mothers' descriptions of the psychological functioning of their children bore no relationship to the self-report of their children during the CAS interview while there was substantial concordance between the reports of supportive mothers and their children.

Impact of Maternal Support

The impact of maternal support on the child's overall psychological functioning was examined relative to six other variables: child's age, gender, estimate of verbal IQ (i.e., score on the Peabody Picture Vocabulary Test-Revised), identity of the perpetrator (parent figure vs other), type of abuse (anal/vaginal penetration vs. other types of sexual contact), and length of abuse (the percentage of life for which the child has been abused). A series of multiple regressions predicting CAS Total Psychopathology scores were run, forcing in maternal support group (None/Low, Ambivalent, High) and the other six predictor variables separately and in various combinations. The results of these analyses confirmed the relative importance of maternal support in predicting the child's psychological functioning. Maternal support was second to the child's gender (female) as the best single predictor of Total Psychopathology ($R^2 = .063$ vs .077). Furthermore, in comparisons of regression models including combinations of two to seven predictor variables, maternal support was always one of the predictor variables included in the model having the highest R^2.

A second issue of interest was whether level of maternal support exerted an influence on child psychopathology independent of the child's placement after the disclosure of incest. As noted earlier, the decision about whether to remove the child from the home after disclosure rested in large measure on the level of support and protection offered by the child's mother. It is possible that the significantly higher level of psychopathology identified in the combined Low Support and Mother Absent group was due, not to the quality of the mother-child relationship, but to the stress and disruption of an out-of-home placement. In an attempt to isolate the influence of maternal support from the effect of out-of-home placement, we focused on the 43 children who had been removed from their homes soon after disclosure.

They were dichotomized into a combined High Support/Ambivalent group ($N = 21$) and Low Support/Mother Absent group ($N = 22$) and their CAS scores were compared using t-tests. Children in the Low Support/Mother Absent group were again found to have significantly higher Total Psychopathology scores than children with ambivalent or supportive mothers (means of 55.0 vs 44.0, $t = -2.23$, $p = .03$). There were similar group differences for the Self-Image and Depression subscales ($p = .03$ and .07 respectively). These results suggest that maternal support has an impact on the child's psychological functioning over and above the impact of the child's removal from the home and alternative placement.

DISCUSSION

These findings parallel the results of other studies (Adams-Tucker, 1982; Faller, 1984; Tufts, 1984) in identifying substantial variability in how mothers respond to reports of incest within their families. The finding that less than one-half of the mothers in our sample could be classified as consistently supportive of their children underscores the overwhelming emotional turmoil most parents feel after a report of sexual abuse. Many others of incest victims experience intense role conflict over their responsibilities and allegiances as a parent versus their responsibilities and allegiances as a spouse. While nearly a quarter of the women sampled in this study resolved this dilemma by siding with their male partners, the majority offered at least ambivalent support to their offspring. We found no relationship between child characteristics and maternal support, in contrast to Tufts (1984) and Lyon and Kouloumpos-Lenares (1987) who found mothers to be more protective of their sons than of their daughters, and of younger rather than of older children. The trend, in our sample, for the 16-to-18 year olds to have the highest level of maternal support is probably confounded by the disproportionate number of biological father perpetrators in this age group.

There was a strong relationship, however, between support and the mother's current relationship with the perpetrator. The high maternal support among women in the ex-spouse subgroup is consistent with the high level of maternal "protectiveness" reported by Faller (1984) and Tufts (1984) among women who had earlier divorced or separated from the perpetrator. In such cases, the limited investment in the relationship with her ex-spouse seems to make the mother's decision about whom to believe and support easier. Our findings further suggest that maternal support is inversely related to the recency, and perhaps intensity, of the mother's relationship with the perpetrator, and that the relationship with a current boyfriend is typically more recent and intense than the other relationships studied. The child's disclosure may represent a threat to the potential for increased emotional and financial security that a new relationship offers compared to the problems and uncertainties of single parenthood. Another reason for lower maternal support in the boyfriend group may be that all of the boyfriends denied involvement, whereas over one-third of the biological fathers admitted their guilt. Thus, no conflict existed in the latter cases about whom to believe, only how to divide allegiance and support.

Like others (Adams-Tucker, 1982; Tufts, 1984), we also found a relationship between low maternal support and psychological disturbance among child victims of incest. In the current sample, level of maternal support was found to be more strongly predictive of the child's initial psychological functioning than were the type or length of the abuse or the perpetrator's relationship to the child. While the Tufts study reported increased behavioral disturbances, our Low Support Group manifested more internalized symptoms (e.g., depression, poor self-image).

The comparisons between child self-report during the clinical interview and maternal report on the CBCL were intriguing. Supportive mothers' reports were surprisingly concordant with those of their children. In meta-analyses of cross-informant agreement, derived from 119 studies of child behavioral and emotional problems, Achenbach, McConaughy, and Howell (1987) found the mean correlation between parent report and mental health worker ratings, including clinical interviews like the CAS, to be .25. The authors interpreted the limited agreement between different informants as evidence of situational specificity and argued for a multiaxial approach to child assessment to highlight variations across situation and interaction partners.

Our findings of a high association between supportive mothers' reports and the clinical interview ($r = .63$) and no association between the clinical interview and the reports of ambivalent and unsupportive mothers suggest alternative interpretations of the limited agreement between parent report and other sources of data on the child. Perhaps, as some studies have suggested (Billings & Moos, 1983; Griest, Forehand, Wells, & McMahon, 1980; Hagman, 1930; Schaefer, Hunter, & Edgerton, 1987), a parent's perception of child behavior and emotional problems may reflect the parent's personality and adjustment more than the child's. Mothers who fail to support their children may be struggling with their own personal problems and consequently out of touch with the distress and emotional needs of their children. It is also possible that the descriptions these mothers provide of their children are consciously or unconsciously distorted in an attempt to shape others' perceptions of their accusing children. These distortions may include attempts to discredit their children as "disturbed" and untrustworthy or to minimize the severity of their children's problems as a way of minimizing the probability or significance of the sexual abuse.

These findings have important implications for research in the field because the CBCL has been a popular measure in studies of the mental health of sexually abused children. Considering the questionable validity of many such maternal reports, the methodology of studies relying exclusively on the CBCL or other parental behavior checklists may be seriously challenged.

Finally, the current study and the Tufts study (1984) demonstrate that negative chain events are set into motion when protective service workers perceive low maternal support. Children with blaming or rejecting mothers are more likely to be removed from their homes; this may entail testimony in juvenile court, changing schools, changing church, and otherwise being removed from familiar activities and friends. Further, any support a child may be receiving from important others, from success in academic or nonacademic activities, or simply from familiar routine may be undermined by removal from home.

The child protective service worker and, to a lesser degree, mental health, legal, and medical professionals, exercise some control over the chain of events following disclosure. The perception of the mother's ability to protect the child will be an important factor in decisions about the child's disposition. It is also likely that societal perception of the mother has some impact on how the mother will respond to this personal crisis. Dietz and Craft (1980) found that most social workers (especially those who read professional literature) believe that mothers are as responsible as perpetrator-fathers for the occurrence of incest, despite evidence that 78% of the mothers are victims of physical abuse by their husbands. This type of bias suggests that a victim's mother may feel blamed rather than supported by intervening professionals. For a confused mother caught in the dilemma of choosing between her adult male partner and her child, a perception of blame may tip the scales in favor of alignment with the more powerful adult male.

Clearly, we need less emphasis on the mother's contribution to the occurrence of incest and more emphasis on her contribution to her child's recovery. Immediate intervention aimed at supporting mothers and helping them to believe, empathize with, and offer consistent emotional support and protection to their children may be the most effective way of reducing the child's emotional stress and disruption following disclosure of incest.

REFERENCES

Achenbach, T., & Edelbrock, C. (1981). Behavioral problems and competencies reported by parents of normal and disturbed children aged 4 through 16. *Monographs of the Society for Research in Child Development, 46* (Serial No. 188).

Achenbach, T., & Edelbrock, C. (1983). *Manual for the Child Behavior Checklist and Revised Child Behavior Profile.* Burlington, VT: Department of Psychiatry, University of Vermont.

Achenbach, T., McConaughy, S., & Howell, C. (1987). Child/adolescent behavioral and emotional problems: Implications of cross-informant correlations for situational specificity. *Psychological Bulletin, 101,* 213–232.

Adams-Tucker, C. (1982). Proximate effects of sexual abuse in childhood: A report on 28 children. *America Journal of Psychiatry, 139,* 1252–1256.

Bagley, C., & Ramsay, R. (1985–86). Disrupted childhood and vulnerability to sexual assault: Long-term sequels with implications for counseling. *Journal of Social Work and Human Sexuality, 4,* 33–47.

Billings, A., & Moos, R. (1983). Comparison of children of depressed and nondepressed parents: A social-environmental perspective. *Journal of Abnormal Child Psychology, 11,* 463–486.

Block, J.H., & Block, J. (1980). The role of ego-control and ego-resiliency in the organization of behavior. In W.A. Collins (Ed.), *Development of cognition, affect, and social relations. The Minnesota symposia on child psychology* (Vol. 13). Hillsdale, NJ: Erlbaum.

Bowlby, J. (1973). *Attachment and loss: Vol. I. Attachment.* NY: Basic Books.

Bretherton, I. (1985). Attachment theory: Retrospect and prospect. In I. Bretherton & E. Waters (Eds.), Growing points of attachment theory and research. *Monographs of the Society for Research in Child Development, 50* (Serial No. 209, Nos. 1–2).

Briere, J., & Runtz, M. (1988). Symptomatology associated with childhood sexual victimization in a nonclinical adult sample. *Child Abuse and Neglect, 12,* 367–379.

Burgess, A.W., & Holmstrom, L.L. (1978). Accessory to sex: Pressure, sex, and secrecy. In A. Burgess, A. Groth, L. Holmstrom, & S. Sgroi (Eds.), *Sexual assault of children and adolescents.* Lexington, MA: Lexington Books.

Cobb, S. (1976). Social support as a moderator of life stress. *Psychosomatic Medicine, 38,* 301–314.

Dean, A., & Lin, N. (1977). The stress buffering role of social support. *Journal of Nervous and Mental Disease, 165,* 403–417.

Dietz, C.A., & Craft, J.L. (1980). Family dynamics of incest: A new perspective. *Social Casework, 61,* 602–609.

Faller, K. (1984, May). *Sexual abuse by caretakers.* Paper presented at National Conference of Family Violence Researchers. Durham, NH.

Freud, A., & Burlingham, D. (1943). *War and children.* London: Medical War Books.

Friedrich, W., Urquiza, A., & Beilke, R. (1986). Behavior problems in sexually abused young children. *Journal of Pediatric Psychology, 11,* 47–57.

Garbarino, J., Guttman, E., & Seeley, J. (1986). *The psychologically battered child.* San Francisco: Jossey-Bass.

Garmezy, N. (1985). Stress resistant children: The search for protective factors. In J. Stevenson (Ed.), *Recent research in developmental psychopathology,* Oxford: Pergamon Press.

Gomes-Schwartz, B., Horowitz, J., & Sauzier, M. (1985). Severity of emotional distress among sexually abused preschool, school-age, and adolescent children. *Hospital and Community Psychiatry, 36,* 503–508.

Griest, D., Forehand, R., Wells, K., & McMahon, R. (1980). An examination of differences between nonclinic and behavior-problem clinic-referred children and their mothers. *Journal of Abnormal Psychology, 89,* 497–500.

Hagman, E. (1930). A study of fears of children of preschool age. *Journal of Experimental Education, 1,* 110–130.

Herman, J. (1981). *Father-daughter incest.* Cambridge: Harvard University Press.

Herman, J., Russell, D., & Trocki, K. (1986). Long-term effects of incestuous abuse in childhood. *American Journal of Psychiatry, 143,* 1293–1296.

Hodges, K. (1987). Assessing children with a clinical research interview: The Child Assessment Schedule. In R.J. Prinz (Ed.), *Advances in behavioral assessment of children and families* (Vol. 3, pp. 203–233). Greenwich, CT: JAI Press.

Hodges, K., & Cools, J. (in press). Structural diagnostic interviews. In A.M. LaGreca (Ed.), *Child assessment: Through the eye of a child.* Newton, MA: Allyn & Bacon.

Hodges, K., Kline, J., Stern, L., Cytryn, L., & McKnew, D. (1982). The development of a child assessment schedule for research and clinical use. *Journal of Abnormal Child Psychology, 10,* 173–189.

Lyon, E., & Kouloumpos-Lenares, K. (1987). Clinician and state social worker: Collaborative skills for child sexual abuse. *Child Welfare, 67,* 517–527.

Main, M., Kaplan, N., & Cassidy, J. (1985). Security in infancy, childhood and adulthood. In I. Bretherton & E. Waters (Eds.), Growing points of attachment theory and research. *Monographs for the Society for Research in Child Development, 50* (Serial No. 209).

Mannarino, A., & Cohen, J. (1986). A clinical-demographic study of sexually abused children. *Child Abuse and Neglect, 10,* 17–23.

Meyer, M. (1985). A new look at mothers of incest victims. *Journal of Social Work and Human Sexuality, 3,* 47–58.

Runyan, D., Everson, M., Edelsohn, G., Hunter, W., & Coulter, M. (1988). Impact of legal intervention on sexually abused children. *Journal of Pediatrics, 113,* 647–653.

Rutter, M. (1979). Protective factors in children's responses to stress and disadvantage. In M.W. Kent & J.E. Rolfe (Eds.), *Primary prevention of psychopathology: Social competence in children* (Vol. 3). Hanover, NH: University Press of New England.

Rutter, M. (1987). Psychosocial resilience and protective mechanisms. *American Journal of Orthopsychiatry, 57,* 316–331.

Schaefer, E., Hunter, W., & Edgerton, M. (1987). Maternal prenatal, infancy, and concurrent predictors of maternal reports of child psychopathology. *Psychiatry, 50,* 320–331.

Simrel, K., Berg, R., & Thomas, J. (1979). Crisis management of sexually abused children. *Pediatric Annals, 8,* 59–72.

Summit, R. (1983). The child sexual abuse accommodation syndrome. *Child Abuse & Neglect, 7,* 177–193.

Tufts' New England Medical Center, Division of Child Psychiatry. (1984). *Sexually exploited children: Service and research project.* Final report for the Office of Juvenile Justice and Delinquency Prevention, U.S. Department of Justice, Washington, DC.

Werner, E., & Smith, R. (1982). *Vulnerable but invincible: A study of resilient children.* New York: McGraw Hill.

White, S., Halpin, B., Strom, G., & Santilli, G. (1986, May). *Behavioral comparisons of young sexually abused, neglected, and nonreferred children.* Paper presented at National Conference on the Sexual Victimization of Children, New Orleans.

Part IV
CLINICAL ISSUES

The publication of DSM-III in 1980 ushered in a new era in child psychiatry. It has become possible to study the clinical characteristics and correlates, natural history and response to treatment of disorders defined in terms of specific behavioral criteria. Entities previously not thought to occur in childhood have been identified and new questions regarding the coexistance of different disorders have arisen as child psychiatrists continue to work toward the development of a meaningful system of classification of disorder. The papers in this section reflect some of these concerns.

Cantwell and Baker report on the stability and natural history of specific DSM-III childhood diagnoses over a four to five-year period. The subjects were 151 children and adolescents whose ages at the time of initial presentation for assessment of speech and/or language disorders were between 2.3 and 15.9 years. The data provide a wealth of information. The persistence of disorder was striking: 87% of children with an initial diagnosis of a behavior disorder; 67% with an emotional disorder; 100% with PDD; 74% with adjustment disorders; and 80% with parent/child problems were still ill at time of follow-up. However, diagnostic stability was found for only infantile autism, attention deficit disorder with hyperactivity, and oppositional disorder. Children initially diagnosed as having attention deficit disorder without hyperactivity, avoidant disorder, separation anxiety disorder, overanxious disorder, and conduct disorder were highly likely to have other different disorders at follow-up. Despite methodologic limitations deriving from the age range of the sample and the fact that all of the subjects had a coexisting speech and language disorder, the findings raise important questions regarding our understanding of specific diagnostic entities and the validity of diagnostic categories as we currently understand them.

In their introduction to the second paper in this section, Russell, Bott, and Sammons provide an overview of the controversies concerning the phenomenology and classification of the severe psychiatric disorders of childhood. For many years broad or unspecified diagnostic criteria for "childhood schizophrenia" were used to identify research subjects, mixing together a variety of psychotic children including those with autism, schizophrenia, mental retardation, organic disorders, and possibly major affective disorder as well.

With the publication of DSM-III, and its revision DSM-III-R, the separation between the pervasive developmental disorders and schizophrenia as it occurs in prepubertal children is clearly established. Russell et al. have used a semistructured interview, the Interview for Childhood Disorders and Schizophrenia to specify the phenomenology of schizophrenia in 35 children between the ages of four and 13 who met strict DSM-III criteria for the disorder. The report is a superb example of a modern clinical study, which includes not only a summary of data of specified reliability but descriptive examples as well. Of particular interest in light of the growing attention being directed toward the study of comorbid conditions is the fact that 24 of the 35 subjects (69%) met DSM-III criteria for additional diagnoses. Moreover, in 30 of 35 (86%) of cases there was a clear history of behavioral disturbance prior to the onset of psychosis. Although the type of premorbid symptoms varied widely, two groups could be identified. Over 40% of the sample had a premorbid history of attentional problems and hyperactivity, complicated in some by conduct disturbances as well. Approximately one-quarter had premorbid histories marked by a variety of developmental abnormalities—echolalia, rituals, tactile sensitivity, flapping—but none were felt to have met full criteria for autism or pervasive developmental disorder. Whether these different prepsychotic symptom patterns have different implications for subsequent course is a matter for future research.

The next three papers address the question of panic disorder in children and adolescence from somewhat different vantage points. Taken as a whole, they expand our awareness of a heretofore unrecognized, or at best underrecognized, disorder in this age group. Ballenger, Carek, Steele, and Cornish-McTighe present clinical vignettes of three children ages seven, eight, and 13, all of whom met DSM-III-R criteria for panic disorder with agoraphobia of mild-to-moderate severity. These children came to be noticed in the course of clinical practice, and structured diagnostic interviews were not employed to make the diagnosis. Although all of children were noted to have features of separation, avoidant, and phobic disorders of childhood, their clinical syndromes were similar to that of the usual adult presentation of panic disorder, and all responded to treatment with imipramine.

From a somewhat different perspective, Moreau, Weissman, and Warner report that seven children and adolescents were found to have panic symptoms in the course of a study of a total of 220 children ages six to 23, who were at high or low risk for depression by virtue of their parent's diagnosis. Information deriving from structured interviews with children and parents, and school and psychiatric records, were reviewed by a child psychiatrist and child psychologist to arrive at a reliable DSM-III diagnosis. Of the seven children who had panic symptoms, six met criteria for panic disorder. Onset was before puberty in four children. All of these children had other diagnoses, most commonly major depression and separation anxiety disorder. No cases of panic disorder were found in children of nondepressed parents. Moreau et al. suggest that a systematic assessment of panic disorder should be part of a general psychiatric workup of children, particularly children whose parents are depressed.

The saliency of this suggestion is underscored by Hayward, Killen, and Taylor, who also found that panic attacks are by no means confined to adults. The lifetime prevalence of panic attacks as determined in the course of brief interviews with 95 9th graders (between the ages of 14 and 16) was found to be 11.6%. Responses to a self-report questionnaire designed to assess depressive symptoms revealed a significant association between the two sets of symptoms.

Adolescence often marks the onset of eating disorders. Fava, Copeland, Schweiger, and Herzog's review of research on neurochemical abnormalities in anorexia nervosa and bulimia nervosa updates this area of research for the general clinician. Understanding the neurochemistry of eating disorders is an important step in the clarification of pathophysiology and the development of more effective treatments. The authors have focused upon the neurotransmitters and neuromodulators that regulate eating behavior. Anorexia nervosa is associated with changes in the noradrenergic, serotonergic, and opiod systems, whereas bulimia nervosa is accompanied by marked alterations in serotonin and norepinephrine activity. Although it is debated whether these neuroendocrine changes are primary or secondary to starvation or marked fluctuations in food intake, it has become increasingly clear that they may contribute to the perpetuation of pathologic eating behavior, and that they also may be responsible for several associated psychiatric symptoms including anxiety and depression.

In the final paper in this section, the issue of comorbidity is addressed, this time in relation to depressive and anxiety disorders in children. Kovacs, Gatsonis, Paulauskas, and Richards report on the co-occurrence of anxiety disorders and major depressive disorder, dysthymic disorder, and adjustment disorder with depressed mood in 104 reliably diagnosed children who ranged in age from eight to 13 years at the time of their enrollment in an ongoing longitudinal study. Forty-one percent were found to have anxiety disorders in conjunction with their index depression. Anxiety disorders were more likely to co-occur with major depression and dysthymia than with adjustment disorder, and the most frequently occurring anxiety diagnosis was separation-anxiety disorder. The results are discussed against the background of the debate about whether, in adults, depression and anxiety are categorically distinct. The authors note that the co-occurrence of separation-anxiety and major depression in this sample of children is of particular interest because of its phenomenologic similarity to the agoraphobia-panic-depression cluster in adults.

16

Stability and Natural History of *DSM-III* Childhood Diagnoses

Dennis P. Cantwell and Lorian Baker

UCLA Neuropsychiatric Institute

Follow-up or natural history outcome data for various DSM-III *child and adolescent psychiatric diagnoses are presented. The data are relevant not only to our understanding of the specific disorders but also to the validity of the* DSM-III *diagnostic categories. "Semi-blind" psychiatric evaluations of 151 children were made as they presented to a community speech/language clinic and again approximately 4 years later. The follow-up data revealed high stability for only three diagnoses: infantile autism, attention deficit disorder with hyperactivity, and oppositional disorder. The data revealed that several of the* DSM-III *subcategories lacked predictive validity. This was true for the distinctions between attention deficit disorder with versus without hyperactivity; and between avoidant, separation anxiety, and overanxious disorders. Surprisingly low stability was found for conduct disorder diagnoses as were surprisingly poor prognoses for parent-child problems and adjustment disorders. Key Words:* DSM-III, *prognosis, validity, attention deficit disorder, conduct disorder.*

Little is known about the natural history (or outcome) of many of the childhood and adolescent psychiatric disorders. Such data are not only necessary to our understanding of the various psychiatric disorders, but also relevant to the establishment of a psychiatric diagnostic classification system.

In a recent publication in the *Journal*, Cantwell and Baker (1988a) discussed the criteria (including reliability, validity, and feasibility) for a successful psychiatric diagnostic classification system. One of the more important criteria is that the diag-

Reprinted with permission from *Journal of the American Academy of Child and Adolescent Psychiatry,* 1989, Vol. 28, No. 5, 691–700. Copyright © 1989 by the American Academy of Child and Adolescent Psychiatry.

nostic categories have external validity, that is, that they can be verified as unique categories by external data. As outlined elsewhere (Cantwell, 1975), various types of data are relevant to the external validity of psychiatric diagnostic categories. These include epidemiological data, family aggregation data, biological and laboratory data, psychosocial data, natural history and outcome data, and response to treatment studies. The present paper presents data of one such type, namely, natural history and outcome data, for various *DSM-III* childhood and adolescent diagnostic categories.

In particular, this paper presents data from a prospective 4- to 5-year follow-up study of a cohort of children drawn from a large community speech and hearing clinic. Six hundred children were seen initially when they presented for assessment of speech and/or language disorders. All were initially under the age of 16 and without significant hearing impairment. The results of the initial psychiatric assessment of these children, presented in the *Journal* and elsewhere (Baker and Cantwell, 1982a, b; Cantwell and Baker, 1980; Cantwell et al., 1979, 1981) revealed a psychiatric illness rate of approximately 50%.

The preliminary results of follow-up evaluations of 300 of these children were presented recently in the *Journal* (Baker and Cantwell, 1987). It was found that the overall prevalence of psychiatric disorder and the overall prevalence of certain specific diagnoses had increased significantly between the initial and follow-up evaluations. However, the specific outcomes for the various initial psychiatric diagnoses were not examined.

The present paper examines 151 of those children who initially had various *DSM-III* childhood psychiatric diagnoses and traces the stability of the various diagnoses found. These data are relevant to the external validity of these *DSM-III* diagnostic categories.

METHOD

The methodology of the studies has been described in previous publications (Baker and Cantwell, 1982a, b, 1987; Cantwell and Baker, 1980, 1985; Cantwell et al., 1979, 1981). Both initial and follow-up evaluations consisted of speech/language assessment, academic achievement testing, and intellectual testing (administered by L.B.) and psychiatric assessment by a board-certified child psychiatrist (D.P.C. or others in initial study; D.P.C. alone in the follow-up study).

Psychiatric diagnoses were made initially and at follow-up using *DSM-III* diagnostic criteria and based on data collected with four types of instruments: parent and child interviews (the DICA, Orvaschel, 1985) and parent and teacher behavior rating scales (two forms of each: Conners, 1973; Rutter et al., 1970). The reliability of the psychiatric diagnosis procedure was tested at the time of the initial study; it was 96% for the presence or absence of psychiatric disorder, and 94% for the specific diagnoses (Cantwell and Baker, 1985). The same procedures were used for the follow-up evaluation, but they were not retested for reliability at that time.

The follow-up psychiatric diagnoses were made "semi-blind" to the initial psychiatric diagnosis. (That is, the clinician did not have the initial evaluation materials and diagnosis available to him. Because of the large number of children in the initial study, most were not remembered by the time of follow-up; however, in a few outstanding cases the child's initial visit and diagnosis were remembered).

Ninety percent of the entire initial sample was seen for follow-up. However, this present paper reports only on 150 cases who had certain specific psychiatric diagnoses initially. The initial diagnoses, and age and sex distributions for these cases, are summarized in Table 1.

The group studied consisted of 151 children, 105 (70%) of whom were males, and 46 (30%) of whom were females. Initially the children ranged in age from 2.3 to 15.9 years (mean age 5.9 years; standard deviation 2.9). At follow-up, the group ranged in age from 5.2 to 20.6 years (mean age 9.7; standard deviation 2.9). Initially, all of the children had some impairment in either speech and/or language functioning. Twenty-three percent of the group had only disorders of speech production; 65% had disorders involving both speech production and language, and 12% of

TABLE 1
Initial Data for Cases Followed

| Diagnosis | N | Age (in years) | | | Sex (% Male) |
		Range	Mean	SD	
ADDH	35	2.3 to 9.6	5.5	1.8	91
ADDNO	5	5.7 to 8.3	6.7	1.2	40
Conduct disorders	9	3.2 to 9.4	5.7	2.0	89
Oppositional disorder	15	3.4 to 13.1	5.4	3.3	80
Total behavioral	64	2.3 to 13.1	5.6	2.3	84
Separation anxiety	9	2.4 to 6.6	3.6	1.3	56
Avoidant disorder	14	3.1 to 9.7	5.0	1.9	43
Overanxious disorder	8	4.0 to 11.2	7.3	2.3	63
Total anxiety	31	2.4 to 11.2	5.2	2.3	48
Affective disorders	7	6.5 to 15.8	10.4	3.9	43
Total emotional	38	2.4 to 15.8	6.1	3.3	58
Adjustment disorders	19	3.0 to 15.8	6.4	4.2	53
Pervasive devel disorder	3	5.4 to 11.8	8.3	3.2	100
Parent-child problem	15	2.8 to 7.7	4.1	1.3	80
Mixed psychiatric diagnoses	12	2.8 to 15.9	8.1	3.8	67
Total cases followed	151	2.3 to 15.9	5.9	2.9	70

the children had disorders involving only language development. The intellectual functioning of the group was within normal limits, and the socioeconomic distribution was approximately one third upper or upper-middle social class level, one third middle-class level, and one third lower- or lower-middle social class level (using Hollingshead two-factor scoring of social class).

The majority of children in the sample (approximately 85%) received at least 4 months of speech/language therapy, either within the school setting, in a private speech clinic setting, or both. Conversely, the majority of children did not receive psychiatric treatments, although 10% of the group had received medication trials (usually under the supervision of a pediatrician) and 15% had had at least one visit with a psychologist, psychiatric, or family therapist.

RESULTS

Outcome of the Behavioral Disorder Diagnoses

The outcome data for all of the cases ($N = 139$) with uncomplicated or "pure" initial diagnoses are summarized in Table 2. The behavioral psychiatric disorders (which include the *DSM-III* diagnostic categories of attention deficit disorders, oppositional disorder, and conduct disorders) are discussed first.

Overall, the behavioral psychiatric disorders were among the most stable categories of diagnoses. Children with early behavioral disorders were highly likely to have some psychiatric disorder 4 to 5 years later. In fact, 87% of those children with behavioral disorders initially were still psychiatrically ill at follow-up. Within the general group of behavioral disorders, however, the various specific diagnostic categories showed a considerable range in stability.

Attention Deficit Disorder with Hyperactivity

Attention deficit disorder with hyperactivity (ADDH) was the most stable subtype of the behavioral disorders. Of the 35 children with this pure diagnosis initially, a total of 28 (or 80%) still had ADDH at follow-up, 23 in pure form, and five with some additional diagnosis. Furthermore, the recovery rate for ADDH was very low; only three of the 35 children (or 9%) were psychiatrically well at follow-up.

The other psychiatric outcomes for the ADDH children were diverse. The most commonly occurring other outcome for the ADDH children was some type of emotional disorder. The emotional disorders included both anxiety disorders (two cases with overanxious disorder, and one case with obsessive compulsive disorder) and affective disorders (one case with dysthymic disorder, three with major depression). Of the six ADDH children who had emotional disorders at follow-up, five had comorbid ADDH diagnoses and only one child had a pure emotional disorder.

TABLE 2

Outcomes for Cases with Pure Initial Disorders

Initial Diagnosis		Well		Same Disorder		Follow-up Status[a] Other Diagnoses (N)				
							Emotional			
	N	N	%	N	%	Behavioral	Anxiety	Affective	PDD	Other
Behavioral										
ADDH	35	3	9	28	80	1	3	4	2	1
ADDNO	5	1	20	0	0	5	0	1	0	0
Conduct	9	3	33	1	11	3	0	0	0	2
Oppositional	15	1	7	6	40	10	1	2	0	1
Total behavioral	64	8	13	35	55	18	3	7	2	5
Emotional										
Avoidant	14	5	36	4	29	3	4	2	0	0
Separation anxiety	9	4	44	1	11	2	3	0	0	0
Overanxious	8	2	25	2	25	3	2	1	0	0
Affective	7	2	29	2	29	1	2	2	1	0
Total emotional	38	13	67	9	24	9	11	5	1	0
Parent/child	15	3	80	0	0	14	1	0	0	3
Pervasive developmental disorder	3	0	0	3	100	0	0	0	0	0
Adjustment disorders with										
Depressed mood	2	2	100	0	0	0	0	0	0	0
Emotional problems	8	2	25	0	0	5	3	0	0	0
Withdrawl	1	0	0	0	0	1	1	0	0	0
Conduct and emotional problems	5	1	20	0	0	4	2	0	0	0
Conduct disorder	2	0	0	0	0	2	1	0	0	0
Atypical disorder	1	0	0	0	0	1	0	0	0	0
Total adjustment disorders	19	5	74	0	0	13	7	0	0	0

[a] Numbers under "Follow-up status" refer to the number of times this diagnosis occurred; hence, due to comorbid diagnoses, these numbers will not tally with the number of children in the N column.

Among the other psychiatric illnesses found in the ADDH children at follow-up were: other behavioral disorders (one case with undersocialized aggressive conduct disorder); pervasive developmental disorders (two cases with infantile autism); and transient tic disorder (one case).

Comorbid diagnoses at follow-up were found in a total of five of the ADDH children; three children had dual diagnoses and two children had triple diagnoses. For all of these children, the comorbid diagnoses consisted of ADDH plus some other associated psychiatric illness. The other associated illnesses were usually emotional disorders (three cases of major depression, and one case each of dysthymic disorder, overanxious disorder and obsessive compulsive disorder). However there was one ADDH child who had ADDH and transient tic disorder at follow-up.

Attention Deficit Disorder without Hyperactivity

As can be seen in Table 2, the psychiatric outcome for attention deficit disorder *without* hyperactivity (ADDNO) showed very different recovery and stability rates from those of ADDH. First, the recovery rate of ADDNO appeared to be higher than for ADDH. One child (constituting 20% of the ADDNO group) was psychiatrically well at follow-up, as opposed to only 9% of the ADDNO group. Unfortunately the ADDNO group was so small (only five cases) that statistical analysis of this comparison was not possible.

ADDNO was the least stable of the behavioral diagnoses. At follow-up, none of the children from the initial ADDNO group had maintained the same diagnoses. However, all four of the ADDNO children who were still psychiatrically ill at follow-up had a diagnosis of ADDH. In addition to the ADDH follow-up diagnosis, one child had two other associated diagnoses at follow-up. These were undersocialized unaggressive conduct disorder, and dysthymic disorder.

Conduct Disorders

Nine children had pure initial diagnoses of conduct disorders. Of these, one had socialized unaggressive conduct disorder, one had undersocialized unaggressive conduct disorder, and eight had undersocialized aggressive conduct disorder. The conduct disorders, as a group, showed a better rate of recovery than either ADDH or ADDNO. Three (33%) of the nine conduct disordered children (two with undersocialized aggressive conduct disorder and one with socialized unaggressive conduct disorder) were well at follow-up.

The conduct disorders were not stable, either as individual diagnoses or as a general group. At follow-up, only one of the children (with initial undersocialized aggressive conduct disorder) still had any conduct disorder diagnosis (in fact, the same diagnosis). Of those conduct disordered children who were still psychiatrically ill at follow-up, three had other behavioral disorders (ADDH), and two had other types of disorders (organic personality syndrome and unspecified psychiatric disorder).

Oppositional Disorder

Oppositional disorder showed the poorest recovery rate of all the behavioral psychiatric disorders. At follow-up, only one of the fifteen oppositional children (7%) had become psychiatrically well.

The oppositional disorder diagnosis showed an intermediate degree of stability over the 4- to 5-year period. Six of the oppositional children (or 40%) retained the same diagnosis at follow-up. However, other behavioral disorders were also common outcomes for those children with initial diagnoses of oppositional disorder. At follow-up, six of the oppositional children had ADDH and four had some type of conduct disorder. Three oppositional children had emotional disorders at follow-up (two had dysthymic disorder and one had overanxious disorder), and one child had organic personality syndrome.

Three of the 15 oppositional children had comorbid diagnoses at follow-up. These were ADDH, oppositional disorder and dysthymic disorder in one case; ADDH and undersocialized conduct disorder in the second case, and ADDH, unaggressive conduct disorder, and dysthymic disorder in the third case.

Emotional Disorder Diagnoses

In contrast to the behavioral psychiatric disorders (which involve overt disturbances in behaviors), the emotional psychiatric disorders involve disturbances of mood or feelings. The emotional psychiatric disorders fall into two major subclasses: anxiety disorders (including separation anxiety disorder, avoidant disorder, and overanxious disorder) and affective disorders (including major depression, dysthymic disorder, cyclothymic disorder, and bipolar disorder). Thirty-eight of the children in this study initially had pure emotional disorders. They were slightly older (aged 2.4 to 15.8 years, $\bar{X} = 6.1$) than the children with pure behavioral disorders (aged 2.3 to 13.1, $\bar{X} = 5.6$), and they were more likely to be girls (58% were males in the emotional group versus 84% in the behavioral group).

In general, the emotional disorders were characterized by higher rates of recovery, and, for those cases who remained psychiatrically ill, lower rates of stability than the behavioral disorders. Within the general category of emotional disorders, the various specific diagnostic categories were less dissimilar with regard to outcome than the various categories of behavioral disorders. The specific categories of emotional disorders are each discussed below.

Avoidant Disorder

The most common of the pure emotional disorders occurring initially was avoidant disorder with 14 cases. These children ranged in age from 3.1 years to 9.7 years ($\bar{X} = 5.0$, SD $= 1.9$) and consisted of eight girls and six boys. At follow-up, these children were most commonly still psychiatrically ill (with only five of the group or 36% being well).

Avoidant disorder was the most stable of the childhood anxiety disorders. At follow-up, four of the avoidant children still had the same diagnosis. This represents 29% of the group of avoidant children, and 44% of the subgroup of avoidant children who had not recovered from psychiatric illness at follow-up.

The most common other follow-up diagnoses for these children were other types of emotional disorders. Four of the initially avoidant children had overanxious disorder at follow-up, and two had dysthymic disorder. Three behavioral disorder diagnoses were found: ADDH, ADDNO, and oppositional disorder.

Of the six avoidant children who were ill at follow-up with other disorders, three had more than one diagnosis. The comorbid psychiatric diagnoses were (1) overanxious disorder, dysthymic disorder, and ADDNO; (2) avoidant disorder and overanxious disorder; and (3) oppositional disorder, dysthymic disorder, and overanxious disorder.

Separation Anxiety Disorder

The group of children with an initial pure diagnosis of separation anxiety disorder consisted of four girls and five boys, aged 2.4 to 6.6 years ($\bar{X} = 3.6$, SD $= 1.3$). At follow-up, four of these children (44% of the group) were psychiatrically well, and one child (11%) still had separation anxiety disorder. These figures represent the highest rate of recovery and the lowest rate of stability of any of the emotional disorders.

Other psychiatric diagnoses at follow-up were approximately equally distributed between anxiety and behavioral disorders. Two children had behavioral disorders (ADDH and ADDNO) and three children had overanxious disorder. Only one of the children with separation anxiety disorder initially had comorbid diagnoses at follow-up. These were ADDNO and overanxious disorder.

Overanxious Disorder

Eight children (three girls and five boys) received pure initial diagnoses of overanxious disorder. These children tended to be older initially (4.0 to 11.2 years, mean age 7.3, SD 2.3) than the other anxiety disordered children. Of all the subgroups of emotionally disordered children, the overanxious group had the lowest recovery rate. Only two overanxious children (or 25%) were psychiatrically well at follow-up.

The stability of the overanxious disorder diagnosis was also quite low. Only two children (25%) continued to have overanxious disorder at follow-up, whereas an equal number had another type of anxiety disorder (avoidant disorder). Other follow-up diagnoses found in the overanxious group were ADDH (one case), ADDNO (two cases), and major depression (one case). Two of the overanxious children received multiple diagnoses at follow-up: avoidant disorder and overanxious disorder in one case, and avoidant disorder and ADDNO in the other.

Affective Disorders

Seven older children (ages 6.5 to 15.8 years, mean age 10.4 years, SD 3.9), consisting of four girls and three boys, had pure initial diagnoses of some type of affective disorder. The specific affective disorder diagnoses found were: major depression (two cases), dysthymic disorder (two cases), cyclothymic disorder (one case), and bipolar disorder (one case).

At follow-up, two of the affective disorder cases (one of major depression and one of dysthymic disorder) had become psychiatrically well and two (one of dysthymic disorder and one of bipolar disorder) were stable. In addition, two cases still had affective disorders, but a different subtype than initially (the initial diagnoses of major depression and cyclothymic disorder both became dysthymic at follow-up).

Other follow-up diagnoses in the affective group included: pervasive developmental disorder, ADDH, overanxious disorder, and avoidant disorder. Although the numbers are too small for statistical analysis, it appears that children with affective disorders may be less likely to develop behavioral disorders than children with anxiety disorders. Conversely, it appears that children with affective disorders may be more likely to have multiple diagnoses at follow-up. Three of the affective disordered children (43%) had comorbid psychiatric disorders at follow-up. Two were cases of initial major depression (one case with ADDH and pervasive developmental disorder at follow-up and the other with dysthymic disorder and overanxious disorder) and one was an initial case of bipolar disorder (with two follow-up diagnoses, bipolar disorder and avoidant disorder).

Parent-Child Problem

The *DSM-III* "V-code" diagnosis of parent-child problem occurred as the single initial diagnosis in 15 young (2.8 to 7.7 years, X̄ 4.1, SD 1.3) children. Three of these children were girls and the remainder were boys. Although parent-child problem is not considered a "true" psychiatric disorder, it is of interest here because the prognosis for these children was as poor or poorer than that for the children with true psychiatric disorders. As can be seen in Table 2, only three of the children with early parent-children problems (or 20%) were found to be psychiatrically well at follow-up.

Of the 12 children with parent-child problem initially who remained psychiatrically ill at follow-up, all but one received a developmental disorder diagnosis. Of the 11 children with parent-child problem initially who had behavioral disorders at follow-up, ten had ADDH, one had ADDNO, and three had secondary diagnoses of oppositional disorder. Other psychiatric disorders found at follow-up included pica (two cases), avoidant disorder (one case) and adjustment disorder with disturbance of conduct and emotions (one case).

Multiple psychiatric diagnoses were very common among the children with initial parent-child problems. One-third of the group had comorbid psychiatric disorders at follow-up: two cases had ADDH and pica, one had ADDH and oppositional disorder, one had ADDNO and oppositional disorder, and one had ADDH, oppositional disorder and avoidant disorder.

Pervasive Developmental Disorders

Three boys received initial diagnoses of infantile autism. Not surprisingly (insofar as *DSM-III* considers the pervasive developmental disorders to be chronic) this group of disorders had the lowest recovery rate (0% were well at follow-up) and the highest stability rate (100%). All three of the autistic children had the same diagnosis at follow-up as initially.

Adjustment Disorders

Nineteen children in the sample had a pure diagnosis of some type of adjustment disorder. These included adjustment disorder with disturbance of conduct (two cases), adjustment disorder with depressed mood (two cases), adjustment disorder with mixed emotional features (eight cases), adjustment disorder with mixed disturbance of emotions and conduct (five cases), adjustment disorder with withdrawal (one case), and adjustment disorder with atypical features (one case).

The adjustment disorders had the lowest stability rate (0%) of any of the psychiatric disorders. The recovery rate for the adjustment disorders was also relatively low (26%).

The outcome data for the children with adjustment disorders were also examined in order to determine if there was any stability in the general types of symptoms, i.e., if children with initial adjustment disorders with emotional symptoms tended to have follow-up emotional diagnoses and if children with initial adjustment disorders with conduct symptoms tended to have follow-up behavioral disorders. In fact, as the data in Table 2 show, there was little correspondence between initial symptomatology and follow-up diagnosis. The adjustment disordered children were most likely to have follow-up diagnoses of behavioral disorders or anxiety disorders, regardless of their specific initial type of adjustment disorder. The follow-up diagnoses of the adjustment disordered children were ADDH (11 cases), oppositional disorder (two cases), overanxious disorder (six cases), and avoidant disorder (one case).

Six of the 19 children (32%) with initial adjustment disorders had comorbid diagnoses at follow-up. These included three cases with ADDH and overanxious disorder, two cases with ADDH and oppositional disorder, and one case with avoidant disorder and overanxious disorder.

Outcome of Cases with Initial Comorbidity

Twelve children had comorbid psychiatric diagnoses initially. The initial and follow-up diagnoses of these cases along with their (initial) age and sex data are summarized in Table 3.

ADDH, the most common of the pure initial diagnoses, was also the most common comorbid diagnosis. Seven children had an initial diagnosis of ADDH along with some other coexisting diagnosis. The outcomes for these seven children largely mirrored those of the children with the pure ADDH diagnoses: low rate of recovery and high rate of stability. Of the seven comorbid ADDH children, none were well at follow-up, and five (71%) had some type of ADD diagnosis at follow-up.

Affective disorders were also common among the initial comorbid group of children. Six children had some type of initial comorbid affective disorder (four with major depression and one each with dysthymic disorder and cyclothymic disorder). As with the children with initial pure affective disorders, these children had follow-up diagnoses most commonly in the behavioral or anxiety disorders groups. None of the children with initial comorbid affective disorders had the same affective diagnosis at follow-up, although there was one child whose initial major depression became dysthymic disorder at follow-up.

DISCUSSION

Attention Deficit Disorder with Hyperactivity

ADDH was one of the most stable disorders seen, with 80% of the ADDH disorder still having the same diagnosis four to five years later. This finding is not surprising in view of the large number of reports of childhood ADDH continuing into adolescence and even adulthood (Amado and Lustman, 1982; Borland and Heckman, 1976; Cowart, 1982; Thorley, 1984; Weiss and Hechtman, 1986).

The other psychiatric disorders that developed in the ADDH children included transient tic disorder, pervasive developmental disorder, anxiety disorders and

TABLE 3
Data for Cases with Initial Comorbid Diagnoses

Initial Diagnoses	Follow-up Diagnoses	Age	Sex
ADDH/separation anxiety	ADDNO	4.3	m
ADDH/major depression	avoidant disorder/ADDNO	10.7	m
ADDH/elective mutism	ADDH/overanxious disorder	2.8	m
ADDH/organic personality syndrome	organic brain syndrome	9.8	m
ADDH/major depression	ADDH/dysthymic disorder	9.0	m
ADDH/major depression	ADDH/overanxious disorder	11.1	m
ADDH/major depression	ADDH	9.6	m
ADDNO/gender identity disorder	ADDH/avoidant/oppositional	8.2	f
Avoidant/cyclothymic disorder	well	8.5	f
Oppositional/overanxious	well	3.2	f
Oppositional/avoidant disorder	elective mutism/oppositional	4.6	f
Dysthymic/parent-child pblm	ADDH/generalized anxiety	15.9	m

depressive disorders. An association between tics and ADDH has been observed in the Comings' research on Tourette syndrome. As reported in Comings and Comings (1987), in the natural course of the disease, in the majority of Tourette syndrome patients, ADDH develops first, then 2.4 years later motor and vocal tics develop. Although the patient in this study developed a transient (motor) tic rather than chronic motor and vocal tics, it is likely that a similar mechanism may be involved. It is relevant to note that this particular patient had not received stimulant medication.

The association between ADDH and anxiety and affective disorders has also been reported in the literature (Biederman et al., 1987; Carlson and Cantwell, 1982; Lahey et al., 1987). The appearance of these disorders at follow-up in certain of the ADDH children, as well as the high frequency of initial comorbid diagnoses of ADDH plus emotional disorders may be relevant to the hypotheses that ADDH children with affective disorders constitute a distinct subgroup (Biederman, et al., 1987). Unfortunately, the numbers of children in this study are too small for statistical comparisons of other background and family variables that could confirm this hypothesis.

The development at follow-up of infantile autism in two of the initially ADDH patients is somewhat surprising, although less so considering that infantile autism is a major cause of speech/language disturbances and that these children were drawn from a speech clinic sample. Both of these patients had been quite young initially (2.3 years and 3.2 years of age), both were boys, and both had severe disturbances in both speech and language. Retrospective examination of these patients' initial charts revealed an inability to test either child using formal procedures due to apathetic noninvolvement in one child and tantrums in the other child. These two cases point out the difficulty of establishing a differential diagnosis between hyperactivity and pervasive developmental disorder in young children. They also confirm the findings of Konno and Ohno's (1981) developmental study of the symptoms of hyperactivity and autism. These authors reported that, according to parental reports, the earliest symptoms in hyperactive children were hyperactivity, followed by temper tantrums and perseveration, whereas the earliest symptom of autistic children was temper tantrums.

Despite a well-documented association between hyperactivity and conduct disorders (Langner et al., 1974; Reeves et al., 1987; Rutter et al., 1970; Sandbert et al., 1980; Werry et al., 1987a), only one of the ADDH children in this study had a conduct disorder at follow-up. Thus, the data from this group of children support those authors arguing for the independence of hyperactivity and conduct syndromes (Loney et al., 1978; Taylor et al., 1986; Taylor, 1988; Trites and Laprade, 1983). Insofar as the children studied were still fairly young at follow-up, it is still possible, however, that conduct disorders may develop in some of these children as they become older and face learning and social difficulties in the school setting that might predispose to later development of conduct disorder.

Attention Deficit Disorder without Hyperactivity

The ADDNO category is a controversial one, and, in fact, the ADDH versus ADDNO dichotomy (as defined in *DSM-III*) is no longer maintained in *DSM-III-R*. The evidence that ADDNO is valid as a psychiatric disorder distinct from ADDH is primarily symptom data having to do with either emotional or cognitive functioning (Berry et al., 1985; Carlson, 1986; Carlson et al., 1987; Edelbrock et al., 1984; King and Young, 1982; Sergeant and Scholten, 1985). However, one recent study (Frank and Ben-Nun, 1988) found that certain neurological correlates did distinguish the two disorders.

The present study is the only one of which the authors are aware that examines the natural history of both ADDH and ADDNO. These data revealed very different recovery and stability rates for the two disorders. The recovery rate for ADDNO was considerably higher than that for ADDH; and the stability rate was considerably lower. Twenty percent of the ADDNO group became well versus 9% of the ADDH group; and 0% of the ADDNO group remained stable versus 80% of the ADDH group. Although these data would appear to argue for the distinctness of the two disorders, closer examination reveals that the outcomes for the two disorders were actually rather similar. In fact, all of the ADDNO children who were still psychiatrically ill at follow-up received a diagnosis of ADDH. Thus, the rate for ADDH at follow-up was exactly the same, (80%), among the children with initial ADDNO as it was for the children with initial ADDH. This suggests that ADDH and ADDNO may not have validity as distinct psychiatric syndromes.

Conduct Disorders

Of the nine purely conduct disordered children in this study, three (33%) recovered and only one (11%) remained conduct disordered at follow-up. These findings contradict the generally held belief that aggressive behaviors and/or conduct disorders in children are relatively stable over time (Halverson and Waldrop, 1976; Kagan and Moss, 1962; Minde and Minde, 1977; Olweus, 1979; Zeitlin, 1986).

Furthermore, the finding has relevance to the validity of the *DSM-III* conduct disorder definition. Rutter and Tuma (1988) have observed that a diagnostic system for childhood psychiatric disorders needs to differentiate between those conduct disorders that constitute transient problems during childhood or adolescence and those that represent the precursors of sociopathic or personality disorders in adult life. The present data would indicate that the definition of conduct disorders provided by *DSM-III* applies to transient childhood problems.

There are two other factors that may be relevant to the observed lack of continuity of conduct disorders in this sample of children. First, the children were very young when first diagnosed (the mean age was 5.7 years), and did not yet manifest some of the more "serious" or "delinquency" symptoms of conduct disorder (such as firesetting, stealing outside the home, mugging, vandalism, or rape). Furthermore, because of the young age of the children initially, they did not display school failure or learning disability, factors which, when present with nondelinquent conduct disorder, are typically associated with persistence (Wolff, 1985).

Finally, it must be remembered that all of the children in this study had, at least initially, some type of speech and/or language dysfunction, and that this dysfunction may have played a role in the outcome and indeed in the diagnosis of these children's psychiatric disorders. With the conduct disorder diagnosis in particular, it is possible the conduct symptomatology manifested by these young children was a response to the frustration of being unable to express themselves due to a language disorder. Although the number of children here is too small for statistical analysis, the raw data do give some support to the hypothesis that frustration/language disorder plays a role in the continuity of the conduct disorder diagnoses. In fact, the three conduct disordered children who became psychiatrically well had speech/language disorders that were milder initially and that had markedly recovered at follow-up. Those conduct disordered children who remained ill at follow-up had more severe speech/language disorders both initially and at follow-up. Thus far, however, there has been only one published study providing any suggestion that improvement in communication is linked with improvement in emotional/behavioral symptoms (Carr and Durand, 1985).

The natural history data for conduct disorder presented here are of particular interest when compared to the natural history data for ADDH and ADDNO. It will be recalled that of those conduct disordered children who were still psychiatrically ill at follow-up, three had other behavioral disorders (ADDH), and two had other types of disorders (organic personality syndrome and unspecified psychiatric disorder).

Thus, although the conduct disordered children did not show stability of the conduct disorder over the four year follow-up period, they did show differential outcomes from the ADDH and ADDNO children. Unlike the children with initial ADDH or ADDNO, none of the initial conduct disordered children had follow-up disorders in the emotional or pervasive developmental categories. Also, unlike a number of the ADDH and ADDNO children, none of the children with initial conduct disorders showed comorbid psychiatric disorders at follow-up.

Oppositional Disorder

Oppositional disorder is one of the less well researched of the *DSM-III* childhood categories. Little empirical data are available regarding the prevalence and incidence of the disorder, or the genetic, neurological, biochemical, or demographic factors that may be associated with it (Paez and Hirsch, 1988). In addition to the lack of established validity, this diagnosis has reliability problems having to do with its distinction from normal developmental behaviors on the one hand and from conduct disorder on the other hand (Rey et al., 1988; Rutter, 1988).

In the present study, oppositional disorder showed a natural history that was quite distinct from that of conduct disorder and from normal development. Oppositional disorder had the poorest recovery rate (7%) of all the behavioral psychiatric disorders. Unlike conduct disorder, oppositional disorder had a relatively high degree of stability (45%) over time. Those oppositional disordered children who developed other psychiatric illnesses at follow-up tended to have other behavioral disorders, either ADDH alone or ADDH plus conduct disorder.

Emotional Disorder Diagnoses (Anxiety Disorders and Affective Disorders)

The natural history data presented here lend additional validity to the already empirically validated (Achenbach and Edelbrock, 1981) "broad band" distinction between emotional and behavioral disorders. The emotional disorders as a group were characterized by higher rates or recovery and lower rates of stability than the behavioral disorders. Although there was little stability for specific subtypes of emotional disorders, there was some stability within the general category of emotional disorders. This finding supports those authors (Rutter and Gould, 1985; Werry et al., 1987b), who suggest that subdivisions between types of emotional disorders are premature.

Children with initial anxiety disorders showed a mild trend towards anxiety disorder at follow-up, but with very limited stability for the particular subtypes of anxiety disorder. Separation anxiety disorder was particularly unstable, with 44% recovering and only 11% remaining stable. The very young age of patients with this diagnosis (this was the youngest diagnosis group with a mean age of 3.6 years) may have played a role in the lack of stability. Even overanxious disorder, which has been thought to be a forerunner of generalized anxiety disorder in adults, was quite unstable (25%). The anxiety disorder data is discussed further elsewhere (Cantwell and Baker, 1988b).

As with anxiety disordered children, the affectively disordered children were most likely to have emotional (rather than behavioral) disorders at follow-up. As with the anxiety disorders, the affective disorders showed both recovery and stability rates of approximately one in three. Almost half of the affectively disordered children had comorbid diagnoses at follow-up. This is in keeping with other studies (Cantwell and Carlson, 1983; Kovacs et al., 1984) that have found that depressive disorder in children frequently occurs with other psychiatric disorders including anxiety disorders and behavioral disorders.

Adjustment Disorders

Adjustment disorders are, by definition, unstable. The *DSM-III* definition of adjustment disorders specifies that these are disturbances that are associated with stressors and will remit either when the precipitating stressor ceases or when a new level of adaptation occurs. Thus, it was not expected that these disorders would show much stability. As expected, none of the adjustment disordered children had retained this diagnosis at follow-up.

However, recovery from adjustment disorders was less common than had been hoped, with only 26% of the adjustment disordered children being well at follow-up. The poor prognosis for the adjustment disordered children in this study replicates the findings of Andreasen and Hoenk (1982) that adjustment disorders are unstable and carry a poor prognosis for children and adolescents. In Andreasen and Hoenk's study, adjustment disordered adolescents and adults were followed five years after initial evaluation. While 71% of the adults were psychiatrically well at follow-up, only 44% of the adolescents were psychiatrically well and 50% had a different diagnosis.

Adjustment disorders appear to be a rather common diagnosis in children and adolescents (Jacobsen et al., 1980; Weiner and DelGaduio, 1976). The findings here indicate that it is often not a self-limiting condition as the *DSM-III* definition implies but can be a serious disorder carrying a poor prognosis. Furthermore, the diversity of outcomes suggests that rather than a single disease entity, adjustment disorders may in fact be precursors or preliminary stages of various other diagnoses. Furthermore, there is an apparent lack of predictive value for the various subclassifications of adjustment disorders. These findings, coupled with the documented lack of reliability for the adjustment disorder diagnoses (Werry et al., 1983) suggest the need for serious reconsideration of this diagnostic category.

Parent-Child Problem

A final comment is necessary regarding the *DSM-III* "V-code" diagnosis parent-child problem. This diagnosis was used in cases where there were problems in parent-child interactions but where the child did not manifest definitive psychiatric illness. Thus, all of these children were clearly without psychiatric illness initially.

Nonetheless, even though parent-child problem is not considered a true psychiatric disorder, its natural history was as poor or poorer than that of many of the true psychiatric disorders. Parent-child problem had a recovery rate of only 20% and a stability rate of 0%. Of 15 children with initial parent-child problem, three were well at follow-up, 11 had a behavioral disorder and one had an adjustment disorder. Among the 11 children with follow-up behavioral disorders, there were 10 cases of ADDH, three cases of oppositional disorder, and one case of ADDNO. Thus, these follow-up data suggest that the parent-child problem may be a precursor to later full-blown behavioral psychiatric disorders.

It has been suggested that these children may have had behavioral disorders initially, i.e., that the diagnostic threshold for ADDH used initially may have been too high. However, retrospective chart review provided no evidence of any behavioral psychiatric illness initially.

A search for common family or background factors revealed no consistent trends in the parent-child group. There was no specific common pattern of family structure, environmental stressors, or family pathology in the group, although there did seem to be somewhat elevated rates of maternal depression (present in five of the 15 mothers) and paternal alcoholism (present in three of the 15 fathers). Nonetheless, fully one half of the parents were psychiatrically well and the majority of families were without psychosocial stressors (other than parent-child conflict). The parental psychiatric diagnoses were the same at follow-up as initially.

Methodological Considerations

There are several possible explanations for the low stability of many of the *DSM-III* childhood diagnoses. First, the *DSM-III* system was developed without detailed consideration of developmental factors in diagnosis. Nonetheless, it is likely that the symptomatology of the various psychiatric disorders will vary for different age levels. The initial diagnoses reported here were made when the majority of children were rather young (approximately half being in the preschool age range). Furthermore, given the young age of the sample, school reports were not available for some of the children, making diagnosis at that time still more difficult. If indeed the low stability of the diagnoses were due to an age factor, the present study may contribute to improved validity for *DSM-IV* by pointing out the need for attention to the developmental factor.

A second explanation of the low stability is that some of the cases may have been misdiagnosed. It has been observed, for example, that the three cases who "developed" pervasive developmental disorder (PDD) are particularly suspicious, given that PDD typically has early onset. However, retrospective examination of these children's charts confirmed that initially none met the diagnostic criteria for PDD. Two were young boys (2.3 and 3.2 years of age) who had marked ADDH and some type of language disorder (the younger child was nonverbal and the older had significant but not gross deficits). The third was an older boy (6.6 years) with clear mood disorder. All three of these children had initial behavioral abnormalities including severe tantrums. None of the children initially had ritualistic behaviors, stereotypic movements, or pervasive lack of responsiveness to people, although these became prominent later on.

Finally, it must be remembered that the sample in this study is an unusual one, neither a clinically-referred sample nor a community sample. By definition, all of the children in the sample had a coexisting speech/language disorder at some point in time. This not only means that reaching an accurate diagnosis is more difficult in these children, but it may also mean that these children are different in other ways. However, given that several researchers have reported a high prevalence of undiagnosed speech/language disorders among both inpatient and outpatient psychiatrically-referred children (Grinnell et al., 1983,

Gualtieri et al., 1983; Love and Thompson, 1988), this difference may be more apparent than real.

CONCLUSION

Although there are certain methodological issues to be considered with regard to this study, the study provides important information about the outcomes of various of the *DSM-III* childhood diagnoses. The follow-up data revealed high stability for only three diagnoses: infantile autism, attention deficit disorder with hyperactivity, and, more surprisingly, oppositional disorder. The study revealed that a number of psychiatric diagnoses lacked predictive validity; that is, children with these disorders were highly likely to have other different disorders at follow-up. This was true for attention deficit disorder without hyperactivity, avoidant disorder, separation anxiety disorder, overanxious disorder, and conduct disorder. The study also revealed surprisingly poor prognoses for parent-child problems and adjustment disorders.

REFERENCES

Achenbach, T. M. & Edelbrock, C. S. (1981), Behavioral problems and competencies reported by parents of normal and disturbed children aged 4 through 16. *Monogr. Soc. Res. Child Dev.*, 46, Serial No. 188.

Amado, H. & Lustman, P. J. (1982), Attention deficit disorders persisting in adulthood. *Compr. Psychiatry*, 23:200–214.

Andreasen, N. C. & Hoenk, P. R. (1982), The predictive value of adjustment disorders. *Am. J. Psychiatry*, 139:584–590.

American Psychiatric Association (1980), *Diagnostic and Statistical Manual of Mental Disorders, 3rd Ed. (DSM-III)*. Washington, DC: APA.

Baker, L. & Cantwell, D. P. (1982a), Developmental, social, and behavioral characteristics of speech and language disordered children. *Child Psychiatry Hum. Dev.*, 12:195–207.

———— ————(1982b), Language acquisition, cognitive development, and emotional disorder in childhood. In: *Children's Language. Volume 3*, ed. K. E. Nelson. Hillsdale, NJ: Lawrence Erlbaum Associates, pp. 286–321.

———— ————(1987), A prospective psychiatric follow-up of children with speech/language disorders. *J. Am. Acad. Child Adolesc. Psychiatry*, 26:546–553.

Berry, C. A., Shaywitz, S. E. & Shaywitz, B. A. (1985), Girls with attention deficit disorder: a silent minority? A report on behavioral and cognitive characteristics. *Pediatrics*, 76:801–809.

Biederman, J., Munir, K., Knee, D. et al. (1987), High rate of affective disorders with probands with attention deficit disorder and in their relatives: a controlled family study. *Am. J. Psychiatry*, 144:330–333.

Borland, B. L. & Heckman, H. K. (1976), Hyperactive boys and their brothers: a 25 year follow-up study. *Arch. Gen. Psychiatry*, 33:669–675.

Cantwell, D. P. (1975), A model for the investigation of psychiatric disorders of childhood: its application in genetic studies of the hyperkinetic syndrome. In: *Explorations in Child Psychiatry*, ed. E. J. Anthony. New York: Plenum, pp. 57–79.

——and Baker, L. (1980), Psychiatric and behavioral characteristics of children with communication disorders. *J. Pediatar. Psychol.*, 5:161–178.

—— ——(1985), Psychiatric and learning disorders in children with speech and language disorders: a descriptive analysis. *Advances in learning and behavioral disabilities*, 4:29–47.

—— ——(1988a), Anxiety disorders in children with communication disorders. *Journal of Anxiety Disorders*, 2:135–146.

—— ——(1988b), Issues in the classification of child and adolescent psychopathology. *J. Am. Acad. Child Adolesc. Psychiatry*, 26:546–553.

—— ——Mattison, R. (1979), The prevalence of psychiatric disorder in children with speech and language disorder. *J. Am. Acad. Child Adolesc. Psychiatry*, 18:450–461.

—— —— ——(1981), Prevalence, type and correlates of psychiatric disorder in 200 children with communication disorder. *J. Dev. Behav. Pediatr.* 2:131–136.

——Carlson, G. A. (1983), *Affective Disorders in Childhood and Adolescence—An Update.* New York: Spectrum Publications.

Carlson, C. L. (1986), Attention deficit disorder without hyperactivity. In: *Advances in Clinical Child Psychology, Vol. 9*, ed. B. Lahey & A. Kazdin. New York: Plenum, pp. 153–175.

——Lahey, B. B., Frame, C. L., Walker, J. Hynd, G. W. (1987), Sociometric status of clinic-referred children with attention deficit disorders with and without hyperactivity. *J. Abnorm. Child Psychol.*, 15:537–547.

Carlson, G. A. Cantwell, D. P. (1982), Suicidal behavior and depression in children and adolescents. *J. Am. Acad. Child Psychiatry*, 21:361–368.

Carr, E. & Durand, V. (1985), The social-communicative basis of behavior problems in children. In: *Theoretical Issues in Behavioral Therapy*, ed. S. Reiss & R. Bootzin. New York: Academic Press.

Comings, D. E. & Comings, B. G. (1987), A controlled study of Tourette's syndrome. I. Attention-deficit disorder, learning disorders, and school problems. *Am. J. Hum. Genet.*, 41:701–741.

Conners, C. K. (1973), Rating scales for use in drug studies with children. *Psychopharmacol. Bull. (Special Issue)*, 24–34.

Cowart, V. S. (1982), ADD: Not limited to children. *JAMA*, 16:248–286.

Edelbrock, C., Costello, A. J. & Kessler, M. D. (1984), Empirical corroboration of the attention deficit disorder. *J. Am. Acad. Child Psychiatry*, 23:285–290.

Frank, Y. & Ben-Nun, Y. (1988), Toward a clinical subgrouping of hyperactive and nonhyperactive attention deficit disorder. Results of a comprehensive neurological and neuropsychological assessment. *Am. J. Dis. child.*, 142:153–155.

Grinnell, S. W., Scott-Hartnett, D. & Glasier, J. L. (1983), Language disorders (Letter to the Editor). *J. Am. Acad. Child Psychiatry*, 22:580–581.

Gualtieri, C. T., Koriath, U., Van Bourgondien, M. & Saleeby, N. (1983), Language disorders in children referred for psychiatric services. *J. Am. Acad. Child Psychiatry*, 22:165–171.

Halverson, C. F. & Waldrop, M. F. (1976), Relations between preschool activity and aspects of intellectual and social behavior at age 7½. *Developmental Psychology*, 12:107–112.

Jacobsen, A. M., Goldberg, I. D., Burns, B. J., Hoeper, E. W., Hankin, J. R. & Hewitt, K. (1980), Diagnosed mental disorders in children and use of health services in four organized health care settings. *Am. J. Psychiatry*, 137:559–565.

Kagan, J. & Moss, H. A. (1962), *Birth to Maturity*. New York: Wiley.

King, C. & Young, R. D. (1982), Attentional deficits with and without hyperactivity: teacher and peer perceptions. *J. Abnorm. Child Psychol.*, 10:483–495.

Konno, Y. & Ohno, K. (1981), A comparative and developmental study of hyperactivity and its related symptoms in autistic and hyperactive children. *Japanese Journal of Special Education*, 19:37–47.

Kovacs, M., Feinberg, T. L., Crouse-Novak, M. A., Paulauskas, S. L. & Finkelstein, R. (1984), Depressive disorders in childhood. I. A. longitudinal prospective study of characteristics and recovery. *Arch. Gen. Psychiatry*, 41:229–237.

Lahey, B. B., Schaughency, E. A., Hynd, G. W., Carlsonk, C. L. & Nieves, N. (1987), Attention deficit disorder with and without hyperactivity: Comparison of behavioral characteristics of clinic-referred children. *J. Am. Acad. Child Adolesc. Psychiatry*, 26:718–723.

Langner, T. S., Gersten, J. C. & Eisenberg, J. G. (1974), Approaches to measurement and definition in the epidemiology of behavior disorders: ethnic background and child behavior. *Int. J. Health Serv.*, 4:483–501.

Loney, J., Langhorne, J. E. & Paternite, C. E. (1978), Empirical basis for subgrouping the hyperkinetic/minimal brain dysfunction syndrome. *J. Abnorm. Psychol.*, 87:431–441.

Love, A. J. & Thompson, M. G. (1988), Language disorders and attention deficit disorders in young children referred for psychiatric services: analysis of prevalence and a conceptual synthesis. *Am. J. Orthopsychiatry*, 58:52–64.

Minde, R. & Minde, K. (1977), Behavioral screening of pre-school children: A new approach to mental health? In: *Epidemiological Approaches to Child Psychiatry*, ed. P. Graham. London: Academic Press, pp. 139–164.

Olweus, D. (1979), Stability of aggressive reaction patterns in males: A review. *Psychol. Bull.*, 86:852–875.

Orvaschel, H. (1985), Psychiatric interviews suitable for use in research with children and adolescents. *Psychopharmacol. Bull.*, 21:737–746.

Paez, P. & Hirsch, M. (1988), Oppositional disorder and elective mutism. In: *Handbook of Clinical Assessment of Children and adolescents*, ed. C. J. Kestenbaum & D. T. Williams, Vol. 2, New York: New York University Press, pp. 800–811.

Rey, J. M., Bashir, M. R., Schawrz, M., Richards, I. N., Plapp, J. M. & Stewart, G. W. (1988), Oppositional disorder: fact or fiction? *J. Am. Acad. Child Adolesc. Psychiatry*, 27:157–162.

Reeves, J. C., Werry, J. S., Elkind, G. A. & Zametkin, A. (1987), Attention deficit, conduct, oppositional, and anxiety disorders in children: II. Clinical characteristics. *J. Am. Acad. Child Adolesc. Psychiatry*, 26:144–155.

Rutter, M. (1988), DSM-III-R: A postcript. In: *Assessment and Diagnosis in Child Psychopathology*, ed. M. Rutter, A. H. Tuma & I. S. Lann. New York: Guilford Press, pp. 453–464.

——Gould, M. (1985), Classification. In: *Child and Adolescent Psychiatry: Modern Approaches*, ed. M. Rutter & L. Hersov. Boston: Blackwell Scientific, pp. 304–324.

——Graham, P. & Yule, W. (1970), *A Neuropsychiatric Study in Childhood*. Lavenham, Suffolk: The Lavenham Press.

——Tizard, J. & Whitmore, K. (1970), *Education, Health, and Behavior*. London: Longman.

——Tuma, A. H. (1988), Diagnosis and classification: Some outstanding issues. In: (Eds.), *Assessment and Diagnosis in Child Psychopathology*, ed. M. Rutter, A. H. Tuma & I. S. Lann. New York: Guilford Press, pp. 437–452.

Sandberg, S. T., Wieselberg, M. & Shaffer, D. (1980), Hyperkinetic and conduct problem children in a primary school population. *J. Child Psychol. Psychiatry*, 21:293–311.

Sergeant, J. A. & Scholten, C. A. (1985), On resource strategy limitations in hyperactivity: cognitive impulsivity reconsidered. *J. Child Psychol. Psychiatry*, 26:97–109.

Taylor, E. (1988), Attention deficit disorder and conduct disorder syndromes. In: *Assessment and Diagnosis in Child Psychopathology*, ed. M. Rutter, A. H. Tuma & I. S. Lann. New York: Guilford Press, pp., 377–407.

——Schachar, R., Thorley, G. & Wieselberg, M. (1986), Conduct disorder and hyperactivity: I. Separation of hyperactivity and antisocial conduct in British child psychiatric patients. *Br. J. Psychiatary*, 149:760–767.

Thorley, G. (1984), Review of follow-up and follow-back studies of childhood hyperactivity. *Psychol. Bull.*, 96:116–132.

Trites, R. & Laprade, K. (1983), Evidence for an independent syndrome of hyperactivity. *J. Child Psychol. Psychiatry*, 24:573–586.

Weiner, I. B. & DelGaudio, A. C. (1976), Psychopathology in adolescence. *Arch. Gen. Psychiatry*, 33:187–193.

Wiess, G. & Hechtman, L. T. (1986), *Hyperactive Children Grown Up: Empirical Findings and Theoretical Considerations*. New York: Guilford Press.

Werry, J. S., Elkind, G. S. & Reeves, J. C. (1987a), Attention deficit, conduct, oppositional, and anxiety disorders in children: III. Laboratory differences. *J. Abnorm. Child Psychol.*, 15:409–428.

——Methven, R. J., Fitzpatrick, J. & Dixon, H. (1983), The interrater reliability of DSM-III in children. *J. Abnorm. Child Psychol.*, 11:341–354.

——Reeves, J. C. & Elkind, G. S. (1987b), Attention deficit, conduct, oppositional, and anxiety disorders in children: I. A review of research on differentiating characteristics. *J. Am. Acad. Child Adolesc. Psychiatry*, 26:133–143.

Wolff, S. (1985), Non-delinquent disturbances of conduct. In: *Child and Adolescent Psychiatry: Modern Approaches* (2nd ed.), ed. M. Rutter & L. Hersov. Oxford: Blackwell Scientific, pp. 400–413.

Zeitlin, H. (1986), *The Natural History of Psychiatric Disorder in Childhood*. New York: Oxford University Press.

17

The Phenomenology of Schizophrenia Occurring in Childhood

Andrew T. Russell, Linda Bott, and Catherine Sammons

Neuropsychiatric Institute, University of California, Los Angeles

Thirty-five children, aged 4 to 13 ($\bar{x}$ = 9.54), meeting strict DSM-III *criteria for schizophrenia, are described. The subjects were diagnosed using a new semistructured interview. All were in the normal range of intelligence (mean IQ = 94) and free of neurological disorders. Characteristic auditory hallucinations were present in 80% and delusions in 63% of the sample. The mean age of onset of psychotic symptoms was 6.9 years. Premorbid histories of attention deficit, conduct disturbance and/or developmental abnormalities were common. The nature and content of psychotic symptoms varied with developmental stage. The phenomenological presentation of the sample was similar to previous studies of young schizophrenic children. Key Words: schizophrenia, structured interviews, hallucination, delusion.*

A small group of severe psychiatric disorders of childhood, often described generically and imprecisely as the "childhood psychoses" or "childhood schizophrenia," have been the focus of research interest out of proportion to their actual prevalence. Yet in the over 40 years since Kanner (1943, 1971) described autism as a diagnostic entity distinct from schizophrenia, many basic questions concerning the phenomenology and classification of these disorders remain unanswered and many controversies unresolved. This is particularly true for schizophrenia, defined with modern (adult) diagnostic criteria, occurring in childhood. Although descriptive

Reprinted with permission from *Journal of the American Academy of Child and Adolescent Psychiatry,* 1989, Vol. 28, No. 3, 399–407. Copyright © 1989 by the American Academy of Child and Adolescent Psychiatry.

Preparation of this manuscript was supported by USPHS grant MH30897 (UCLA Child Psychiatry Clinical Research Center).

Special thanks to Nancy Wainwright, who prepared the manuscript and tables, and Delores Adams, Donald Guthrie, Ph.D., and Sandra Perdue, O.P.H., who provided statistical assistance.

and phenomenological research focusing on autism has been relatively extensive, there are few careful descriptive studies of schizophrenia with an onset in the pre-adolescent years.

There are several reasons for the relative lack of useful phenomenological research with schizophrenic children. A major problem has been sample heterogeneity. For many years broad or unspecified diagnostic criteria for "childhood schizophrenia" were used to identify research subjects. These studies undoubtedly mixed together a variety of psychotic children, including those with autism, schizophrenia, mental retardation, organic disorders and, perhaps, major affective disorder (Prior and Werry, 1986). The influential work of Kolvin et al. (Kolvin, 1971; Kolvin et al., 1971a–e) and Rutter (1972) led to the renewed realization that autism and schizophrenia should be considered as separate disorders; this is reflected in current diagnostic nomenclature (*DSM-III-R*) and research. Complicating the picture further is the recognition that symptoms previously thought to be characteristic of schizophrenia occur in a variety of disorders in young children. Major depressions in childhood are often accompanied by hallucinations and delusions (Chambers et al., 1982). Recent studies have also described small samples of children who exhibit "psychotic" symptoms (e.g., auditory hallucinations) but who do not meet criteria for schizophrenia or other psychoses (Garralda, 1984a, b; Burke et al., 1985; Kotsopoulos et al., 1987). Current research therefore requires very detailed phenomenological distinctions and makes comparison with older descriptive research very difficult.

Another barrier to useful diagnostic research is the rarity of the disorder. The prevalence rate for autism has been estimated to be between 4 and 5 per 10,000, and schizophrenia occurring in childhood is probably even less common (Tanguay and Asarnow, 1985). Prospective studies have thus required large referral centers and major time commitments to gather samples of a useful size.

A third significant research problem has been the lack of standardized diagnostic instruments geared to the disorders of autism, schizophrenia, and schizophrenic spectrum disorders in children. For example, structured and semistructured diagnostic interviews have recently been employed in diagnostic research with children with the goals of achieving broad symptomatic coverage and increasing diagnostic reliability (Gutterman et al., 1987). Yet the majority of these instruments have been designed for epidemiological studies and do not cover psychotic symptoms in sufficient depth for a detailed phenomenological study focusing on schizophrenia in childhood. Until the present study, a structured diagnostic interview had not been specifically developed for use with a large population of psychotic children.

A review of the childhood psychosis literature reveals only a few studies that have attempted to systematically describe the phenomenology of schizophrenia occurring in childhood while at the same time using modern (*DSM—III* or related) criteria (Chambers, 1986; Prior and Werry, 1986). In a now classic study reported in 1971,

Kolvin and Colleagues (Kolvin, 1971: Kolvin et al., 1971 a–e) described 33 children with "late onset psychosis" (schizophrenia) and compared them with a sample of "infantile psychosis" (autistic) children. Kolvin et al. used Schneiderian criteria, which are similar to but not identical with *DSM-III* criteria. Cantor et al. (1982) described 11 children and 19 adolescents with childhood schizophrenia. Cantor utilized a special set of diagnostic criteria that emphasize physical and neuromuscular characteristics, but all subjects had to meet *DSM-III* criteria (excluding deterioration) first. Green et al. (1984) reported on 24 schizophrenic children (*DSM-III* criteria) hospitalized at Bellevue hospital and also compared them with a sample of autistic children.

The present study complements and expands on this previous work. Under the auspices of the University of California at Los Angeles (UCLA) Child Psychiatry Clinical Research Center (CPCRC), a sample of 35 preadolescent children meeting strict *DSM-III* criteria for schizophrenia were interviewed and diagnosed over a 3½-year period. The subjects described in this report were recruited as part of a larger study conducted by the CPCRC, which focused on children of normal intelligence meeting *DSM-III* criteria for schizophrenia, schizotypal personality disorder, or infantile autism. Some of the 35 children have been subjects in previously reported CPCRC research (J. Asarnow and Ben-Meir, in press; J. Asarnow et al., in press; R. Asarnow et al., 1987; Caplan et al., 1988; Strandburg et al., 1987; Watkins et al., 1988).

An important feature of the present study is the development and use of a semistructured diagnostic interview by the authors in an attempt to systematically elicit a wide variety of symptoms and to maximize diagnostic reliability.

METHOD

The Interview Instrument

Development

The diagnoses were based on a semistructured interview, the Interview for Childhood Disorders and Schizophrenia (ICDS), compiled and developed by the authors (copies of the instrument and methods of administration are available from the authors). The ICDS was developed in 1983 after the authors examined the then available structured and semi-structured interviews for children. It was felt that no one of the interviews examined contained inquiries that sufficiently addressed the diagnoses of principal interest to the research project: schizophrenia, schizophrenic spectrum disorder (schizotypal personality disorder), and autism. In compiling the ICDS, it was decided to include in-depth inquiries concerning symptoms of the target diagnoses and a relatively less detailed inquiry (yet sufficient to make a *DSM-III* diagnosis) into a broader range of other childhood disorders. A related decision was to use, whenever possible, intact sections and questions from previously developed interviews of known reliability. During the development phase several versions and revisions were piloted until the basic format and content was determined.

Contents

The resulting instrument consists of questions from a variety of sources but is largely based on the Kiddie-Schedule for Affective Disorders and Schizophrenia-Present State version (K-SADS-P) (Puig-Antich and Chambers, 1978; Chambers et al., 1982) and the Diagnostic Interview for Children and Adolescents (DICA) (Herjanic and Campbell, 1977; Welner et al., 1987). The entire psychosis section of the K-SADS-P was used to cover major psychotic symptoms. It addresses hallucinations and delusions in great depth and allows distinctions to be made concerning the type, frequency, and severity of these symptoms. Sections of the DICA were incorporated to cover, in somewhat less detail, a variety of other diagnostic entities including affective disorders, ADD/H, conduct disorder, oppositional disorder, obsessive compulsive disorder, phobia, and overanxious disorder. Questions and sections taken from both instruments were essentially unaltered and are easily identified by letter codes. Questions relating to schizotypal disorder were adapted from the appropriate section of the Interview Schedule for Children (ISC) (Kovacs, 1978) and the UCLA Schizophrenia Interview (Fish, unpublished manuscript, 1982). Slightly modified items from the Developmental Inventory for Children (Ornitz et al., 1978) were included to allow a more in-depth coverage of autism and pervasive developmental disorder. New questions on dysthymic disorder were adapted directly from the *DSM-III* symptom criteria for that disorder.

Parallel versions of the interview were developed for use with parents and children. The parent version includes additional diagnostic sections that primarily depend on parental recall, e.g., autism and pervasive developmental disorder.

Use of the Interview

The ICDS is intended for use with children aged 6 to 18 years. The interviewers, clinicians experienced in working with children and sensitive to developmental issues, modified the wording of questions as necessary based upon the child's age and level of understanding. They were also free to modify the order of the interview to better follow material spontaneously introduced by the child. The interview ambience was informal to engage the child in conversation and to encourage elaboration of responses. Every attempt was made to obtain a sufficient amount of information and specific examples before scoring the symptom as present or absent.

Establishment of Interrater Reliability

To establish interrater reliability, one author (A.T.R.) reviewed the child and parent videotaped interviews and independently made symptom ratings and diagnoses at each step of the diagnostic protocol (see below). Fifteen consecutive cases were rated in this fashion with full interrater agreement on final diagnoses in 85% of the cases. Periodic interrater reliability was then checked throughout the remainder of the project to preclude interrater drift. In total, 102 cases were interviewed using the described protocol and formal reliability was measured in 23 cases. Using the kappa statistic to account for chance agreement, interrater reliability on final diagnosis was satisfactory ($\kappa = 0.88$). Seven of the 35 schizophrenic children described here were part of the reliability study with independent agreement on the diagnosis of schizophrenia in all seven cases. There was disagreement between schizotypal personality disorder and schizophrenia in one additional case. That case received a final research diagnosis of schizotypal personality disorder. At the *DSM-III* criteria level, interrater agreement on the core *DSM-III* symptoms of schizophrenia was also relatively high, i.e., characteristic delusions (any type), $\kappa = 1.0$; characteristic auditory hallucinations; $\kappa = 0.69$; thought disorder, $\alpha = 0.86$; blunted or inappropriate affect, $\kappa = 0.56$; and disorganized behavior, $\kappa = 0.47$.

Recruitment and Screening of Subjects

Subjects were recruited from a variety of sources. These included the child inpatient and outpatient programs at the UCLA Neuropsychiatric Hospital and the UCLA pediatric clinics. Community sources included selected classrooms of the Los Angeles County Schools program for severely emotionally disturbed students. Other referrals came from private practitioners and community mental health agencies familiar with the CPCRC program. Screening consisted of determining whether potential subjects met exclusionary and inclusionary criteria. Potential subjects were *not* recruited for research if any of the following conditions existed: age under 5 or over 14; WISC-R full-scale IQ score less than 70; onset of the disorder after the 11th birthday; diagnosed seizure disorder or medications for seizures within past 6 months; other diagnosed neurological/medical disorder affecting the central nervous system; hearing deficit greater than 40 decibels in either ear; vision deficit greater than 20/60 with correction. Inclusionary criteria included the probable presence of symptoms within the past year consistent with *DSM-III* criteria for schizophrenia, schizotypal personality disorder, or autism. Evidence for the latter were gathered by review of current records and discussions with clinicians, teachers, and caretakers. Positive findings were then arrayed on a form that was made available to the interviewers prior to the diagnostic phase.

Description of the Sample

The sample consists of 35 children (24 males, 11 females), with a mean age of 9.54 years (range 4 years, 9 months to 13 years, 3 months; SD = 2.07). All children were interviewed and diagnosed by the authors and met strict *DSM-III* criteria for schizophrenia. The 35 children came from a group of 102 children who met screening criteria and were interviewed over a 3½-year period. Subjects had WISC-R full-scale IQ scores ranging from 76 to 114 (mean 94, SD = 10.5). Twenty-two of the subjects were Caucasian, seven were black, and four were Hispanic; all were English speaking. Using the Hollingshead method of calculating socioeconomic status, seven of the families were from class I, 12 from class II, 8 from III, 3 from IV, and 5 from V (Hollingshead, 1958). At the time of diagnosis, 23 of the subjects were inpatients, seven were outpatients at the UCLA Neuropsychiatric Institute, and five were attending educational programs for the severely emotionally disturbed. Eleven of the 35 children (31%) were receiving phenothiazine medication (Mellaril = 10, Thorazine = 1) at the time of assessment. The mean dosage was 143 mgm/day (range 50 to 375). None of the children were obviously sedated and the authors did not feel the medication significantly interfered with the diagnostic assessment.

Diagnostic Protocol

Parents and children were interviewed independently on videotape, using the ICDS, by two of the authors, a clinical social worker (C.S.) and a child psychologist (L.B.), respectively. After the completion of the interview (sometimes more than one session was required), each interviewer rated *DSM-III* criteria as absent, likely or suspected, or definitely present and made Axis I and II diagnoses. The two interviewers then met and made *DSM-III* criteria ratings and diagnoses combining data from both the parent and child interviews. A third set of ratings and diagnoses were then completed after reviewing all collateral information. This information included previous records, school and teacher reports, psychological testing, etc. Finally, the two interviewers met with the third author (A.T.R., a child psychiatrist) to establish the final symptom ratings and the CPCRC research diagnosis. In this session, interview and collateral material and key portions of the videotape were again reviewed. Through this detailed process consensus ratings and diagnoses for all the cases reported here were obtained.

RESULTS

Associated Diagnoses

Twenty-four of the 35 subjects met *DSM-III* criteria for diagnoses in addition to schizophrenia. These are listed in Table 1. Special note should be made of the nine cases who met criteria for a major depressive episode. In all these cases, the onset of the depressive syndrome occurred after the onset of the characteristic schizophrenic syndrome or was brief in duration compared to the psychotic symptoms. According to *DSM-III* guidelines, these patients received a diagnosis of atypical depression. The category of atypical depression was used rather than schizoaffective disorder (which has no operational criteria in *DSM-III*), because the depressive symptoms occurred within a longer and persistent course of psychotic symptoms. The four cases with a diagnosis of dysthymia met *DSM-III* criteria for that disorder, including symptom duration of at least 1 year. Three of the four had depressive symptoms of long duration that preceded the onset of the psychosis. In the fourth case the onset was difficult to determine. In all these individuals the schizophrenic symptoms, once present, dominated the clinical picture and, for that reason, the category of schizoaffective disorder was inappropriate.

Schizophrenic Symptoms

To meet criteria for a diagnosis of schizophrenia, *DSM-III* requires the presence of at least one of three major positive symptoms, characteristic delusions, characteristic auditory hallucinations, and/or marked thought disorder. The latter must be associated with either blunted, flat or inappropriate affect, delusions or hallucinations, or catatonic or grossly disorganized behavior. Table 2 lists all 35 schizophrenic subjects by increasing age and indicates the presence or absence (rated definitely present or absent) of these symptoms. Visual and other types of hallucinations (e.g., somatic) are also listed although they are not part of the *DSM-III* criteria for schizophrenia. As noted in Table 3, auditory hallucinations was the most common major positive symptom in our sample (80%), followed by delusions (63%), and marked thought disorder (40%). Twenty-three children (66%) exhibited more than one of the three major symptoms. Of the remaining 12 children who exhibited only one major

TABLE 1
Associated Diagnoses

Diagnosis	Frequency
Conduct disorder	10
Atypical depression	9
Dysthymia	4
Enuresis/encopresis	5
Sexual/physical abuse	2
Elective mutism	1
Separation anxiety disorder	1
Oppositional disorder	1

Note: $N = 24$.

positive symptom, five experienced auditory hallucinations, four were thought disordered, and three were delusional. All 35 subjects exhibited a marked deterioration from a previous level of functioning. This was verified in the present sample by parental report and manifested by either the need for acute psychiatric hospitalization or, in the case of the severely emotionally disturbed schoolchildren, by a marked deterioration of behavior within the school setting. All exhibited signs of the illness (prodromal and/or acute) for over 6 months.

The subjects who were rated as having only one major positive symptom (e.g., hallucinations, delusions, or thought disorder) presented some differential diagnosis problems. For example, one 8.3-year-old boy (Table 2) was rated as only having def-

TABLE 2
Schizophrenic Symptom Presentation

Subjects (N = 35)		Hallucinations			Delusions[b]	Thought Disorder	Disorganized Behavior	Affective Disturbance
Age	Sex	Auditory[a]	Visual	Other				
4.9	f	+		+	+	+		+
5.1	m	+	+	+				+
7.2	f					+		+
7.3	m	+			+	+		
7.8	m	+			+	+		+
8.0	m	+	+		+	+	+	+
8.0	m	+					+	+
8.2	m	+	+		+	+	+	+
8.3	f					+	+	+
8.3	m				+			
8.3	f	+	+	+	+			+
8.4	f	+	+	+	+			+
8.6	m					+	+	+
8.7	m	+						+
8.7	f	+			+			+
9.2	m	+				+		+
9.3	m	+			+			
9.4	m	+				+	+	+
9.5	m				+		+	
9.7	f	+	+	+	+	+	+	+
9.9	m	+		+	+	+		
10.0	m	+	+	+	+	+		+
10.6	f	+	+				+	+
10.11	m		+			+	+	+
11.0	m	+			+		+	
11.2	m	+			+			+
11.4	f	+			+		+	+
11.6	m	+	+		+		+	
11.9	m	+			+			
11.11	m	+	+					+
11.11	f	+			+			+
12.0	m	+						
12.2	m	+	+	+	+			+
13.3	f				+		+	+
13.3	m	+	+		+			+

[a] *DSM-III* (p. 189): diagnostic criteria A, 4–5.
[b] *DSM-III* (p. 189): diagnostic criteria A, 1–3.

inite persecutory delusions; this raised the issue of whether he met criteria for paranoid disorder rather than schizophrenia. However, a variety of auditory hallucinations (including a voice telling him to jump off a cliff) were rated as "suspected or likely." They had been reported previously, although at the time of interview the boy was quite guarded. In addition, he was observed on the unit to be probably responding to command hallucinations. For this reason it was felt that a diagnosis of schizophrenia was more appropriate than paranoid disorder.

A similar problem presented itself with a 12.0-year-old boy who only received a "definitely present" rating on a wide variety of characteristic auditory hallucinations (including conversing) but presented with a relatively normal affect. However, he also expressed odd and magical thinking that fell just short of being rated as definitely delusional. Because of his overall presentation it was felt that a diagnosis of schizophrenia, as opposed to atypical psychosis, was warranted.

Hallucinations

A wide variety of hallucinations was noted in the research sample (Table 4). "True" hallucinations were carefully distinguished from other phenomenon such as imaginary companions and hypnogogic experiences (Egdell and Kolvin, 1972). It was not uncommon for a single child to exhibit several types of auditory and other kinds of hallucinations (Table 2). However, nonauditory hallucinations were never noted without accompanying auditory hallucinations. To give a sense of the kinds of symptoms reported by the subjects, some examples of auditory hallucinations follow.

Auditory—unrelated to affective state: a girl reported the voice of a dead baby brother saying "I love you sister," "sister I am going to miss you"; a second child reported the kitchen light saying to do things and "to shut up"; another

TABLE 3
Symptomatic Presentation of Schizophrenic Children

	N	Percentage
Hallucinations (auditory)	28	80
Delusions	22	63
Thought disorder	14	40
Hallucinations and delusions	19	54
Hallucinations and thought disorder	10	29
Delusions and thought disorder	0	–
Hallucinations, delusions, and thought disorder	8	23

Note: N = 35.

child stated "everything is talking, the walls, the furniture, I just know they're talking."

Command: a boy stated, "I once heard a noise coming from the south and the east, one told me to jump off the roof and one told me to smash my mom"; another child heard "good" voices say things like "help your mom with dinner"; another child heard a man's voice saying "murder your stepfather" and "go play outside."

Conversing: a child stated, "I can hear the devil talk—God interrupts him and the devil says 'shut up God' "; another child described voices of various animals talking softly with each other (about child).

Religious: one child heard God's voice saying, "sorry D., but I can't help you now, I am helping someone else."

Persecutory: a boy described monsters calling him "stupid F.," and saying they will hurt him; another child reported voices calling him bad names, and threatening that if he doesn't do what he is told something bad will happen to him.

Commenting: a boy described voices commenting on how he was feeling or what he was doing, e.g., "You're feeling excited today"; another child reported an angel saying "You didn't cry today."

The ICDS elicits four types of nonauditory hallucinations—visual, tactile, olfactory, and somatic. While visual hallucinations were noted in over one-third of the sample, the other types were uncommon. Some examples of each type follow.

Visual: A child saw a ghost (man) with red, burned and scarred face on multiple occasions and in different locations; another reported, "If I stare at the wall I

TABLE 4
Frequency of Hallucinations in Schizophrenic Population

Types of Hallucinations	N	Percentage Schizophrenic Subjects with Symptoms
Nonaffective auditory	28	80
Command	24	69
Visual	13	37
Conversing voices	12	34
Religious	12	34
Persecutory	9	26
Commenting voices	8	23
Tactile	6	17
Olfactory	2	6
Somatic	2	6

Note: N = 35.

see monsters coming toward me" (child was noted to react to visual hallucinations while hospitalized).

Tactile: a boy felt the devil touching him and moving his body "so he can make me come and live with him"; another child felt snakes and spiders on his back (and was so convincing he was taken to the emergency room by his parents).

Somatic: a child reported feeling an angel, babies, and devil inside her arm, and that she could feel them fighting.

Delusions

In the course of the diagnostic assessment, delusions were rated as definitely present in 22 of the 35 subjects. The relative frequency of the different types of delusions is shown in Table 5. Overall, a wide variety of delusions were elicited, with no particular type predominating. As with hallucinations, it was not uncommon for a single child to describe several different types of delusional beliefs. Some examples follow.

Bizarre: a child believed that there were "memory boxes" in his head and body and reported that he could broadcast his thoughts from his memory boxes with a special computer using radar tracking; a boy was convinced he was a dog and was growing fur, and on one occasion, refused to leave a veterinarian's office unless he received a shot.

Persecutory: a child believed his father had escaped from jail and was coming to kill him; a girl believed that the "evil one" was trying to poison her orange juice.

TABLE 5
Frequency of Delusions in Schizophrenic Population

Types of Delusions	N	Percentage Total Schizophrenic Population
Persecutory	7	20
Somatic	7	20
Bizarre	6	17
Reference	5	14
Grandiose	4	11
Thought insertion	4	11
Control/influence	3	9
Mind reading	3	9
Thought broadcasting	2	6
Thought control	1	3
Religious	1	3

Note: N = 35.

Somatic: one subject believed that there were boy and girl spirits living inside his head, "they're squishing on the whole inside, they're touching the walls, the skin"; a boy described "waste" produced when the good and bad voices fought with each other; the "waste" came out of his feet when he swam in chlorinated pools.

Reference: a girl believed that people outside of her house were staring and pointing at her trying to send her a message to come outside, she also believed that people on the TV were talking to her because they used the word "you."

Grandiose: a boy had the firm belief that he was "different" and able to kill people, he felt that when "God zooms through me [him]" he became very strong and developed big muscles.

Thought Disorder

Fourteen of 35 subjects (40%) were rated as exhibiting incoherence or *marked* loosening of associations, illogical thinking, or poverty of context of speech accompanied by affect disturbance, delusions or hallucinations, or disorganized behavior. It should be noted, however, that *DSM-III* criteria requires a judgment concerning the severity of thought disorder. Another seven subjects received a "suspected or likely" rating for thought disorder as opposed to a "definite" rating. These latter children had disturbances of form of thought but not severe enough to meet the authors' interpretation of the *DSM-III* criteria of "marked." If the suspected or likely ratings are combined with the definite ratings, 60% of the research sample could be described as showing some evidence of thought disorder. These results and the whole issue of rating thought disorder in children is considered in the discussion section. Whenever thought disorder was noted on interview, a verbatim transcript of an illustrative portion of the dialogue was made. An example from the interview of a 7-year-8-month-old boy follows:

> I used to have a Mexican dream. I was watching TV in the family room. I disappeared outside of this world and then I was in our closet. Sounds like a vacuum dream. It's a Mexican dream. When I was close to that dream earth I was turning upside down. I don't like to turn upside down. Sometimes I have Mexican dreams and vacuum dreams. It's real hard to scream in dreams.

Age and Mode of Onset

Based on a review of the child and parent interviews and all collateral information, an estimate was made of the age of onset of the disorder. Onset was defined as the emergence of psychotic symptoms that met *DSM-III* criteria and were described with enough clarity that they would be rated by the authors as "definitely present." In other words, the definite onset of characteristic delusions, hallucinations, or formal thought disorder was rated. Using this criteria, the mean age of onset was 6.9 yrs, with a range of 3 to 11 years.

Similarly, the onset of significant nonpsychotic behavioral and psychiatric symptomatology was rated. In 30 of 35 subjects (86%) there was a clear history of behavioral and psychiatric disturbance prior to the onset of psychosis. This history was obtained from parent and/or collateral information. The mean age of onset for the nonpsychotic premorbid symptoms was 4.6 years with a range of 3 to 9 years. In five subjects behavioral symptoms were judged to appear approximately the same time as psychotic symptoms.

The type of premorbid symptoms reported varied widely, but a few patterns emerged, fourteen subjects (40%) had a premorbid history of attentional problems and hyperactivity suggestive of attention deficit disorder and six had a history of a stimulant drug trial. The ADDH group overlapped with six children (17%) with significant premorbid conduct disturbance, e.g., aggression, truancy, fire setting. Seventy-five of those with a premorbid history of ADDH and/or conduct disturbance were boys. Another group of nine children (26%) had premorbid histories marked by a variety of developmental abnormalities seen in children with pervasive developmental disorder, e.g., echolalia, rituals, tactile sensitivity, flapping. None of these children, however, met full criteria for autism or pervasive developmental disorder. The remaining children exhibited a wide variety of less specific behavioral and emotional symptoms.

Developmental Trends

The age distribution of the sample suggests that it is rare for very young children to present with a symptomatic picture that meets full *DSM-III* criteria for schizophrenia. Only five of the subjects were under the age of 8 at the time of diagnosis. The incidence of the disorder seems to be relatively stable during latency, but, as noted by others (Loranger, 1984), shows a dramatic increase in adolescence. The fact that only three subjects were age 12 or older most likely is an artifact of the exclusionary criteria, i.e., 12- and 13-year-olds were not accepted into the project unless the onset of the disorder occurred before the age of 11. These results must be interpreted with caution as the study was not an epidemiological sampling of a total population.

A visual inspection of Table 2 suggests that the frequency of occurrence of the major symptoms does not vary greatly by age. For example, young children with schizophrenia were as likely to report delusions as older schizophrenic children. The one exception to this generalization is that none of the children age 11 or older exhibited *marked* formal thought disturbances. It is unclear whether this is an artifact of the sample or whether older children, with more sophisticated language skills, were able to compensate better for underlying disturbance in their thought processes, at least during the interview itself.

A somewhat different question is whether the nature or content of the psychotic symptomatology varies with developmental stage. Not surprisingly, it does. Generally it was noted that as age increased, both hallucinations and delusions tended to be more complex and elaborate. The authors feel this is not only because older children are better able to describe their symptoms but also because more complex hallucinations and delusions are part of the natural course of the illness. In addition, the "content" of the symptoms in this largely latency age sample differed considerably from what one sees in adolescents or adults. For example, persecutory and other delusions tended to be simple, e.g. "my parents want to kill me," "people want to hurt me." More elaborate and "fixed" delusions, not infrequently reported by adult patients, were uncommon. Many childhood themes emerged in psychotic forms. The source of auditory hallucinations were often animals (pets or toys). Monster themes were common. Primitive somatic beliefs, both in the form of hallucinations and delusions (see above for examples) were also relatively common. Sexual themes were rare. In short, the content of the psychotic symptoms in our sample reflected the developmental level of the subjects.

DISCUSSION

To put the results in perspective, it is important to compare and contrast the findings with the small number of previous phenomenological studies of schizophrenia occurring in childhood. Such comparisons are particularly important with rare disorders in that they help establish descriptive validity and point the way to further research that can resolve discrepancies and ambiguities.

The prior studies most directly comparable to the present study are the Kolvin and colleagues 1971 study (Kolvin, 1971; Kolvin et al., 1971a–e) and one by the Bellevue group (Green et al., 1984). Table 6 presents a summary of demographic and symptom data from these two studies and the present study (UCLA/CPCRC study). Diagnosis before the age of 8 was unusual and occurred for only three subjects in the Bellevue study and five subjects in the present study.

All three studies show a positive male to female ratio but somewhat less than reported for autism. The proportion of racial groups varied among the three studies, probably reflecting their cachement areas. Similarly, social class data must be interpreted with caution because of possible referral artifact. The issue of whether childhood onset schizophrenia is related to socioeconomic status (as is adult schizophrenia) must await large scale epidemiological studies.

In spite of the somewhat different demographic characteristics, diagnostic methods, and diagnostic criteria used in the three studies, the phenomenological similar-

TABLE 6
Characteristics of Schizophrenic Children in Three Centers

	Kolvin et al. (1971) Study (N = 33)	Green et al. (1984) Study (N = 24)	UCLA/CPCRC (Present) Study (N = 35)	Significance
AGE				
Mean (SD)	11.1[a]	9.96 (±1.63)	9.54 (±2.07)	NS
Range	(5–15)	(6.7–11.11)	(4.9–13.3)	
SEX				
Male	24	15	24	
Female	9	9	11	
Ratio (M:F)	2.66:1	1.67:1	2.2:1	NS
RACE				
Caucasian	33	4	22	$\chi^2 = 42.63^b$
Black	0	13	7	$p = <0.005$
Hispanic	0	6	4	
Asian	0	1	0	
SES				
I & II	5 (16%)	0	19 (54.0%)	$\chi^2 = 31.6$
III	12 (37%)	4 (16.6%)	8 (23.0%)	$p = <0.005$
IV & V	16 (47%)	20 (83.3%)	5 (14.0%)	
IQ				
N	30	24	34	NS[c]
Mean	85.9	88.5 (±16.0)	94 (±10.5)	
range	<69–>110	65–125	76–114	
Symptomatic presentation				
Auditory hallucinations	7 (81.8%)	19 (79.2%)	28 (80.0%)	NS
Visual hallucinations	10 (30.3%)	11 (45.8%)	13 (37.0%)	NS
Delusions	19 (57.6%)	13 (54.2%)	22 (63.0%)	NS
Thought disorder	20 (60%)	24 (100%)	14 (40.0%)	$\chi^2 = 22.3$
				$p < 0.005$

[a] Estimated from tabular data "age of recognition of psychosis."

[b] Caucasian compared with all others.

[c] Green vs. UCLA only; Kolvin study not compared.

Note: NS = nonsignificant.

ities among the three research samples are striking. The most commonly reported symptom is auditory hallucinations, present in four-fifths of the subjects in all three studies. Visual hallucinations were noted in 30 to 45% of the children. Visual hallucinations were always associated with auditory hallucinations with the exception of a single case reported by Green et al. (1984). The frequency of delusions was also strikingly similar, varying between 54 and 63% of the samples. The present study and the Kolvin et al. 1971 study also report frequencies for specific types of delusional thinking. At this level of analysis there are some differences. For example, Kolvin et al. report 21% of their sample reported thought deprivation (withdrawal), 18% thought insertion, and 21% thought broadcasting. The comparable frequencies for these Schneiderian symptoms in the present study were 0%, 11%, and 6%, respectively.

The most important difference between the otherwise quite similar samples was the reported prevalence of thought disorder. The Bellevue study (Green et al., 1984) reported that all subjects met *DSM-III* criteria for disturbances in form of thought, i.e., "incoherence, marked loosening of associations, markedly illogical thinking or marked poverty of content of speech." Kolvin et al. reported that 60% of subjects showed "disorder of association," 51% "talking past the point," 45% "derailment," and 24% dereistic thinking. As noted previously, in the present study only 40% were judged to meet *DSM-III* criteria, while an additional 20% exhibited less severe disturbances in form of thought. There are several possible reasons for these apparent phenomenological differences among the three samples. The first is interpretation variance. Andreasen (1979) has pointed out that definitions of "thought disorder" (a term she would like to see abandoned) vary greatly. This problem is compounded by difficulties rating disturbances of thinking in a reliable fashion. These issues are even more apparent when trying to diagnose disturbances of form of thought in young children. A second possible problem, alluded to previously, is that *DSM-III* requires a severity distinction that is not operationally defined. In short, each of the three studies may have been rating similar phenomenon in a different fashion. Of course the three samples may indeed have shown real differences on this variable, although the similarities in other aspects of the phenomenological picture tend to argue against this interpretation. The whole issue of thought disorder in psychotic and nonpsychotic children is currently the subject of extensive research, which may lead to more reliable ways of measuring this variable (Caplan et al., 1988).

In summary, three independent studies, using different methodologies and slightly different diagnostic criteria, have identified three groups of similar children with symptoms closely resembling those seen in adult schizophrenia. As Kraepelin (1919), a small proportion of schizophrenics indeed experience the onset of their disorder in childhood. As Kolvin et al. (Kolvin 1971; Kolvin et al. 1971a–e), Rutter (1972), and Green et al. (1984) emphasized, these children differ both phenomenologically and in other ways from children with infantile autism.

Yet a few cautions are in order and many research questions remain (Beitchman, 1983). As pointed out by Prior and Werry (1986) and alluded to by Kolvin et al. (Kolvin, 1971; Kolvin et al., 1971a–e), there is the problem of circularity. Children with hallucinations, delusions, and thought disturbance were found because those symptoms formed the selection criteria. More research is required to establish to what extent these symptoms are independently associated with schizophrenia or occur in children with other disorders. Chambers et al. (1982) described hallucinations in children with major affective disorder and, as mentioned previously, others have reported hallucinations in children falling into other diagnostic groupings (Garralda, 1984a,b). To partially answer this question, the authors plan to use the diagnostic protocol and the ICDS to blindly evaluate groups of children (e.g., conduct disorder) that have been previously and rigorously diagnosed using other protocols of known reliability.

Similarly, other aspects of schizophrenia occurring in childhood need careful examination. Very little is known about the longitudinal course of this disorder and to what extent it is contiguous with adult schizophrenia (Beitchman, 1983, Eggers, 1978; Kydd and Werry, 1982). Premorbid characteristics of these children need further examination, particularly the still controversial issue as to what extent children who develop schizophrenia may initially exhibit symptoms characteristic of autism (Petty et al., 1984, Watkins et al., 1988). The psychobiological substrate underlying schizophrenia in childhood is yet another area that is receiving intensive, ongoing investigation (Asarnow et al., 1986).

Underlying all of the above research efforts will be the need to reliably identify and diagnose children with schizophrenia occurring in childhood. To establish diagnostic homogeneity, careful and detailed phenomenological distinctions will be required. An important feature of the study reported here has been the use of a detailed semistructured diagnostic interview, the ICDS. The authors were surprised by the extent that patient and direct questioning of these young and very disturbed children yielded useful and detailed symptomatic data. Of great importance was the fact the parents were often unaware of important symptoms that, as a result, could only be elicited by direct questioning of the child. Of course, the reliability of structured interviewing of young children is in itself an important research question (Edelbrock et al., 1985). The authors have not yet evaluated test-retest reliability of the diagnostic interview or protocol, and need to do so.

In spite of the rarity of the disorder and research problems noted above, the study of schizophrenia occurring in childhood is of vital importance. As with adults, these children are highly disturbed, and the children and their families suffer intensely. We have little systematic knowledge about treatment, including the degree to which these children respond to psychotropic medication. To prescribe appropriate treatment, we need to be able to carefully distinguish schizophrenic children from children suffering from other disorders with psychotic symptoms, especially major affective disorder. As with adults, this distinction is not always an easy task. Finally, by studying schizophrenia in its earliest form, we may better understand etiological and treatment issues pertinent to adult forms of the disorder.

REFERENCES

Andreasen, N. C. (1979), Thought, language, and communication disorders. I. Clinical assessment, definition of terms, and evaluation of their reliability. *Arch. Gen. Psychiatry,* 36:1315–1321.

Asarnow, J. R. & Ben-Meir, S. (1988), Children with schizophrenia spectrum and depressive disorders: a comparative study of onset patterns, premorbid adjustment, and severity of dysfunction. *J. Child Psychol. Psychiatry,* 29:477–488.

———Goldstein, M. J. & Ben-Meir, S. (1988), Parental communication deviance in childhood onset schizophrenia spectrum and depressive disorders. *J. Child Psychol. Psychiatry* 29:825–838.

———Sherman, T. & Strandburg, R. (1986), The search for the psychobiological substrate of childhood onset schizophrenia. *J. Am. Acad. Child Psychiatry,* 26:601–604.

———Tanguary, P. E., Bott, L. & Freeman, B. J. (1987), Patterns of intellectual functioning in non-retarded autistic and schizophrenic children. *Journal of Psychology and Psychiatry,* 28:273–280.

Beitchman, J. H. (1983), Childhood schizophrenia: a review and comparison with adult onset schizophrenia. *Psychiatr. J. Univ. Ottawa,* 8:(2)25–37.

Burke, P., Delbeccaro, H., McCauley, E. & Clark, C. (1985) Hallucinations in children. *J. Am. Acad. Child Psychiatry,* 24:71–75.

Cantor, S., Evans, J., Pearce, J. & Pezzot-Pearce, T. (1982) Childhood schizophrenia: present but not accounted for. *Am. J. Psychiatry,* 139:758–762.

Caplan, R., Guthrie, D., Fish, B., Tanguay, P. E. & David-Lando, G. (1989), The Kiddie Formal Thought Disorder Rating Scale. *J. Am. Acad. Child Adolesc. Psychiatry,* 28:408–416.

Chambers, W. (1986), Hallucinations in psychotic and depressed children. In: *Hallucinations in children,* ed. D. Pilowsky & W. Chambers. Washington DC: American Psychiatric Press.

———Puig-Antich, J., Tabrizi, M. & Davies, M. (1982), Psychotic symptoms in prepubertal major depressive disorder. *Arch. Gen. Psychiatry,* 39:921–927.

Edelbrock, C., Costello, A. J., Dulcan, M. K., Kalas, R. & Conover, N. C. (1985), Age differences in the reliability of the psychiatric interview of the child. *Child Dev.,* 56:365–375.

Egdell, H. G. & Kolvin I. (1972), Childhood hallucinations. *J. Child Psychol. Psychiatry,* 13:279–287.

Garralda, M. (1984a), Hallucinations in children with conduct and emotional disorders: I. The clinical phenomena. *Psychol. Med.,* 14:589–596.

_____(1984b), Hallucinations in children with conduct and emotional disorders: II. The follow-up study. *Psychol. Med.,* 14:597–604.

Green, W., Campbell, M., Hardesty, A. et al. (1984), A comparison of schizophrenic and autistic children. *J. Am. Acad. Child Psychiatry,* 23:399–409.

Gutterman, E. M., O'Brien, J. D. & Young, J. G. (1987), Structured Diagnostic Interviews for Children and Adolescents: current status and future directions. *J. Am. Acad. Child Adolesc. Psychiatry,* 26:621–631.

Herjanic, B. & Campbell, W. (1977), Differentiating psychiatrically disturbed children on the basis of a structured interview. *J. Abnorm. Child Psychol.,* 5:127–134.

Hollingshead, A. B. & Redlich, F. (1958), *Social Class and Mental Illness.* New York: Wiley.

Kanner, L. (1943), Autistic disturbances of affective contact. *Nervous Child,* 2:217–250.

_____(1971), Childhood psychosis: a historical overview, *Journal of Autism and Childhood Schizophrenia,* 1:14–19.

Kolvin, I. (1971), Studies in the childhood psychoses: I. Diagnostic criteria and classification. *Br. J. Psychiatry,* 118:381–384.

_____Ounsted, C., Humphrey, M. & McNay, A. (1971a), Studies in the childhood psychoses: II. The phenomenology of childhood psychoses. *Br. J. Psychiatry,* 118:385–395.

_____ _____Richardson, L. M. & Garside, R. F. (1971b), Studies in the childhood psychoses: III. The family and social background in childhood psychoses. *Br. J. Psychiatry,* 118:396–402.

_____Garside, R. F. & Kidd, J. S. H. (1971c), Studies in the childhood psychoses: IV. Parental personality and attitude and childhood psychoses. *Br. J. Psychiatry,* 118:403–406.

_____Ounsted, C. & Roth, M. (1971d), Studies in the childhood psychoses: V. Cerebral dysfunction and childhood psychoses. *Br. J. Psychiatry,* 118:407–414.

_____Humphrey, M. & McNay, A. (1971e), Studies in the childhood psychoses: VI. Cognitive factors in childhood psychoses. *Br. J. Psychiatry,* 118:415–419.

Kovacs, M. (1978), *The Interview Schedule for Children (ISC)* (10th Revision). Pittsburgh: University of Pittsburg School of Medicine.

Kotsopoulos, S., Kanigsberg, J., Cote, A. & Fiedorowicz, C. (1987), Hallucinatory experiences in nonpsychotic children *J. Am. Acad. Child Adolesc. Psychiatry,* 26:375–380.

Kraepelin, E. (1919), *Dementia Praecox and Paraphrenia.* Translated by R. M. Barclay from the 8th German Edition of the *Textbook of Psychiatry.* Edinburgh: Livingstone.

Kydd, R. R. & Werry, J. S. (1982), Schizophrenia in children under 16 years. *J. Autism Dev. Disord.,* 12:343–357.

Loranger, A. W. (1984), Sex difference in age at onset of schizophrenia. *Arch. Gen. Psychiatry,* 41:157–161.

Ornitz, E. M., Guthrie, D. & Farley, A. J. (1978), The early symptom of childhood autism. In: *Cognitive Defects in the Development of Mental Illness,* ed. G. Serban. New York: Bruner-Mazel.

Petty, L. K., Ornitz, E. M., Michelman, J. D. & Zimmerman, E. G. (1984), Autistic children who become schizophrenic. *Arch. Gen. Psychiatry,* 41:129–135.

Prior, M. & Werry, J. S. (1986), Autism, schizophrenia, and allied disorder. In:

Psychopathological Disorder of Childhood, 3rd Ed., ed. H. C. Quay & J. S. Werry. New York: Wiley.

Puig-Antich, J. & Chambers, W. (1978), *The Schedule for Affective Disorders and Schizophrenia for School-Aged Children (Kiddie-SADS).* New York: New York State Psychiatric Association.

Rutter, M. (1972), Childhood schizophrenia considered. *Journal of Autism and Childhood Schizophrenia,* 2:315–337.

Strandburg, R. J., Marsh, J. T., Brown, W. S., Asarnow, R. F., & Guthrie, D. (1987), P3, PCA and schizophrenia: amplitude or latency? In: *Current Trends in Event-Related Potential Research* (EEG Suppl. 40), ed. R. Johnson, Jr., J. W. Rohrbaugh & R. Parasuraman. New York: Elsevier Science Publishers B. V.

Tanguay, P. & Asarnow R. (1985), Schizophrenia in children. In: *Psychiatry,* ed. R. Michaels & J. O. Cavenar. New York: Lippincott.

Watkins, J., Asarnow, R. & Tanguay, P. (1988), Symptom development in childhood onset schizophrenia. *J. Child Psychol. Psychiatry,* 29:865–878.

Welner, Z., Reich, W., Herjanic, B., Jung, K. G. & Amado, H. (1987), Reliability, validity, and parent-child agreement studies of the Diagnostic Interview for Children and Adolescents (DICA). *J. Am. Acad. Child Adolesc. Psychiatry,* 26:649–653.

18

Three Cases of Panic Disorder With Agoraphobia in Children

**James C. Ballenger, Donald J. Carek, Jane J. Steele,
and Denise Cornish-McTighe**

Medical University of South Carolina, Charleston

The authors report three cases of panic disorder with agoraphobia in children, with characteristic panic attacks, separation anxiety, and fear and avoidance of crowds and public places. The panic and agoraphobic symptoms responded to medications effective with agoraphobic adults, i.e., imipramine and alprazolam.

It is increasingly apparent that psychiatric illnesses previously thought to be specific to adulthood can begin in childhood.[1-3] Anxiety disorders such as panic disorder and agoraphobia are rarely diagnosed in children, although the diagnosis of separation anxiety is commonly made. Even though there is evidence that panic disorder and agoraphobia are familial[4,5] and many agoraphobic adults retrospectively report symptoms as children, few clinicians or investigators have studied these disorders in children.[6-8] We report here three children with typical panic attacks and agoraphobic fears and avoidance in an effort to stimulate further discussion of the childhood form of panic disorder.

CASE REPORTS

Case 1

Ann, 8 years old, presented with a 6-month history of abdominal pain and nonspecific fear that occurred in crowded places. Ann avoided school activities and family outings because of her fear of going into crowded areas. On one occasion

Reprinted with permission from *American Journal of Psychiatry,* 1989, Vol. 146, 922–924. Copyright © 1989 by the American Psychiatric Association.

when on a trip with her family, she ran out of a building after she experienced a panic attack in a cafeteria line. Panic attacks, accompanied by shortness of breath, palpitations, abdominal pain, and a feeling of being "out of control," occurred as often as twice a day, especially when she was away from the home. Ann frequently called from school, asking to be taken home, and protested when she was encouraged to attend activities with peers away from the home. Her abdominal pain and unwillingness to eat in the cafeteria at school led to a 5-lb weight loss in 3 months. She denied feelings of depression, worthlessness, or hopelessness. Her panic attacks and persistent fear of having more attacks would have met adult criteria (*DSM-III-R*) for panic disorder with agoraphobia of moderate severity. Ann's mother, successfully treated with alprazolam for panic disorder with extensive phobic avoidance (*DSM-III-R*), felt that her daughter's symptoms paralleled her own and brought her for treatment.

Treatment with alprazolam, in combination with imipramine for almost a year, resulted in complete remission of symptoms. Alprazolam was tapered and discontinued easily, and Ann was treated with imipramine (75 mg at bedtime) alone for 2 additional years. She was seen in individual supportive psychotherapy every 1 to 2 weeks during most of this time. When imipramine was discontinued she developed transient somatic symptoms, but these cleared and she did well. However, 5 months after imipramine was discontinued she experienced a full relapse, was retreated with imipramine (75 mg/day), and recovered in several weeks. After an additional 2 years of successful drug treatment and supportive psychotherapy, medication was tapered and discontinued at the end of a school year. Ann did well initially but began having spontaneous panic attacks approximately 5 months later, after returning to the stress of school. Imipramine treatment was restarted, and there was complete improvement of symptoms with 75 mg/day. Supportive psychotherapy and family sessions, as well as simple relaxation techniques, were included as adjuncts to drug treatment. Ten months later Ann continued to take the medication, the frequency of supportive psychotherapy sessions had decreased, and she remained symptom free despite major stressors within her family. Medication taper was again planned at the end of the school year.

Case 2

Alan, 13 years old, developed the fear that he would faint in school or other public places after having felt faint in the lunch line at school. He began to experience sudden episodes of palpitations and increased perspiration accompanied by the fear that he would faint or "lose control" in class, the mall, or church. At those times he was noted to look pale and to feel cold and "clammy." Examination by a cardiologist resulted in the diagnosis of mitral valve prolapse, but this was not felt to account for his symptoms. Because of his attacks, Alan avoided crowds, especially in malls and large school functions. He would attend church services only if he could sit in the back of church so that he could leave quickly if he became anxious. He met adult criteria (*DSM-III-R*) for panic disorder with agoraphobia of moderate severity.

Alan was treated with alprazolam, 1.0 mg twice daily, and imipramine, 125 mg at bedtime, and experienced complete remission of his symptoms. After 4 months alprazolam was reduced to 0.5 mg twice a day. After 8 months alprazolam was tapered and discontinued without reappearance of symptoms, and imipramine was reduced to 75 mg/day. Imipramine was discontinued after a total of 12 months of treatment without return of symptoms.

Alan was seen in psychotherapy a total of 14 times over the initial 7 months. An attempt was made to engage him in reflective psychotherapy, but this was largely unsuccessful. Over the next 6 months he was seen four times to determine "how things were going," for general support, and to check on his medications. It was our impression that his improvement was primarily related to the medications.

Case 3

Cathy, 11 years old, had always had a problem with separation, avoided sleepover parties, and disliked it when her parents went out. She began having abdominal pain when she changed to a new school. Several visits to her pediatrician resulted in no diagnosis, and an upper gastrointestinal series was normal. While in school, she began to have spontaneous panic attacks that were characterized by the sudden feeling that she was going to die, trembling, sweaty hands, tingling in her legs, and dizziness. Afterward, she worried that "something might happen to me." Although Cathy had been active and independent during the summer, after school began she spent less time with friends and did not want to be left alone. Consequently, she often accompanied her mother on errands but would have panic attacks in stores. She called her mother frequently from school, asking to be taken home. She met adult criteria (*DSM-III-R*) for panic disorder with agoraphobia of mild severity. Cathy was awakened at night by abdominal pain and lost 5 lb. She denied feeling sad or worthless. The only family history of psychiatric problems was depression in her maternal grandmother.

Cathy was treated successfully with 75 mg/day of imipramine, which effectively blocked her panic attacks. Despite occasional complaints of stomachaches when she was under stress, she returned to activities she had been avoiding. Sessions with the patient and her parents provided education about anxiety disorders and focused on helping the parents encourage appropriate separation. Imipramine was tapered after 2 years, and there was no known relapse over 27 months.

DISCUSSION

There is a relative dearth of information and clinical investigation concerning panic disorder and agoraphobia in childhood, although Gittelman-Klein and Klein first suggested in 1973 that separation anxiety in childhood was closely related to adult agoraphobia.[9,10] The children we have described met adult criteria (*DSM-III-R*) for panic disorder with varying degrees of agoraphobia. Although we did not use structured diagnostic interviews with these children, we came to know them well through extensive clinical contact, generally over several years. Although they had features of separation, avoidant, and phobic disorders of childhood, their clinical syndromes appeared very similar to the usual adult presentation of panic disorder, and we feel it is most appropriate to conceptualize them as having the same syndrome. This conclusion is further supported by the fact that they appeared to respond to treatment "like adults" (e.g., to the same medications).

There are several reasons why the presence of panic disorder and agoraphobia in children may be underappreciated, other than the belief that they do not occur until early adulthood. Avoidant behavior in children may be more difficult to recognize because children are protected and dependent and underlying anxiety may remain unchallenged and therefore unexposed. There is a relatively greater diagnostic awareness of depression in children than of anxiety. A child's tearful, sad, forlorn appearance may distract examiners from the underlying anxiety that becomes evident only on closer scrutiny. In addition, children may be even more prone than adults to emphasize their physical symptoms (e.g., cases 1 and 3) over their anxiety and avoidance symptoms. Correct recognition of this disorder in children is probably quite important because it would better allow early detection and intervention, which should help prevent the patterns of chronic avoidance and lowered self-esteem that individuals with untreated panic disorder frequently develop.

These three children responded to treatment with resolution of their panic and avoidance symptoms and with resumption of age-appropriate activities. Although each of the children was seen in psychotherapy by psychotherapy-oriented clinicians, there was clear consensus among us that symptom resolution was primarily related to the medications. This impression was based on both the time course of symptom resolution and the two relapses in patient 1 when medication was discontinued and the subsequent good responses when medication was reinstituted.

Obviously, many of the issues raised by this preliminary report now require rigorous study. However, it is our hope that our description of the symptom patterns and successful treatment of these children will stimulate others to explore the nature of these symptoms and this disorder in children.

REFERENCES

1. Cytryn L, McKnew DH Jr, Bartko JJ, et al: Offspring of patients with affective disorders, II. J Am Acad Child Psychiatry 1982; 21:389–391

2. Beardslee WR, Bemporad J, Keller MB, et al: Children of parents with major affective disorder: a review. Am J Psychiatry 1983; 140:825–832

3. Rapoport JL: The Boy Who Couldn't Stop Washing: The Experience and Treatment of Obsessive-Compulsive Disorder. New York, EP Dutton, 1989

4. Crowe RR, Noyes R, Pauls DL, et al: A family study of panic disorder. Arch Gen Psychiatry 1983; 40:1065–1069

5. Harris EL, Noyes R, Crowe RR, et al: Family study of agoraphobia: report of a pilot study. Arch Gen Psychiatry 1983; 40:1061–1064

6. Berg I: School phobia in children of agoraphobic women. Br J Psychiatry 1967; 128:86–89

7. Weissman MM, Leckman JF, Meukanjos KR, et al: Depression and anxiety disorders in parents and children. Arch Gen Psychiatry 1984; 41:845–852

8. VanWinter JT, Stickler GB: Panic attack syndrome. J Pediatr 1984; 105:661–665

9. Gittelman-Klein R, Klein D: School phobia: diagnostic considerations in light of imipramine effects. J Nerv Ment Dis 1973; 156:199–215

10. Gittelman-Klein R: Pharmacotherapy and management of pathological separation anxiety. Int J Ment Health 1975–1976; 4:255–271

19

Panic Attacks in Young Adolescents

Chris Hayward, Joel D. Killen, and C. Barr Taylor

Stanford University School of Medicine, California

The lifetime prevalence of interview-determined four-symptom panic attacks in 95 ninth graders was 11.6%. Those with panic attacks were significantly more depressed, were significantly more likely to have separated or divorced parents, and tended to be more likely to have tried cigarette smoking.

Although adults with panic attacks often report experiencing their first panic episode during adolescence[1], little is known about the frequency of panic attacks in this age group. Moreau et al.[2] have described six cases of panic disorder that began in childhood and adolescence; however, there have been no population-based studies of panic attacks in adolescents.[3] In this study, we interviewed a sample of ninth graders to determine the prevalence of panic attacks in young adolescents. We also explored the relationship between panic attacks in adolescents and both substance use and depression.

METHOD

Ninth-grade students (N = 106) from three physical education classes in a suburban high school near a large northern California city were asked to complete a survey questionnaire and participate in a structured psychiatric interview. The racial composition of the school is 59.8% white, 21.2% Asian, 15.0% Hispanic, 3.3% black, and 0.7% other. Three classes were randomly selected from a total of six physical education classes in the ninth

Reprinted with permission from *American Journal of Psychiatry,* 1989, Vol. 146, No. 8, 1061–1062. Copyright © 1989 by the American Psychiatric Association.

Supported by grant HL-32185 from the National Heart, Lung, and Blood Institute and by grant MH-16744 from NIMH.

The authors thank John Mix for help in conducting the study and Guangrui Zhu, Danyang Zhang, and Beth Sherman for technical assistance.

grade. Passive consent was obtained from the parents and written informed consent was obtained from the students.

The questionnaire included questions about ethnicity, parents' marital status, and substance use and the depression scale from the SCL-90-R.[4] Cigarette smoking, marijuana use, and alcohol use were categorized as "never used," "experimental use" (use of the substance less than once a week), and "regular use" (use of the substance weekly or daily).

Interviews lasting 5–15 minutes were conducted privately by a psychologist or a doctoral candidate in psychology who used the panic disorder section of the Structured Clinical Interview for *DSM-III-R* Disorders (SCID).[5] Only the panic section of the SCID was used because of the time limitation in the classroom. If a student responded affirmatively to the SCID screening question about sudden fright, the interviewer then determined if the fright was spontaneous and not due to phobic stimuli (social or simple) and did not occur in situations in which most people might experience some fear or autonomic stimulation, such as when taking an examination or during exercise. If so, the interviewer proceeded with the other SCID questions about panic attacks. The primary investigator (C.H.) later determined if the subject had experienced a panic attack as defined in *DSM-III-R*. Possible medical conditions and drug use associated with panic attacks were not assessed.

Ninety-five of the 106 students who received the questionnaire also participated in the structured psychiatric interview. Because of the time constraints of class periods, 11 students were not interviewed. The completion rates for those who both received the questionnaire and were interviewed (N = 95) were 98% (N = 93) for the substance use questions and 82% (N = 78) for the SCL-90-R depression scale. Of those interviewed, 52% (N = 49) were boys and 48% (N = 46) were girls; their mean age was 14.5 years (range, 14–16). With respect to ethnicity, 48.4% identified themselves as white, 20.0% as Asian, 14.7% as Hispanic, 6.3% as black, 3.2% as Native American, and 5.4% as other (total = 98%; some subjects did not answer question).

For data analysis the sample was divided into those who had experienced a panic attack, including a symptom-limited attack (which has fewer than four symptoms), and those who had not. Chi-square analysis with Yates' correction was used to compare the two groups with respect to substance use; experimental and regular users were combined for this analysis. Group differences in marital status of the parents were also tested with Yates-corrected chi-square analysis. The Student's t test was used to test for group differences on the depression scale of the SCL-90-R.

RESULTS

Those who experienced at least one four-symptom panic attack constituted 11.6% (N = 11) of the sample (N = 95), 17.4% (N = 8) of the girls and 6.1% (N = 3) of the boys. An additional 3.2% (N = 3) of the sample, all boys, reported experiencing at least one symptom-limited panic attack. Thus, there were 14 students who had experienced a panic attack of any kind and 81 who had not. As indicated in Table 1, significantly more of the panic attack group than the no panic attack group had parents who were divorced or separated; in addition, there was a tendency for more of the panic attack group than the no panic attack group to have tried smoking cigarettes, and there were no significant differences between the groups with respect to marijuana use and alcohol use. The panic attack group had significantly higher mean ±SD scores on the depression scale of the SCL-90-R (1.4±0.8, N = 13) than the no panic attack group (0.82±0.7, N = 65) (t = 2.6, df = 76, p<0.05).

DISCUSSION

The results of this study confirm that panic attacks are not confined to adults. The 11.6% lifetime prevalence rate of four-symptom panic attacks we observed in adolescents is high compared with the 9.7% lifetime rates for panic attacks in adults found in the Epidemiologic Catchment Area Program study.[6] Other population-based studies have reported prevalence rates between 11% and 35% for panic attacks in adults (7–9). Telch et al. (unpublished paper), using a questionnaire, assessed 2,375 college students and observed that approximately 12% had experienced unexpected panic attacks in their lifetimes. Clearly, the observed

TABLE 1
Substance Use and Parental Divorce or Separation Among Ninth
Graders With and Without Panic Attacks[a]

Variable	Panic		No Panic	
	N	%	N	%
Cigarette use[b]				
Never used	3	23	42	53
Experimental or regular use	10	77	38	48
Marijuana use				
Never used	8	61	54	68
Experimental or regular use	5	39	25	32
Alcohol use				
Never used	3	23	13	17
Experimental or regular use	10	77	65	83
Parental separation or divorce[c]				
Yes	8	61	22	29
No	5	39	54	71

[a] Not all adolescents answered every question on the questionnaire.
[b] $\chi^2 = 2.8$, df=1, p<0.10.
[c] $\chi^2 = 3.9$, df=1, p<0.05.

frequency of panic attacks varies according to the method of assessment, number of symptoms required for the diagnosis, time period considered, and the population studied. Caveats in interpreting the prevalence rate we found include the possible recall bias in the assessment of lifetime prevalence rates and the as yet unstudied comparability of a shortened interview with the standard structured diagnostic interview.

In children and in adults there is considerable comorbidity between anxiety and depression.[10] The significant association that we found between panic attacks in young adolescents and a self-report measure of depression suggests that panic attacks and depression probably overlap in adolescents as well. Future community-based studies of panic attacks in adolescents should formally assess depression to better distinguish between these two disorders.

The finding that the parents of those having experienced a panic attack are more likely to be divorced or separated is consistent with a theory of panic attacks which suggests that early loss, or sensitivity to separation, may be a risk factor for the later development of panic attacks. We do not know the temporal relationship between the parental separation and the reported panic attacks in this study.

We also found a possible association between cigarette smoking and panic attacks. Panic attacks may predispose adolescents to smoke cigarettes, or, alternatively, smoking withdrawal may have triggered panic episodes. With respect to the negative finding regarding alcohol use, ninth graders may be too young to exhibit the frequently observed relationship in adults between anxiety disorders and alcohol abuse.

REFERENCES

1. Von Korff MR, Eaton WW, Keyl PM: The epidemiology of panic attacks and panic disorder. Am J Epidemiol 1985; 122:970–981
2. Moreau DL, Weissman M, Warner V: Panic disorder in children at high risk for depression. Am J Psychiatry 1989; 146:1059–1060
3. Orvaschel H, Weissman MM: Epidemiology of anxiety disorders in children: a review, in Anxiety Disorders of Childhood. Edited by Gittelman R. New York, Guilford Press, 1986
4. Derogatis LR: SCL-90-R: Administration, Scoring, and Procedures Manual, II. Towson, MD, Clinical Psychometric Research, 1983
5. Spitzer RL, Williams JBW, Gibbon M: Structured Clinical Interview for DSM-III-R (SCID). New York, New York Psychiatric Institute, Biometrics Research, 1987
6. Eaton WW, Dryman A, Weissman MM: Panic and phobia, in Psychiatric Disorders of America. Edited by Robins LN, Reiger DA. New York, Free Press (in press)
7. Wittchen HU: Epidemiology of panic attacks and panic disorders, in Panic and Phobias:

Empirical Evidence of Theoretical Models and Longterm effects of Behavioral Treatments. Edited by Hand I, Wittchen HU. New York, Springer-Verlag, 1986

8. Salge RA, Beck JG, Logan AC: A community survey of panic. J Anxiety Disorders 1988; 2:157–167

9. Norton GR, Harrison B, Hauch J, et al: Characteristics of people with infrequent panic attacks. J Abnorm Psychol 1985; 94:216–221

10. Puig-Antich J, Rabinovich H: Relationship between affective and anxiety disorders in childhood, in Anxiety Disorders of Childhood. Edited by Gittelman R. New York, Guilford Press, 1986

20

Panic Disorder in Children at High Risk for Depression

Donna L. Moreau, Myrna Weissman, and Virginia Warner

New York State Psychiatric Institute

While conventional clinical wisdom has been that panic disorder does not occur in children, evidence derived from structured diagnostic interviews suggests that panic disorder, similar in symptom pattern to the adult disorder, does occur in children and can occur before puberty.

Conventional clinical wisdom has been that panic disorder does not occur in children (1). Recently, there have been isolated clinical reports on the existence of panic disorder in children (2, 3). However, with the exception of the two cases reported by Vitiello et al. (3), the diagnoses have not been based on structured diagnostic interview.

Although small studies have been conducted (4, 5), to our knowledge there have been no large epidemiological studies of children or adolescents that used *DSM-III* criteria to determine the prevalence of psychiatric disorders, including panic disorder. However, a recent study by Hayward et al. (6) of 95 ninth-grade high school students found, on the basis of clinical interview, that the lifetime prevalence of four-symptom panic attacks was 11.6%. Epidemiological studies of adults who retrospectively reported their age at onset of panic disorder suggest that onset of panic disorder can be quite early. Results from the National Institute of Mental Health Epidemiologic Catchment Area Study showed a peak onset of panic disorder between the ages of 15 and 19 years, with onset before puberty in some cases (7).

Retrospectively taken childhood histories of adults with panic disorder, studies of the parents of children with anxiety disorders, and studies of children with depressed

Reprinted with permission from *American Journal of Psychiatry*, 1989, Vol. 146, No. 8, 1059–1060. Copyright © 1989 by the American Psychiatric Association.

Supported in part by NIMH grants MH-36197 and MH-28274 from the Affective and Anxiety Disorders Research Branch and by grant 86-213 from the John D. and Catherine T. MacArthur Foundation Mental Health Research Network.

...d anxious parents lend support to an association between adult and childhood forms of anxiety disorders. Specifically, studies of adults with panic disorder have found cases of onset of panic disorder in childhood or early adolescence (8).

This paper presents symptom and diagnostic data on seven children with panic attacks. Six of these children met *DSM-III* criteria for panic disorder on the basis of direct, structured diagnostic assessment with the Schedule for Affective Disorders and Schizophrenia for School-Age Children, Life-Time Version (Kiddie-SADS-L).

METHOD

The subjects were part of a study of 220 children, ages 6 to 23 years, who were at high or low risk for depression by virtue of their parents' diagnosis. Children of depressed parents were matched by age and sex to children of nondepressed parents. Detailed methodology is presented elsewhere (9). Because this study determined age at onset of psychiatric disorders on the basis of retrospective report, subjects included individuals up to 23 years of age. Subjects and their parents were interviewed separately with the Kiddie-SADS-L during the initial assessment by a trained interviewer with clinical experience. At 2-year follow-up the children were interviewed again with the Kiddie-SADS-L. *DSM-III* diagnoses of children were made by a child psychiatrist and a child psychologist on the basis of all available information from both interviews, as well as school and psychiatric records where available; the child psychiatrist and psychologist were blind to the parents' clinical condition. Agreement between the psychiatrist and psychologist was excellent (kappa = 0.69 for anxiety disorders in the 220 children) (10).

RESULTS

Of the 220 children, four girls and three boys, who ranged in age from 11 to 23 years at the time of initial assessment, were found to have panic symptoms (see Table 1). Six of the seven children met the criteria for panic disorder. One child did not have panic attacks with sufficient frequency to meet the diagnostic criteria. The age at onset of panic disorder ranged from 5 to 18 years. In four cases onset was before puberty.

During the first interview, four of the children recalled panic symptoms, all of which had occurred within 1 year of the interview, and five of the parents reported previous panic symptoms in their children. During the follow-up interview, two of the subjects were still experiencing panic attacks. Only subjects who were currently symptomatic reported panic symptoms at the follow-up interview.

Symptoms were similar to those found in adults with panic disorder (see Table 1). Feelings of panic, anxiety, or fear occurred suddenly and were accompanied by multiple physical and psychological symptoms. All of the children reported shortness of breath, and the majority had palpitations. Symptoms reported by half of the subjects included sensations of chest pain, choking, dizziness, sweating, trembling, or fainting; fears of death; and feelings of unreality. The mean number of symptoms for each subject was 6.1

All of the children had other diagnoses, most commonly major depression and separation anxiety disorder. The onset of panic disorder either occurred in conjunction with separation anxiety disorder or major depression or followed the onset of separation anxiety disorder by at least several months. Although several of the subjects used illicit drugs and alcohol, only one met the criteria for substance abuse. Four of the seven children had at least one parent with panic disorder in addition to depression. All cases of panic disorder were found in the children at high risk for depression; no cases were found in the children of nondepressed parents.

DISCUSSION

The findings suggest that panic disorder does occur in children and can occur before puberty. The symptom pattern and high comorbidity with major depression

TABLE 1
Age, Age at Onset, Symptoms, and Comorbidity in Seven Children With Panic Symptoms

Item	Patient						
	1	2	3	4	5	6	7
Age (years)							
At second interview	17	20	11	18	23	14	11
At onset of panic	9	18	5	10	12	13	6
Sex	M	F	M	F	F	F	M
Symptoms							
Shortness of breath	+	+	+	+	+	+	+
Palpitations	+	+	+	+	+	+	
Chest pain	+	+		+	+		
Choking		+		+	+		
Dizziness		+		+	+		
Sweating		+		+		+	
Trembling			+		+	+	
Fears of death	+		+		+	+	
Faintness	+		+	+	+		
Feelings of unreality				+		+	+
Tingling					+		+
Hot and cold flashes					+		
DSM-III diagnoses							
Most common							
Panic disorder		+	+	+	+	+	+
Major depression	+	+		+	+	+	
Separation anxiety disorder	+		+	+	+		+
Total	5	4	5	3	3	2	2

are similar to those found in adults. It must be noted that the children we studied did not represent a probability sample of a community. Because panic disorder occurred in the children of depressed parents and not those of nondepressed parents, the frequency with which the disorder occurred is probably exaggerated.

In this study we used the child psychiatrist's and psychologist's best estimate, based on multiple sources of information, to determine the child's diagnosis. Agreement between psychiatrists was excellent. There were discrepancies between parents' and children's reports, however. Parents were more consistent than the children in reporting past episodes of panic. Of the four children who reported panic symptoms, all either were experiencing symptoms at the time of the interview or had experienced symptoms within a year of the interview. The children were able to report the phenomenology of panic attacks when they were symptomatic, but in their retrospective reports they failed to note past panic episodes that the parents reported.

These findings, if replicated, would suggest that systematic assessment of panic disorder should be part of a general psychiatric workup of children, particularly children at risk by virtue of depression in the parent. A host of questions remain. We do not know the continuity of childhood panic disorder into adulthood, the clinical course or its impact on development, or the actual prevalence. While there is good evidence for the efficacy of pharmacologic and behavioral treatment of panic disorder in adults (11), the efficacy of these treatments in children is unknown.

REFERENCES

1. Gittelman-Klein R, Klein DF: Adult anxiety disorders and childhood separation anxiety, in Handbook of Anxiety, vol 1: Biological and Cultural Perspectives. Edited by Roth M, Noyes R Jr, Burrows GD. New York, Elsevier, 1988
2. Van Winter JT, Stickler GB: Panic attack syndrome. J Pediatr 1984; 105:661–665
3. Vitiello B, Behar D, Wolfson S, et al: Panic disorder in prepubertal children (letter). Am J Psychiatry 1987; 144:525–526
4. Anderson JC, Williams S, McGee R, et al: DSM-III disorders in preadolescent children. Arch Gen Psychiatry 1987; 44:69–81
5. Kashani JH, Orvaschel H: Anxiety disorders in mid-adolescence: a community sample. Am J Psychiatry 1988; 145:960–964
6. Hayward C, Killen JD, Taylor CB: Panic attacks in young adolescents. Am J Psychiatry 1989; 146:1061–1062
7. Von Korff MR, Eaton WW, Keyl PM: The epidemiology of panic attacks and panic disorder: results of three community surveys. Am J Epidemiol 1985; 122:970–981
8. Sheehan DV, Sheehan KE, Minichiello WE: Age of onset of phobic disorders: a reevaluation. Compr Psychiatry 1981; 22:544–553

9. Weissman MM, Leckman JF, Merikangas KR, et al: Depression and anxiety disorders in parents and children. Arch Gen Psychiatry 1984; 41:845–852

10. Weissman MM: Psychopathology in the children of depressed parents: direct interview studies, in relatives at Risk for Mental Disorders. Edited by Dunner DL, Gershon ES, Barrett JB. New York, Raven Press, 1988

11. Frances AJ, Hales RE (eds): American Psychiatric Press Review of Psychiatry, vol 7. Washington, DC, American Psychiatric Press, 1988

PART IV: CLINICAL ISSUES

21

Neurochemical Abnormalities of Anorexia Nervosa and Bulimia Nervosa

Maurizio Fava and Paul M. Copeland
Massachusetts General Hospital, Boston
Ulrich Schweiger
Max Planck Institute of Psychiatry, Munich, West Germany
David B. Herzog
Massachusetts General Hospital, Boston

The authors review the research on anorexia nervosa and bulimia nervosa, emphasizing the neurotransmitters and neuromodulators that regulate eating behavior. Anorexia nervosa is associated with changes in the noradrenergic, serotonergic, and opioid systems; bulimia nervosa is accompanied by marked alterations in serotonin and norepinephrine activity. These neurochemical changes may perpetuate pathological eating behavior and may be responsible for several associated psychiatric symptoms, including anxiety and depression. The authors also summarize studies of several drugs that are used in the treatment of eating disorders and are known to modify neurotransmitter activity. Understanding the neurochemistry of eating disorders seems crucial for the rational development of both psychopharmacological and behavioral treatments.

Anorexia nervosa and bulimia nervosa are syndromes characterized by gross disturbances in eating behavior that share underlying concerns for dieting and weight regulation.

According to *DSM-III-R*, anorexia nervosa is characterized by refusal to maintain body weight over minimal norms, weight more than 15% below expected body weight, intense fear of gaining weight or becoming fat, disturbance of body image, and, in females, absence of at least three consecutive expected menstrual cycles.

Reprinted with permission from *American Journal of Psychiatry*, 1989, Vol. 146, No. 8, 963–971. Copyright © 1989 by the American Psychiatric Association.

Bulimia nervosa, according to *DSM-III-R*, involves recurrent episodes of binge eating occurring at least twice a week for 3 months, a feeling of lack of control over eating behavior during the binges, persistent overconcern with body shape and weight, and the use of self-induced vomiting, laxatives, diuretics, dieting, or vigorous exercise to prevent weight gain.

Although these two disorders are considered to be two distinct entities, stringent attempts by patients with anorexia nervosa to limit food intake may be interrupted at times by episodes of bulimia; it also appears that the proposed distinction between bulimic patients with and without anorexia nervosa is not supported by a rigorous analysis of their demographic, clinical, and psychometric features.[1] Therefore, it is quite possible that psychoneuroendocrinological correlates of these two disorders may overlap.

Neurochemical alterations may have a pathophysiological role in these disorders. Several CNS neurotransmitters and neuromodulators are known to be involved in the regulation of eating behavior in animals and have been implicated in symptoms such as depression and anxiety often observed in patients with eating disorders. Since neurochemical changes in patients with anorexia nervosa or bulimia nervosa may precede, accompany, or follow behavioral changes, it is difficult to assess what role these changes play in the etiology and maintenance of these disorders. The effects of weight loss on the CNS are quite marked and may confound the interpretation of the data. The study of neurochemical alterations in eating disorders can delineate secondary endocrine and metabolic changes that represent some of the biochemical substrates for the physical complications in anorexia nervosa and bulimia nervosa and may, in turn, facilitate and reinforce abnormal patterns of eating behavior. Neurochemical research may also contribute to understanding the pathophysiology of eating disorders, and this knowledge could potentially benefit various nonsomatic (e.g., behavioral and psychotherapeutic) treatment modalities in addition to leading to the development of more successful psychopharmacological treatment for these disorders.

In this paper, we will review studies on noradrenergic, serotonergic, dopaminergic, and opioid systems; on the neuromodulators corticotropin-releasing hormone (CRH), vasopressin (antidiuretic hormone) (ADH), and cholecystokinin; and on some brain metabolic and morphologic measures in patients with eating disorders. Furthermore, we will highlight some of the studies on drug therapy of eating disorders with reference to the effects of these agents on neurotransmitters and neuromodulators.

NEUROTRANSMITTER SYSTEMS

Noradrenergic

The noradrenergic system has been implicated in the pathogenesis of anorexia nervosa[2] and is likely to be involved in the physiological regulation of feeding behavior at the CNS level.[3] For example, application of α_2-adrenergic agonists to the paraventricular nucleus of the rat hypothalamus produces pronounced hyperphagia,[4] and application of β-adrenergic agonists to the perifornical region of the hypothalamus inhibits feeding.[5] Several studies suggest that the noradrenergic system provides important neural substrates for anxiety[6] and depression.[7] These affective states are observed frequently in patients with anorexia nervosa and bulimia nervosa.[8] Activation of the locus ceruleus, the major norepinephrine cell group in the mammalian brain, may be associated with anxiety[9]; starvation may decrease central and, in particular, locus ceruleus norepinephrine activity with subsequent reduced anxiety.[10] Decreased sympathetic activity may also decrease metabolic rate[11] and protect the anorexia nervosa patient by decreasing nutrient requirements.

Central norepinephrine metabolism has been extensively studied in anorexia nervosa either directly by looking at CSF concentrations of norepinephrine and/or its major metabolite, 3-methoxy-4-hydroxyphenyl-glycol (MHPG), or indirectly by measuring peripheral (plasma or urinary) MHPG concentrations, which partly reflect central norepinephrine metabolism. Studies of patients with anorexia nervosa[2, 12–19] have consistently found lower than normal concentrations of urinary and plasma MHPG and of CSF norepinephrine and MHPG, suggesting that norepinephrine turnover is reduced in anorexia nervosa. This finding may be secondary to the starvation state, since plasma norepinephrine and urine MHPG levels increase to near-normal levels after weight gain.[12] In addition, urinary MHPG excretion is best predicted by percentage of body fat in both normal and anorectic women.[19] When patients with anorexia nervosa are studied after mild nutritional rehabilitation[20] or in the early stages of weight gain, norepinephrine and MHPG values tend to be in the normal range.[21] However, anorectic patients who have recovered their normal weight for a mean$\pm$SD of 20 ± 7 months had a 50% lower CSF norepinephrine level than normal control subjects[20]; therefore, a pervasive defect in norepinephrine metabolism may be a "trait" marker of anorexia nervosa.

Indirect evidence of lower levels of peripheral norepinephrine concentration comes from a greater number of platelet α_2-adrenergic receptor binding sites in patients with anorexia nervosa.[17,22,23] When these patients regained 10% of their weight, the platelet α_2-adrenergic receptor binding sites stabilized at normal levels.[22] Mikhailidis et al.[23] also found greater platelet aggregation and thromboxane A_2 release in response to epinephrine in patients with anorexia nervosa compared with normal control subjects. Following weight gain these responses normalized.

Postsynaptic α_2-receptor activity has been evaluated in patients with anorexia nervosa by examining the growth hormone (GH) response to stimulation with the α_2-adrenergic receptor agonist clonidine. However, the interpretation of this test in patients with anorexia nervosa is complicated by the finding that these patients have an abnormal GH secretion secondary to reduced levels of somatomedin C. The GH response to clonidine challenge was found to be normal in low-weight patients with anorexia nervosa but was diminished during nutritional rehabilitation and weight gain.[10] Presynaptic α_2-receptor sensitivity (as assessed by clonidine-induced decreases in plasma MHPG) was found to be higher than normal in low-weight patients with anorexia nervosa but decreased to the normal range during refeeding.[10] A higher level of presynaptic inhibitory α_2-adrenergic receptor sensitivity would possibly potentiate a decrease in central norepinephrine release.

Several studies found altered noradrenergic function in bulimia nervosa as well. During the first week after hospital admission patients with bulimia nervosa had a blunted rise in plasma norepinephrine concentration on standing.[24] Even after 3 weeks of treatment in a clinical research inpatient unit, without binge eating and purging, these patients had significantly lower resting plasma levels of norepinephrine.[25] In addition, bulimic patients had a higher number of platelet α_2-adrenergic receptors.[22]

Bulimic patients have a significantly lower resting pulse, systolic blood pressure, and plasma norepinephrine than control subjects. In response to increasing doses of intravenous infusion of the β-adrenergic agonist isoproterenol, patients with bulimia nervosa show greater sensitivity to the chronotropic effects of isoproterenol, reaching a pulse increase of 25 beats per minute at a significantly lower drug dose than control subjects.[26] This last finding probably reflects greater sensitivity of cardiovascular β-adrenergic receptors, which may be induced by decreased release of catecholamines.

Serotonergic

Animal studies have shown that serotonin plays an inhibiting role in feeding behavior.[27] This neurotransmitter acts on the ventromedial hypothalamus, which is considered a satiety system.[27] The relevance of the serotonergic system in eating disorders may be linked to the observation that patients with eating disorders often present with depression, anxiety,[8] and obsessive-compulsive features and that this system seems to play an important role in other psychiatric disorders, including depression,[28] obsessive-compulsive disorder,[29] and anxiety.[30]

The results of the studies on serotonergic activity in patients with anorexia nervosa are somewhat conflicting. In fact, although Gerner et al.[21] reported that CSF levels of the serotonin metabolite 5-hydroxyindoleacetic acid (5-HIAA) and of tryptophan, a precursor of serotonin, were no different in patients with anorexia nervosa than in normal control subjects, Kaye et al.[20] found that underweight anorectic patients had CSF 5-HIAA levels that were 20% lower than normal and that these levels normalized after weight recovery. In addition, platelet serotonin uptake did not differ between anorectic patients and normal control subjects.[31,32]

Serotonin metabolism has been extensively studied in patients with bulimia nervosa. Normal-weight bulimic subjects have a blunted L-tryptophan-induced rise of plasma prolactin levels compared with control subjects.[33] Bulimic patients who became satiated and stopped binge eating and vomiting had an increase in their plasma L-tryptophan-large neutral amino acids ratio, but the plasma L-tryptophan-large neutral amino acids ratio did not increase in bulimic patients who did not feel satiated by binge eating and vomiting.[34] Since large neutral amino acids compete with L-tryptophan for the same carrier system to cross the blood-brain barrier, the plasma L-tryptophan-large neutral amino acids ratio is considered the most important factor determining transport of tryptophan from plasma into the CNS.[35] Greater CNS concentrations of L-tryptophan lead to an increase in serotonin synthesis. These observations are consistent with the hypothesis that increased brain serotonin turnover contributes to satiety. Weight-restored anorectic patients with bulimia have been found to have smaller probenecid-induced increases of CSF levels of 5-HIAA than weight-restored nonbulimic anorectic patients, suggesting decreased serotonergic release in bulimia.[36]

Dopaminergic

In animal studies, the central administration of low doses of dopamine and dopamine agonists stimulates feeding and administration of higher doses inhibits feeding, probably through the perifornical lateral hypothalamus.[3,37] The dopaminergic system appears to be closely linked to the opioid system in the neuroregulation of eating, since naloxone, an opioid antagonist, inhibits dopamine stimulation of feeding[37] and dopamine antagonists inhibit opioid-stimulated feeding.[38]

The results of the studies on dopamine metabolism in anorexia nervosa are inconsistent. In one study,[20] underweight anorectic patients had CSF levels of the dopamine metabolite homovanillic acid (HVA) that were 30% lower than normal, but their HVA levels returned to normal shortly after weight recovery. In two other studies,[19,21] however, the CSF level of HVA in underweight anorectic women and normal control subjects did not differ.

Opioid

In animal experiments, naloxone administration decreased feeding in rats following food deprivation[39] and central administration of the endogenous κ-opioid agonists dynorphin and α-neo-endorphin enhanced feeding.[37] Moreover, in normal humans, the administration of the κ-opiate agonist butorphanol tartrate can increase food intake[40] and naloxone seems to reduce food intake.[41]

Gerner and Sharp[42] found that CSF β-endorphin immunoreactivity among moderately underweight anorectic patients was not different from that of normal subjects. Other researchers found that CSF opioid activity, measured by a radioreceptor assay, was higher in patients with anorexia nervosa than in normal control subjects or in the same patients after weight restoration.[43]

Kaye et al.[44] found by radioimmunoassay that levels of β-lipotropin, ACTH, β-endorphin, and the N-terminal fragment of pro-opiomelanocortin in the CSF were significantly lower in extremely underweight anorectic patients but normalized after weight restoration. These authors concluded that a reduction in concentration of these pro-opiomelanocortin peptides occurs as a consequence of weight loss and malnutrition in patients with anorexia nervosa. Furthermore, values of β-endorphin in CSF were found to be less than 1% of the values for total opioid activity measured by the radioreceptor assay; therefore, these pro-opiomelanocortin peptides could not account for the higher levels of CSF opioid activity in anorectic patients.[44]

Unfortunately, most of the research studies on bulimia nervosa have examined only peripheral levels of opioids that do not predict central opioid activity. Waller et al.[45] noted that baseline plasma β-endorphin immunoreactivity in bulimic patients was significantly lower than in control subjects. Immunoreactivity also correlated inversely with the severity of bulimic symptoms.[45] In contrast, the plasma β-endorphin levels of a smaller group of bulimic subjects were higher than those of control subjects throughout a 5-hour study period and did not respond to glucose ingestion; analysis of variance of repeated measures revealed a significant overall difference between the bulimic subjects and the control subjects.[46]

NEUROMODULATORS

CRH

Believed to be the principal substance regulating pituitary corticotropin (ACTH) release, CRH can reduce starvation-induced feeding after central administration in the rat.[47] Adrenal demedullation partially diminishes this effect, indicating that the peripheral release of epinephrine may play a role in CRH-induced feeding inhibition.[48]

The mean concentration of immunoreactive CRH in the CSF of seven patients with anorexia nervosa was significantly higher than that of 11 subjects with cervical spondylosis.[49] CSF levels of CRH in patients with anorexia nervosa were significantly higher than those of normal control subjects but subsequently fell to normal when the patients were fed again. This fall paralleled the normalization of their plasma cortisol levels.[50] This is an interesting finding, since higher levels of CSF CRH have also been found in depressed patients in two studies[51,52] but not in another one.[53]

Vasopressin

Since patients with anorexia nervosa often have polyuria, the role of vasopressin in this disorder has been investigated. In four subjects with anorexia nervosa studied before correction of weight loss, the response of plasma arginine vasopressin to hypertonic saline was abnormal.[54] In one of these subjects, the plasma concentration of arginine vasopressin increased subnormally relative to the plasma sodium concentration, whereas in the other three it fluctuated erratically with no relation to plasma sodium concentrations. These defects persisted 3 to 4 weeks after recovery of body weight in the three patients studied.[54]

Cholecystokinin

Cholecystokinin is a 33-amino-acid polypeptide released from the intestine after eating. Its exogenous administration reduces food intake in rats, sheep, and monkeys, and its slow intravenous infusion reduces food intake in humans.[55–57] It appears that both the nucleus tractus solitarius and the paraventricular nucleus of the hypothalamus play important roles in the inhibitory action of systemic cholecystokinin on eating.[58,59]

A recent study[60] showed that both the total integrated plasma cholecystokinin response to a mixed-liquid meal and the postprandial peak plasma cholecystokinin levels were significantly lower in a group of bulimic women than in normal control subjects. Postprandial satiety was also significantly reduced in the bulimic women. In five bulimic patients the satiety response and the postprandial cholecystokinin response to eating increased significantly after an open trial of tricyclic antidepressants.[60]

METABOLIC AND MORPHOLOGIC BRAIN CHANGES

Investigators have also considered the role of altered energy metabolism and morphologic changes in the brains of anorectic patients. Positron emission tomography (PET) both during the anorectic state and after weight gain has been used to study regional cerebral glucose metabolism. Caudate metabolism was found to be significantly greater bilaterally during the anorectic state than after weight gain.[61] Since a greater percentage of neurons in the caudate nucleus of monkeys responds to the appearance of food in conditioned tasks than after unconditioned stimuli,[62] it has been hypothesized that caudate nuclei may play an important role in integrating environmental influences with cognitive processing to form the subject's individual motor response.[61] It has also been suggested that global brain hypermetabolism with accentuation in the caudate nuclei may correlate with the clinical observation of greater vigilance and performance in anorectic patients.[61]

Morphologic changes in the brain have been documented in patients with anorexia nervosa by transmission computerized tomography (CT).[63,64] More recently, Krieg et al.[65] showed that 82% of 50 patients with anorexia nervosa had enlarged outer CSF spaces that normalized after weight gain.

DRUG THERAPY OF EATING DISORDERS

Some of the neurochemical abnormalities observed in eating disorders may be particularly relevant to the mechanism of action of those psychotropic drugs which have been used successfully in the treatment of these disorders. In fact, although the mechanism of action of most psychotropic drugs is still unknown, in vitro and in vivo studies have shown that these drugs can affect many neurotransmitter and neuromodulator systems. To date, no drug has been consistently effective in the treatment of anorexia nervosa, including antipsychotic and anticonvulsant drugs.[66–68] The best studied and most promising psychotropic agents in bulimia nervosa are the tricyclic antidepressants (desipramine and imipramine) and the monoamine oxidase inhibitors (MAOIs) (phenelzine).

Antidepressants

Tricyclic antidepressants have been found to have numerous in vivo and in vitro effects on central neurotransmitters, including block of amine uptake and decrease in sensitivity of presynaptic (and postsynaptic) α_2-adrenergic receptors and in sensitivity of β-adrenergic receptors.[69] In a placebo-controlled study of anorectic patients, clomipramine was not associated with greater weight gain or improved eating behavior at 8-week, 1-year, and 4-year follow-ups,[70] and amitriptyline failed to differ from placebo in the treatment of 25 anorectic patients.[71] Double-blind, placebo-controlled studies in bulimic patients have shown that both imipramine[72] and desipramine[73] are significantly superior to placebo in reducing binge eating and purging behavior but that amitriptyline is not.[74]

Newer antidepressants have variable effects on neurotransmission: nomifensine is a potent blocker of norepinephrine uptake and has some effect on the uptake of dopamine; bupropion may be metabolized to amphetamines and also has some effect on uptake of dopamine; fluoxetine seems to be a relatively selective blocker of uptake of serotonin; and trazodone seems to have some serotonin-uptake-blocking effect.[69] The only controlled study on the effects of one of these newer antidepressants in the treatment of bulimia[75] showed that bupropion had a greater effect than placebo. Uncontrolled trials suggested the efficacy of nomifensine,[76] fluoxetine,[77] and trazodone.[78]

Some putative antidepressants (mianserin and cyproheptadine) have serotonin-receptor-blocking effects, although mianserin also appears to block the uptake of norepinephrine.[69] A double-blind study of 72 patients with anorexia nervosa[79] showed that cyproheptadine had a marginal effect on decreasing the number of days necessary to achieve a normal weight but increased treatment efficacy significantly in the nonbulimic subgroup of these patients when compared with amitriptyline and placebo. Mianserin did not prove superior to placebo in reducing bulimic symptoms in a controlled trial on patients with bulimia nervosa,[80] although the dose used was only 60 mg/day, which may be low.

MAOIs are antidepressant agents that inhibit an enzyme important for the inactivation of endogenous monoamines. No controlled studies have been reported on the use of these antidepressants in the treatment of anorexia nervosa. In an open study of only six anorectic patients,[81] treatment with isocarboxazid was associated with partial improvement in eating behavior. In bulimia nervosa, phenelzine was significantly superior to placebo in a double-blind trial with 50 women,[82] and isocarboxazid appeared to be more helpful on most eating behavior measures than placebo in a double-blind study of 24 bulimic patients.[83]

Lithium can inhibit the release of norepinephrine and dopamine and can increase the release of serotonin. A placebo-controlled trial with anorectic patients[84] showed that lithium may augment weight gain in patients treated with behavioral modification, but the results were not clinically meaningful. Preliminary findings on 13 patients with bulimia nervosa participating in an 8-week, double-blind, placebo-controlled trial of lithium[85] showed no difference between lithium and placebo.

Other Drugs

Oral naltrexone, a long-acting opiate antagonist, appeared to have a positive effect in six of eight patients in an uncontrolled trial.[86] In a 6-week controlled study of 16 subjects with bulimia nervosa,[87] high-dose oral naltrexone induced a significant reduction in frequency of binge eating or purging and low-dose oral naltrexone had no significant effects on these behaviors.

Fenfluramine, a sympathomimetic amine that increases central serotonin turnover, appeared to be effective in treating bulimia nervosa in a controlled study with desipramine.[88]

L-Tryptophan, which is a seotonin precursor, did not appear to be effective in treating bulimia in a double-blind, placebo-controlled trial.[89]

Clonidine, a preferential α_2-adrenergic receptor agonist, had no effect on eating behavior in a double-blind, placebo-controlled trial.[90]

DISCUSSION

Table 1 summarizes the results of animal studies on the effects of neurotransmitters and neuromodulators on feeding behavior. Tables 2 and 3 summarize the results of studies on neurochemical abnormalities in anorexia nervosa and bulimia nervosa, respectively.

Anorexia nervosa seems to be associated consistently with lower concentrations of norepinephrine and MHPG in the CSF and with a higher platelet α_2-adrenergic receptor number and greater sensitivity, suggesting a reduced norepinephrine ac-

TABLE 1

Summary of Animal Studies on the Effects of Neurotransmitter and Neuromodulator
Administration on Feeding Behavior

Item	Findings	Implications
Neurotransmitter system		
Noradrenergic and adrenergic	Application of α_2-adrenergic receptor agonist to the paraventricular nucleus produces hyperphagia; application of β-adrenergic receptor agonist to the perifornical region of the hypothalamus inhibits feeding (4, 5)	Stimulates or inhibits feeding, depending on the area of the brain
Serotonergic	Serotonin inhibits feeding by acting on the ventromedial hypothalamus (27)	Inhibits feeding
Dopaminergic	Central administration of low doses of dopamine stimulates but high doses inhibit feeding by acting on the perifornical hypothalamus (3, 37)	Stimulates or inhibits feeding, depending on the amount of neurotransmitter
Opioid	Administration of opioid antagonist (naloxone) decreases feeding following food deprivation (39)	Stimulates feeding
	Central administration of κ-opioid agonists enhances feeding (37)	Stimulates feeding
Neuromodulators		
CRH	Central administration reduces starvation-induced feeding (42)	Inhibits feeding
Cholecystokinin	Systemic administration inhibits feeding (55, 58, 59)	Inhibits feeding

TABLE 2
Summary of Studies on the Neurochemical Abnormalities in Anorexia Nervosa

Item	Findings	Implications
Neurotransmitter system		
Noradrenergic and adrenergic	Lower norepinephrine and MHPG in plasma, urine, and CSF (2, 12–19)	Less norepinephrine turnover
	Greater number of platelet α_2-adrenergic receptor binding sites (17, 22, 23)	Less norepinephrine activity
Serotonergic	Normal CSF 5-HIAA (21)	Normal serotonin turnover
	Lower CSF 5-HIAA (20)	Less serotonin turnover
Dopaminergic	Normal CSF HVA (19, 21)	Normal dopamine turnover
	Lower CSF HVA (20)	Less dopamine turnover
Opioid	Greater CSF total opioid activity measured by radio-receptor assay (43)	Greater opioid activity
	Normal CSF β-endorphin in extremely underweight patients (42)	Normal β-endorphin turnover
	Reduced CSF β-endorphin in extremely underweight patients (44)	Less β-endorphin turnover
Neuromodulators		
CRH	Higher CSF levels of immunoreactive CRH (49, 50)	Greater turnover
Vasopressin	Subnormal or erratic response to hypertonic saline (54)	Dysregulation in secretion

TABLE 3

Summary of Studies on the Neurochemical Abnormalities in Bulimia Nervosa

Item	Findings	Implications
Neurotransmitter system		
Noradrenergic and adrenergic	Higher number of platelet α_2-adrenergic receptor binding sites (22)	Less norepinephrine activity
	Reduced resting levels of plasma norepinephrine and blunting in the rise of plasma norepinephrine on standing (24, 25)	Less norepinephrine turnover
Serotonergic	Smaller probenecid-induced increases of CSF 5-HIAA in weight-restored bulimic anorectic patients than in nonbulimic anorectic patients (36)	Less serotonin turnover
	Absent rise in plasma L-tryptophan–large neutral amino acids in bulimic patients who did not feel satiated after a binge (34)	Less serotonin turnover
Neuromodulator		
Cholecystokinin	Reduced total integrated plasma response to eating and peak plasma response after eating (60)	Impaired secretion in response to a meal

tivity and turnover. The findings of the studies on serotonergic and dopaminergic activity in patients with anorexia nervosa are variable. Patients with anorexia nervosa also seem to have elevated CSF total opioid activity and elevated CSF levels of CRH, together with abnormalities in the secretion of vasopressin.

Bulimia nervosa is accompanied by lower than normal peripheral and, perhaps, central noradrenergic function with more than the usual number of platelet α_2-adrenergic receptor binding sites. Less serotonergic activity in bulimia nervosa is suggested by the finding that weight-restored anorectic patients with bulimia have lower probenecid-induced CSF levels of the serotonin metabolite 5-HIAA than weight-restored nonbulimic anorectic patients. Finally, patients with bulimia nervosa seem to have an impaired secretion of cholecystokinin in response to a meal.

These neurochemical abnormalities could have implications in the psychopharmacological approach to the treatment of eating disorders. In fact, psychotropic drugs are known to affect various neurotransmitter and neuromodulator systems and, although no drug has been consistently effective in the treatment of anorexia nervosa, numerous psychotropic drugs (particularly tricyclic antidepressants and MAOIs) appear to be promising agents in the treatment of bulimia nervosa.

It appears that patients with abnormal eating behavior have important changes in CNS neurotransmitter and neuromodulator systems that are known to modulate hypothalamic-pituitary function and may therefore underlie such physical manifestations of eating disorders as osteoporosis, infertility, and amenorrhea that are intimately connected with the neuroendocrine apparatus.[91]

Changes in hypothalamic-pituitary function may be secondary to the patient's dieting and caloric deprivation. Studies indicate that refeeding and weight gain ameliorate these neuroendocrine changes, suggesting that they are secondary either to weight loss or to caloric deprivation.[92] A longitudinal study of 24 inpatients with anorexia nervosa demonstrated a normalization of all the neuroendocrine abnormalities (higher cortisol secretion, cortisol nonsuppression in response to dexamethasone, and abnormal 24-hour plasma luteinizing hormone pattern) after 10% weight gain.[93] The authors concluded that the dysfunctions in the hypothalamic-pituitary-adrenal/gonadal axes of these patients have little specificity for this disease and are mainly a consequence of nutritional factors and starvation.[93] However, it is also possible that certain neuroendocrine abnormalities may be secondary to abnormal eating behaviors such as intermittent starvation or marked fluctuation in food intake.

Even if we assume that the neurochemical and neuroendocrine changes associated with eating disorders are secondary to dieting and caloric deprivation, it is possible that these changes may in turn perpetuate the pathological behavior and be responsible for a number of psychiatric symptoms.[94] In one study,[95] voluntarily starving subjects manifested many psychological symptoms seen in anorexia nervosa, including disturbed mood and altered eating behavior. In 64 patients with anorexia nervosa, body weight and β-hydroxybutyric acid, a good indicator of caloric restriction, were significantly correlated with mood and neurovegetative aspects of depression when the effects of diagnostic group and specific psychopathology were controlled.[96] These findings suggest that at least some depressive symptoms in eating disorders are related to low body weight, dieting, and starvation. Animal experiments have shown that starvation causes a decrease in noradrenaline turnover in the CNS of the rat,[97] and changes in central noradrenergic metabolism have been implicated in depression.[7]

Finally, it has been postulated that CNS changes may precede the onset of abnormal eating behavior,[98] and the neurochemical abnormalities observed in the patient with an eating disorder may therefore be primary.

It is apparent that further research on the neurochemistry of eating disorders is crucial to the understanding of the pathophysiology of these disorders and to the development of more effective pharmacological and cognitive-behavioral treatments.

REFERENCES

1. Garner DM, Garfinkel PE, O'Shaughnessy M: The validity of the distinction between bulimia with and without anorexia nervosa. Am J Psychiatry 1985; 142:581–587

2. Halmi KA, Dekirmenjian J, Davis JM, et al: Catecholamine metabolism in anorexia nervosa. Arch Gen Psychiatry 1978; 41:350–355

3. Leibowitz SF: Neurochemical systems in the hypothalamus: control of feeding and drinking behavior and water-electrolyte excretion, in Handbook of the Hypothalamus, vol 3, part A: Behavioral Studies of the Hypothalamus. Edited by Morgane PJ, Panksepp J. New York, Marcel Dekker, 1980

4. Leibowitz SF, Brown LL: Histochemical and pharmacological analysis of noradrenergic projections to the paraventricular hypothalamus in relation to feeding stimulation. Brain Res 1980; 201:289–314

5. Leibowitz SF, Brown LL: Histochemical and pharmacological analysis of catecholaminergic projections to the perifornical hypothalamus in relation to feeding inhibition. Brain Res 1980; 201:315–345

6. Charney DS, Heninger GR: Noradrenergic function and the mechanism of action of antianxiety treatment, I: the effect of long-term imipramine treatment. Arch Gen Psychiatry 1985; 42:473–481

7. Price LH, Charney DS, Rubin AL, et al: Alpha-2-adrenergic receptor function in depression. Arch Gen Psychiatry 1986; 43:849–858

8. Herzog DB, Norman DK: Subtyping eating disorders. Compr Psychiatry 1985; 4:375–380

9. Redmond DE, Hyang YH: New evidence for a locus coeruleus-norepinephrine connection with anxiety. Life Sci 1979; 25:2149–2162

10. Kaye WH, Gwirtsman HE, Lake CR, et al: Disturbances of norepinephrine metabolism

and alpha-2-adrenergic receptor activity in anorexia nervosa: relationship to nutritional state. Psychopharmacol Bull 1985; 21:419–423

11. Landsberg L, Young JB: Diet-induced changes in sympathoadrenal activity: implications for thermogenesis and obesity. Obesity and Metabolism 1981; 1:5–33

12. Gross HA, Lake CR, Ebert MH, et al: Catecholamine metabolism in primary anorexia nervosa. J Clin Endocrinol Metab 1979; 49:805–809

13. Van Loon GR: Abnormal catecholamine mechanisms in hypothalamic-pituitary disease. Metabolism 1980; 57(suppl 1):911–914

14. Abraham SF, Beumont PJV, Cobbin DM: Catecholamine metabolism and body weight in anorexia nervosa. Br J Psychiatry 1981; 138:244–247

15. Gerner RH, Gwirtsman HE: Abnormalities of dexamethasone suppression test and urinary MHPG in anorexia nervosa. Am J Psychiatry 1981; 138:650–653

16. Riederer P, Toifl K, Kruzik P: Excretion of biogenic amine metabolites in anorexia nervosa. Clin Chem Acta 1982; 123:27–32

17. Luck P, Mikhailidis DP, Dashwood MR, et al: Platelet hyperaggregability and increased alpha-adrenoceptor density in anorexia nervosa. J Clin Endocrinol Metab 1983; 57:911–914

18. Biederman J, Herzog DB, Rivinus TM, et al: Urinary MHPG in anorexia nervosa patients with and without a concomitant major depressive disorder. J Psychiatr Res 1984; 18:149–160

19. Johnston JL, Leiter LA, Burrow GN, et al: Excretion of urinary catecholamine metabolites in anorexia nervosa: effect of body composition and energy intake. Am J Clin Nutr 1984; 40:1001–1006

20. Kaye WH, Ebert MH, Raleigh M, et al: Abnormalities in CNS monoamine metabolism in anorexia nervosa. Arch Gen Psychiatry 1984; 41:350–355

21. Gerner RH, Cohen DJ, Fairbanks L, et al: CSF neurochemistry of women with anorexia nervosa and normal women. Am J Psychiatry 1984; 141:1441–1444

22. Heufelder A, Warnhoff M, Pirke KM: Platelet alpha-2-adrenoceptor and adenylate cyclase in patients with anorexia nervosa and bulimia. J Clin Endocrinol Metab 1985; 61:1053–1060

23. Mikhailidis DP, Barradas MA, De Souza V, et al: Adrenaline-induced hyperaggregability of platelets and enhanced thromboxane release in anorexia nervosa. Prostaglandins Leukot Med 1986; 24:27–34

24. Pirke KM, Pahl J, Schweiger U, et al: Metabolic and endocrine indices of starvation in bulimia: a comparison with anorexia nervosa. Psychiatry Res 1985; 15:33–39

25. Kaye WH, Gwirtsman HE, Lake CR: Noradrenergic disturbances in normal weight bulimia, in CME Syllabus and Scientific Proceedings in Summary Form, 139th Annual Meeting of the American Psychiatric Association. Washington, DC, APA, 1986

26. Jimerson DC, George DT, Kaye WH, et al: Norepinephrine regulation in bulimia, in Psychobiology of Bulimia. Edited by Hudson JI, Pope HG Jr. Washington, DC, American Psychiatric Press, 1987

27. Hoebel BG, Leibowitz SF: Brain monoamines in the modulation of self-stimulation, feeding and body weight. Res Publ Assoc Nerv Ment Dis 1981; 59:103–142

28. Heninger GR, Charney DS, Sternberg DE: Serotonergic function in depression: prolactin

response to intravenous tryptophan in depressed patients and healthy subjects. Arch Gen Psychiatry 1984; 41:398–404

29. Zohar J, Mueller EA, Insel TR, et al: Serotonergic responsivity in obsessive-compulsive disorder: comparison of patients and healthy controls. Arch Gen Psychiatry 1987; 44:946–951

30. Traber J, Davies MA, Dompert WU, et al: Brain serotonin receptors as a target for the putative anxiolytic TVXQ7821. Brain Res Bull 1984; 12:741–744

31. Weizman R, Carmi M, Tyano S, et al: High affinity [3H]imipramine binding and serotonin uptake to platelets of adolescent females suffering from anorexia nervosa. Life Sci 1986; 38:1235–1242

32. Zemishlany Z, Modai I, Apter A, et al: Serotonin (5-HT) uptake by blood platelets in anorexia nervosa. Acta Psychiatr Scand 1987; 75:127–130

33. Brewerton TD, George DT, Jimerson DC: Neuroendocrine response to L-tryptophan in bulimia, in CME Syllabus and Scientific Proceedings in Summary Form, 139th Annual Meeting of the American Psychiatric Association. Washington, DC, APA, 1986

34. Kaye WH, Gwirtsman HE, Brewerton TD, et al: Bingeing behavior and plasma amino acids: a possible involvement of brain serotonin in bulimia nervosa. Psychiatry Res 1988; 23:31–43

35. Wurtman RJ: Nutrients that modify brain function. Sci Am 1982; 246(4):50–59

36. Kaye WH, Ebert MH, Gwirtsman HE, et al: Differences in brain serotonergic metabolism between nonbulimic and bulimic patients with anorexia nervosa. Am J Psychiatry 1984; 141:1598–1601

37. Essatara MB, Morley JE, Levine AS, et al: The role of the endogenous opiates in zinc deficiency anorexia. Physiol Behav 1984; 32:475–478

38. Morley JE, Levine AS, Yim GKW, et al: Opioid modulation of appetite. Neurosci Biobehav Rev 1983; 7:281–305

39. Holtzman SG: Behavioral effects of separate and combined administration of naloxone and d-amphetamine. J Pharmacol Exp Ther 1974; 189:51–60

40. Morley JE, Parker S, Levine AS: Effect of butorphanol tartrate on food and water consumption in humans. Am J Clin Nutr 1985; 43:1175–1178

41. Cohen MR, Cohen RM, Pickar D, et al: Naloxone reduces food intake in humans. Psychosom Med 1985; 7:132–138

42. Gerner RH, Sharp B: CSF beta-endorphin-immunoreactivity in normal, schizophrenic, depressed, manic and anorexic subjects. Brain Res 1982; 237:244–247

43. Kaye WH, Pickar D, Naber D, et al: Cerebrospinal fluid opioid activity in anorexia nervosa. Am J Psychiatry 1982; 139:643–645

44. Kaye WH, Berrettini WH, Gwirtsman HE, et al: Reduced cerebrospinal fluid levels of immunoreactive pro-opiomelanocortin related peptides (including beta-endorphin) in anorexia nervosa. Life Sci 1987: 41:2147–2155

45. Waller DA, Kiser SR, Hardy BW, et al: Eating behavior and plasma beta-endorphin in bulimia. Am J Clin Nutr 1986; 44:20–23

46. Fullerton DT, Swift WJ, Getto CJ, et al: Plasma immunoreactive beta-endorphin in bulimics. Psychol Med 1986; 16:59–63

47. Morley JE, Levine AS: Corticotrophin releasing factor, grooming and ingestive behavior. Life Sci 1982; 31:1459–1464

48. Gosnell BA, Morley JE, Levine AS: A comparison of the effects of corticotropin releasing factor and sauvagine on food intake. Pharmacol Biochem Behav 1983; 19:771–775

49. Hotta M, Shibasaki T, Masuda A, et al: The responses of plasma adrenocorticotropin and cortisol to corticotropin-releasing hormone (CRH) and cerebrospinal fluid immunoreactive CRH in anorexia nervosa patients. J Clin Endocrinol Metab 1986; 62:319–324

50. Kaye WH, Gwirtsman HE, George DT, et al: Elevated cerebrospinal fluid levels of immunoreactive corticotropin-releasing hormone in anorexia nervosa: relation to state of nutrition, adrenal function, and intensity of depression. J Clin Endocrinol Metab 1987; 64:203–208

51. Nemeroff CB, Widerlov E, Bissette G, et al: Elevated concentrations of corticotropin releasing factor-like immunoreactivity in depressed patients. Science 1984; 226:1342–1343

52. Banki CM, Bissette G, Arato M, et al: CSF corticotropin-releasing factor-like immunoreactivity in depression and schizophrenia. Am J Psychiatry 1987; 144:873–877

53. Roy A, Pickar D, Paul S, et al: CSF corticotropin-releasing hormone in depressed patients and normal control subjects. Am J Psychiatry 1987; 144:641–645

54. Gold PW, Kaye W, Robertson GL, et al: Abnormalities in plasma and cerebrospinal-fluid arginine vasopressin in patients with anorexia nervosa. N Engl J Med 1983: 308:1117–1123

55. Gibbs J, Young RC, Smith GP: Cholecystokinin decreases food intake in rats. J Comp Physiol Psychol 1973; 84:488–495

56. Kissilef HR, Pi-Sunyer FX, Thornton J, et al: C-Terminal octapeptide of cholecystokinin decreases food intake in man. Am J Clin Nutr 1981; 34:154–160

57. Smith GP, Gibbs J: The satiety effect of cholecystokinin: recent progress and current problems. Ann NY Acad Sci 1985; 448: 417–423

58. van der Kooy D: Area postrema: site where cholecystokinin acts to decrease food intake. Brain Res 1984; 295:345–347

59. Crawley JN, Kiss JZ: Paraventricular nucleus lesions abolish the inhibition of feeding induced by systemic cholecystokinin. Peptides (Fayetteville) 1985; 6:927–935

60. Geracioti TD, Liddle RA: Impaired cholecystokinin secretion in bulimia nervosa. N Engl J Med 1988; 319:683–688

61. Herholz K, Krieg JC, Emrich HM, et al: Regional cerebral glucose metabolism in anorexia nervosa measured by positron emission tomography. Biol Psychiatry 1987; 22:43–51

62. Rolls ET: Feeding and reward, in The Neural Basis of Feeding and Reward. Edited by Hoebel BG, Novin D. Brunswick, Maine, Haer Institute, 1982

63. Sein P, Searson S, Nicol AR: Anorexia nervosa and pseudoatrophy of the brain (letter). Br J Psychiatry 1981; 139:257–258

64. Kohlmeyer K, Lehmkuhl G, Poutska F: Computed tomography of anorexia nervosa. Am J Neuroradiol 1983; 4:437–438

65. Krieg JC, Backmund H, Pirke KM: Endocrine, metabolic, and brain morphological

abnormalities in patients with eating disorders. Int J Eating Disorders 1986; 5:999–1005

66. Vandereycken W, Pierloot R: Pimozide combined with behavior therapy in the short-term treatment of anorexia nervosa: a double-blind placebo-controlled cross-over study. Acta Psychiatr Scand 1982; 60:446–451

67. Wermuth BM, Davis KL, Hollister LE, et al: Phenytoin treatment of the binge-eating syndrome. Am J Psychiatry 1977; 134:1249–1253

68. Kaplan AS, Garfinkel PE, Darby PL, et al: Carbamazepine in the treatment of bulimia. Am J Psychiatry 1983; 140:1225–1226

69. Baldessarini RJ: Chemotherapy in Psychiatry: Principles and Practice, revised ed. Cambridge, Harvard University Press, 1985, pp 130–234

70. Crisp AH, Lacey JH, Crutchfield M: Clomipramine and "drive" in people with anorexia nervosa: an inpatient study. Br J Psychiatry 1987; 150:355–358

71. Biederman J, Herzog DB, Rivinus TM, et al: Amitriptyline in the treatment of anorexia nervosa: a double-blind, placebo-controlled study. J Clin Psychopharmacol 1985; 5:10–16

72. Pope HG, Hudson JI, Jonas JM, et al: Bulimia treated with imipramine: a placebo-controlled double-blind study. Am J Psychiatry 1983; 140:554–558

73. Hughes PL, Wells LA, Cunningham LJ, et al: Treating bulimia with desipramine: a placebo-controlled double blind study. Arch Gen Psychiatry 1985; 43:182–186

74. Mitchell JE, Groat R: A placebo controlled double blind trial of amitriptyline in bulimia. J Clin Psychopharmacol 1984; 4:186–193

75. Horne RL, Ferguson JM, Pope HG, et al: Treatment of bulimia with bupropion: a multicenter controlled trial. J Clin Psychiatry 1988; 49:262–266

76. Pope HG Jr, Herridge PL, Hudson JI, et al: Treatment of bulimia with nomifensine. Am J Psychiatry 1986; 143:371–373

77. Freeman CPL, Hampson M: Fluoxetine as a treatment for bulimia nervosa. Int J Obesity 1987; 11(suppl 3):171–177

78. Pope HG, Hudson JI, Jonas JM: Antidepressant treatment of bulimia: preliminary experience and practical recommendations. J Clin Psychopharmacol 1983; 3:274–281

79. Halmi KA, Eckert E, LaDu TJ, et al: Anorexia nervosa: treatment efficacy of cyproheptadine and amitriptyline. Arch Gen Psychiatry 1986; 43:177–181

80. Sabine ET, Yonaie A, Forringten AT, et al: Bulimia nervosa: a placebo controlled double-blind therapeutic trial of mianserin. Br J Clin Pharmacol 1983; 15:195S–202S

81. Kennedy SH, Piran N, Garfinkel PE: Monoamine oxidase inhibitor therapy for anorexia nervosa and bulimia: a preliminary trial of isocarboxazid. J Clin Psychopharmacol 1985; 5:279–285

82. Walsh BT, Gladis M, Roose SP, et al: Phenelzine vs placebo in 50 patients with bulimia. Arch Gen Psychiatry 1988; 45:471–475

83. Kennedy S, Piran N, Garfinkel PE: Isocarboxazid in the treatment of bulimia (letter). Am J Psychiatry 1986; 143:1495–1496

84. Gross HA, Ebert MH, Faden VB, et al: A double-blind controlled trial of lithium carbonate in primary anorexia nervosa. J Clin Psychopharmacol 1981; 1:376–381

85. Hsu GLK, Clement L, Santhouse R: Treatment of bulimia with lithium: a preliminary study. Psychopharmacol Bull 1987; 23:45–48

86. Luby ED, Marrazzi MA, Kinzie J: Treatment of chronic anorexia nervosa with opiate blockade (letter). J Clin Psychopharmacol 1987; 7:52–53

87. Jonas JM, Gold MS: The use of opiate antagonists in treating bulimia: a study of low-dose versus high-dose naltrexone. Psychiatry Res 1988; 24:195–199

88. Blouin AG, Blouin JE, Perez EL, et al: Treatment of bulimia with fenfluramine and desipramine, in CME syllabus and Scientific Proceedings in Summary Form, 140th Annual Meeting of the American Psychiatric Association. Washington, DC, APA, 1987

89. Krahn D, Mitchell J: Use of L-tryptophan in treating bulimia (letter). Am J Psychiatry 1985; 142:1130

90. Casper RC, Schlemmer FR, Javaid JI: A placebo-controlled crossover study of oral clonidine in acute anorexia nervosa. Psychiatry Res 1987; 20:249–260

91. Copeland PM, Herzog DB: Menstrual disturbances in bulimia, in Psychobiology of Bulimia. Edited by Hudson JI, Pope HG Jr. Washington, DC, American Psychiatric Press, 1987

92. Wakeling A: Neurobiological aspects of feeding disorders. J Psychiatr Res 1985; 19:191–201

93. Fichter MM, Doerr P, Pirke KM, et al: Behavior, attitude, nutrition and endocrinology in anorexia nervosa. Acta Psychiatr Scand 1982; 66:429–444

94. Ploog D: The importance of physiologic, metabolic and endocrine studies for the understanding of anorexia nervosa, in The Psychobiology of Anorexia Nervosa. Edited by Pirke KM, Ploog D. Berlin, Springer-Verlag, 1984

95. Keys A, Brozek J, Henschel A, et al: The Biology of Human Starvation. Minneapolis, University of Minnesota, 1950

96. Laessle R, Schweiger U, Pirke KM: Depression as a correlate of starvation in patients with eating disorders. Biol Psychiatry 1988; 23:719–725

97. Schweiger U, Warnhoff M, Pirke KM: Brain tyrosine availability and the depression of central nervous norepinephrine turnover in acute and chronic starvation in adult male rats. Brain Res 1985; 335:207–212

98. Donohoe TP: Stress-induced anorexia: implications for anorexia nervosa. Life Sci 1984; 34:203–218

22

Depressive Disorders in Childhood IV. A Longitudinal Study of Comorbidity With and Risk for Anxiety Disorders

Maria Kovacs

University of Pittsburgh School of Medicine

Constantine Gatsonia

Harvard Medical School

Stana L. Paulauskas

Ohio State University, Columbus

Cheryl Richards

University of Pittsburgh School of Medicine

As part of a longitudinal nosologic study of major depressive disorder (MDD), dysthymic disorder (DD), and adjustment disorder with depressed mood (ADDM) in a school-age cohort, we examined the prevalence and clinical consequences of comorbid anxiety disorders. We also estimated the risk of a first anxiety disorder and examined its predictors. Of 104 cases, 41% had anxiety disorders in conjunction with their index depression, which was more likely with MDD and DD than with ADDM. The age-corrected risk of a first anxiety disorder was 0.47 up to age 18 years. Separation-anxiety disorder was the most frequent diagnosis of anxiety, followed by overanxious disorder of childhood. Among the MDD cases with comorbidity, the anxiety disorder preceded

Reprinted with permission from *Archives of General Psychiatry*, 1989, Vol.46, 776–782. Copyright © 1989 by the American Medical Association.

This investigation was supported by grant MH-33990 from the National Institute of Mental Health, Health and Human Services Administration, Bethesda, Md; support was also provided by the W.T. Grant Foundation.

Jack Paradise, MD, from the Children's Hospital in Pittsburgh, gave us access to the pediatric ambulatory clinic cases. Alka Indurkhya and Robert Hollis were responsible for the computer analyses, many individuals provided clinical and technical support throughout the years of this project, and Tammy J. Denk provided clerical assistance.

the depression about two thirds of the time and often persisted after the depression remitted. The effect of comorbid anxiety disorder on the length of index MDD depended on the presence of other clinical features, but it did not seem to affect the risk of subsequent MDD or the course of DD or ADDM. Concurrent maternal psychopathology and poor physical health increased the risk of anxiety disorder in the children, but a history of prior separation from parental figures did not seem to have an effect.

Depressive disorders and anxiety disorders frequently occur contemporaneously.[1-5] This fact and the symtomatic overlap between these two types of conditions have posed dilemmas for psychiatric nosology and clinical management.

The classification problem has revolved around the question of whether the two disorders are separate from each other.[4-7] When they are viewed as categorically distinct, both are diagnosed even when they occur simultaneously. Alternatively, if they are considered as phases of one underlying psychopathologic dimension, the single diagnosis at any point in time reflects the observed "ratio of anxiety to depressive symptoms."[7] The Dimensional approach to these conditions is also exemplified by Bowlby's[8,9] formulation that separation-anxiety disorder merging into clinical depression represents pathologic forms of the sequence of response to disrupted attachment bonds.

In contrast to the nosologic debates that have surrounded this issue in adult psychiatry, relatively little attention has been paid to the theoretical aspects of how to classify comorbid depression and anxiety among children.[10] Instead, various practical solutions have been proposed. One approach has been to create a new diagnostic category such as "phobic depression" for some forms of coexisting anxiety and despondency.[2] According to another approach, anxiety is an age-specific feature of childhood depression and should not be separately diagnosed.[11,12] The most recent trend has been to assign a particular case all the diagnoses that are warranted, resulting in estimates that about 40% to 75% of children and adolescents with depressive disorders also qualify for a diagnosis of some type of anxiety disorder.[3,13,14]

The clinical issues raised by the presence of both syndromes have involved questions about the type and focus of treatment and whether single vs dual diagnoses carry differential prognostic information. Research on adults has documented that comorbidity influences the choice of pharmacotherapy[4-6,15,16] and that the rate of recovery among adults with uncomplicated depression seems to be better than recovery among those with anxiety disorders or mixed states.[15,17,18] However, there is no comparable body of information on depressed juveniles. It is not known, for example, whether an anxiety disorder complicates the course of a depressive disorder in children.

In our article, we address the topic of comorbid depressive and anxiety disorders using data on a sample of depressed children who have been participating in a longitudinal nosologic investigation. The comorbidity of interest was approached from the categorical stance to make it possible to examine the following issues: (1) the prevalence and correlates of comorbid anxiety disorders among clinically referred depressed children: (2) the time-dependent risk of anxiety disorder in this population; (3) the chronology of the anxiety disorder with respect to the onset of the depression; (4) the effect of comorbid anxiety on recovery from a depression and on the risk of its recurrence; and, finally (5) whether maternal characteristics and historic variables, which reflect parental unavailability,[8,9] contribute to anxiety and depressive disorders developing among the children. Information about these issues should shed light on the implications of comorbid depression and anxiety in juvenile populations.

SUBJECTS AND METHODS

Design

Our study was a longitudinal investigation with multiple assessments. Cases were recruited through the child psychiatry clinic of the University of Pittsburgh (Pa) and the general medical clinic of the Children's Hospital of Pittsburgh; a few cases were made available to us through other avenues. The sites contributed, respectively, 82%, 16%, and 2% of the sample described in this article. To be considered for the study, the children had to meet the following demographic criteria: 8 to 13 years old, not mentally retarded, no major systemic medical illness, ambulatory psychiatric and medical status, lives with parent(s) or legal guardian(s), and resides within commuting distance of greater Pittsburgh. Written consents were obtained from parent(s) and children for the intake interview, an initial 5-year follow-up period, and then for a second 5-year follow-up.

The study includes a depressed group (N = 142), only a portion of whom are described in our article for technical reasons, and a nondepressed psychiatric comparison group (N = 49), relatively few of whom had anxiety disorders. As described elsewhere,[19–21] subjects were recruited in two phases, and their suitability for the study was determined by our research staff. The protocol stipulated three postintake assessments in the first study year and no more than two interviews every year thereafter. At each assessment, families were provided a monetary reimbursement.

Psychiatric Evaluations and Diagnosis

At each clinical assessment, the parent was first interviewed alone about the child, then the child was interviewed separately by the same clinician. These evaluations were conducted with the semistructured, symptom-oriented Interview

Schedule for Children and its addenda. The interviewers were mental-health professionals who were fully affiliated with this project and were trained in individually supervised interviews.

Diagnosis was based on the clinician's final single ratings of each symptom based on data supplied by both parent and child. The reliability of these ratings has been reported.[22] The assessments were routinely reviewed by the clinicians, and the diagnoses were consensually assigned. All diagnoses conformed to the *DSM-III* criteria,[23] with the further provision that at least three pertinent symptoms be present for a diagnosis of adjustment disorder.

Irrespective of the type of depressive disorder, if a child's history and presentation indicated one or more anxiety disorders, all pertinent diagnoses were assigned. We have illustrated elsewhere our approach to diagnosing concurrent disorders that had overlapping and similar symptoms.[19,21]

Definition of Onset and Recovery From a Disorder

For the chronology of disorders, parental report was relied on most heavily. The onset of a disorder was dated to the time when, according to all indicators, the child had the full syndromatic picture, not just prodromal or subclinical symptoms. Offset, or recovery, was operationally defined as the absence of the relevant symptoms or, at most, one remaining clinically significant symptom, and few, if any, subclinical symptoms of the pertinent syndrome and the maintenance of the foregoing state for at least a 2-month interval. If the subject recovered from an episode but was later found to have become symptomatic in less than 2 months, he or she was viewed as still in the previous episode of illness. If a major depressive disorder (MDD) was superimposed on a dysthymic disorder (DD), we "offset" the MDD when the child no longer had those depressive symptoms by virtue of which he or she initially met criteria for the major depression, although the baseline DD could be (and often was) present. Similar rules were used if a separation-anxiety disorder was superimposed on an overanxious disorder.

If an onset or offset date could not be readily determined, a calendar interval was delimited, during which the problems emerged or remitted, respectively (e.g., "between Christmas and Easter"). The date in question was then operationally set at the midpoint of that interval. Onset and offset dates were also reviewed and consensually assigned by the research clinicians. All available information was utilized to assure maximum precision in the dating of disorders.

Developmental and Sociodemographic Data Ascertainment

The structured Intake General Information Sheet was used with the parents to gather demographic information as well as data on separations and parental hospitalizations throughout the child's development. At subsequent evaluations, this sheet was replaced by the Follow-up General Information Sheet, which duplicated the items of the former sheet, except that the data covered only the time since the last research contact, including interim maternal health and hospitalizations. The Follow-up General Information Sheet therefore provided a continuous record of non-clinical events over the length of the study.

The Assessment of Parental Psychopathologic Symptoms

Parental depression and anxiety were rated at each interview via the 24-item Hamilton Psychiatric Rating Scale for Depression (HAMD)[24,25] and the 14-item Hamilton Psychiatric Rating Scale for Anxiety (HAM-A).[25,26] These evaluations were done by a clinician independently of and "blinded" to the evaluation of the child, except in the case of personnel shortage. On the basis of an observer independently completing the scales, interrater reliability was high; the intraclass correlation coefficient was .98 for the HAM-D (n = 58) and was .96 (n = 57) for the HAM-A.

Parents also completed, independently of the rest of the protocol, the 21-item Beck Depression Inventory (BDI) and the 90-item Symptom Checklist (SCL-90). The BDI total score reflects the severity of depressive symptoms[27]; the SCL-90 quantifies overall psychopathology.[25,28] On each of the four scales described above, the higher the score, the more severe the symptomatology that is being assessed.

Statistical Methods

Cross-classified categorical data were analyzed via χ^2 tests; Yates' correction was used if the expected cell frequency was less than 5. Since the latter is often too conservative, Fisher's Exact Test was also used for some 2 × 2 tables.[29] Odds ratios were calculated for 2 × 2 tables; for a table with entries (a, b, c, d), the odds ratio equals ad/bc. Univariate and step-wise multivariate logistic-regression analyses were used to assess the effects of continuous or categorical covariates on categorical responses. Between-group differences on continuous variables were examined via the Kruskal-Wallis nonparametric test or the *t* test. To account for the effects of multiple, simultaneous comparisons, Bonferroni's inequality was used[30]; for sets of comparisons, the overall α was held at .05, thereby making the *P* level required for individual contrasts more stringent.

Recovery from the index episode of depressive disorder and the risk of a subsequent episode were examined using techniques from survival analysis.[31,32] These techniques can accommodate the fact that, in a longitudinal study, some subjects drop out before the outcome of interest occurs and others may not have experienced the outcome by the last observation point.

The impact of covariates on "time to criterion" (recovery or recurrence) was assessed using Cox's[33] regression analysis, which yields an estimate of the coefficient and its SE for each covariate. A positive coefficient indicates that higher values of the covariate are associated with an increased hazard rate and, consequently, with a shorter time to criterion. Computations were done via the BMDP statistical package.[34]

Cohort

The first 104 consecutive patients of the depressed cohort, on whom this article is based, entered the study between April 1978 and October 1984. Clinical follow-up interviews up to January 8, 1987, were used in the analyses. Up to that time, the mean follow-up interval for this group was 3 years (range, 0 to 8 years), including 11 patients who were dropouts (follow-up range, 0 to 44 months) and 7 who had been unavailable for follow-up because they moved (follow-up range, 2 to 36 months).

The index depression, which was diagnoses at study entry or during the first 6 months of diagnostic verification, was used for initial case classification. It was distributed as follows: 46 children had MDD, 23 had DD, 16 had both an MDD and a concurrent DD or "double depression" (MDD/DD), and 19 children had adjustment disorder with depressed mood (ADDM).

The demographic characteristics of the 104 children were similar to those reported for a smaller portion of our sample.[19,20] The sex distribution was even (52 boys and 52 girls); the mean age at study entry was 11.2 years (SD, 1.7 years; range, 8.0 to 13.9 years); and the ethnic distribution was 58% white, 38% black, 4% biracial, and 1% other. Socioeconomic status according to Hollingshead's Two Factor Index of Social Position (unpublished copyrighted manuscript, 1957) was as follows: category I (highest), 5%; category II, 8%; category III, 22%; category IV, 36%; and category V, 30%; thus suggesting that, compared with the general population, the lowest socioeconomic status was overrepresented. At study entry, 26% of these children lived with both biologic parents, but altogether 49% lived in two-parent households (biologic and stepparent). The average household had 4 persons (range, 2 to 11 persons), and 57% of the heads-of-household were gainfully employed.

At study intake, one third of the sample had a history of outpatient mental health treatment; 6% had had pharmacotherapy; and 4% had been hospitalized in the past for psychiatric reasons. Subsequently, 69% (72/104) of the patients received psychosocial treatment during the index episode of depression (63% of the MDD cases, 75% of the MDD/DD cases, 83% of the DD cases, and 63% of the ADDM cases). The durations, formats, and orientations of the interventions were highly variable. Pharmacotherapy during the index depression was reported for 7 MDD cases (6.7% of the sample), all of whom received tricyclic antidepressants (for 1 case, this occurred before the study intake). Two children with DD received minor tranquilizers (before intake) during their dysthymia. On the basis of the information, the dosages and durations of the pharmacotherapy were diverse.

RESULTS

Prevalence of Anxiety Disorders

Comorbid Anxiety Disorders. During the index episodes of depression, 43 (41%) of the 104 children had anxiety disorders (Table 1), which accounted for a large portion of the rate of overall psychiatric comorbidity at intake. Three of the cases with comorbid anxiety also had a prior episode of anxiety disorder. The most frequent comorbid anxiety (32 instances) was separation-anxiety disorder, followed by overanxious disorder of childhood (17 instances). Panic disorder and other forms of anxiety were infrequent (Table 2)

Anxiety Disorders Anytime During the Study. Examination of the postintake clinical course revealed that there were 5 cases who had anxiety disorders during their index depression and subsequent new episodes of anxiety. There were 3 children who were free of anxiety during their index depressions, but who developed an anxiety disorder later. Therefore, a total of 46 cases (44%) had at least one episode of anxiety disorder any time during study observation.

Age-Dependent Risk of Anxiety Disorder. The foregoing prevalence figures do not take into consideration that, because the lengths of observation varied for the cases, they had been at risk for the outcome of interest for unequal time periods, and there were dropouts from the study before the possible occurrence of the outcome of interest. Both of these factors were accounted for by estimating the cumulative probability of the first episode of anxiety disorder developing as a function of age using the Kaplan-Meier estimator.[32] As shown in Figure 1, the lifetime risk of an anxiety disorder developing up to age 18 years is .47 in this cohort, with a cluster of onsets between ages 9 to 11 years. Thus, among children with depression, if an anxiety disorder develops, it is likely to do so relatively early, certainly by age 12 years.

Correlates of Comorbid Anxiety Disorders

Demographics. The 43 children with comorbid anxiety disorders did not differ from the rest of the sample in regard to sex distribution ($\chi^2 = 0.36$, $df = 1$) and socioeconomic status ($\chi^2 = 2.51$, $df = 4$). However, childen who had comorbid anxiety disorders were younger when they became depressed (mean, 9.6 years; SD, 1.8 years) as compared with the age at onset of depression for the rest of the sample (mean, 10.5 years; SD, 1.9 years; $t = 2.36$, $df = 102$, $P = .02$). White children were three times more likely to have comorbid anxiety disorders than black children

TABLE 1
Psychiatric Comorbidity in Index Depressive Disorders*

Index Depressive Disorder	Proportion of Cases With Comorbid Disorders			
	Anxiety Disorders†			Any Disorder
	1	≥2	Any	
Major depressive disorder (n = 46)	.35	.13	.48 (22)	.83 (38)
Major depressive and dysthymic disorder (n = 16)	.31	.19	.50 (8)	.75 (12)
Dysthymic disorder (n = 23)	.22	.17	.39 (9)	.83 (19)
Adjustment disorder with depressed mood (n = 19)	.16	.05	.21 (4)	.58 (11)
Total sample (n = 104)	.28 (29)	.13 (14)	.41 (43)	.77 (80)

*Excluding *DSM-III* "V"-codes; parenthetic entries are frequencies.
†If a subject had more than one type of anxiety disorder in index depression, each was tallied; if a subject had multiple episodes of same anxiety disorder, that anxiety disorder was tallied only once.

TABLE 2
Types of Comorbid Anxiety Disorders in Index Depressive Disorders*

Anxiety Disorders	Depressive Disorders†				Total Sample (N = 104)
	MDD (n = 46)	MDD/DD (n = 16)	DD (n = 23)	ADDM (n = 19)	
Separation-anxiety disorder	.41	.31	.30	.05	.31 (32)
Overanxious disorder	.13	.31	.17	.11	.16 (17)
Phobic disorder	. . .	. . .	. . .	.05	.01 (1)
Obsessive-compulsive disorder	. . .	. . .	.04	.05	.02 (2)
Panic disorder	. . .	. . .	.09	. . .	.02 (2)
Atypical disorder	.04	. . .	. . .	. . .	.02 (2)
Cases with any anxiety disorder‡	.48 (22)	.50 (8)	.39 (9)	.21 (4)	.41 (43)

*Data given in proportions. If a subject had more than one type of anxiety disorder in index depression, each was tallied; if a subject had multiple episodes of the same anxiety disorder, that anxiety disorder was tallied only once; parenthetical entries are frequencies.

†MDD indicates major depressive disorder; DD, dysthymic disorder; and ADDM, adjustment disorder with depressed mood.

‡Because a subject could have more than one type of anxiety disorder, the sums of proportions with anxiety per index depression exceed the number of cases with anxiety disorder.

(odds ratio $= 3.1$, $\chi^2 = 6.6$, $df = 1$, $P = .01$). The foregoing comparisons were also carried out separately for the probands with major affective disorders (i.e., excluding the adjustment disorders), yielding similar results.

Type of Depression. Major affective disorder (major depression or dysthymia) as compared with ADDM was three times more likely to be associated with comorbid anxiety (odds ratio $= 3.2$, $\chi^2 = 3.95$, $df = 1$, $P < .05$). This trend parallels the finding that the major affective disorders had a higher rate of any psychiatric comorbidity than did ADDM (odds ratio $= 3.1$, Fisher's Exact Test $P = .038$). The small number of ADDM cases with comorbid anxiety disorders precluded a detailed analysis of how the types of anxiety may be related to the three types of depression.

The Role of Maternal Psychopathology and Health

We used two time frames to investigate the relationship of contemporaneous maternal psychopathology and physical health to anxiety in the offspring, namely, the entire observation period and only the period of the index episode of depression. The findings were similar for both sets of analyses; therefore, only the results for the entire observation period are reported.

For each mother, the maximum and the median of each scale of psychopathology (SCL-90, BDI, HAM-D, and HAM-A) were selected over the follow-up. These

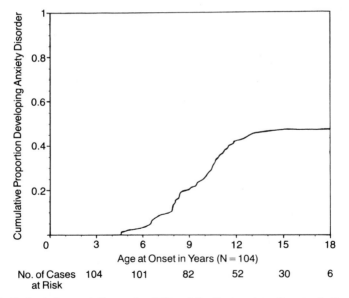

Figure 1. Estimated cumulative probanbility of the first anxiety disorder in the cohort as a function of age.

summary indexes capture the variables' extreme values and centers of distribution, respectively. Assessment data obtained repeatedly on the physical health of the mothers, quantified each time from 1 (excellent) to 4 (poor) on the Intake General Information Sheet and the Follow-up General Information Sheet item, were averaged for each case. Similarly, the number of medical hospitalizations during the study was summarized for each mother as 0 (none), 1 (one), and 2 (two or more).

The general finding was that higher levels of maternal psychopathology, and, to a lesser degree, poor maternal health, were associated with a greater likelihood of anxiety disorder in the offspring. The results of the nonparametric univariate comparisons are presented in Table 3. The *P* values for all maternal psychopathology indexes were significant even after accounting for multiple comparisons.[30]

With multivariate logistic regression, several models were also examined in which measurements of maternal psychopathology and health were the independent variables, while controlling for possible confounders such as age at intake, sex, and

TABLE 3

Comparisons of Maternal Characteristics for Children Grouped According to Whether They Had an Anxiety Disorder Anytime During Follow-up

	Rank Sum†	
Maternal Variable*	**Cases With No Anxiety (n = 58)/ Cases With Anxiety (n = 46)**	**P‡**
BDI total score		
Maximum	2133.5/2717.5	.0017
Median	2159.5/2691.5	.0031
SCL-90 total score		
Maximum	2155.0/2696.0	.0029
Median	2174.5/2676.5	.0044
HAM-D total score		
Maximum	2155.5/2695.5	.0029
Median	2126.6/2724.5	.0014
HAM-A total score		
Maximum	2138.5/2712.5	.0019
Median	2182.0/2669.0	.0052
Maternal physical health, average rating	2288.0/2563.0	.0414
Maternal medical hospitalization of 0, 1, or 2 or more	2409.0/2442.0	.2112

*BDI indicates Beck Depression Inventory; SCL-90, 90-item Symptom Checklist; HAM-D, 24-item Hamilton Psychiatric Rating Scale for Depression; and HAM-A, 14-item Hamilton Psychiatric Rating Scale for Anxiety.

†Ranks are computed on the pooled set of measurements and are then separately summed for the two groups. Higher ranks indicate higher values on the corresponding maternal variable.

‡Using the Kruskal-Wallis method.

socioeconomic status. The results reinforce those derived from the univariate analyses. For example, when the maximum HAM-D score was the only independent variable in the model, its coefficient was .084 (SE = .026, P = .0005). When sex, age at intake, and socioeconomic status were also entered into the model (as possible confounders), the coefficient of the maximum HAM-D score did not change appreciably (coefficient = .087, SE = .027, P = .0005), while only age at intake approached significance as a further predictor of anxiety (for age in months, coefficient = −.024, SE = .012, P = .04). When each of the other maternal psychopathology scales was used instead of the maximum HAM-D, the results were similar, which was not unexpected because the various scales were highly intercorrelated. Combinations of two or more of these scores as independent variables did not provide models with appreciably better predictive ability.

Maternal physical health was also an important predictor of anxiety disorder in the offspring. In a logistic-regression model with maternal physical health and maternal hospitalizations as independent variables and sex, age at intake, and socioeconomic status as covariates, the significant predictors were maternal physical health (coefficient = .97, SE = .49, P = .04) and age at intake (coefficient = −.028, SE = .012, P = .01). However, when the maximum HAM-D score was added to the model, maternal physical health was no longer a significant predictor (new coefficient = .66, SE = .53, P = .21).

The Chronology of Comorbid Anxiety Disorders

The timing of the comorbid anxiety disorders with respect to the onset of the index depressions is given in Table 4. If the onsets (or offsets) of the anxiety and depressive disorders occurred within 2 months of each other, they were considered as contemporaneous to provide for a margin of error in those data.

Among the 30 cases that had major depression and comorbid anxiety (irrespective of whether dysthymia was present), the anxiety disorders predated the major depression about two thirds of the time, while they emerged together with or secondary to MDD in the remaining one third of the cases. However, among the nine cases with DD and comorbid anxiety, only for two did the anxiety disorder start before the DD. It was six times more likely for the anxiety disorder to have predated the MDD than the DD (odds ratio = 6, Fisher's Exact Test P = .036).

Recovery from the comorbid anxiety disorders did not parallel recovery from the depressions (Table 4). When comorbid anxiety disorders occurred with major depression, the odds were roughly even that the anxiety disorder would or would not (12 vs 17) persist after the MDD remitted. Probably partly as a function of the protracted course of DD, the anxiety disorder persisted longer than the dysthymia for only about one fourth of the cases (odds ratio = 0.40, Fisher's Exact Test P = .26).

TABLE 4

Patterns of Onset and Recovery of Comorbid Anxiety Disorders in
Index Depressive Disorders*

Index Depressive Disorder With Anxiety Comorbidity	Onset of Anxiety Disorder		Recovery From Anxiety Disorder	
	Predates Onset of Depression	Follows Onset of Depression	Before or With Recovery From Depression	After Recovery From Depression
Major depressive disorder (n=30)	19	11	17†	12†
Dysthymic disorder (n=9)	2	7	7	2

*Data given in frequencies. If there was more than one anxiety disorder in index depression, only the chronologically earlier one was tallied. All cases of major depressive disorders with comorbidity were tallied in the major depressive group, irrespective of whether there was a concurrent dysthymia. Index cases of adjustment disorder with depressed mood are not shown because only four had comorbid anxiety disorders.

†One case was not tallied because neither disorder had yet remitted.

The Effect of Comorbid Anxiety Disorders on the Course of the Depressions

We examined whether comorbid anxiety disorders affected the duration of the index depressive episodes. For cases with major depression, we also examined the impact of comorbid anxiety disorders on the length of time between recovery from the index MDD and the next episode of MDD. Demographic and clinical factors that have[19] or could have an impact on illness duration served as covariates, including age at onset of depression, sex, socioeconomic status, whether the depression in question was primary (that is, no other psychiatric illness temporally preceded it), and whether the patient received psychotropic medication or psychotherapy during the index depression. For MDD cases, a concurrent dysthymia (WDD) was also a covariate.

For each type of index depression, separate univariate Cox regression analyses were carried out first, and then alternative multivariate models were examined. Only up to five variables (including interactions) were used in a model because of the small sample sizes.

MDD. With univariate analyses, comorbid anxiety disorders did not emerge as affecting the length of the index episode of MDD. Only three variables reached significance: having a primary depression, having had medication, and the presence of WDD ($P = .0038$, $P = .0002$, and $P = .0373$, respectively). Having received medication was associated with a longer episode, but this covariate was not further pursued because only 7 of 62 patients had been so treated.

The effect of comorbid anxiety disorders on MDD duration became important in the multivariate models. The variables of WDD, primary depressive illness, comorbid anxiety disorders, and the interaction of comorbid anxiety disorders-by-WDD were all significant in the regression analyses, whereas all other interactions, as well as age, sex, socioeconomic status, and having received psychotherapy, failed to make a notable contribution. The most parsimonious model is presented in Table 5. The assumption of proportional hazards (necessary for the Cox regression analysis) was checked via graphical techniques and was found to be approximately true.

The regression coefficients in Table 5 should be interpreted in terms of their directions rather than by their numeric values. Additionally, because we used a stringent definition of primary vs secondary depressive disorders, it was not possible for a case to have both primary major depression and a preexisting DD. Therefore, it was necessary to include in the model both primary depressive illness and WDD and their interactions with comorbid anxiety disorders (despite that for one of these interactions, $P = .14$).

The results in Table 5 suggest that the possible effects of comorbid anxiety on the length of the episode of major depression depend on whether the major depression is primary and on whether the child has an underlying DD. There are three groups of children with MDD: (1) those with primary MDD (primary = 1, WDD = 0); (2)

TABLE 5

Effect of Comorbid Anxiety Disorder and Covariates on Time to Recovery From Major Depressive Disorder*

Covariate	Coefficient	SE	P
Comorbid anxiety disorder			
(0 = no, 1 = yes)	− 0.78	0.42	.07
Primary MDD (0 = no, 1 = yes)	− 1.40	0.47	.003
Underlying dysthymic disorder			
(WDD, 0 = no, 1 = yes)	− 0.54	0.48	.26
Comorbid anxiety disorder by			
WDD interaction	2.25	0.72	.002
Comorbid anxiety disorder by			
primary MDD interaction	0.98	0.65	.14

*Results were obtained using multivariate Cox regression analysis (n = 62). MDD indicates major depressive disorder. WDD indicates MDD with concurrent dysthymia.

those with secondary MDD and no dysthymia (primary = 0, WDD = 0); and (3) those with secondary MDD and also dysthymia (primary = 0, WDD = 1).

The presence of comorbid anxiety had a negligible effect on the length of the index MDD episode for the first group of children; it tended to lengthen the episode of MDD for the third group. To illustrate the effect of comorbid anxiety, we estimated that in group 2, the median depressive episode length in the presence of anxiety was 9.8 months (SE = 1.5) vs 5.2 months (SE = 2.8) when there was no anxiety. The effect in group 3 was in the opposite direction—the median MDD episode for cases with anxiety was 3.6 months (SE = 1.0) vs 9.67 months (SE = 2.0) for those without anxiety. These median estimates and their SEs should be interpreted cautiously in view of the small sizes of the subgroups.

For cases that recovered from their index major depressive episodes (n = 51), there was some indication that comorbid anxiety in the index depression predicted a longer interval before the next MDD (comorbid anxiety disorder coefficient = −.8, SE = .47, P = .083). When age at intake was included in the model, it emerged as a significant covariate (for age in months, coefficient = .028, SE = .013, P = .02), suggesting that older children would go into a new episode somewhat faster than younger ones. However, WDD, primary major depression, and their interaction with comorbid anxiety disorders had no apparent effect.

DD and ADDM. The foregoing results did not, in general, hold for the diagnosis of DD (n = 39). Comorbid anxiety did not seem to affect the length of dysthymia, either by itself or in conjunction with covariates. The P value for comorbid anxiety disorder exceeded .6 in all the regressions we examined.

Similar findings were obtained when the length of ADDM was examined (n = 19). Neither comorbid anxiety nor its interactions with other covariates played a role in the duration of the index episodes of ADDM. However, both the DD and the ADDM sample sizes were small, and, thus, the statistical power is low.

Life Events During Development and Anxiety Disorders

To test the hypothesis that a history of separation from caretakers increases the likelihood of anxiety disorders, five variables were used, namely, separation from mother, separation from father, major medical hospitalization of the child, psychiatric hospitalization of the mother, and psychiatric hospitalization of the father. These events occurred before study entry, as coded on the Intake General Information Sheet (recorded as having or not having taken place during successive developmental stages). Information on each variable was summarized (as "yes" and "no") for the period spanning the child's birth to 8 years of age. Alternately, each covariate was divided into two categories that reflected the history up to age 4 years and from age 5 years onward, respectively. However, the results were similar for both methods of categorization.

When all 104 cases were used, 2×2 cross-tabulations of each index of separation by the presence of anxiety disorder in the proband yielded nothing of note. For example, the largest χ^2 value (for history of separation from mother) was only 2.17 ($df = 1$, $P = .14$). In multivariate logistic-regression analyses that used demographic covariates (e.g., sex, socioeconomic status), as well as interactions (e.g., sex of child by history of separation from the mother), none of the variables reflecting separation proved to be a predictor of an anxiety disorder in the proband during study observation. Similar results were obtained when the children were grouped by type of index depressive disorder.

COMMENT

Using data on children with depressive disorders who had been studied prospectively, we found that contemporaneous anxiety disorders occur at a high rate and that the anxiety disorders develop relatively early. The effect of anxiety disorder on recovery from the index depression depends on the type of depression and other clinical features. In most instances of MDD, the contemporaneous anxiety disorder antedated the onset of the MDD, and the anxiety disorder often persisted beyond the episode of depression. Maternal psychopathology and poor physical health were more prevalent in the subset of depressed cases with anxiety disorder than in the rest of the depressed sample, but historic variables did not explain the presence of anxiety disorders in this cohort.

Prevalence Rates

The implications of psychiatric comorbidity depend partly on the rate at which the diagnoses of interest co-occur. According to our findings, cross-sectional rates of anxiety disorders ranged between 41% and 44% in this depressed sample. These figures are in line with both earlier and more recent reports on the high frequency of comorbid anxiety among depressed children, adolescents, and young adults.[2,3,10,13,14,35,36]

An anxiety disorder is the most prevalent comorbid condition among depressed youths as compared with conduct disorder, which is the second most common comorbid diagnosis, occurring among less then 20% of the patients.[21] In all likelihood, the prevalence of anxiety disorder among depressed children also exceeds the base rate of diagnosable anxiety in the general pediatric population (which has yet to be verified[37]). What remains to be explored is whether the high rate of concurrent anxiety is specific to the affective disorders or if it accompanies other major juvenile psychopathology as well.

Developmental Considerations

Aspects of our study are also relevant to developmental psychopathology. First, it seems that among depressed juveniles, anxiety disorders declare themselves before adolescence since cross-sectional rates of anxiety disorder, determined at earlier points during the subject's development, did not appreciably differ from the age-corrected cumulative risk, computed up to age 18 years (.47). Second, separation-anxiety disorder, which was the most frequent diagnosis in this sphere, is typically seen before adolescence.[38]

The association in this population between earlier age and anxiety-depression comorbidity is further supported by the finding that comorbidity in the proband was related to maternal dysfunction. During younger ages, while a child is more dependent on maternal care, a pattern of maternal unavailability and inconsistency (as suggested by psychological problems and poor physical health), may threaten the child's sense of stable attachment and create anxiety and depression.[8,9] The finding that among two thirds of the cases of major depression with anxiety, the anxiety preceded the onset of the depression also offers some support for Bowlby's theory of the chronology of these conditions.[8,9] Should our results be confirmed by others, the implications would be that efforts at prevention or early remediation of depressive disorders in juveniles should take into account maternal functioning.

Nosologic and Clinical Issues

A nosologic issue, which has been long debated in adult psychiatry, is whether depression and anxiety are categorically distinct.[4-7] Evidence in support of this position derives from some studies of clinical course, differential pharmacologic response, and familial aggregation. But there are other clinical studies of adult probands and psychologic[8,9] and neurophysiologic[39] theories to support the contention that depression and anxiety are parts of a single underlying process, and that in the usual course of events, anxiety temporally precedes depression.

The fact that for most of our cases with MDD the anxiety disorder antedated and dovetailed into the depression offers some support for the unidimensional hypothesis. However, the frequent persistence of anxiety after the depression remitted and the lack of the above-noted temporal sequencing of anxiety with respect to the onset of dysthymia support the categorical approach to these entities. It is also possible that an anxiety disorder that precedes the depression (as suggested by the unidimensional position) is nosologically different from one that appears with, or subsequent to, the onset of the depression. A more detailed study with a considerably larger sample size than ours would be needed to test this proposition. Pending further information, we continue to favor the categorical approach that dictates that contemporaneous depression and anxiety be diagnosed separately.

The implications of the results for the validity of the diagnoses of depression in childhood must also be considered. Together with information previously reported,[19-21,40] the evidence is accumulating that major depression and dysthymia are diagnostic entities within the same general domain and are distinct from the adjustment disorders and nonaffective conditions. This distinction is further accentuated by the finding that comorbid anxiety disorders tended to aggregate with major depression and dysthymia rather than with ADDM.

The clinical ramifications of comorbidity are far from simple. The finding that the comorbidity of interest is associated with earlier age of onset of depression could suggest that this dual diagnosis signals greater vulnerability. With regard to prognosis, when comorbidity is examined from the perspective of primary vs secondary disorder, the latter distinction seems to have implications beyond the chronologic information it conveys.[41,42] For instance, when the MDD was the primary diagnosis, its duration was not affected by comorbid anxiety disorder. However, in cases of secondary major depression, the MDD was briefer when the child also had comorbid anxiety and dysthymia, suggesting at least two explanations. The combination of double depression[43] and anxiety disorder could represent a "neurotic," labile, or unstable depression that may be associated with more rapid recovery. But the shorter resolution time of MDD in this situation could also be an artifact; return to a symptomatic baseline (as suggested by the presence of "anxious dysthymia") may be easier than recovery to an asymptomatic level.

Finally, the data raise the question as to whether the psychiatric disorders we examined in childhood persist into the adult years. The co-occurrence of separation anxiety and major depression in our sample is particularly interesting because of its phenomenologic similarity to the agoraphobia-panic-depression cluster in adults. Longer follow-up may provide definitive data about the presumed links between childhood separation anxiety and adult agoraphobia and depression.[44,45]

Methodologic Issues and Constraints

We conclude with remarks on the generalizability of our findings and the possibility of type I error. Although controversy exists about the reliability with which the various anxiety disorders can be differentiated from each other,[4] our data and the work of Last and associates[46] suggest that the differentiation is possible in clinical samples. However, replication in nonreferred samples is needed.

Another methodologic issue is that rates of disorder comorbidity probably vary as a function of the population from which the samples are drawn. Thus, it is important that our sample was obtained from a clinically referred population and that children were recruited because they had a diagnosable depression. Anxiety was neither a study inclusionary nor an exclusionary criterion. Additionally, cases of lower socioeconomic status were somewhat overrepresented in the study compared with the general population. Further information on comorbidity rates in other types of clinical samples and in nonreferred or privately referred samples would broaden our understanding of population-specific variations in coexisting depression and anxiety.

Although it has been suggested[47] that comorbidity could be an artifact of the *DSM-III*, a number of facts argue against this possibility. First, the co-occurrence of anxiety among children with depression has been reported as far back as the 1960s.[2,12] Second, the concept of primary vs secondary psychiatric disorders, which is an alternative way to describe multiple illnesses in the same individual, also predates the *DSM-III*. Moreover, if comorbidity is entirely an artifact of diagnostic conventions, there should be no meaningful differences in course and outcome of patients with single, as opposed to multiple, conditions. However, our findings on the effect of comorbid anxiety disorder on the duration of major depression should be replicated using larger samples to ensure greater statistical precision.

Finally, some of the negative findings, including the failure to detect an effect for a history of separation from parents on the development of anxiety in the proband, could reflect that our indexes and measurements were not sufficiently sensitive. Other effects may not have been detected because of the relatively small sizes of some diagnostic subgroups. Therefore, replication of this study would be important.

REFERENCES

1. Agras S. The relationship of school phobia to childhood depression. *Am J Psychiatry.* 1959;116:533–536.
2. Frommer EA. Depressive illness in childhood. *Br J Psychiatry.* 1968;2(special issue):117–136.
3. Kashani JH, Carlson GA, Beck NC, Hoeper EW, Corcoran CM, McAllister JA, Fallahi C, Rosenberg TK, Reid JC. Depression, depressive symptoms, and depressed mood among a community sample of adolescents. *Am J Psychiatry.* 1987;144:931–934.

4. Brier A, Charney DS, Heninger GR. The diagnostic validity of anxiety disorders and their relationship to depressive illness. *Am J Psychiatry.* 1985;142:787–797.

5. Stavrakaki C, Vargo B. The relationship of anxiety and depression: a review of the literature. *Br J Psychiatry.* 1986;149:7–16.

6. Derogatis LR, Klerman GL, Lipman RS. Anxiety states and depressive neuroses. *J Nerv Ment Dis.* 1972;155:392–403.

7. Dealy RS, Ishki DM, Avery DH, Wilson LG, Dunner DL. Secondary depression in anxiety disorders. *Comp Psychiatry.* 1981;22:612–618.

8. Bowlby J. *Attachment and Loss. Separation: Anxiety and Anger, II.* New York, NY: Basic Books Inc Publishers; 1973.

9. Bowlby J. *Attachment and Loss. Loss: Sadness and Depression, III.* New York, NY:Basic Books Inc Publishers; 1980.

10. Stavrakaki C, Vargo B, Boodoosingh L, Roberts N. The relationship between anxiety and depression in children: rating scales and clinical variables. *Can J Psychiatry.* 1987;32:433–439.

11. Renshaw DC. Suicide and depression in children. *J School Health.* 1974;44:487–489.

12. Toolan JM. Depression in children and adolescents. *Am J Orthopsychiatry.* 1962;32:404–414.

13. Weissman MM, Leckman JF, Merikangas KR, Gammon GD, Prusoff BA. Depression and anxiety disorders in parents and children. *Arch Gen Psychiatry.* 1984;41:845–852.

14. Weissman MM, Gammon GD, John K, Merikangas KR, Warner V, Prusoff BA, Sholomskas D. Children of depressed parents. *Arch Gen Psychiatry.* 1987;44:847–853.

15. McNair DM, Fisher S. Separating anxiety from depression. In: Lipton MA, DiMascio A, Killam KF, eds. *Psychopharmacology: A Generation of Progress.* New York, NY:Raven Press;1978:1411–1418.

16. Fawcett J, Kravitz HM. Anxiety syndromes and their relationship to depressive illness. *J Clin Psychiatry.* 1983;44:8–11.

17. Coryell W, Noyes R, Clancy J. Panic disorder and primary unipolar depression: a comparison of background and outcome. *J Affective Disord.* 1983;5:311–317.

18. Schapira K, Roth M, Kerr TA, Gurney C. The prognosis of affective disorders: the differentiation of anxiety states from depressive illnesses. *Br J Psychiatry.* 1972;121:175–181.

19. Kovacs M, Feinberg TL, Crouse-Novak MA, Paulauskas SL, Finkelstein R. Depressive disorders in childhood, I: a longitudinal prospective study of characteristics and recovery. *Arch Gen Psychiatry.* 1984;41:229–237.

20. Kovacs M, Feinberg TL, Crouse-Novak M, Paulauskas SL, Pollock M, Finkelstein R. Depressive disorders in childhood, II: a longitudinal study of the risk for a subsequent major depression. *Arch Gen Psychiatry.* 1984;41:643–649.

21. Kovacs M, Paulauskas S, Gatsonis C, Richards C. Depressive disorders in childhood, III: a longitudinal study of comorbidity with and risk for conduct disorders. *J Affective Disord.* 1988;15:205–217.

22. Kovacs M. The Interview Schedule for Children (ISC). *Psychopharmacol Bull.* 1985;21:991–994.

23. American Psychiatric Association. *Diagnostic and Statistical Manual of Mental Disorders, Third Edition.* Washington, DC: American Psychiatric Association; 1980.

24. Hamilton M. Development of a rating scale for primary depressive illness. *Br J Soc Clin Psychol.* 1967;6:278–296.

25. Guy W. *ECDEU Assessment Manual for Psychopharmacology Revised, 1976.* US Dept of Health, Education, and Welfare publication ADM 76–338.

26. Hamilton M. Diagnosis and rating of anxiety. *Br J Psychol.* 1967;3(special issue):76–79.

27. Beck AT, Beamesderfer A. Assessment of depression: the Depression Inventory. In: Pichot P, ed. *Psychological Measurements in Psychopharmacology.* New York, NY: S Karger AG; 1974;7:151–169.

28. Lipman RS, Covi L, Shapiro AK. The Hopkins Symptom Checklist (HSCL): factors derived from the HSCL-90. *J Affective Disord.* 1979;1:9–24.

29. Bishop YMM, Feinberg SE, Holland SE. *Discrete Multivariate Analysis: Theory and Practice.* Cambridge, Mass: The MIT Press; 1984.

30. Snedecor GW, Cochran WG. *Statistical Methods.* 7th ed. Ames, Iowa: Iowa State University Press; 1980.

31. Kalbfleish JD, Prentice RL. *The Statistical Analysis of Failure Time Data.* New York, NY:John Wiley & Sons Inc; 1980

32. Kaplan EL, Meier P. Nonparametric estimation from incomplete observations. *J Am Stat Assoc.* 1958;53:457–481.

33. Cox DR. Regression models and life-tables. *J R Stat Soc.* 1972;34:187–220.

34. Dixon WJ, Brown MB, Engelman L, Frane JW, Hill MA, Jennrich RI, Toporek JD, eds. *BMDP Statistical Software Manual.* Berkeley, Calif: University of California Press; 1985.

35. Puig-Antich J, Rabinovich H. Relationship between affective and anxiety disorders in childhood. In: Gittelman R, ed. *Anxiety Disorders of Childhood.* New York, NY: Guilford Press; 1986:136–156.

36. Geller B, Chestnut EC, Miller MD, Price DT, Yates E. Preliminary data on *DSM-III* associated features of major depressive disorder in children and adolescents. *Am J Psychiatry.* 1985;142:643–644.

37. Gittelman R. Childhood anxiety disorders: correlates and outcome. In: Gittelman R, ed. *Anxiety Disorders of Childhood.* New York, NY: Guilford Press; 1986:101–125.

38. American Psychiatric Association. *Diagnostic and Statistical Manual of Mental Disorders, Revised Third Edition.* Washington, DC: American Psychiatric Press; 1987.

39. Gray JA. *The Neuropsychology of Anxiety.* New York, NY: Oxford University Press Inc; 1982.

40. Kovacs M, Gatsonis C. Stability and change in childhood-onset depressive disorders: longitudinal course as a diagnostic validator. In: Robins LN, Fleiss JL, Barrett JE, eds. *The Validity of Psychiatric Diagnosis.* New York, NY: Raven Press; 1989:57–75.

41. Andreasen NC, Winokur G. Secondary depression: familial, clinial, and research perspectives. *Am J Psychiatry.* 1979;136:62–66.

42. Friedman RC, Hurt SW, Clarkin JF, Corn R. Primary and secondary affective disorders in adolescents and young adults. *Acta Psychiatr Scand.* 1983;67:226–235.

43. Keller MB, Shapiro RW, Lavori PW, Wolfe N. Recovery in major depressive disorder: analysis with the life table and regression models. *Arch Gen Psychiatry.* 1982;39:905–910.

44. Klein DF. Anxiety reconceptualized. *Comp Psychiatry.* 1980;21:411–427.

45. Gittelman R, Klein DF. Relationship between separation anxiety and panic and agoraphobic disorders. *Psychopathology.* 1984;17(suppl 1):56–65.

46. Lastk CG, Hersen M, Kazdin AE, Finkelstein R, Strauss CC. Comparison of *DSM-III* separation anxiety and overanxious disorders: demographic characteristics and patterns of comorbidity. *J Am Acad Child Adolesc Psychiatry.* 1987;26:527–531.

47. Klerman GL. Approaches to the phenomena of co-morbidity. In: Maser JD, Cloninger CR, eds. *Comorbidity in Anxiety and Mood Disorders.* Washington, DC: American Psychiatric Press. In press.

Part V

ISSUES IN TREATMENT

As diagnostic specificity has increased so too has the attention being given to the effectiveness of treatments targeted toward specific symptoms and disorders. As treatments that clearly specify procedures and goals and objectively evaluate outcomes, behavioral therapies are an excellent example of systematically directed interventions.

In the first paper in this section, Werry and Wollersheim provide an encyclopediac review of behavior therapy with children and adolescents over the past 20 years. Specific techniques are described including classical conditioning methods, operant techniques, cognitive-behavioral techniques, and social skills training, and their application to specific DSM-III-R disorders is critically considered.

A thoughtful discussion concludes that precise indications for behavior therapy, its comparative efficacy, and relationship to other forms of psychotherapy and other treatments remain to be demonstrated. They further suggest that these uncertainties stem to a great extent from the relatively poor state of research in other forms of psychotherapy. It is impossible to determine whether any other treatment is as good as behavioral methods for the treatment of a number of disorders including tics, habits, and ADHD because the results are unchallenged by comparable data on other psychotherapies. What, Werry and Wollersheim ask, should an honest therapist then advise parents? Recalling that in medicine practitioners usually recommend treatments with proven efficacy, resorting to others only in the face of treatment failure, they wonder how many child psychiatrists would be equal to this ethical challange?

The data presented by Pliska begin to point the way toward greater specificity of pharmacologic treatments for attention deficit hyperactivity disorder. A well planned and carefully executed study has examined the effect of the comorbidity of overanxious disorder and attention deficit hyperactivity disorder on response to methyphenidate as well as on laboratory measures of behavior and cognition. Forty-three children between seven and 10 years of age participated in a four-week, double-blind medication trial. Thirty children met DSM-III-R criteria for ADHD alone, and 13 met DSM-III-R criteria for overanxious disorder as well. Subjects with comorbid anxiety had a significantly poorer response to stimulant medication than those without anxiety. Only four (30.8%) of the comorbid group were considered to be responders, as compared with 26 (86.7%) of the nonanxiety subjects. Subjects without comorbid anxiety were significantly more likely to show no improvement on placebo and dramatic reductions of both teacher and laboratory ratings of inattention, overactivity, and aggression on stimulant. Subjects with anxiety showed only a modest nonsignificant improvement with treatment overall. A number were placebo responders.

Although the number of children in the comorbid group is small, these data raise interesting questions regarding the pharmacological treatment of children with symptoms of both ADHD and anxiety, as well as the underlying nature of their disorder. As one-third of the comorbid subjects did respond to stimulant, the authors caution that their results should not be interpreted as suggesting that ADHD children with comorbid anxiety should never be treated with stimulant medication. However, it may be anticipated that in two-thirds of such cases this treatment may not be effective. The data suggest that children who meet criteria for ADHD and an anxiety disorder are a distinct subgroup. Whether they are a sub-type of ADHD or whether they are children with primary anxiety disorders who develop secondary inattentiveness will require further study to resolve.

The paper by Leonard, Swedo, Rapoport, Koby, Lenane, Cheslow, and Hamburger is a report of a 10-week, double-blind crossover trial of clomipramine and desipramine in treatment of OCD. It is representative of the increasingly sophisticated approach to the evaluation of the effectiveness of pharmacologic interventions for specific clinical disorders.

The trial was undertaken because previous studies demonstrating the effacy of clomipramine relative to placebo were not truly "blind," as most participants were aware of anticholenergic side effects while on active drug. The comparison with another antidepressant obviates this problem. Further, the use of a comparison antidepressant addresses the question of what component of the obsessional response might be mediated by a nonspecific antidepressant or anxiolytic effect. The findings are unequivical. Clomipramine was clearly superior to desipramine in significantly reducing obsessive-compulsive symptoms in 48 children and adolescents with severe primary obsessive-compulsive disorder. Clinical response to clomipramine was not related to age of onset, duration and severity of illness, type of symptom or plasma drug concentrations. Almost two-thirds of patients who received clomipramine as their first active treatment showed at least some sign of relapse during desipramine treatment. The authors interpret the findings further documenting the specificity of the antiobsessional effect of clomipramine and caution clinicians as to the need for maintenance treatment.

Noting that as many as 30% of children with ADDH who are treated with stimulants fail to respond, Biederman, Baldessarini, Wright, Knee, and Harmatz undertook an examination of the effectiveness of a tricyclic antidepressant drug, desipramine. Sixty-two clinically referred patients, (42 children and 20 adolescents) 69% of whom had previously responded poorly to psychostimulant treatment participated in a six-week, randomized placebo-controlled trial. Both previously treatment resistant patients and patients who had never received stimulant medication showed clinical and statistically significant behavioral improvement when on desipramine as contrasted with placebo, and the drug was well tolerated even at the relatively high doses used. Although an examination of the relationship of response/non-response to the presence or absence of comorbid conditions would have further strengthened the study, the findings are of importance in guiding clinical practice. The data of this study adds to clinical experience and other shorter-term trials in indicating that desipramine is a viable alternative in the pharmacologic treatment of ADHD for many children who have failed to respond to stimulant medication, or for whom a long-acting medication is preferable.

23

Behavior Therapy with Children and Adolescents: A Twenty-Year Overview

John Scott Werry

University of Auckland, New Zealand

Janet P. Wollersheim

University of Montana, Missoula

A twenty-year overview of behavior therapy with children and adolescents is presented. The various techniques and their application to relevant major DSM-III-R *categories are critically discussed. It is concluded that behavior therapy has made great progress and has proven applications in child and adolescent disorders but that its precise roles, comparative efficacy, and complementarity to other forms of psychotherapy and other treatments remain to be demonstrated. Much uncertainty stems from the relatively poor state of research in other forms of psychotherapy. Key words: behavior therapy, children, adolescence, psychiatric disorders, psychotherapy.*

PART I. OVERVIEW AND PRINCIPLES

Introduction and Historical Review

Two decades ago, while coworkers at the University of Illinois, the authors published a review of the then-emerging behavior therapy ". . . to acquaint child therapists with some of the concepts and techniques . . . to offer illustrative case studies, and to indicate what [they] believe[d] to be the pertinence of behavior therapy in the remediation of the psychopathology of childhood" (Werry and Wollersheim, 1967, p. 346). At the time, behavior therapy was little understood, not well accepted, and

Reprinted with permission from *Journal of the American Academy of Child and Adolescent Psychiatry,* 1989, Vol. 28, No. 1, 1–18. Copyright © by the American Academy of Child and Adolescent Psychiatry.

oftentimes rejected in the psychiatric community. Today it is a rare psychiatrist who does not have some understanding of its principles and procedures, assets, and limitations.

Since the mid-1960s, behavior therapy has experienced significant and ongoing changes in definition, theory, principles, and techniques. The purpose of this review is to describe what behavior therapy in the arena of child and adolescent psychopathology is today: to outline its current principles and techniques, to comment upon its effectiveness, assets, and limitations, and finally, to highlight what seem to be its future directions.

O'Leary and Wilson (1987, p.1) point out that behavior therapy has a long past but a short history. Many principles and techniques were published during the first part of the twentieth century, before World War II; yet behavior therapy did not emerge as an explicit and systematic body of knowledge distinct from the then-prevailing psychodynamic model until the late 1950s. The publication of the now classical book by Wolpe (1958) and the volume of case studies by Ullmann and Krasner (1965) did much to popularize behavior therapy. The growth has been escalating year by year.

Emerging as the application of learning theory to psychopathology, treatments at first focused either upon the classical or *respondent* conditioning paradigms of Pavlov or upon *operant* conditioning and its reinforcement technology (Skinner, 1938). Learning theory was a major preoccupation of American experimental psychology at the time, and both approaches were derived from animal experiments. By nature of their human subjects, however, clinical behaviorists had to turn their attention to problems of greater breadth and complexity. Consequently, the scope and definitions of behavior therapy began to change (Wollersheim, 1980). Clinical researchers were struggling to discover where internal, complex processes, such as thinking and similar mental processes so essential to other psychotherapies, could fit into the behavioral model. Wollersheim (1970), in an early effort to fit cognitive factors into the treatment of obesity, termed this a *cognitive behavioral approach*, a term now in common parlance. Thus, definitions of behavior therapy were gradually expanded to include not just the principles of animal learning or conditioning but also concepts from human-related branches of experimental psychology, such as social and cognitive psychology. There was the rational-emotive therapy of Albert Ellis (1962) and then the cognitive therapy of Aaron Beck (1967). Terms such as *systematic rational restructuring* (Goldfried et al., 1974) and *cognitive behavior modification* (Meichenbaum, 1979) began to appear with increasing frequency. Although some have viewed the attempts to integrate cognitive and behavioral perspectives with enthusiasm (Mahoney, 1977), others (Wolpe, 1978) have decried efforts, believing that they represent a regression to the state of psychotherapy at which behavior therapy broke away and that they threaten the very distinctiveness of behavior therapy. It is a fact, though, that whatever the outcome of this intimate courtship, there are now some definitional ambiguities *vis-à-vis* other psychotherapies. Indeed, some cognitive-behavioral treatments, such as depression, have some clear similarities to psychodynamic approaches (Wollersheim, 1980). Wilson (1978) defines the essential, common core of behavior therapy as commitment to measurement, methodology, concepts, and procedures from experimental psychology. This definition, however, does not necessarily define clear boundaries, since, in theory at least, other forms of psychotherapy could be equally derived. It is more their too slowly fading *resistance* to science that allows behavior therapy to assume a distinctive look at the moment.

Increasingly, clinicians favor the use of pragmatic combinations of viewpoints and therapies tailored to the specific needs of individual patients (Garske, 1982) in what may be called patient-oriented (versus therapist-oriented) treatment. In research and theory, though, different models continue to be heuristic, but it is not surprising that in our groping toward a more comprehensive, more scientifically robust way of looking at psychotherapy, there is some movement toward ecumenism. What makes this even more valid is the repeated finding that, independent of their theoretical underpinnings, therapies seem to share a common efficacy; this is rather more striking than any specificities (Casey and Berman, 1985; Garfield and Bergin, 1986).

Definition

For the purposes of this review, behavior therapy will be defined as:

> Those treatments that utilize the principles and terms of learning theory and allied aspects of experimental psychology *and* that are committed to explicit specification of treatment procedures and goals and to the objective evaluation of therapeutic outcomes.

The commonly used terms *behavior modification* and *cognitive-behavioral approach,* which represent the extremes of focus between overt behavior and internalized processes, will both be subsumed under behavior therapy.

Theoretical Considerations

In 1967, we saw the unifying conceptual approach of behavior therapy to be derived from the field of learning as viewed and researched in experimental psychology. This is still true today, but it is important to note that, like the field of learning itself, contemporary behavior therapy has no single, simple theoretical underpinning.

Neobehaviorist Approaches

Neobehaviorist approaches are derived from the stimulus response models of learning of Pavlov, Hull, Miller, Mowrer, and Guthrie. Conditioning (or the control of specific stimuli over behavior), rather than cognitions or internal mediating processes, is employed as the explanatory process.

Classical, respondent, or Pavlovian conditioning. The processes concern the linking of conditional stimuli to naturally occurring reflex arcs by simple, immediately preceding association. The organism is passive or a victim of circumstances, as it were. This model is particularly applicable to emotional disorders.

Operant conditioning. Skinner's (1938) approach is still much in evidence and is sometimes referred to as *applied behavioral analysis.* As the term *operant* suggests, it is assumed that the organism has some choice and the behavior operates actively on the environment. Within this framework, the focus is on overt, observable behavior, the eliciting stimuli preceding it, and the reinforcing events, positive or negative, following it.

Cognitive Behavioral Approaches

A newer mode emphasizes internal, cognitive processes as controlling or mediating both normal and maladaptive experience and behavior. Therapists not only assess overt behavior as do neobehaviorists but also explore thinking processes accompanying the problem behavior or emotional experience.

Social Learning Models

Bandura (1969, 1977) did much to integrate the diverse approaches within behavior therapy (including the three described above) into a consistent theoretical system that recognized different levels of behavioral regulation, ranging from pairing of stimuli and responses to cognitive processes. In his highly influential *self-efficacy* theory, Bandura (1977) added a quaintly old-fashioned American value system to a social learning model: one *can* do something to better oneself (the value) and the path is via social learning (the technology). This perspective highlights the human capacity for self-direction and stresses the reciprocal interaction among behavior, environment, and cognitive factors in psychological functioning. In many ways, Bandura is to Skinner and Pavlov as Sullivan was to Freud.

Summary

In 1967, it was relatively easy for the present authors to delineate differences between behavior and other psychotherapies, but the base has become so broadened beyond the stimulus-response, neobehaviorist one that in 1988 it is not easy. Indeed, Davison and Neale (1986) suggest that behavior therapy is now identified as much by its epistemological dedication to the search for rigorous standards of proof as by alignment with any set of concepts.

Techniques of Behavior Therapy

Only those behavior techniques in wide use are described. Full details can be sought in the citations and monographs devoted exclusively to behavior therapy with children and adolescents, such as Mash and Terdal (1981), Ollendick and Cerny (1981), Ross (1981), Bornstein and Kazdin (1985), and Hersen and Van Hasselt (1987). As is true of most treatment methods, adolescents have received less attention and their management has been sought under the management of older children and adults, although the situation is changing (e.g., Hersen and Van Hasselt, 1987).

Classical (Respondent) Conditioning Methods

Systematic desensitization and implosion (flooding) are conditioning methods and, as such, are viewed as most appropriate for the treatment of emotional states, particularly fear and anxiety (see below). Their use in minors, however, has not been researched as thoroughly as has their use in adults. Briefly, these techniques expose the child to the anxiety arousing stimuli in fact and/or imagination. Systematic desensitization does this gradually and only after having taught the child relaxation as a counter-phobic device. On the other hand, implosion provides rapid exposure, rather akin to "throwing the child in at the deep end" (see Ollendick, 1986; Strauss, 1987). Understandably, the latter has not been very attractive to child therapists.

Operant Techniques. Operant techniques have received extensive application and are, by far, still the most widely used. The events immediately preceding a behavior (eliciting stimuli) and/or those immediately after (reinforcing or punishing contingencies) are systematically manipulated so as to change the target behavior. Operant techniques have been used widely in parent management programs (Ross, 1981; Patterson et al., 1982) and inpatient (Quay, 1986), school (MacMillan and Morrison, 1986), and community settings. They have been applied to a wide range of behaviors, from psychotic and self-mutilating, through simple problems of eating, elimination, and tantrums, to more complex social behaviors. Some particular operant techniques deserve mention:

Shaping involves applying positive reinforcement to behavior that is somewhat less than acceptable and gradually rewarding as it gets closer and closer to the final form. This process, of course, is elemental to skill acquisition, as in learning to read and write.

Chaining combines simple behaviors, learned successively, into a complex sequence or skill through stimulus and contingency management. It has been used, for example, to teach retarded persons quite complex assembly line skills.

Discrimination learning concentrates more on teaching the child to recognize cues by differential reinforcement of those to which the child should respond and no reward, or even punishment, for those that should evoke no or a different response. Thus a child is taught that talking at the table will receive adult attention but that talking while the caregiver is on the telephone will not.

Fading involves introducing a stimulus that aids the elicitation of a desired but difficult to produce behavior (prompting), then gradually fading it out. For example, in remedial education (Etzel and LeBlanc, 1979) different colored letters may be used initially for different sounds.

Contingency management, as the name suggests, relies on the systematic control of the consequences of the behavior to be changed through such devices as contracts, token economies, points, star charts, and so on. Such programs often employ not only techniques to facilitate the development of behaviors but also procedures aimed at reducing or eliminating inappropriate behavior. Because of the popularity of the method, a number of sub-techniques has evolved. *Extinction* involves abolishing the naturally occurring reinforcers maintaining a behavior, most often attention from adults or peers (e.g., Kazdin, 1975). In *overcorrection* the undesired behavior invokes extra effort to remedy its negative consequences. For example, encopresis may require the child to wash the soiled underwear. *Response cost* (a variant of fining) involves withdrawing previously acquired rewards contingent upon inappropriate behavior, as in docking an adolescent's allowance after curfew violation. *Time out,* strictly speaking, means removing the opportunity to earn rewards; it has come to imply removing not the rewards but the child from a desirable environment to a less attractive one. As such, it is more suited to children than large, strong, resistive adolescents. Good discussion of this widely misunderstood technique can be found in MacDonough and Forehand (1973) and Forehand and MacDonough (1975).

Punishment means the application of an aversive or unpleasant contingency to undesired behavior, and there is a significant body of research relating to its effectiveness and its limitations (Johnston, 1972; Harris and Ersner-Hershfield, 1978). Although parents ordinarily use physical punishment freely, professionals are, of course, subject to ethical constraints and the acceptable forms are usually disapproval and seclusion or banishment. The use of physical punishment, including the notorious electric shock, is defensible only under very special, rarely occurring situations where life or limb is seriously at risk and when alternative methods have failed (see Ollendick, 1986). It has to be remembered that, in many cases, the alternative will be high, chronic doses of unpleasant, dulling, neuroleptic medication, and that there are now less objectionable alternatives to shock (see autism below). Although techniques such as overcorrection, response-cost, and time-out are given euphemistic names and bland technical rationales, the reality of their administration in practice is that they are but forms of punishment and should be so regarded.

Cognitive-Behavioral Techniques

The newer cognitive-behavioral methods are rather more diffuse and difficult to describe but they are united in the attempt to change behavior and feelings by changing thinking patterns. They involve procedures such as active instruction in alternative solutions to problems (e.g., nonconfrontational methods in aggression), covert self-instruction (e.g., getting hyperactive children to say to themselves "stop, look, listen" before acting), reframing events, challenging maladaptive beliefs, and encouraging children to develop more optimistic or reasonable attitudes about situations that distress them. The links to traditional psychotherapies are obvious. Additional details and supporting data can be found in Kendall and Hollon (1979), Emery et al. (1981), Kendall and Norton-Ford (1982), Bornstein and Kazdin (1985), and Hersen and Van Hasselt (1987).

Social Skills Training

This treatment has received much attention from behavior therapists, but like Bandura's (1977) social learning/self-efficacy model from which it derives, it is really a composite of many different techniques (from models described above), used in varying combinations, all with a particular focus on social skills (Hops et al., 1985; Christoff and Myatt, 1987). As a result, it has been applied across a wide variety of disorders that are accompanied by or that result in social skills deficits. It is particularly important in rehabilitative programs for those with serious disabilities. Children and adolescents are taught, individually or in groups, social stress management, how to make friends, to cooperate, to converse, to be assertive, and to initiate specified social behaviors. Techniques are often highly didactic and include role-playing, social reinforcement, token rewards, modeling procedures, self-instruction training, problem-solving, and systematic desensitization. Positive short-term benefit has been claimed, but proper substantiation of this is awaited, as is the demonstration of long-term gains. Despite this, there are a number of procedures that have sufficient face validity to be worthy of trial with specific social disabilities (Hops et al., 1985; Emmelkamp, 1986; Christoff and Myatt, 1987).

Effectiveness and Efficiency

In the authors' 1967 review (Werry and Wollersheim, 1967), most of the data offered stemmed from uncontrolled case studies. Although such still abound today, they are increasingly being matched by proper evaluations—at least in adults (Agras, 1987). The lag in behavior therapy with children and adolescents merely reflects a more general shortfall in all treatment for children and adolescents (except possibly in pharmacotherapy, where the task is somewhat easier). Nevertheless, the evidence for the efficacy and efficiency of behavior therapy and its wide range of techniques is impressive (see below; Casey and Berman 1985; Hersen and Van Hasselt, 1987; O'Leary and Wilson, 1987). Furthermore, the dogged insistence of behavior therapists on evaluation has produced a wealth of clinical measurement techniques (see Mash and Terdal, 1981; Merluzzi et al., 1981; Bornstein and Kazdin, 1985; Hersen and Van Hasselt, 1987) that could be useful in other psychotherapies should their coyness about evaluation be overcome.

Although as a general proposition it can be said that behavior therapy is effective, it is still not possible to say how it compares with other treatments as to efficacy, cost, and time. In their review of psychotherapies with children, Casey and Berman (1985) concluded that all methods were superior to no treatment. While behavior therapy seemed to be more effective than other methods, this advantage disappeared when the problems treated and/or the outcome measures were more encompassing than mere symptoms. It may well be that the posited nonspecific factors common to all psychological treatment (Garfield and Bergin, 1986), such as the reinforcing qualities of the therapist, are most powerful and account for many of the similarities in outcome (see Fisher and Wollersheim, 1986).

As a group, behavior therapists have probably addressed far more attention to Paul's (1967) oft-quoted dictum that research with psychotherapy should address *what* treatment, *by whom, for whom, for what* specific problem, and *under what* circumstances. The *by whom* is a particularly interesting issue and includes training. This is discussed below, but it is our impression that behavior therapy is still largely done by psychologists. If this is so, there seems no good reason other than tradition for their preference for traditional psychotherapies, particularly since, so far, intensive training often required by such psychotherapies has not emerged as a powerful variable in efficacy of psychotherapy (Berman and Norton, 1985).

PART II. APPLICATION TO SPECIFIC *DSM-III-R* DISORDERS

In this section *DSM-III-R* is followed as far as possible. *DSM-III-R* does not always sit well with behavior therapy because of its *problem-oriented* approach. Indeed, Werry and Wollersheim followed the latter in 1967, but in 1988 it is simply not appropriate to ignore the major thrust of psychiatric classification, which is *disorder-oriented.* Nevertheless, there are many occasions when the disorder model is not appropriate (e.g., V-codes or simple management problems) or where the data available simply do not allow it. In these instances, these problems have been put with the classes of disorder with which they are most often associated and are noted in discussions of other disorders where they may also occur.

Developmental and Speech Disorders

Mental Retardation

Mental retardation is an area that, sadly, has been ignored by most child psychiatrists, despite the fact that treatment of mental retardation calls for a set of skills that they, among physicians, are more likely to have (Corbett, 1985). As a result, and also because they have always had a strong interest and legitimate role in its diagnosis, psychologists have dominated treatment. Perhaps because of this, there is no single area in child or adolescent psychopathology that has attracted so much interest from behavior therapists. Thus, it would be impossible to do justice here to the magnitude, ingenuity, and complexity of the field. Almost every method of behavioral treatment has been applied to practically every problem or psychiatric disorder in the retarded. Thus, it is a microcosm of the field of behavior therapy as a whole; even complex cognitive methods have been employed and some of the work aimed at skills development is quite surprisingly sophisticated.

Problems may be grouped into externalizing/disruptive; internalizing; stereotypies; sexuality; self-care; language and academic skills; and living, social, and vocational skills. Most of these are covered elsewhere in this review. Useful overviews of the role of behavior therapy in the mentally retarded may be found in Matson and McCartney (1981), Whitman et al., (1983), and Whitman and Johnston (1987). Interested readers might also like to look at specialized journals in mental retardation to get some perspective on just how advanced is the state of behavior therapy in this area.

In summary it would be fair to say that behavioral methods have dominated nonpharmacological management of psychopathology of the mentally retarded in North America since 1967, with considerable reported success and some outstanding contributions to research and clinical methodology in behavior therapy. It is certainly an area with which child psychiatrists should be familiar.

Autistic Disorder and Other Pervasive Developmental Disorders

DSM-III-R defines autism in terms that really only more precisely define and quantify Kanner's original triad of grossly impaired social relatedness (autism), language deficits, and ritualistic/obsessional behavior. Among numerous useful reviews of behavioral treatment in this disorder are those by Devany and Nelson (1986), Ollendick (1986), and Harris and Handelman (1987). The latter points out that autism and severe mental retardation share a lot of management problems, so that there is a great deal of overlap in methods used in the two disorders. It is pleasing to see that two of the early behavioral investigators (Lovaas and DeMyer) who figured in the Werry and Wollersheim (1967) review, have devoted much of their professional careers to the study of this disabling and distressing disorder.

Methods used have been virtually restricted to the simple operant or behavior modification, primarily shaping and contingency management (Ollendick, 1986). Lovaas brought notoriety to and widespread rejection of behavior therapy in autism through the use of physical punishment—electric shock for severe self-mutilating rituals. Though he quickly abandoned shock despite its efficacy, he continues to use slaps to the legs to get the child's attention (Lovaas, 1987). There was a similar, if less intense, reaction to his making the children earn their food mouthful by mouthful, which was seen by some as punitive but by Lovaas as the only way to get the attention of the severely autistic children with whom he worked. Others (see Winton and Singh, 1983; Ollendick, 1986; Harris and Handleman, 1987) have sought alternatives to draconian punishment for ritualistic behaviors. Some of these alternatives are physical exercise, shutting out any resultant reinforcing sensory stimuli (such as noise), invoking passive movements incompatible with the injurious or disturbing one, or application of mild discomforts such as cold water mist to the face or briefly interrupting vision. The ethical aspects of punishment are well examined by Ollendick (1986).

It would be a gross disservice to Lovaas, however, to overemphasize the punishment aspects of his method when the essence lies elsewhere: (1) in carefully focused interventions for distracting behaviors (e.g., gaze avoidance) inhibiting social learning, (2) in shaping up social behavior and language, (3) in intensity of treatment (40 hours/week) by carefully trained therapists, (4) in extension of treatment by parents in as much of the rest of the child's waking hours as practicable, (5) in careful evaluation of progress by behavior observations.

Though one may still have mixed feelings about some aspects of Lovaas' methods, there are no properly controlled/documented success rates in autism in children under the age of 4 with mental ages of at least 11 months (his selective criteria) that can compete with his. Lovaas (1987) reports the staggering outcome of a 50% "recovery" rate, defined as normal IQs and language by age 6. Two less intensively treated groups (10 hours/week) had a more usual result of best level of IQ attained (again in 50%) of only around 70, and still markedly abnormal language. As can be imagined, this study is far from perfect and doubts must remain, but the method and its results cannot be ignored. It is interesting to note, however, that Devany, a former coworker of Lovaas', is less enthusiastic and points out that Lovaas' treatment methods are largely unsuccessful for severely retarded, older autistic children and those whose parents cannot carry on the treatment program (Devany and Nelson, 1986). Also, in some cases, enormous effort is expended to produce results of dubious utility, such as parrot-like language. What this possibly illustrates is some kind of threshold effect, whereby those autistic children with certain minimal levels of brain function are most likely to benefit from intensive treatment. Lovaas' work may have important, if rather unpalatable, cost/benefit implications.

Academic Skills Disorders

It is not easy to review academic skills disorders, partly because of the chaotic state of nosology and partly because of serious disagreements between physicians, psychologists, and parents who embrace the "disease" model and educators who think more in learning terms. Another problem for a reviewer is that it is difficult to decide what is behavior therapy and what is normal educational practice. The behavioral approach arising in the 1960s has had a profound effect on education (see Klein, 1979) so that a wide variety of behavioral techniques, such as contingency management, feedback, modeling, and self-recording is now part and parcel of education (see Treiber and Lahey, 1985; Shapiro, 1987). Operant procedures, primarily contingency management, have been shown to be helpful in individual remedial education of children with learning disabilities involving one or more of the three Rs (Shapiro, 1987), but the generalizability of this to the classroom and the durability and the specificity of the treatment seem less well studied.

Lately, cognitive behavior therapy has been added to the list of behavioral methods (see Wong, 1985; Abikoff, 1987). It has been subject to rather more carefully-controlled studies, especially in children with attention-deficit hyperactive disorder (ADHD), but results are mostly negative (Abikoff, 1987). This and studies on the effect of drugs and learning (Werry, 1988) suggest that success claimed for any treatment program may come largely from elevation of performance of *existing* rather than acquisition of *new* academic skills. Another problem is that a number of approaches, such as perceptual-motor and attentional training, focus on skills antecedent or only presumptively related to academic learning that may well not be influenced. All this seems to be part of a more general problem affecting all types of remedial education, which is that this by now rather substantial industry is long on enthusiasm and self-proclaimed efficacy but very short on hard evaluative data (Gittelman, 1985). Some of the problem lies in inherent complexity of the process of learning (see Wong, 1985), but even so, studies such as that by Gittleman and Feingold (1983) and those of cognitive behavior therapy (Abikoff, 1987) show that it is possible to properly evaluate programs.

In summary, while there are clear, if limited, benefits from behavioral methods (Shapiro, 1987), some skepticism toward *all* remedial educational programs is needed unless evaluative data attesting to real skill acquisition and its durability is provided (see Gittelman, 1985).

Language and Speech Disorders

Language and speech disorders are of interest to child psychiatrists because they are clearly associated with childhood psychopathology (Beitchman et al., 1986). Here the concern is primarily with disorders of expression and articulation such as dyslalia, cluttering, and stuttering. In their review, DiLorenzo and Matson (1987) make a distinction between linguistic treatment methods for stuttering aimed at speech patterns, most of which are based on trying to introduce rhythmicity, and what they see as true behavior therapy aimed at etiological or aggravating psychopathology.

The linguistic methods, however, owe much to behavior therapists who introduced earphone metronomes and delayed auditory feedback, both of which are not only very (though not completely) successful but are portable and thus can be used in the environments most prone to evoke stuttering. The disadvantage of these methods is that the resulting speech lacks variability and naturalness; it is also possible to get the same results without the apparatus (DiLorenzo and Matson, 1987). Other more truly behavioral methods include anxiety reduction (see internalizing disorders above), operant, biofeedback, and breathing techniques. As DiLorenzo and Matson (1987) point out, all methods have some success, which suggests a degree of empirical groping as yet somewhat distant from a satisfactory theory or etiology.

Disruptive (Externalizing) Disorders

The disruptive disorders encompass a wide variety of behaviors that violate laws, social norms, or more localized (e.g., family) codes of conduct. Since they cause distress primarily to the external environment, they are also known, especially by psychologists, as *externalizing* disorders.

Attention-Deficit Hyperactive Disorder

It is of interest to note that ADHD did not merit a separate entry in the Werry and Wollersheim 1967 review and, in fact, only one study was mentioned. Although Reatig's (1984) bibliography (1976 through 1984) lists over 600 articles, it is surprising that there are only about 50 articles on behavioral approaches, most by a handful of investigators. This is probably artifactual to some extent, since the bibliography was selective and because behavior therapists have been resistant to diagnostic categories, preferring to target problem behaviors such as hyperactivity.

Exactly what is ADHD is a vexatious issue (see Prior and Sanson, 1986; Werry et al., 1987), but this discussion shall include only studies in which children exhibit the key chronic symptoms of inattention, impulsivity, and hyperactivity and in which behavior therapy has been aimed specifically at these symptoms. Commonly associated symptoms of oppositional/conduct and learning problems not necessary for the diagnosis are covered elsewhere in this review.

A most practical, readable, if somewhat optimistic overview and treatment manual for clinicians interested in behavioral methods in ADHD is the monograph by Barkley (1981), which also addresses assessment and other treatments in general.

From various reviews (Barkley, 1981; Ross and Ross, 1982; Devany and Nelson, 1986; Abikoff, 1987; Rapport, 1987), it is apparent that two behavioral methods have predominated in ADHD. The first, also the oldest, is contingency management: rewards, such as praise, checkmarks or tokens, for desired behavior; and punishment, usually ignoring, sometimes fines (*response cost*), or isolation/seclusion (erroneously euphemized as *time out*). This approach has been modestly successful but is beset with the usual problems of any treatment; decaying interest by both adult and child, lack of generalization outside the situation in which it is applied, and greater success where the child's behavior is more closely supervised and restricted (as in the classroom) than at home or play. This approach has won wide acceptance, especially in educational and clinical settings, but few see it as a complete treatment in itself (Barkley, 1981).

The second method is the cognitive approach, which has tended to have a higher profile lately. It stems partly from general dissatisfaction with simplistic externalized methods, such as contingency management, partly from the popularity of Douglas' (1972) view of ADHD as being an inability to "stop, look and listen," and partly from highly charismatic exponents such as Meichenbaum (1979). As so often happens with treatments, enthusiasm has far outstripped evaluation. In his careful review, which also gives details of the procedures, Abikoff (1987) concluded that studies were inconclusive as far as any effect on attention and impulsivity were concerned, which is disappointing—if not lethal to the treatment—in view of their primary role in ADHD. Not surprisingly, there were no effects on academic performance either.

ADHD is one of the few areas in which possible synergistic interactions between behavior therapy and medication have been explored, since the well-demonstrated value of stimulants in ADHD means that any behavior therapist is going to have to work in conjunction or in comparison with medication. One of the earliest and best of these studies is that by Gittelman-Klein et al. (1976); it failed, however, to show any synergism, and this has been the general pattern since (Brown et al., 1986; Rapport, 1987).

Behavior therapy, especially contingency management, has proved to have a useful, if restricted and possibly rather temporary, role in ADHD. Like medication, it should be only one aspect of a multimodal approach. While Abikoff (1987) and

Whalen et al. (1985) counsel not to abandon cognitive behavior therapy, and Rapport (1987) argues for a potentially much more effective role for behavioral approaches in general in ADHD, their prescriptions for how to achieve this are daunting and call for another decade of research before there is much likelihood of a flow-on to clinicians. In the meantime, enthusiasts (whatever their persuasion) who claim to have the answer for this chronic, disabling, and complex disorder should be viewed with suspicion.

Conduct and Oppositional-Defiant Disorders

Long-term follow-up studies of conduct disordered children show that those with more clinically severe forms have a greater likelihood of maladjustment in adolescence and adulthood (Robins, 1979; Wells and Forehand, 1985; Kazdin, 1987; Kazdin et al., 1987) so that effective treatment is a matter of some importance. Oppositional-defiant disorders do not involve such severe degrees of antisocial behavior, but the difference is largely one of degree, not of type (see Werry et al., 1987), and so all additional references to conduct disorder will include them.

Good reviews of the behavioral treatment of the conduct disorders can be found in Ollendick (1986), Wells and Forehand (1981, 1985), Kazdin (1987), and Kazdin et al. (1987). Four major approaches dominate: behavioral contracting, conflict-resolution skills training, token economies in the home, and training parents to reprogram the social environment. The latter has received the most attention and is often combined with token economies with children and with contracting with adolescents. The effectiveness of parent training programs has been demonstrated in a number of studies by Patterson and colleagues (Wiltz and Patterson, 1974; Patterson et al., 1982), but they have also demonstrated that treatment must be open-ended and adjusted to the specific characteristics of each family. In a move that will appeal to all clinicians, whatever their persuasion, they have further noted that important "treatment ingredients" also lie in direct attention to marital and other parent problems and in clinical skill in dealing with resistance (Patterson and Fleishman, 1979; Patterson et al., 1981). Cognitive behavioral approaches, such as having therapists align themselves with the legitimate goals of the children and then instructing them in problem solving and impulse control necessary to achieve such goals, have also been used to a limited degree (Templeman and Wollersheim, 1979).

Stealing has received specific attention (Reid and Patterson, 1976; Reid et al., 1980). An important feature of this program lies in making the focus not *detection* of stealing, which is often infeasible, but rather *suspicion* of stealing, e.g., the position of any item that cannot be adequately explained. In what may seem a travesty of Anglo-American justice, such suspicion is treated as stealing, as is credible accusation by a reliable other. A mild consequence, such as 1 or 2 hours of chores, is invoked and implemented immediately and consistently.

Aggressive behavior is treated by emphasizing acceptable punishment for it, rewarding incompatible, desirable alternatives, and ignoring some kinds of minor behaviors, since most conduct disordered youth have a wide variety of annoying behaviors and it would be unfeasible and undesirable to punish all of them. That this approach can be successful is shown by Baum and Forehand (1981).

Oppositional and minor problems such as tantrums, swearing, noncompliance, arguing, and blaming others are most often treated by parent programs derived from operant conditioning (Wells and Forehand, 1985; Kazdin et al., 1987).

School problems are typical in conduct disorders where, in addition, academic difficulties also occur. Treatment goals in schools can be divided into three types: better interpersonal behavior, increased motivation for and compliance with learning, and benefit through remedial education. There is considerable evidence that antisocial behavior in the classroom can be changed with behavioral programs that generally reward appropriate behavior and/or use punishment or time-out as well (O'Leary and Wilson, 1987) and which give attention to remedial education (see Treiber and Lahey, 1985).

Delinquency, an increasing problem, is usually handled by methods already mentioned, but because delinquent young persons are usually deficient in other skills such as social, academic, and vocational ones, attention is given to these, as well as to law-breaking, e.g., court-directed peer counseling, family involvement, job training, and education (Slack, 1960; Schwitzgebel and Kolb, 1964). While such programs have reported some success, they have not succeeded reliably in their original goals of reducing criminal behavior (Lemert, 1981).

The best-known and evaluated behavioral treatment for delinquency is the Achievement Place approach, a family-type residential program for predelinquents. The first such home was started in Lawrence, Kansas in 1967, and there are now 150 such houses in the United States (Howard et al., 1982). In these programs, delinquent behavior is seen as a result of inadequate social learning, and desirable behavior is encouraged through the use of a detailed token reinforcement program (Phillips et al., 1971). Gradually, immediate concrete rewards are replaced by rewards that are both more naturally occurring and more remote in time. Research has shown that during their stay in Achievement Place homes, youth evidenced fewer official and self-reported offenses than those placed in other homes but that, sadly, 1 year after discharge, these differences had disappeared (Kirigin et al., 1982). This has forced focus now upon after-care as well, so that parents and foster parents can continue the strategies used during the Achievement Place stay.

In the reviews, Kazdin (1987), Kazdin et al. (1987), and Wells and Forehand (1985) detail the various behavioral treatment methods for conduct disorders and problems and illustrate their beneficial effects in a way not possible here; but they also cast a gloomy picture of the failure of these effects to persist or to influence long-term outcome when the conduct disorder is of any severity. The picture with milder problems—especially oppositional behavior within families and class-rooms—is more favorable, though long-term studies are lacking. Kazdin et al., Wells, and Forehand suggest that there is thus an urgent need for early intervention, preferably with "non-adjudicated" children still living with their families. A similar view has been espoused for the related area of drug abuse (see below). Also, Kazdin et al. (1987) adopt the very reasonable view that combining individually effective treatments (e.g., parent training and cognitive methods) should be investigated to see whether the power and durability of the effect can be increased, which their pilot study suggested could well be done. So while there are grounds for using behavior therapy in conduct disorders, short-term objectives are more reasonable than definitive cure. Behavior therapy, however, is no more unsuccessful than other forms of treatment (Kazdin et al., 1987).

Anxiety Disorders and Problems

In contrast to children with disruptive disorders, whose behavior can be evaluated and readily identified by others, those with anxiety/emotional problems are liable to be overlooked, particularly if the methods of diagnosis rely heavily on reports by others (Anderson et al, 1987). Complaints are typically tenseness, fears, worries, unhappiness, physical symptoms, and feeling inferior and/or rejected. Though it has been said that, apart from monosymptomatic phobias, these problems tend to pass with time and to have relatively few implications for the psychopathology of adult life (Kohlberg et al., 1972; Thomas, 1979; Robins, 1979), there is now reason to doubt the validity of this conclusion (Gittelman, 1986). As Weiner (1982) has noted, a good recovery rate is not a perfect one, and residual problems may continue, if only at a subclinical level. Furthermore, appropriate treatment at the time the problems are manifest may bring about speedier recovery and reduce the amount and duration of distress to all involved. Thus, it is no surprise to find that the overwhelming majority of clinicians believe that such problems should and can be treated by psychotherapeutic methods (Koocher and Pedulla, 1977).

Any review of behavioral psychotherapy in anxiety disorders is beset by two major problems. The first is that most of the work has been done in nonclinical or subclinical samples (Strauss, 1987); therefore, it is hard to know what the implications are for those children and adolescents seen by mental health professionals. As Casey and Berman (1985) point out in their review of psychotherapies with children, the apparent superiority of behavioral methods may relate to just this sort of nonclinical sampling. The second is that, perhaps more than in any other area reviewed here, problems rather than disorders have been the focus. While this may be seen as a perverse tendency for behaviorists to swim against the taxonomic current, it has to be remembered that research into childhood anxiety disorders is surprisingly scanty and that *DSM-III* categories are largely unvalidated (Gittelman,

1986; Quay and La Greca, 1986; Strauss, 1987). Excellent reviews can be found in Morris and Kratochwill (1983), Wells and Vitulano (1984), Ollendick (1986), Carlson et al, (1986), and Strauss (1987).

Methods of Behavioral Treatment of Anxiety

Although the respondent, Pavlovian, or passive conditioning model often fits anxiety better than any other model, methods have not been as dominated by it as has the adult area. Instead, several approaches, well described in the reviews above, are used, often in combination.

Systematic desensitization is the graduated exposure, in fact or in imagination, to the feared/phobic object(s) in the context of incompatible or attenuating procedures such as relaxation or the comforting presence of a trusted other.

Implosion (flooding), by far the most rapid and cost/effective method used in adults, has understandably found little enthusiasm in those who work with children, though it has been used occasionally (Strauss, 1987).

Operant derivatives seek to identify and modify the factors that elicit, contribute to, or maintain the maladaptive anxiety-related behavior (Siegel and Ridley-Johnson, 1985) through stimulus-control, as in prompting and fading, behavior shaping, and/or contingency management, with strong incentives/rewards for mastery of anxiety.

Social learning, primarily modeling using adults or peers either in person or on videos, to show mastery over the feared object/situation has understandably been prominent. Not surprisingly, research suggests that models who show initial anxiety and reluctance are likely to be more successful than those who "don't turn a hair" (Thelen et al., 1979).

Cognitive methods embody a more general strategy of self-control that aims to help individuals become their own therapists by learning specific responses, mostly self-exhortation and self-reassurance. Hopefully, the methods will modify maladaptive responses in the stressful situation. Where the child or adolescent lacks specific skill for mastery, these will be taught.

While success has been claimed with all these methods and with most areas, reviewers all express concern about the lack of well-designed studies and have to conclude that although behavior therapy looks promising, it cannot yet be endorsed without qualification.

Specific Anxiety Disorders

Simple phobias and fears. Most work with anxiety in children has been done in the area of simple phobias and fears, but it is also the least clearly clinical area, since many of the children do not have anything other than simple fears. Davison and

Neale (1986) have noted that clinicians have, by and large, built upon traditional folk wisdom. Exposure (i.e., extinction) is generally agreed to be the most effective method of treatment, and parents are encouraged to expose the child gradually while assisting in various ways to help the child inhibit anxiety and prevent that mortal enemy of successful management of anxiety, avoiding or escaping from the feared situation. Obviously, this is how most parents teach their children confidence intuitively, and only the failures come to clinicians. It is not surprising either that clinicians, in turn, claim great success in treating fears with behavioral methods (see reviews cited above and Morris and Kratochwill, 1983).

Separation anxiety disorder and school phobia. School refusal can be readily found in the behavioral literature as a discrete problem. Even though *DSM-III-R* eschews the term school *phobia* in favor of diagnosis of the causal disorder, separation anxiety disorder is usually considered to be the most important. Separation anxiety and school refusal come in two forms (Kennedy, 1965), roughly coinciding with before and after adolescence. In the first, the problem is simple, often acute, and the families are often healthier. These are easily treated by forced separation procedures (Kennedy, 1965; Yates, 1970; Baker and Willis, 1978), such as leaving the child with other than the attachment figure or firmly sending the child back to school, though most other methods, such as systematic desensitization, have been used (e.g., Lazarus and Abramovitz, 1962; Morris and Kratochwill, 1983; Ollendick, 1986; Strauss, 1987).

Later childhood and adolescence seem to bring a far more pervasive and difficult school phobia, which may derive from separation anxiety only in part. In fact, Kennedy (1965) some time ago referred to this as "way-of-life phobia" and it may well have more in common with avoidant disorder/personality and agoraphobia than separation anxiety disorder, even though the ticket of entry is usually school refusal. This crippling disorder has been poorly studied and evidence to support effective treatment is lacking.

Obsessive compulsive disorder. While many adults with obsessive compulsive disorder report that their first episode occurred in childhood or adolescence, they also report that usually no clinical contact occurred. Evidence as to how many children/adolescents with obsessive compulsive attacks or symptoms before maturity go on to develop the adult disorder is gravely deficient, and what there is raises serious doubts about any inexorability (Berg et al., 1986; Rapoport, 1986). None of the reviews cited above addresses the behavioral treatment of this disorder in children or adolescents specifically. One way to extrapolate is to suggest that the techniques used in other anxiety disorders should be helpful, but the literature in adults supports this contention only with a very few techniques (Emmelkamp, 1986). In any case, Berg et al. (1986) query whether many obsessions/compulsions before adulthood should even be regarded as an anxiety disorder. A more viable extrapolation is to suggest that the standard behavioral methods used in adults with obsessive compulsive disorders should be applicable to children and adolescents. These adult techniques are based primarily on response prevention, which is far easier to apply, and they are more effective with compulsions than with obsessions without compulsions (*thought stopping*) (Emmelkamp, 1986). Cognitive behavioral methods are in their infancy and so cannot be evaluated, but McFall and Wollersheim (1982) have employed a method in adolescents that uses self-instruction to challenge obsessions. There are others also.

Behavior therapy for anxiety disorders has been most successful in nonclinical populations and for relatively minor fears and phobias. Good evaluative studies of its use in other areas are lacking, but there are some promising techniques and initial indications. Behavior therapy research accurately reflects the underdeveloped state of the field of anxiety disorders in childhood and adolescence, including problems associated with the undemonstrated validity of the *DSM-III-R* diagnoses (Quay and LaGreca, 1986; Stauss, 1987).

Eating Disorders and Obesity

Disorders of Infancy and Early Childhood

Those eating disorders affecting infants and toddlers include rumination, pica, and food fads. All of these have been the subject of behavioral interventions, mostly within the operant/contingency management approach. There is little systematic literature—most reports are only case studies (Winton and Singh, 1983; Starrin and Fuqua, 1987). While success has been claimed (case studies seldom are negative, perhaps because of publication trends), Winton and Singh (1983) suggest that for the best-studied disorder, rumination, there is little to indicate what treatment is most effective. Food fads may be best viewed as part of the general class of oppositional behavior that is dealt with above. More details of the state of and types of behavior therapy in these disorders can be found in the detailed critical review by Starin and Fuqua (1987); although it addresses the developmentally disabled, it has clear implications for and utility in normal infants.

Anorexia Nervosa and Bulimia

Anorexia nervosa and bulimia did not merit mention in 1967 (Werry and Wollersheim, 1967). There can be little doubt that these two disorders have become much more prominent, even faddish, in the past decade or so. In his review, Hsu (1986) defines three different treatment objectives in anorexia: treatment of physical complications; weight restoration; and attitudinal change. Most of the behavioral literature has focused on weight gain, possibly because it provides a simple explicit goal that fits well with the zeitgeist of behavior therapy. The core of the behavioral approach, which Hsu claims has been widely adopted, is the operant one of control of privileges (including the powerful ones of visitors and physical activity) that are contingent on weight gain. However, there is usually a large cognitive behavioral component as well—planning around objectives, diet, routines, etc.—with frequent feedback. Some therapists have added anxiety-control methods such as desensitization (e.g., Ollendick, 1986). As with other treatment methods, there are claims of success in the majority of patients—as far as significant weight gain is concerned.

There are few studies of comparative behavioral approaches (e.g., lenient vs restrictive programs) and those that exist, like those that compare behavioral with other approaches, do not support the hypothesis that any method is superior to any other (Hsu, 1986; Harris and Phelps, 1987). This leads to the uncomfortable possibilities that either everyone is doing the same thing (Hsu defines eight principles common to all treatments) or that anorexia runs its own course independently. The latter possibility is somewhat discounted by controlled studies showing that weight gain can be influenced directly be behavioral methods, though such controlled studies numbered only five of a total of 32 in the review by Harris and Phelps (1987).

While successful in weight restoration in a large majority of cases, behavioral methods have had far less success in weight *maintenance* (Harris and Phelps, 1987). This problem is not peculiar to behavioral methods, however, (Hsu, 1986). There is general recognition that various personality and attitudinal changes are necessary for weight maintenance, and these, so far, have been poorly addressed by behavioral methods. Most behavior therapists, like all good clinicians, spend a lot of time working with their patients on these problems. A recent study by Hall and Crisp (1987) suggests psychotherapy may be better in this area, though it is less successful than dietary-focused advice in weight gain. If so, there is a glimmer of hope that all treatments may not in fact be equivalent but indeed have specific effects and different roles.

Bulimia is only of relatively recent interest and tends to affect an older age group (16 to 24 years) than anorexia (Harris and Phelps, 1987). It can be associated with anorexia but is usually not. Reviews (Huon and Brown, 1984; Hsu, 1986; Harris and Phelps, 1987) suggest that while behavior methods—mostly of a cognitive nature as would be expected in usually older and self-referred patients—have been used, and success has been claimed (e.g., Fairburn, 1981; Lacey, 1983; Leitenberg et al., 1984), much more work is needed to define efficacy and relevance.

Obesity

While obesity is not a true eating disorder in that overeating is not necessarily a feature after it is well-established (Werry, 1986), it is convenient to group it with anorexia and bulimia. Its management objectives are qualitatively similar, just polar opposites—to create a state of (negative) energy balance by restricting food intake and increasing physical activity. It is only recently that increased activity has become generally recognized as being as important as restricting calories (Spence, 1986; Foreyt and Cousins, 1987). Behavioral methods (Wells and Copeland, 1985) are similar to those used in anorexia, except that hospitalization is less often invoked, which means that parents have had to be more often involved right from the start. The poor results from early studies (Spence, 1986), which used primarily operant methods focused on weight loss, have led to the addition of cognitive methods aimed at eating habits and situations and activity level. Many obese children are rejected by peers (but by no means in all sociocultural groups—see Kaplan and Wadden [1986]). They also lack social skills and may have a very poor self-image (Korsch, 1986). Hence, attention is usually given to these areas, too (Foreyt and Cousins, 1987). Attempts have been made, especially with adolescents, to use modeling and social pressure through groups methods, some operating in school. One interesting result of parental involvement is that parents were found to lose weight too. This was often to the detriment of weight loss in their adolescent children, who did better treated apart (Brownwell et al., 1983). While behavioral programs have had some success, it has been only modest in degree and good studies are not numerous (Wells and Copeland, 1985; Spence, 1986). The same remarks could, of course, be made about all approaches to obesity (Brownwell et al., 1983; Korsch, 1986).

Tic Disorders

As Werry and Wollersheim's 1967 review shows, tic disorders were among the first disorders to be treated by behavioral methods. This may have been because of the ease with which tics can be measured and counted, something which has always appealed to behaviorists. Methods were respondent at first, then operant, then cognitive, and finally became multimodal. Not surprisingly, the application of behavioral methods to Tourette's disorder has risen in frequency with increased recognition of the disorder.

In their comprehensive review, Azrin and Peterson (in press) found 31 studies of behavioral treatment in Tourette's syndrome, and the methods of treatment seemed to resemble those reported for tics. Massed practice (i.e., voluntarily performing the tic) achieved about a 50% reduction in 50% of cases, which is similar to that for tics in general. Contingency management, especially positive reinforcement for not twitching, was reasonably effective in children but was generally only one component of treatment in most studies and very difficult to evaluate. Teaching incompatible behaviors, primarily relaxation, achieved only temporary relief, whereas self-monitoring seemed quite effective in the few children in which it was tried.

Habit reversal, a composite technique developed by Azrin and Peterson (in press), uses a combination of incompatible, competing, active motor behaviors, cognitive procedures, and relaxation and is described as "highly successful."

Review of behavioral treatment of tics (Azrin and Peterson, in press; Turpin, 1983) shows results similar to those achieved with Tourette's syndrome, i.e., modest success from most methods. In one comparative study, however, habit reversal was found to be outstandingly successful, much more so than massed practice (Azrin et al., 1980). This latter study is also unique in that it is one of the very few in Tourette's and/or tic disorders that involved more than one or two subjects.

In summary, Azrin's multimethod habit reversal technique may hold substantial promise for the treatment of Tourette's and tic disorders but requires further evaluation, especially in children, where it may not be so easy to apply.

Elimination Disorders

Enuresis

The alarm, bed buzzer, or conditioning treatment of enuresis had already established itself as the most effective of any in 1967, and the subsequent two decades have merely confirmed its success (Doleys, 1977; Dische et al., 1983). Perhaps because of this, interest has waned somewhat, though the use of electrodes in sanitary pads adherent to the child's pants has greatly improved the apparatus and made it more child- and less bed-bound. There are still a significant number of failures and relapses after successful treatment (Doleys, 1977; Dische et al., 1983), however, and the loss of interest in additional research is hardly justified. Efforts to improve success rates have focused partly on intensifying the program in the so called dry bed approach, which required overloading the bladder to produce frequent wetting and resetting an alarm and reloading the bladder every time wetting occurs. This has not proved superior to the standard, much more simple program and can engender considerable resistance (Bollard, 1982; Berg, in press). It is now recognized that many failures are due to poor motivation, disorganization, and psychopathology in child or parent (Dische et al., 1983), so that most other developments have been aimed at these problems. In view of the proved efficacy and practicality of the bed buzzer (Doleys, 1977; Dische et al., 1983), it is surprising how few mental health professionals seem to use it.

The value of the alarm in diurnal enuresis has also been demonstrated, although a comparative study suggested its value is more as a reminder to go to the toilet than as a true operant contingency to wetting itself (Berg, in press). Other methods include bladder training in which the child is loaded up with fluid and then taught to practice increasing the time and volume of urine passed. This technique is successful in achieving its immediate objectives and possibly may be helpful in diurnal enuresis. It is without effect on nocturnal enuresis (Doleys, 1977), although using it in conjunction with the alarm in the minority of enuretic children who also have a small bladder capacity may have some value (Berg, in press).

Operant methods such as star charts and other rewards probably have little value beyond that of placebo but may be useful to maintain motivation when used with the bed buzzer. Their drawback is that they may convey the impression that the child can control the wetting if enough effort is made.

Encopresis

Encopresis is a very disabling and not uncommon disorder in children (Werry, 1986). Although behaviorists (as well as others) have written freely on this disorder, claiming great success for each particular method, there is a conspicuous dearth of proper clinical trials. Consequently, it is impossible to properly evaluate the value of behavioral or any other treatment in the disorder (Werry, 1986). One controlled study (Berg et al., 1983) did show that laxatives added nothing to a behavioral program, but since there was no untreated or other-treated group, this tells little of the efficacy of the behavioral program itself.

Speech Disorders

See Developmental Disorders subsection, *Language and Speech Disorders.*

Other Disorders-Stereotypy/Habit Disorders

Stereotypy/habit disorders have been discussed to some degree under autism and mental retardation, where they are frequent and may be mutilating or life-threatening, justifying heroic techniques in some cases (Ollendick, 1986). This is seldom, if ever, the case in normal children whose stereotypies such as rocking, thumb-sucking, head-banging, and slavish attachment to cuddly toys or blankets are minor annoyances to parents. Most such stereotypies disappear before age 5 (Werry et al., 1983). There are few good studies on how to deal with normal children's habits, despite the fact that, while they are of concern in only a small percentage of the population, the number of children affected are considerably higher than those who are autistic/mentally retarded. The persistent undesirable habits likely to need treatment are public genital self-stimulation, nail-biting, severe head-banging, or thumb-sucking (which some believe may cause orthodontic problems [Werry et al. 1983; Christensen and Sanders, 1987]). There is no reason to suppose that these stereotypies would respond any differently to behavior therapy with normal children than with autistic or mentally retarded children. There, successful methods have included developing alternative incompatible behaviors offering the same kind of sensory stimulation as the stereotypy and contingency management techniques, including punishments ranging from reprimand to overcorrection and, occasionally, physical means (but see Harris and Handelman [1987] for "creative alternatives to punishment"). The reviews by LaGrow and Repp (1984) and Whitman and Johnston (1987) cover this area in more detail.

One habit that is fairly typical of the group and illustrates the techniques is thumb-sucking; it is worth discussing in more detail because there are more data. In particular, a study by Christensen and Sanders (1987) models how treatment should be evaluated, addressing not only comparative efficacy but also generalization and durability. Two techniques have predominated in the management of thumb-sucking. One is operant, primarily contingency management (escalating reinforcement for not sucking) and the other is Azrin et al.'s (1980) habit reversal (see tics above). Christensen and Sanders (1987) showed that both techniques were superior to no treatment and that improvement was substantial, generalized across environments, and sustained, although not complete. Parents preferred habit reversal, probably because it generates less oppositional behavior than the more directive differential reinforcement of other incompatible behaviors.

Organic Disorders

Those organic disorders of greatest interest here are not the life-threatening acute ones such as deliria but those that result in residual disability and psychopathology after nonprogressive, nonfatal brain disorders. The most important affecting children are due to malformations/genetic disorders, perinatal anoxia, and (for adolescents) head injury. There is nothing specific to brain injury in the behavioral procedures used, which apply to similar types of symptoms whatever the cause. For example, when the residue is primarily cognitive/intellectual, the behavioral methods most applicable are those described under mental retardation and specific academic skill disorders. When the problems are behavioral or affective, the methods for externalizing disorders or anxiety would be most appropriate. A clinical example is provided by McCabe and Green (1987), who describe the treatment of three head injured adolescents in which behavior therapy, primarily contingency management, was used mainly for impulsive, aggresive behavior that was making other rehabilitative treatment difficult.

Schizophrenia

Schizophrenia is rare before puberty, and, although interest is growing, there is remarkably little about adolescent schizophrenia per se (Prior and Werry, 1986). There is, however, a significant literature on the behavioral treatment of schizophrenia in adults with some substantial benefits shown for isolated, disabling symptoms and less, certainly, for general rehabilitation and community management (e.g., Falloon et al., 1982). In 1983 the American Academy of Child Psychiatry recognized the need for child and adolescent psychiatrists to accord serious psychiatric disorder a high priority; it is hoped that studies of behavioral methods developed in adults will begin to be studied in adolescents with schizophrenia. Also important is the area of children and adolescents at risk for schizophrenia, and it is possible that this active area of research (Prior and Werry, 1986) will yield important behavioral intervention programs derived from behavioral technologies of stress management and social skills training described elsewhere in this review.

Mood Disorders

Mood disorders are not given a specific category for children and adolescents in *DSM-III-R*. With only minor modifications, they are classified with, and by the same criteria as, the adult disorders. The diagnostic criteria for depression and mania are still somewhat controversial in children and, to a lesser extent, in adolescents (Graham, 1974; Lefkowitz and Burton, 1978; Quay and LaGreca, 1986; Pataki and Carlson, in press), but there is general agreement that depression does occur in children and mania and depression occur in adolescents. The controversy about prevalence and treatment and relationship to adult forms is much more substantial (Graham, 1974; Anderson et al., 1987; Pataki and Carlson, in press). Another problem is the rarity with which depression occurs in isolation. Children with depression often show several other *DSM-III-R* disorders (Anderson et al., 1987) and will appear to be miserable, oppositional, unsuccessful, unlucky children.

Unlike prevalence and diagnosis, treatment of children with mood disorders has received little systematic attention, particularly with respect to nonpharmacological methods. Kaslow and Rehm (1985) recommend that if depressed children show symptoms associated with other disorders (e.g., school phobia, enuresis, hyperactivity, disruptive problems, poor social skills), and if these disorders seem primary, then treatment should focus on the primary disorders rather than the depression (which may then remit as a consequence). If the depression is primary, then it should receive attention. However, reports of behavioral treatment of depression in children and adolescents are infrequent (Kolko, 1987). Thus, we must turn to the adult literature to see what are the prospects, if any, for children and adolescents.

Behavioral treatment for depressed adults has been shown to be effective and with few side effects (Emmelkamp, 1986; O'Leary and Wilson, 1987), although Emmelkamp is careful to specify mild to moderate depression. The procedures are derived from different behavioral models of depression. Some are operant and encourage patients to engage in behaviors more likely to bring positive reinforcement (Lewinsohn et al., 1982); some (perhaps most) are cognitive, designed to change pessimistic views of oneself and the world (Beck, 1976); others involve composite self-control techniques such as self-monitoring, self-evaluation, and self-reinforcement (Rehm, 1981). These techniques appear most promising for adolescents but their application in children requires tailoring them to their cognitive level. Efforts so far have been only preliminary (Kolko, 1987).

So far, mania seems to have escaped behavior therapy, for adults and children, and the mainstay remains pharmacological.

Behavioral methods have had a role in the treatment of depression in adults, and, although effort so far has been minimal, there is no good reason that the methods could not be adapted for children and adolescents. No one behavioral method is clearly more effective than any other (Emmelkamp, 1986), and there are strong resemblances to other kinds of psychotherapy. Perhaps behavior therapists are not considering depression in the *DSM-III* sense, where most psychiatrists would want to try pharmacotherapy first. Perhaps they are interpreting depression to mean depressive symptoms and/or personality traits, not an acutely-onsetting, time-limited disorder with strict, rather severe, criteria.

Psychoactive Substance Disorders

Normal Substance Use in Children and Adolescents

There is enormous public concern with both grossly abnormal uses of legal drugs such as alcohol and use of illegal substances such as cannabis, cocaine, hallucinogens, and so on. But the long-term health risks of *any* use of tobacco and alcohol, to say nothing of the short-term risks of mortality and morbidity in adolescence from alcohol-related motor vehicle accidents, makes health professionals interested in ways to prevent children and adolescents from starting to use these two substances. Behavioral programs of this nature will be discussed below, since they are variations on strategies for prevention of drug abuse in general.

Substance Disorders

Abuse and dependency. Both abuse and dependency are of great interest, but acute intoxication (with alcohol) is much more serious in terms of immediate threat to life and limb in adolescence because of its involvement in motor vehicle accidents.

Alcohol/drug dependency affects only a minority of children and adolescents and the percentage involved with illegal drugs has been declining since about 1978 (see Horan and Straus, 1987). Alcohol abuse/dependency and tobacco dependency dwarf all other drug problems, though it cannot be said that in the United States, stimulant (including cocaine), opiate, and other illegal drug uses are insignificant—just that they attract a disproportionate degree of public attention.

Treatment programs for alcohol and drug abusing adolescents are said to be reasonably successful (Dishion et al., in press)—in the two-thirds who remain in the programs—but most adolescents with such problems are never seen and the dropouts are likely to be the most severely affected. Some programs are so restrictive that it is a wonder they get any adolescents at all (Horan and Straus, 1987). Although most programs have rather pragmatic approaches, behavioral principles are often prominent: decreasing immediate reinforcing properties of the substance (through antabuse, methadone, aversive smoking); reinforcing abstinence; teaching alternative successful social behaviors; social learning by modeling from high status, nonabusing peers; and cognitive behavioral approaches such as self-help, self-programming, etc. (Horan and Straus, 1987). While there are promising leads, skeptics would require better evidence of a durable effect than is presently offered.

Preventive programs. Preventive programs are popular and numerous for illegal drugs, but tobacco is attracting increasing attention. Only a handful of the programs offer an interpretable evaluation, and few or none use drug *use* (as opposed to *information* about drugs) as their outcome criterion or assess long-term evaluation. It is possible to say only that there are promising leads, many of them behavioral, but no proven methods (Peterson and Roberts, 1986; Horan and Straus, 1987).

The uncertain or indifferent results of focused programs and the fact that all forms of drug use and abuse are part of a more general pattern of maladaptation and unsuccessfulness among young people have led to attempts to identify what these behavioral patterns are and the factors that lead to them. Primary (though not alone) among these are conduct disorders/behaviors (Jessor and Jessor, 1975; Dishion et al., in press), and among the processes causing them, parenting styles (Dishion et al., in press). Peer models are also very important, but these do not assume their role until late childhood or adolescence when, in the view of Dishion et al., it is already too late to bring about effective preventive programs.

Dishion et al. (in press) argue for a strategy that begins in childhood and that capitalizes on the research, such as that by Patterson and coworkers (Patterson, 1982) (see also Wells and Forehand, 1985), showing what causes and cures the prodromal behaviors of aggressiveness, oppositional-defiances, and antisocial acts. Because only a minority of children are at serious risk, it is not efficient to aim such programs at the entire population. Dishion et al. (in press) propose a "three gate" model. In the first, teachers screen the entire child population and those children who display risk behaviors at school are identified. These children are then subject to an additional screening by a parent (telephone) report, and those identified by both screens then have a third screen, a structured child and family interview. While the above screening has been used by Patterson and the Oregon Social Learning Center group successfully to identify and treat children with conduct type problems (largely through changing parenting styles along dimensions of discipline, monitoring, positive reinforcement, problem solving, and involvement), it is not empirical demonstration but logical deduction that suggests such strategies may be successful in preventing alcohol, tobacco, and drug abuse. It can be said that this approach is more "data driven" and logical than most other preventive programs, even though doubts remain about success with more severe conduct disorders, with disorganized families, and in the longer term.

Behavioral methods figure large in the treatment and prevention of substance use and disorders and offer promise, but firm proof of their value is awaited.

Somatoform and Dissociative Disorders

Despite a substantial adult literature devoted to somatoform, especially pain disorder, studies in children and adolescents are surprisingly sparse (Goodyer, 1981; Volkmar et al., 1984; Werry, 1986; Williamson et al., 1987). It is not unexpected to find that behavioral studies of child and adolescent treatment are even fewer, mostly single case studies of isolated symptoms such as blindness, limping, aphonia, abdominal pain, etc. treated primarily by operant methods (contingency management) (Williamson et al., 1987). There are a few controlled studies, however, some with large groups of children, of the management of headache. All use a variant of progressive relaxation combined with biofeedback called *autogenic training*. Andrasik et al. (Williamson et al., 1987) and Labbe and Williamson (1984) found a reasonably durable, significant clinical improvement in 80% of children and adolescents, while untreated controls showed little change. Larsson et al. (1982) confirmed the value of relaxation in adolescents and found in addition, that it could be self-taught with tapes and a manual, as well as at school, just as effectively as by a therapist.

In summary, the frequency and medical importance of these disorders is not matched by studies of their treatment of any kind, though there is reason to believe that behavioral methods could be quite effective. Only headache has received any serious attention, where behavior therapy has been shown to be clearly worthwhile.

Sleep Disorders

Sleep disorders are frequent in children before 2 years and common before age 5; they cause a great deal of parental distress and conflict (Richman et al., 1985; Werry, 1986). Because of their clear association with child and family psychopathology, they are of interest to mental health professionals. The more common disorders are resisting going to bed and/or settling down to sleep and, most troublesome, nightwaking. None fits well into any category of sleep disorder as classified in *DSM-III-R*. Etiology is poorly understood, though. In a view held by many professionals but few parents, Richman et al. (1985) postulated nightwaking to be failure to learn to settle while alone, prolonged by reinforcement through parental concern and attention, rather than anxiety or not needing continuous sleep. There is little doubt that behavioral methods are widely employed (Seymour et al., 1982; Clements et al., 1986), but there are few systematic studies of their efficacy (Richman et al., 1985). Richman et al. (1985) used an approach based on operant methods of contingency management (withdrawing attention for waking and giving it for staying quiet/ asleep) and some shaping of appropriate bedtime behaviors. Emphasis was put on careful assessment, individualization of treatment, and shaping rather than the more draconion flooding technique of "let the child cry" (Seymour et al., 1982). In Seymour et al.'s (1982) study of 35 children, most achieved complete or marked and durable improvement in six or fewer treatments. However, the study was uncontrolled and the children and parents were a well-motivated, mentally healthy group. A number of techniques developed in adults (Richman et al., 1985; Clements et al., 1986), such as relaxation, paradoxical intention (trying to stay awake), might be suitable for older children and adolescents, less than 10% of whom have significant sleep problems (Simonds and Parraga, 1982), a figure well below that of infants and toddlers (Werry, 1986).

Psychological Factors Affecting Physical Conditions

Along with the somatoform and allied disorders, psychosomatics is burgeoning and is now known as behavioral medicine. As the name suggests, it is largely dominated by behaviorally oriented psychologists and boasts a journal and a society of its own. Behavioral medicine is also concerned with prevention and health promotion. This concern is filtering down to pediatrics, enough to make it impossible to do other than indicate where to find more information and make some summary statements. Certain disorders of long-standing interest to child psychiatry, because of their frequency, chronicity, disability, and problems of compliance with medical treatment for chronic illnesses such as asthma, diabetes, eczema, and epilepsy, seem to have attracted the most attention from behavior therapists (Balaschak and Mostofsky, 1981; Melamed and Johnson, 1981; Williamson et al., 1987). There has been emphasis on cognitive approaches of self-recording, understanding of the illness/treatment, and stress management. However, there is an absence of good studies by which to evaluate the value of behavioral treatment. In the area of prevention/health promotion, a number of programs aimed at nutrition, dental care, and smoking, again largely cognitive, have been described by Peterson and Roberts (1986), but evaluation of these programs is sketchy.

In summary, in this most important area of behavioral medicine, it is again disappointing to find that single case studies, enthusiasm, and description dominate over hard data by which to evaluate the worth of behavior therapy. However, this is not confined to behavior therapy, as is shown by the thoughtful review of intervention in the psychosocial consequences of childhood cancer by Van Dongen-Melman and Sanders-Woudstra (1986).

CONCLUSIONS

In 1967, Werry and Wollersheim described the distinguishing features of behavior therapy as: functional and empirical orientation; adherence to learning theory; and active, systematic manipulation of the behavior of the patient, family, and therapist. These features are still clearly evident, but behavior therapy has some newer dimensions, most conspicuously a concern with internal process in the cognitive-behavioral approach. The latter should make it more acceptable to those who tended to dismiss it in 1967 as simplistic, denying the complexity of human behavior (as opposed to animal behavior). Nevertheless, behavior therapy is still basically a reductionistic approach with a deep suspicion of what it cannot see, objectify, measure, or treat strictly as an intervening variable. However, anyone who watches behavior therapists at work or reads their case studies knows that behavior therapy explains only part of what goes on and that variables that are essential to engage and keep patients in any therapy are equally integral to it, if seldom described.

Behavior therapy has grown and is thriving; many references are new reviews of substantial numbers of studies in small areas rather than the studies themselves. However, this growth would seem not to have been at the expense of traditional insight or more subjective treatments. For example, family therapy, which started at approximately the same time, flourishes as well. It is therefore appropriate to ask once again "where the proper place for behavior therapy lies among the *therapies* of child [and adolescent] psychopathology" (Werry and Wollersheim, 1967; p. 365). Werry and Wollersheim (1967) suggested that behavior therapy was the treatment of choice for isolated or isolatable symptoms, where the consumer prefers a symptom-oriented approach, where clinical conditions such as chronological or mental age or lack of insight require a simple approach, and where trained therapists are scarce and it is necessary to use untrained caregivers such as parent, nurses, or teachers to do the treatment. None of these indications appears to have changed, but the sophistication of behavior therapy has been growing and it is now more difficult to say where its real limits are and to explain why one should choose another modality in preference. For example, it cannot any longer be said that insight is beyond behavior therapy, though psychoanalysts may criticize the superficiality of what cognitive behavior therapists call self-control, self-monitoring, and so on. Neither is working with the whole family nor a systems approach, as the work of Patterson (1982) shows. Conversely, some of the above specificities of behavior therapy have also been eroded to some degree, i.e., most other psychotherapies favor problem-oriented approaches (Garfield and Bergin, 1986; Kovacs and Paulauskas, 1986). There is the unpalatable and often denied fact that untrained therapists do as well as trained ones in psychotherapy (Berman and Norton, 1985), so this apparent difference from behavior therapy is also questionable. There are some other differences between behavior therapy and other psychotherapies, too; there are few graphs of the type that abound in behavior therapy articles found in family or individual psychotherapy journals. Though behavior therapy has retained emphasis on measuring both process and outcome, the authors cannot accept that this is a *necessary* distinction from other therapies. It is true that the simplistic conceptualization of the behavioral approach does lend itself rather better to measurement than other approaches. However, parents, teachers, and children have little difficulty in stating precisely what problems they have and want fixed, although they may not agree among themselves as to what these problems are or which should have priority (Anderson et al., 1987). Surely, lack of evaluating is one of the less defensible aspects of nonbehavioral therapies (Casey and Berman, 1985; Kovacs and Paulauskas, 1986). Assertion and charisma are poor ways to establish efficacy in a professional field.

One disappointing aspect of behavior therapy over the past 20 years is its tendency to be almost as profession-bound as it was in 1967 (e.g., Andrews and Hadzi-Pavlovic, 1988). While most child psychiatrists may have heard of behavior therapy and often recommend it for problems such as the refeeding phase of treatment in anorexia (Hsu, 1987), they would usually turn to psychologists to plan and execute the therapy. This would be quite legitimate if delegation were based on lack of time and/or cost, restricting child psychiatrists to diagnosis, consultation, or treatments such as pharmacotherapy that require a medical license, but the authors believe these do not prevent the direct use of behavior therapy by child psychiatrists. Instead, tradition seems to favor other forms of psychotherapy. As a profession that is ostensibly rooted in science, child psychiatry cannot easily explain away its seeming preference for traditional forms of psychotherapy, particularly when the behavioral approach has been so clearly more fulfilling of the fundamental ethos of medicine, which requires proof of efficacy and safety before promulgation. This is a challenge for directors of training in child psychiatry.

Perhaps, then, these issues of specificities should be left and other questions raised. First, is behavior therapy more cost-effective, and if so, for what disorders/problems? These questions are not easy to answer, partly because of the reluctance of nonbehavioral therapies to provide evaluative data on children and adolescents (Casey and Berman, 1985; Kovacs and Paulauskas, 1986). For example, only a handful of the 80-odd acceptable studies reviewed by Casey and Berman (1985) were other than behavioral. What data there are, nearly all from adults, does not sustain the hypothesis that there are remarkable differences in efficacy across treatments, although there is evidence that behavioral methods are superior for *discrete problems* such as phobias or enuresis (Casey and Berman, 1985; Lambet et al., 1986; Doleys, 1977). This lack of a clear overall advantage, especially in more global areas of function, causes behavior therapists great distress as they try to explain away the results. In his presidential address to the Association for the Advancement of Behavior Therapy, Agras (1987) pointed out the flawed methodology in most comparative data and, in his view, the logical ridiculousness of the now popular meta-analysis that pools data across very different studies. One is reminded of a similar outcry 30 years ago when Levitt (1957) claimed to show that psychotherapy with children was no better than spontaneous remission without treatment. However, just as it now seems that Levitt was wrong (Casey and Berman, 1985; Kovacs and Paulauskas, 1986), so it may well prove with the current apparent lack of advantage to behavior therapy.

A rather more telling point in favor of behavior therapy is that there are a number of problems/disorders where it is impossible to determine whether any other treatment is as good as behavioral methods because the results are unchallenged by any comparable data on other psychotherapies (for example, tics, habits, stereotypies, self-mutilation, ADHD, and so on). What should the honest therapist then advise parents? In medicine, the position would usually be to advise taking the treatment that has demonstrated its efficacy and safety and to resort to the others only if the proven treatment should fail. How many child psychiatrists would be equal to this ethical challenge?

Behavior therapy with children is not without its problems, however, some of which are clear from this review and some enuciated by critics from within the disipline. One of the latter is Ollendick (1986) who raises the issue of effectiveness. While behavior therapy has been conscientious about evaluation, much of the data are derived from single case studies and imperfectly or poorly executed designs. In general, these studies have not shown that any improvement was specifically due to treatment rather than to placebo or expectancy effects or to the mere passage of time. Fortunately, the number of such studies is decreasing relative to good studies (Agras, 1987). A second problem noted by Ollendick (1986) is that of maintenance of improvement with time and its generalizability outside the narrow situation in which the treatment is often done. Most studies cannot shed light on these two issues. There is the problem of outcome measures, as well, which Ollendick, like Casey and Berman (1985), sees as often narrow, trivial, or ignoring of system effects. Ollendick (1986) also points to the problem of cost-effectiveness and the failure to move much beyond the traditional therapist-bound treatment that can never hope to reach more than a handful of the total of children and adolescents who need help.

To Ollendick's list could be added the important areas/disorders that have been largely neglected by behavior therapists, such as psychological factors affecting many physical illnesses, psychoses of adolescence, organic brain disorders, and so on. And last, there is still an irritating degree of zealotism and arrogance in some behavior therapists who would dismiss all nonbelievers as fools and charlatans. This pays little credence to the enormous complexity and severity of many of the problems that are brought to child psychiatrists and other mental health professionals. Often these problems are not sensible of a simple solution and call for multimodal, multidisciplinary approaches with limited goals. Finally, in defense of behavior therapy, it must be said that all the problems outlined above are present in all other psychotherapeutic approaches—only more so. It is a curious paradox that behavior therapy, which recoils at the concept of insight, may, in fact, have considerably more insight into its own shortcomings.

REFERENCES

Abikoff, H. (1987), An evaluation of cognitive behavior therapy for hyperactive children. In: B. B. Lahey & A. E. Kazdin, (Eds.), *Advances in clinical child psychology*, (Vol. 10), ed. B. B. Lahey & A.E. Kazdin. New York: Plenum Press, pp. 171–216.

Agras, W. S. (1987), Presidential address: so where do we go from here? *Behavior Therapy*, 18:203–217.

American Academy of Child Psychiatry, (1983), *Child psychiatry: a plan for the coming decades*. Washington, D. C.: AACP, pp. 57–65.

Anderson, J. C., Williams, J. McGee, R. & Silva, P. (1987), DSM-III disorders in preadolescent children. *Arch. Gen. Psychiatry*, 44:69–76.

Andrews, G. & Hadzi-Pavlovic, D. (1988), The work of Australian psychiatrists, circa 1986. *Aust. N. Z. J. Psychiatry*, 22:153–165.

Azrin, N. H., & Peterson, A. L. (in press), Behavior therapy for Tourette's Syndrome and tic disorders. In: *Tourette's and tic disorders: A treatment manual*. ed. D. J. Cohen, J. F. Leckman, & R. D. Brunn. Washington, D. C.: American Psychiatric Association Press.

_____ Nunn, R. G. & Frantz, S. E. (1980), Habit reversal versus negative practice treatment of nervous tics. *Behavior Therapy* 11:169–178.

Baker, H. & Willis, U. (1978), *School phobia: classification and treatment.* Br. J. Psychiatry, 132:492–499.

Balaschak, B. A. & Mostofsky, D. I. (1981), Seizure disorders. In: *Behavioral assessment of children's disorders*, ed. E. J. Mash & L. G. Terdal. New York: Guilford Press, pp. 601–637.

Bandura, A. (1969), *Principles of behavior modification*. New York: Holt, Rinehart & Winston.

_____ (1977), Self-efficacy: toward a unifying theory of behavioral change. *Psychol. Rev.*, 84:191–215.

Barkley, R. A. (1981), *Hyperactive children: a handbook for diagnosis and treatment*. New York: Guilford Press.

Baum, C. G. & Forehand, R. (1981), Long-term follow-up assessment of parent training by use of multiple outcome measures. *Behavior therapy*, 12:643–652.

Beck, A. T. (1967), *Depression: causes and treatment.* Philadelphia: University of Pennsylvania Press.

_____ (1976), *Cognitive therapy and the emotional disorders*. New York: International Universities Press.

Beitchman, J. H., Nair, R., Clegg, M., Ferguson, B. & Patel, P. G. (1986), Prevalence of psychiatric disorders in children with speech and language disorders. *J. Am. Acad. Child Psychiatry*, 25:528–535.

Berg, C., Zahn, T. P., Behar, D. & Rapoport, J. L. (1986), Childhood obsessive-compulsive disorder. In: *Anxiety disorders of childhood*, ed. R. Gittelman. New York: Guilford, pp. 126–135.

Berg, I. (in press), Elimination disorders. In: *Handbook of studies in child psychiatry*, ed. B. Tonge, G. D. Burrows & J. S. Werry. Amsterdam: Elsevier.

—— Forsythe, I., Holt, P. & Watts, J. (1983), A controlled trial of "Senokot" in faecal soiling treated by behavioural methods. *J. Child Psychol. Psychiatry*, 24:543–550.

Berman, J. S. & Norton, N.C. (1985), Does professional training make a therapist more effective? *Psychol. Bull.*, 98:401–404.

Bollard, J. (1982), A 2-year follow-up of bedwetters treated by dry bed training and standard conditioning. *Behav. Res. Ther.*, 20:571–580.

Bornstein, P. H. & Kazdin, A. E. (1985), *Handbook of clinical behavior therapy with children*. Homewood, Ill.: Dorsey Press.

Brown, R. T., Borden, K. A., Wynne, M. E., Schleser, R. & Clingerman, S. R. (1986), Methylphenidate and cognitive therapy with ADD children. *J. Abnorm. Child Psychol.*, 14:481–497.

Brownwell, K. D., Kelman, J. H. & Stunkard, A. J. (1983), Treatment of obese children with and without their mothers. *Pediatrics*, 71:515–523.

Carlson, C. L., Figueroa, R. G. & Lahey, B. B. (1986), Behavioral therapy for childhood anxiety disorders. In: *Anxiety disorders of childhood*, ed. R. Gittleman. New York: Guilford, pp. 204–232.

Casey, R. J. & Berman, J. S. (1985), The outcome of psychotherapy with children. *Psychol. Bull.*, 98:388–400.

Cass, L. k. & Thomas, C. B. (1979), *Childhood psychopathology and later adjustment*. New York: Wiley.

Christensen, A. P. & Sanders, M. (1987), Habit reversal and differential reinforcement of other behaviors in the treatment of thumbsucking. *J. Child Psychol. Psychiatry*, 28:281–295.

Christoff, K. A. & Myatt, R. J. (1987), Social isolation. In: *Behavior therapy with children and adolescents*, ed. M. Hersen & V. B. Van Hasselt, New York: Wiley, pp. 512–535.

Clements, J., Wing, L. & Dunn, G. (1986), Sleep problems in handicapped children—a preliminary study. *J. Child Psychol. Psychiatry*, 27:399–408.

Corbett, J. A. (1985), mental retardation—psychiatric aspects. In: *Child and adolescent psychiatry—modern approaches, (2nd Ed.)*, ed. M. Rutter & L. Hersov, Oxford: Blackwell, pp. 661–678.

Davison, G. C. & Neale, J. M. (1986), *Abnormal psychology: an experimental clinical approach*. New York: Wiley.

Devany, J. M. & Nelson, R. O. (1986), Behavioral approaches to treatment. In: *Psychopathological disorders of childhood* (3rd ed.), ed. H. C. Quay & J. S. Werry. New York: Wiley, pp. 523–559.

DiLorenzo, T. M. & Matson, J. L. (1987), Stuttering. In: *Behavior therapy with children and adolescents*, ed. M. Hersen & V. B. Van Hasselt. New York: Wiley, pp. 263–278.

Dische,. S., Yule, W., Corbett, J. & Hand, D. (1983), Childhood nocturnal enuresis. *Dev. Med. Child Neurol.*, 25:67–80.

Dishion, T. J., Reid, J. B. & Patterson, G. R. (in press), Empirical guidelines for a family intervention for adolescent drug use. In: *The family context of adolescent drug use*, ed. R. H. Coombs. New York: Haworth Press.

Doleys, D. M. (1977), Behavioral treatments for nocturnal enuresis in children. *Psychol. Bull.*, 84:30–54.

Douglas, V. I. (1972), Stop, look and listen: the problem of sustained attention and impulse control in hyperactive children. *Canadian Journal of Behavioural Science*, 4:259–276.

Ellis, A. (1962), *Reason and emotion in psychotherapy.* New York: Stuart.

Emery, G., Hollon., S. G. & Bedrosian, R. C., eds. (1981), *New directions in cognitive therapy.* New York: Guilford Press.

Emmelkamp, P. M. G. (1986), Behavior therapy with adults. In: *Handbook of psychotherapy and behavior change.* (3rd Ed.), ed. S. L. Garfield & A. E. Bergin. New York: Wiley, pp. 385–442.

Etzel, B. C. & LeBlanc, J. M. (1979), The simplest treatment alternative. *J. Autism Dev. Disord.*, 9:361–383.

Falloon, I. R. H., Boyd, J. L., McGill, C. W., Razani, J., Moss, H. B. & Gilderman, A. M. (1982), Family management in the prevention of exacerbations of schizophrenia. *New Engl. J. Med.*, 306:180–183.

Fairburn, C. G. (1981), A cognitive behavioral approach to the management of bulimia. *Psychol. Med.*, 11:707–711.

Foreyt, J. P. & Cousins, J. H. (1987), Obesity. In: *Behavior therapy with children and adolescents*, ed. M. Hersen & V. B. Van Hasselt. New York: Wiley, pp. 485–511.

Fisher, D. A. & Wollersheim, J. P. (1986), Social reinforcement: a treatment component in verbal self-instruction. *J. Abnorm. Child Psychol.*, 14:38–41.

Forehand, R. & MacDonough, S. (1975), Response contingent timeout. *European Journal of Behavioural Analysis and Modification*, 1:109–115.

Garfield, S. L. & Bergin, A. E. (1986), *Handbook of psychotherapy and behavior change* (3rd ed.), New York: Wiley, pp. 12–13.

Garske, J. P. (1982), Issues regarding effective psychotherapy. *Critical issues, developments, and trends in professional psychology*, ed. J. McNamara & A. Barclay. New York: Praeger.

Gittelman, R. (1985), Controlled trials of remedial approaches to reading disability. *J. Child Psychol. Psychiatry*, 26:843–846.

—— (1986), *Anxiety disorders of childhood.* New York: Guilford, pp. 101–125.

—— Feingold, I. (1983), Children with reading disorders—I. Effects of reading instruction. *J.Child Psychol. Psychiatry*, 24:167–191.

Gittelman-Klein, R., Klein, D. G., Abikoff, H., Katz, S., Gloisten, A. C. & Kates, A. W. (1976), Relative efficacy of methylphenidate and behavior therapy in hyperkinetic children. *J. Abnorm. Child Psychol.*, 4:361–379.

Goodyer, I. (1981), Hysterical conversion reactions in childhood, *J. Child Psychol. Psychiatry*, 22:179–188.

Goldfried, M. R., Decenteco, E. T. & Weinberg, L. (1974), Systematic rational restructuring as a self-control technique. *Behavior Therapy*, 5:247–254.

Graham, P. (1974), Depression in prepubertal children. *Dev. Med. Child Neurol.*, 16:340–349.

Hall, A. & Crisp, A. (1987), Brief psychotherapy in the treatment of anorexia nervosa. *Br. J. Psychiatry*, 151:185–191.

Harris, S. L. & Ersner-Hershfield, R. (1978), Behavioral suppression of seriously disruptive behavior in psychotic and retarded patients. *Psychol. Bull.*, 85:1352–1375.

_____ Handelman, J. S. (1987), Autism. In: *Behavior therapy with children and adolescents.* ed. M. Hersen & V. B. Van Hasselt. New York: Wiley, pp. 224–240.

Harris, F. C. & Phelps, C. F. (1987), Anorexia and bulimia. In: *Behavior therapy with children and adolescents*, ed. M. Hersen & V. B. Van Hasselt. New York: Wiley, pp. 465–484.

Hersen, M. & Van Hasselt, V. B. (1987), *Behavior therapy with children and adolescents.* New York: Wiley.

Hops, H., Finch, M. & McConnell, S. (1985), Social skills deficits. In: *Handbook of clinical behavior therapy with children*, ed. P. H. Bornstein & A. E. Kazdin. Homewood, Ill.: Dorsey Press.

Horan, J. J. & Straus, L. K. (1987), Substance abuse. In: *Behavior therapy with children and adolescents*, ed. M. Hersen & V. B. Van Hasselt. New York: Wiley Interscience, pp. 440–464.

Howard, J. R., Jones, R. R. & Weinrott, M. R. (1982), Cost-effectiveness of teaching family programs for delinquents. *Evaluation Review*, 6:173–201.

Hsu, L. K. G. (1986), The treatment of anorexia nervosa. *American Journal of Psychiatry*, 143:573–581.

Huon, G. F. & Brown, L. B. (1984), Bulimia: the emergence of the syndrome. *Aust. N. Z. J. Psychiatry*, 24:113–126.

Jessor, R. & Jessor, S. L. (1975), Adolescent development and the onset of drinking. *J. Stud. Alcohol*, 36:27–51.

Johnston, J. M. (1972), Punishment of human behavior. *American Psychologist*, 27:1033–1054.

Kaplan, K. M. & Wadden, T. A. (1986), Childhood obesity and self-esteem. *J. Pediatr.*, 109:367–372.

Kaslow, N. J. & Rehm, L. (1985), Conceptualization, assessment and treatment of depression in children. In: *Handbook of clinical behavior therapy with children*, ed. P. H. Bornstein & A. E. Kazdin. Homewood, Ill.: Dorsey Press.

Kazdin, A. E. (1975), *Behavior modification in applied settings*, (1st Ed.). Homewood, Ill.: Dorsey Press.

_____ (1987), *Conduct disorder in childhood and adolescence.* Newberry Park, Cal.: Sage.

_____ Esveldt-Dawson, K., French, N. H. & Unis, A. S. (1987), Effects of parent management and problem solving skills training combined in the of antisocial child behavior. *J. Am. Acad. Child Adolesc. Psychiatry*, 26:416–424.

Kennedy, W. A. (1965), School phobia: rapid treatment of fifty cases. *J. Abnorm. Psychol.*, 70:285–289.

Kendall, P. C. & Hollon, S. D., eds. (1979), *Cognitive-behavioral interventions: theory, research, and procedures.* New York: Academic Press.

—— Norton-Ford, J. D. (1982), *Clinical psychology: scientific and professional dimensions.* New York: Wiley.

Kirigin, K. A., Braukman, C. J., Atwater, J. D. & Wolf, M. M. (1982), An evaluation of teaching family (Achievement Place) group homes for juvenile offenders. *J. Appl. Behav. Anal.*, 15:1–16.

Klein, R. D. (1979), Modifying academic performance in the grade school classroom. In: *Progress in behavior modification*, Vol. 10, ed. M. Hersen, R. Eisler & P. M. Miller. New York: Academic Press, pp. 292–321.

Kohlberg, L., LaCrosse, J. & Ricks, D. (1972), The predictability of adult mental health from childhood behavior. In: *Manual of child psychopathology*, ed. B. B. Wolman. New York: McGraw-Hill.

Kolko, D. J. (1987).Depression. In: *Behavior therapy with children and adolescents*, ed. M. Hersen & V. B. Van Hasselt. New York: Wiley, pp. 137–183.

Koocher, G. P. & Pedulla, B. M. (1977), Current practices in child psychotherapy. *Professional Psychology*, 8:275–287.

Korsch, B. (1986), Childhood obesity. *J. Pediatr.*, 109:299–300.

Kovacs, M. & Paulauskas, S. (1986), The traditional psychotherapies. In: *Psychopathological disorders of childhood*, (3rd Ed.), ed. H. C. Quay & J. S. Werry. New York: Wiley, pp. 496–522.

Labbe, E. E. & Williamson, D. A. (1984), Treatment of childhood migraine using autogenic feedback training. *J. Consult. Clin. Psychol.*, 52:968–976.

Lacey, J. H. (1983), Bulimia nervosa, binge eating, and psychogenic vomiting. *Br. Med. J.*, 1:1609–1613.

LaGrow, S. J. & Repp, A. C. (1984), Stereotypic responding: a review of intervention research. *Am. J. Ment. Defic.*, 88:595–609.

Larsson, B., Daleflod, B., Hakansson, L. & Melin, L. (1987), Therapist-assisted versus self-help relaxation treatment of chronic headache in adolescents. *J. Child Psychol. Psychiatry*, 28:127–136.

Lazarus, A.A. & Abramovitz, A. (1962), The use of emotive imagery in the treatment of children's phobias. *Journal of Mental Science*, 108:191–195.

Lefkowitz, M. M. & Burton, N. (1978), Childhood depression: a critique of the concept. *Psychol. Bull.*, 85:716–726.

Lemert, E. M. (1981), Diversion in juvenile justice: what hath been wrought. *Journal of Research in Crime and Delinquency*, 28:685–695.

Leitenberg, H., Gross, J., Peterson, J. & Rosen, J. C. (1984), Analysis of an anxiety model and the process of change during exposure plus response prevention treatment of bulimia nervosa. *Behav. Ther.*, 15:3–20.

Levitt, E. E. (1957), The results of psychotherapy with children. *J. Consult. Clin. Psychol.*, 21:189–196.

Lewinsohn, P. M., Sullivan, J. M. & Grosscup, S. J. (1982), Behavior therapy. In: *Short-*

term psychotherapies for the depressed patient, ed. A. J. Rush. New York: Guilford Press.

Lovaas, O. I. (1987), Behavioral treatment and normal educational and intellectual functioning in young autistic children. *J. Consult. Clin. Psychol.*, 55:3–9.

MacDonough, T. S. & Forehand, R. (1973), Response-contingent timeout. *J. Behav. Ther. Exper. Psychiatry*, 4:231–236.

MacMillan, D. L. & Morrison, G. M. (1986), Educational intervention. In: *Psychopathological disorders of childhood* (3rd Ed.), ed. H. C. Quay & J. S. Werry. New York: Wiley, pp. 583–621.

Mahoney, M. J. (1977), Reflections on the cognitive-learning trend in psychotherapy. *Am. Psychol.*, 32.

Mash, E. J. & Terdal, L. G. (1981), *Behavioral assessment of childhood disorders.* New York: Guilford.

Matson, J. L. & McCartney, J. R. (1981), *Handbook of behavior modification with the mentally retarded.* New York: Plenum.

McCabe, R. J. R. & Green, D. (1987), Rehabilitating severely head-injured adolescents: three case reports. *J. Child Psychol. Psychiatry*, 28:111–126.

McFall, M. E. & Wollersheim, J. P. (1982), Cognitive behavior therapy for obsessive-compulsive neurosis. In: *Therapies for adults: depressive anxiety and personality disorders*, ed. H. L. Millman, J. T. Huber, & D. R. Diggins. Washington, D. C.: Jossey-Bass Publishers.

Meichenbaum, D. H. (1979), Teaching children self-control. In: *Advances in child clinical psychology* (Vol. 2), ed. B. B. Lahey & A. E. Kazdin. New York: Plenum.

Melamed, B. G. & Johnson, S. B. (1981), Chronic illness. In: *Behavioral assessment of childhood disorders*, ed. E. J. Mash & L. G. Terdal. New York: Guilford Press, pp. 529–572.

Merluzzi, T. V., Glass, C. R. & Genest, M. (1981), *Cognitive assessment.* New York: Guilford Press.

Morris, R. J. & Kratochwill, T. R. (1983), *Treating children's fears and phobias.* New York: Pergamon Press.

O'Leary, K. D. & Wilson, G. T. (1987), *Behavior therapy* (2nd Ed.). Engelwood Cliffs, N.J.: Prentice-Hall.

Ollendick, T. H., (1986), Behavior therapy with children and adolescents. In: *Handbook of psychotherapy and behavior change* (3rd Ed.), ed. S. L. Garfield & A.E. Bergin. New York: Wiley, pp. 525–564.

—— Cerny, J. A. (1981), *Clinical behavior therapy with children.* New York: Plenum Publishing.

Pataki, C. S. & Carlson, G. A. (in press), Affective disorders. In: *Handbook of studies in child psychiatry*, ed. B. Tonge, G. D. Burrows & J. S. Werry. Amsterdam: Elsevier.

Patterson, G. R. (1982), *Coercive family process.* Eugene, Ore.: Castalia.

—— Fleischman, M. J. (1979), Maintenance of treatment effects. *Behav. Ther.*, 10:168–185.

—— Reid, J. B. & Chamberlain, P. (1981), *Beyond technology.* Paper presented at the XII Annual Banff International Conference on Behavior Modification, Banff, Alberta.

_____ Chamberlain, P. & Reid, J. B. (1982), A comparison evaluation of a parent-training program. *Behav. Ther.*, 13:638–650.

Paul, G. L. (1967), Strategy of outcome research in psychotherapy. *J. Consult. Clin. Psychol.*, 42:109–119.

Peterson, L. & Roberts, M. C. (1986), Community intervention and prevention. In: *Psychopathological disorders of childhood.* (3rd Ed.), ed. H. C. Quay & J. S. Werry. New York: Wiley, pp. 622–660.

Phillips, E. L., Philipps, E. A., Fixen, D. L. & Wolfe, M. M. (1971), Achievement Place: modification of the behaviors of predelinquent boys within a token economy. *J. Appl. Behav. Anal.*, 4:45–59.

Prior, M. & Sanson, A. (1986), Attention deficit disorder with hyperactivity. *J. Child Psychol. Psychiatry*, 27:307–319.

_____ Werry, J. S. (1986), Autism, schizophrenia and allied disorders. In: *Psychopathological disorders of childhood*, (3rd Ed.), ed. H. C. Quay & J. S. Werry. New York: Wiley, pp. 156–210.

Quay, H. C. (1986), Residential treatment. In: *Psychopathological disorders of childhood* (3rd Ed.), ed. H. C. Quay & J. S. Werry. New York: Wiley, pp. 558–582.

_____ LaGreca, A. M. (1986), Disorders of anxiety, withdrawal and dysphoria. In: *Psychopathological disorders of childhood*, ed. H. C. Quay & J. S. Werry, New York: Wiley, pp. 73–110.

Rapoport, J. L. (1986), Childhood obsessive compulsive disorder. *J. Child Psychol. Psychiatry*, 27:289–298.

Rapport, M. D. (1987), Attention deficit disorder with hyperactivity. In: *Behavior therapy with children and adolescents*, ed. M. Hersen & V. B. Van Hasselt. New York: Wiley Interscience, pp. 325–361.

Reatig, N. (1984), Attention deficit disorder. *Psychopharmacol. Bull.*, 20:693–718.

Rehm, L. P. (1981), A self-control therapy program for treatment of depression. In: *Depression: behavioral and directive intervention strategies*, ed. J. F. Clarkin & H. I. Glazer. New York: Garland Press.

Reid, J. B. & Patterson, G. R. (1976), The modification of aggression and stealing behavior of boys in the home setting. In: *Behavior modification*, ed. A. Bandura & E. Ribes-Inesta. Hillsdale, N.J.: Lawrence Erlbaum Associates.

_____ Hinojosa-Rivera, G. & Lorber, R. (1980), *A social learning approach to the outpatient treatment of children who steal.* Unpublished manuscript, Oregon Social Learning Center, Eugene, Oregon.

Richman, N., Douglas, J., Hunt, H., Lansdown, R. & Levere, R. (1985), Behavioural methods in the treatment of sleep disorders—a pilot study. *J. Child Psychol. Psychiatry*, 26:581–590.

Robins, L. (1979), Follow-up studies. In: *Psychopathological disorders of children*, (2nd Ed.), ed. H. C. Quay & J. S. Werry. New York: Wiley.

Ross, A. (1981), *Child behavior therapy.* New York: Wiley.

Ross, D. M. & Ross, S. A. (1982), *Hyperactivity.* (2nd Ed.). New York: Wiley Interscience, pp. 250–275.

Schwitzgebel, R. & Kolb, D. A. (1964), Inducing behaviour change in adolescent delinquents. *Behav. Res. Ther.*, 1:297–304.

Seymour, F. W., Bayfield, G., Brock, P. & During, M. (1982), Management of nightwaking in young children. *Australian Journal of Family Therapy*, 4:217–223.

Shapiro, E.S. (1987), Academic problems. In: *Behavior therapy with children & adolescents*, ed. M. Hersen & B. V. Van Hasselt. New York: Wiley, pp. 362–284.

Siegel, L. J. & Ridley-Johnson, R. (1985), Anxiety disorders of childhood and adolescence. In: *Handbook of clinical behavior therapy with children*, ed. P. H. Bornstein & A. E. Kazdin. Homewood, Ill.: Dorsey Press.

Simonds, J. F. & Parraga, H. (1982), Prevalence of sleep disorders and sleep behaviors in children and adolescents. *J. Am. Acad. Child Adolesc. Psychiatry*, 21:383–388.

Skinner, B. F. (1938), *The behavior of organisms*. New York: Appleton-Century-Crofts.

Slack, C.W. (1960), Experimenter-subject psychotherapy. *Mental Hygiene*, 44:238–256.

Spence, S. H. (1986), Behavioural treatments of childhood obesity. *J. Child Psychol. Psychiatry*, 27:447–445.

Starin, S. P. & Fuqua, R. W. (1987), Rumination and vomiting in the developmentally disabled. *Res. Dev. Disabil.*, 8:575–606.

Strauss, C. (1987), Anxiety. In: *Behavior therapy with children and adolescents*, ed. M. Hersen & V. B. Van Hasselt. New York: Wiley, pp. 109–136.

Templeman, T. L. & Wollersheim, J. P. (1979), A cognitive-behavioural approach to the treatment of psychopathy. *Psychotherapy Theory Research and Practice*, 16:132–139.

Thelen, M., Fry, R. A., Fehrenback, P. A. & Frautschi, N. M. (1979), Therapeutic video-tape and film modeling. *Psychol. Bull.*, 86:701–720.

Treiber, F. A. & Lahey, B. B. (1985), A behavioural model of academic remediation with learning disabled children. In: *Handbook of clinical behavior therapy with children*, ed. P. H. Bornstein & A. E. Kazdin, Homewood, Ill.: Dorsey Press.

Turpin, G. (1983), The behavioral management of tic disorders., *Advances in Behavioral Research and Therapy*, 5:203–245.

Ullman, L. P. & Krasner, L. (1965), *Case studies in behavior modification*. New York: Holt, Rinehart & Winston.

Van Dongen-Melman, J. E. W. M. & Sanders-Woudstra, J. A. R. (1986), Psychosocial aspects of childhood cancer. *J. Child Psychol. Psychiatry*, 27:145–180.

Volkmar, F. R., Poll, J. & Lewis, M. (1984), Conversion reactions in childhood and adolescence. *J. Am. Acad. Child Psychiatry*, 23:424–430.

Weiner, I. B. (1982), *Child and adolescent psychopathology*. New York: Wiley.

Wells, K. C. & Copeland, B. C. (1985), Childhood and adolescent obesity. *Prog. Behav. Modif.*, 19:145–176.

――― Vitulano, L. A. (1984), Anxiety disorders in childhood. In: *Behavioral theories and treatment of anxiety* ed. S. M. Turner. New York: Plenum, pp. 413–433.

――― Forehand, R. (1981), Childhood behavior problems in the home. In: *Handbook of clinical behavior therapy*, ed. S. M. Turner, K. S. Calhoun & H. E. Adams. New York: Wiley.

――― (1985), Conduct and oppositional disorders. In: *Handbook of clinical behavior therapy with children*, ed. P. H. Bornstein & A. E. Kazdin. New York: Dorsey Press.

Werry, J. S. (1986), Physical illness, symptoms and allied disorders. In: *Psychopathological disorders of childhood* (3rd Ed.), ed. H. C. Quay & J. S. Werry. New York: Wiley, pp. 424–430.

_____ (1988), The effect of drugs on learning and cognitive function in children. *J. Child Psychol. Psychiatry*, 29:129–141.

_____ Carlielle, J. & Fitzpatrick, J. (1983), Rhythmic motor activities in children under five. *J. Am. Acad. Child Adolesc. Psychiatry*, 22:172–179.

_____ Reeves, J. C. & Elkind, G. S. (1987), Attention deficit, conduct, oppositional and anxiety disorders in children I. *J. Am. Acad. Child Adolesc. Psychiatry*, 26:127–132.

_____ Wollersheim, J. P. (1967), Behavior therapy with children. *J. Am. Acad. Child Psychiatry*, 6:346–370.

Whalen, C. K., Henker, B. & Hinshaw, S. P. (1985), Cognitive behavioral therapies for hyperactive children. *J. Abnorm. Child Psychol.*, 13:391–410.

Whitman, T. L. & Johnston, M. B. (1987), Mental retardation. In: *Behavior therapy with children & adolescents*, ed. M. Hersen & V. B. Van Hasselt. New York: Wiley, pp. 184–223.

_____ Scibak, J. & Reid, D. H. (1983), *Behavior modification with the severely and profoundly retarded*. New York: Academic Press.

Wilson, G. T. (1978), On the much discussed nature of the term "behavior therapy." *Behav. Ther.*, 9:89–98.

Wiltz, W. A. & Patterson, G. R. (1974), An evaluation of parent training procedures designed to alter inappropriate aggressive behavior of boys. *Behav. Ther.*, 5:215–221.

Williamson, D. A., McKenzie, S. J., Goreczny, A. J. & Faulstich, M. (1987), Psychophysiological disorders. In: *Behavior therapy with children and adolescents*, ed. M. Hersen & V. B. Van Hasselt. New York: Wiley, pp. 279–300.

Winton, A. S. W. & Singh, N. N. (1983), Rumination in pediatric populations. *J. Am. Acad. Child Psychiatry*, 22:269–275.

Wollersheim, J. P. (1970), The effectiveness of group therapy based upon learning principles in the treatment of overweight women. *J. Abnorm. Psychol.*, 76:462–474.

_____ (1980), Direct cognitive therapies. In: *Direct cognitive therapies: psychological and philosophical foundations and implications*, chair, H. E. Wilson. Symposium presented at the convention of the Rocky Mountain Psychological Association, Las Vegas, Nevada.

Wolpe, J. (1958), *Psychotherapy by reciprocal inhibition*. Stanford, Cal.: Stanford University Press.

_____ (1978), Cognition and causation in human behavior and its therapy. *Am. Psychol.*, 33:436–446.

Wong, B. Y. L. (1985), Issues in cognitive-behavioral interventions in academic skill areas. *J. Abnorm. Child Psychol.*, 13:425–442.

Yates, A. J. (1970), *Behavior Therapy*. New York: Wiley.

24

Effect of Anxiety on Cognition, Behavior, and Stimulant Response in ADHD

Steven R. Pliszka

The University of Texas Health Science Center, San Antonio

The effect of the comorbidity of overanxious disorder (ANX) in attention deficit hyperactivity disorder (ADHD) on laboratory measures of behavior, cognition, and stimulant response was examined. Seventy-nine children who met DSM-III-R *criteria for ADHD were tested further for an oppositional defiant disorder (ODD), conduct disorder (DC), or ANX. Subjects with comorbid ANX showed less impulsiveness on a laboratory measure of behavior and had longer, sluggish reaction times on the Memory Scanning Test than those without ANX. ADHD subjects with comorbid ANX were less frequently diagnosed as CD. Forty-three of the subjects completed a double-blind trial of methylphenidate; subjects with comorbid anxiety had a significantly poorer response to the stimulant than those without anxiety, while the comorbidity of ODD or CD did not affect stimulant response. The results suggest that ADHD with comorbid ANX may represent children with primary anxiety who develop secondary inattentiveness, or they may represent a different subtype of ADHD, perhaps similar to the condition of attention deficit disorder without hyperactivity under* DSM-III. *Key Words: ADHD, anxiety, stimulant response.*

It is generally accepted that attention deficit hyperactivity disorder (ADHD) is a heterogeneous disorder. Indeed, separating ADHD from other childhood mental disorders on objective measures of psychopathology has proved difficult, even when relatively "pure" diagnostic groups are compared. Werry et al. (1987) compared children with attention deficit disorder (ADD), children with ADD plus conduct dis-

Reprinted with permission from *Journal of American Academy of Child and Adolescent Psychiatry,* 1989, Vol. 28, No. 6, 882–887. Copyright © 1989 by the American Academy of Child and Adolescent Psychiatry.

order (CD), children with anxiety disorder, and normal controls on a large number of laboratory measures of cognition and behavior, many of which have been widely used in research on ADHD over the years. On the vast majority of the measures, few differences emerged between the psychiatric groups, especially after the effects of age, socioeconomic status, and intelligence were controlled for.

Further evidence of heterogeneity among the diagnostic groups comes from several studies showing marked overlap of both anxiety and conduct disorders with ADHD. Using structured psychiatric interviews to assess a community sample, Anderson et al. (1987) found that about 47% of children with ADD had a coexisting conduct or oppositional disorder, while about 26% of children with ADD had a coexisting anxiety or phobic disorder. A small group (18%) of the ADD children met criteria for both a conduct and an anxiety disorder, and children with mixed disorders were far more likely to have been referred to mental health clinics. Very similar figures emerged from a Puerto Rico epidemiological study (Bird et al., 1988). Strauss et al. (1988) found that 34.6% of preadolescent children with anxiety disorders met criteria for ADD.

In routine clinical situations this overlap of diagnosis is often reduced by the clinician interpreting the inattention, conduct, or anxiety symptoms as primary. Thus, a clinician presented with anxiety in a child who meets criteria for ADHD may conclude that the anxiety symptoms are secondary to the problems the child is experiencing because of his disruptive behavior. On the other hand, a child with an anxiety disorder may have symptoms of inattention or hyperactivity, but these may be seen as stemming from the anxiety. From a research perspective, however, there are no agreed upon rules for making such a determination. In rare cases, the parent and child may be able to state the precise time course of the different symptoms, allowing the clinician to rule out one or the other of the disorders. Most of the time, however, the use of structured or semistructured clinical interviews will require making several diagnoses.

Issues regarding the comorbidity of anxiety and ADHD are complex, and little direct research on this problem is available. Lahey and colleagues (1983, 1985, 1987) examined clinical differences between children diagnosed as ADD with and without hyperactivity, thereby shedding some light on this issue. Lahey et al. (1983) found children identified as ADD without hyperactivity to be more anxious, shy, and socially withdrawn than control children. A follow-up study (Lahey et al., 1985) found that compared to controls and ADD children with hyperactivity, ADD children without hyperactivity showed a sluggish, drowsy cognitive tempo and, unlike the hyperactive group, were not more impulsive than controls. Both ADD groups are equally inattentive compared to controls. A study of clinic referred children (Lahey et al., 1987) confirmed that ADD children without hyperactivity showed less impulsivity and a more sluggish cognitive tempo than ADD children with hyperactivity. Of particular interest, the ADD without hyperactivity groups had a higher prevalence of anxiety and depressive disorders. The conduct problems in the ADD without hyperactivity group were much less severe than those in the ADD with hyperactivity group. The advent of *DSM-III-R* has shifted the focus of research away from the hyperactive/nonhyperactive distinction, but the above findings suggest there is a population of children who are inattentive, but not impulsive or motorically active, and who may show higher levels of anxiety or depression. Zahn et al. (1975) and Taylor et al. (1987) both showed that higher levels of "emotional problems" (i.e., anxiety and depressive symptoms) in children undergoing a medication trial were associated with a poorer response to stimulants. This further suggests that children with comorbid ADHD and anxiety are a unique subtype.

This study examined the effect of the comorbidity of anxiety in ADHD on a number of laboratory measures of behavior, cognition, and stimulant response. Werry et al. (1987) found that seat activity and restlessness, both before and during a cognitive task, discriminated different diagnostic groups, regardless of IQ. Milich et al. (1983) developed a method of directly observing ADHD behaviors (off task, fidgeting, out of seat, etc.) during an academic task, which discriminated ADHD children from both controls and conduct disordered children. Barkley (1987) modified this system to one in which the child, alone in a room, performs arithmetic problems for a specified time while an observer rates ADHD behaviors according to a set protocol. Since such a method correlates with teacher rating of hyperactivity and conduct problems (Barkley et al., 1988), it seemed a reasonable measure of motor restlessness and impulsivity.

Van der Meere and Sergeant (1987, 1988) examined attentional deficits in behaviorally disordered children using the paradigm of Sternberg (1969). In the paradigm, effortful mental processing is operationalized by the reaction time needed to perform a task. For instance, a subject can be asked to remember one, two, or four letters. Next, he or she is shown a display of four letters and then asked to say whether or not one of the letters he/she memorized is present or absent. As the load increases from one to four, the subject must spend more time examining the display before responding. Thus reaction time can be plotted against load, revealing a linear, increasing function. Two variables are produced: the reaction time intercept, and the slope of the reaction time-memory load function. According to Sternberg (1969), the slope of the line represents the efficiency of mental processing, while the intercept represents input and output factors. Sergeant and Scholten (1983), as well as van der Meere and Sergeant (1987; 1988), have shown that children identified as hyperactive show no differences in slope of the reaction time-memory load function but show marked differences in the intercept. They conclude that children with ADHD do not show deficits in effortful mental processing per se but have difficulty organizing a motor output. A cognitive task similar to that used by van der Meere and Sergeant (1987) was used in this study, based on the reasoning that if ADHD children with different comorbidities showed only differences in intercept, similar to the findings in the above study, this would suggest that differences between the groups were of a quantitative nature only. If, on the other hand, there were differences in the slope, this would suggest that one of the comorbid groups showed a deficit in effortful mental processing, a qualitatively different deficit than the one van der Meere and Sergeant (1987, 1988) have shown in their hyperactive subjects.

METHOD

Subjects and Diagnostic Interview

Subjects had been referred to a community child mental health clinic for treatment of disruptive behavior at home or school. Children whose teacher had rated them as higher than one standard deviation from the mean for their age and sex on the Inattention Overactivity (I/O) factor of the Iowa Conners Teacher Rating Scale (CTRS) (Loney and Milich, 1982) were referred for evaluation of ADHD. The Iowa CTRS is a 10-item scale which yields a *t*-score for an I/O factor, and an Aggression (AGG) factor. The I/O factor consists of five items: Fidgets; Hums and makes other odd noises; Excitable, impulsive; Inattentive; and Fails to finish things he starts. The AGG factor also has five items: Argues; Acts "smart"; Temper outbursts and unpredictable behavior; Defiant; and Uncooperative. Both parent and child were interviewed by the same clinician, and all interviews were performed by the author or by a psychiatric resident directly under his supervision. During the clinical interview, all major symptom areas in *DSM-III-R* were explored. For externalizing symptoms, greater weight was placed on parental report of behavior at home and school. Parental report of serious difficulties with inattentiveness, impulsivity, hyperactivity and conduct problems were sufficient to diagnose the child as ADHD or CD, even if the child denied the symptoms during his or her interview. Subjects who expressed transient anxiety or depression about consequences of punishment for misbehavior were not considered to meet criteria for an overanxious disorder (ANX). In order to meet criteria for an ANX, the child had to report the symptoms him/herself. Occasionally, parents would report the child was very anxious or had "low-self-esteem," while the child denied all such symptoms. Such subjects were not diagnosed as having an ANX. Careful questioning of these parents often revealed that they were interpreting oppositional behavior (i.e., throwing a tantrum when pushed to do homework) as a lack of self-confidence or underlying unhappiness. This report concerns 79 children (74 boys, 5 girls) who met *DSM-III-R* criteria for ADHD and thus were candidates for a stimulant trial. None met criteria for any psychotic or depressive disorder. Subjects were free of medication, as well as any other medical disorder, and all were attending local public schools. Twenty-two (27.8%) of the sample met criteria for ANX as well as ADHD.

Laboratory Measures

A research assistant, blind to the clinical data, performed the following measures as part of the child's evaluation:

1. The child was placed in an observation room with a one-way mirror where he or she performed arithmetic problems (set at his/her own grade level) for 15 minutes. The observer rated the following behaviors according to the method described by Barkley (1987): Off task, Fidgeting, Vocalizes, Plays with Objects, and Out of Seat. Off task behavior was defined as breaking eye contact with the worksheet for longer than 3 seconds. A fidget was defined as a motor movement which resulted in a change in the position of the trunk or legs. Hence, simple foot tapping or leg vibration was not coded as a fidget. A vocalization was defined as any audible sound other than a cough or sneeze. The 15-minute period was divided into 30 thirty-second intervals; the end of each interval was signaled to the observer by means of a tape recorder. If one of the five behaviors occurred during the 30-second interval, the observer recorded it; if the behavior occurred multiple times during the interval, it was still only recorded once. A score for each behavior was obtained by summing the number of intervals in which the behavior occurred, dividing by 30, and expressing this number as a percentage. A total ADHD behavior score was obtained by summing the total number of intervals in which a behavior occurred in all five categories and dividing by 150; this was also expressed as a percentage. The author trained both research assistants used in the study; interrater reliability between them was calculated using the number of agreements divided by the total possible number of occurrences. Interrater reliability for the five coded behaviors ranged from 0.81 to 1.0.

2. *The Memory Scanning Test (MST)*. The version described by Swanson and Cantwell (1986) was used. The child memorized four numbers, and then the computer presented one of three possible displays: a number by itself, a number within a 4×4 matrix of letters, or a number within a 4×4 matrix of numbers. The child had to scan the display and determine if one of the numbers he/she memorized at the start of the task was present or not, then he/she had to press a "yes" or "no" button. Twelve trials were presented in each of the distractor conditions: six with the target present, and six with the target absent. The task lasted approximately 10 to 15 minutes, depending on the child's cognitive tempo. Reaction times in each of the three "yes" conditions were assessed. The task is easier when the display load is smallest, (the no distractor condition) and there is increasing difficulty in the dissimilar distractor and similar distractor conditions, respectively. The effect of codiagnosis of ANX, distractor type, and the codiagnosis by distractor type interaction on reaction time were examined.

Stimulant Trial

Upon completion of the baseline assessment, a double-blind trial of methylphenidate was offered to families as a more accurate method to assess their child's response to medication. Participating in the double-blind phase involved weekly testing, and the clinic did not have sufficient staff to perform the double-blind trial on all subjects. Also, some families were judged to be too dysfunctional to be able to complete the trial. Of the 79 families, five refused stimulant treatment altogether, and 28 families either were not offered or declined the double-blind treatment. These children were treated with an open trial of methylphenidate. Of the 46 families who started the double-blind trial, three dropped out before completing it; thus 43 of the subjects (30 without ANX, 13 with ANX) completed the 4-week trial. *T*-tests between subjects completing the double-blind trial and the remaining 36 did not reveal any significant differences in age or in baseline Iowa CTRS scores. There was no difference in the distribution of ANX in the two groups.

Each subject was placed on 4 weeks of medication. The first week was always placebo, and ratings from this week were not used in data analyses. The remaining 3 weeks were randomized into placebo, low (0.25 to 0.40 mg/kg) and high (0.45 to 0.70 mg/kg) dose methylphenidate; each subject served as his or her own control. For children weighing less than 25 kg, the low and high doses were 5 and 10 mg; for children over that weight, the two dose conditions were 10 and 20 mg. The doses are those typically used in clinical practice and similar to those used by Barkley et al. (1988). That study showed such doses, given for 1-week periods, resulted in robust changes not only in teacher ratings, but on an observation room task similar to one used here. The child, his or her parents, teachers, and the research assistant were all blind to the drug status. All medication was given at 7 A.M. and 12 noon except on Saturday as noted below. At the end of each week, the teacher filled out the Iowa CTRS (both I/O and AGG factors) rating the child's behavior for that week. On Saturday mornings the research assistant repeated the observation room measure. The Saturday morning dose was adjusted so that it occurred 90 minutes before the measure was taken.

Data Analysis

The baseline Iowa CTRS factors, subject age, and the scores from the observation room task were compared in subjects with and without ANX via two-tailed Student *t*-tests. The prevalence of the diagnosis of oppositional defiant disorder (ODD) or CD was contrasted in the two groups via chi-square tests. For the MST, a 2 (ANX present or absent) × 3 (no distractor, dissimilar distractors, similar distractors) repeated measures ANOVA was performed. In order to determine the effect of the comorbidity of ANX on stimulant response a 2 (ANX present or absent) × 4 (baseline, placebo, low dose methylphenidate, high dose methylphenidate) repeated measures ANOVA was performed on the teacher's weekly Iowa CTRS ratings (both factors) and the child's weekly scores on the observation room ratings. Pairwise *t*-tests with alpha adjustment using the Bonferroni correction were used to compare the individual groups when the main effect was significant. The comparisons chosen were: baseline vs. placebo, placebo vs. low dose methylphenidate, placebo vs. high dose methylphenidate, and low vs. high dose methylphenidate for both the ANX and non-ANX conditions. Finally, subjects were categorically defined as stimulant responders or nonresponders if, during at least one of the stimulant weeks, they showed a decrease of one standard deviation on the Iowa CTRS I/O relative to both the baseline and placebo weeks. A chi-square test was then used to contrast the number of stimulant responders in the ANX and non-ANX groups.

RESULTS

Table 1 shows the results for the baseline measures. The groups were not different in age. ADHD subjects with ANX were rated significantly lower on the Iowa CTRS I/O factor than those without ANX, though the mean score for both groups was well into the disturbed range. There was a trend for the comorbid group to be rated as less oppositional and defiant on the AGG factor, though this did not reach significance. On the observation room measure, ADHD subjects with ANX were significantly less off task, and there were strong trends for them to play with objects less and to

TABLE 1
Differences in Clinical and Laboratory Measures of Behavior in
ADHD Children with and without Comorbid Anxiety

Measure	Anxiety Present	Anxiety Absent	p
Age	$9.0^a (1.1)^b$	8.9 (1.9)	0.78
Iowa CTRS			
I/O	69.2 (6.9)	72.9 (7.1)	0.05
A	62.0 (16.0)	68.8 (16.1)	0.10
Observation room ratings			
Off task	14.9 (20.8)	30.8 (26.5)	0.01
Fidget	64.9 (22.5)	65.4 (25.1)	0.94
Vocalizes	23.1 (24.2)	30.3 (26.3)	0.26
Objects	1.5 (4.4)	6.7 (13.6)	0.08
Out of seat	0.8 (2.9)	6.5 (14.8)	0.08
Total	21.0 (10.4)	28.2 (12.6)	0.02
% with ODD	54.5	59.6	0.87
% with CD	0	33.3	0.03

[a] Values for Anxiety without parentheses are means.
[b] Values in parentheses are standard deviations.

remain seated longer. Vocalizing and fidgeting did not distinguish the groups. When the five behaviors were combined to yield a total ADHD behavior score, the comorbid group performed significantly better. Oppositional defiant disorder (ODD) was equally prevalent in both groups. No subject with comorbid ANX had a diagnosis of CD, as opposed to a third of the non-ANX group who met criteria for CD, a highly significant difference ($\chi^2 = 4.78$, $df = 1$, $p < 0.03$).

The effect of comorbid ANX on the MST reaction time is shown in Figure 1. The effect of distractor type on reaction time was highly significant ($F = 22.51$, $df = 2$, 104, $p < 0.0001$); that is, as more distractors are present, reaction time increases as the subject spent more time scanning the display. The main effect of ANX was not significant. On the other hand, the diagnosis by distractor type interaction was highly significant ($F = 3.72$, $df = 2$, 104, $p < 0.03$). This shows that as the display load increased, the comorbid group had a marked increase in their reaction time, whereas those without ANX became more impulsive.

The effects of the comorbidity of ANX on measures of stimulant response was examined next; this is shown in Table 2. For the Iowa CTRS I/O ratings, the main effect of drug status was highly significant ($F = 89.06$, $df = 3,123$, $p < 0.0001$), while the main effect of ANX was not. There was, however, a significant drug by diagnosis interaction ($F = 4.72$, $df = 3$, 123, $p < 0.01$). Pairwise comparisons showed that placebo and baseline scores for the non-ANX subjects were not significantly different from each other but were significantly higher than either of the two drug conditions, which were not, in turn, different from each other. On inspection of the data, it appears that the comorbid group is improving with a decline in I/O ratings while on placebo and another decline on drug. However, none of the pairwise comparisons were significant for this group. When subjects were classified as responders or nonresponders according to the difference between drug and placebo I/O scores, only 4 (30.8%) of the comorbid group were considered to be responders,

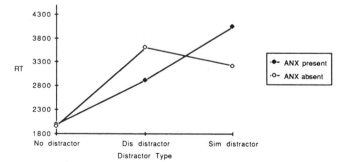

Figure 1. Effect of distractor type on reaction time in the Memory Scanning Test in anxious and nonanxious ADHD subjects.

TABLE 2

Effects of Stimulant Treatment on Anxious and Nonanxious Subjects with ADHD

Measure	Diagnosis	Baseline	Placebo	MPH (Low)	MPH (High)
I/O*	Anxious[c]	69.7 (5.3)	61.5 (11.0)	55.7 (6.7)	53.5 (8.0)
	Nonanxious[a]	72.8 (6.9)	69.3 (9.2)	54.9 (9.4)	50.1 (8.5)
AGG*	Anxious[c]	60.3 (11.8)	59.2 (13.2)	56.5 (12.7)	55.5 (11.8)
	Nonanxious[b]	65.8 (16.1)	62.6 (16.1)	52.7 (10.6)	48.2 (8.6)
Total ADHD* behavior	Anxious[c]	21.1 (10.4)	17.3 (10.0)	17.3 (8.7)	16.2 (8.2)
	Nonanxious[a]	24.2 (10.5)	25.2 (15.3)	14.5 (12.5)	13.8 (8.8)

Note: Values without parentheses are means; values with parentheses are standard deviations.

* The main effect of drug was significant ($p < 0.001$); the drug by diagnosis interaction was significant ($p < 0.01$). The main effect of anxiety was not significant.

[a] Baseline scores not different from placebo, both are significantly higher ($p < 0.5$) than the two drug conditions, which are not different from each other.

[b] The high dose of MPH is significantly lower than the other three conditions, which are not different from each other.

[c] No differences across groups.

while 26 (86.7%) of the 30 non-ANX subjects were responders, a highly significant difference ($\chi^2 = 13.4$, $df = 1$, $p < 0.001$). Due to the smaller size of the comorbid group, the four responders had a sufficiently robust response to stimulant to result in a mean reduction in I/O scores on drug relative to placebo, though as pointed out earlier, the pairwise comparisons did not reach significance. The smaller number of clinically defined responders in the comorbid group tends to rule out the possibility that a significant difference between placebo and drug in this group was not detected by the conservative Bonferroni correction. ODD and CD were combined to analyze the effect of these diagnoses on stimulant response. ODD and CD were distributed equally among responders and nonresponders ($\chi^2 = 0.86$, $df = 1$, NS).

With regard to the Iowa CTRS ratings on the AGG factor, drug effect was again significant ($F = 21.62$, $df = 3, 123$, $p < 0.0001$), and there again emerged a strong drug by diagnosis interaction ($F = 3.98$, $df = 3, 123$, $p < 0.001$). Pairwise comparison showed no differences across drug conditions for the comorbid group, while in the non-ANX group, there was a significant difference between the high dose of methylphenidate and the other three conditions which were not different from each other.

Figure 2 shows the effect of the comorbidity of ANX on subjects performance on the observation room task across the drug conditions. The main effect of drug was significant ($F = 16.71$, $df = 3, 123$, $p < 0.0001$), as was the drug by diagnosis interaction ($F = 4.18$, $df = 3, 123$, $p < 0.01$). Pairwise comparisons revealed that the comorbid group showed no significant reduction of ADHD behavior on active drug relative to placebo while subjects without ANX did.

DISCUSSION

These data show there is considerable heterogeneity among subjects with ADHD depending on the presence or absence of an ANX. The presence of a comorbid ANX tended to attenuate the teacher ratings of inattention and overactivity, as well

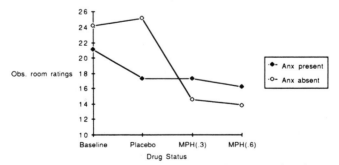

Figure 2. Effect of methylphenidate on observation room ratings in anxious and nonanxious ADHD subjects.

as those of oppositional behavior and defiance, though the ratings clearly remained in the disturbed range. No subject in the comorbid group had a diagnosis of CD, though they showed an equal prevalence of ODD relative to subjects without an ANX. This is consistent with the finding of Lahey et al. (1987) that children with ADD without hyperactivity (who had a higher incidence of anxiety and depressive disorders) tended to have milder conduct problems. On the observation room measures, those with comorbid anxiety had lower overall ratings, in particular, they were much less likely to be off task. In this method, off task behavior is rated by the observer as the child breaking eye contact with his or her paper. A child who is daydreaming, or internally distracted, without making a motor response (i.e., shifting head and eyes) would not be rated as off task using this method. The other items measure discrete motor acts (playing with objects, out of seat, etc.). Thus, this technique is essentially a measure of impulsivity and motor behavior. Perhaps the group with comorbid anxiety is similar to the ADD without hyperactivity group in the studies by Lahey et al. (1985, 1987) who showed less impulsivity, and more anxiety and social withdrawal, than controls or subjects with ADD with hyperactivity.

The results on the MST are interesting in view of the work of van der Meere and Sergeant (1987, 1988). The task used, while similar, differed from the one in their studies, and the task duration was much shorter as well. Also, the studies of van der Meere and Sergeant (1987, 1988) compared children identified as hyperactive to controls, while this study contrasted two different subtypes of children with ADHD; thus, comparisons between the studies should be made with caution. Van der Meere and Sergeant (1987, 1988) have consistently found differences in reaction time intercept, but not in reaction time-memory load slope, between hyperactives and controls. They have argued that this rules out deficits of effortful mental processing in hyperactivity, and implicates input or output factors, particularly in the organization of a motor response. Whatever the merits of this argument, this study found that ADHD subjects with and without an ANX showed highly significant differences in the reaction time-display load slope. As the display load became more difficult (similar distractors), the comorbid group became much slower to respond. According to the model of Sternberg (1969), this would implicate information processing difficulties in this group, a qualitatively different type of deficit from that found between hyperactives and controls by van der Meere and Sergeant (1987, 1988). The slower reaction times in the comorbid group is also suggestive of the "sluggish cognitive tempo" found by Lahey et al. (1987) in subjects with ADD without hyperactivity, who, as was pointed out earlier, had higher levels of anxiety and depression.

The finding of a less robust stimulant response in subjects with comorbid ANX is striking. Subjects without comorbid anxiety showed no improvement on placebo and showed dramatic reductions of teacher ratings of inattention, overactivity, and aggression on stimulant; a similar pattern of findings was found with regard to independently gathered observation room ratings during an academic task. Subjects with

ANX showed only a modest, nonsignificant improvement with treatment overall, and this was only noted in terms of the teacher I/O ratings. No change in the observation room ratings or teacher AGG ratings was noted for the comorbid group. There was no evidence that subjects with ANX worsened on stimulant. A number of these subjects were placebo responders; that is, their ratings declined from baseline, but they did as well on placebo as on stimulant. About a third of the comorbid group were determined to have responded well to stimulant, and continued treatment with methylphenidate. Thus the results should not be interpreted to suggest that ADHD children with comorbid anxiety should never be treated with stimulant medication, but it does suggest that in two-thirds of such cases, it may be ineffective. Whether the comorbid group would respond better to antidepressant medication as suggested by Pliszka (1987) remains a subject for further study.

These data strongly suggest that children who meet criteria for ADHD and an ANX are not children who simply have become "demoralized" due to frequent conflicts with parents and teachers. The data suggest they are a distinct subgroup. It is unclear from this data whether children with comorbid ADHD and ANX form a separate subtype of ADHD, similar to the *DSM-III* diagnosis of ADD without hyperactivity, or whether this is a group of children with primary anxiety disorders who develop secondary inattentiveness. Irritability associated with anxiety may lead to oppositional behavior and temper tantrums, and the presence of these symptoms may lead parents and teachers to report inattention and overactivity when these symptoms may not be objectively present. Future studies are needed to resolve this issue. Comparisons to normal controls and children with "pure" anxiety disorders are needed. Family studies, as well as follow up studies of the comorbid group, would also be useful in this regard. If children with comorbid ADHD and ANX have a higher level of relatives with anxiety or affective disorders, or if they themselves develop such disorders in later life, then one could conclude that the comorbid group should be classified as primary anxiety disorders. This study strongly suggests that it is important to control for the presence of anxiety disorders in research on ADHD.

REFERENCES

Anderson, J. C., Williams, S., McGee, R. & Silva, P. A. (1987), DSM-III disorders in pre-adolescent children: prevalence in a large sample from the general population. *Arch. Gen. Psychiatry,* 44:69–76.
Barkley, R. A. (1987), The assessment of attention deficit hyperactivity disorder. *Behavioral Assessment,* 9:207–233.
———Fischer, M., Newby, R. F. & Breen, M. J. (1988), Development of a multimethod clinical

protocol for assessing stimulant drug response in children with attention deficit disorder. *Journal of Clinical Child Psychology.* 17:14–24.

Bird, H. R., Canino, G., & Rubio-Stipec, M. (1988), Estimates of the prevalence of childhood maladjustment in a community survey in Puerto Rico. *Arch. Gen. Psychiatry,* 45:1120–1126.

Lahey, B. B., Schaughency, E. A., Strauss, C. D. & Frame, C. L. (1983), Are attention deficit disorders with and without hyperactivity similar or dissimilar disorders? *J. Am. Acad. Child Psychiatry,* 23:302–310.

——Frame, C. L. & Strauss, C. C. (1985), Teacher ratings of attention problems in children experimentally classified as exhibiting attention deficit disorder with and without hyperactivity. *J. Am. Acad. Child Psychiatry,* 24:613–616.

——Hynd, G. W., Carlson, C. L. & Nieves, N. (1987), Attention deficit disorder with and without hyperactivity. *J. Am. Acad. Child Adolesc. Psychiatry,* 26:718–723.

Loney, J. & Milich R. (1982), Hyperactivity, inattention and aggression in clinical practice. In: *Advances in Developmental and Behavior Pediatrics Vol 3,* ed. M. Wolraich & D. K. Routh. Grerenwich, CT:JAI, pp. 113–147.

Milich, R., Loney, J. & Landau, S. (1982), Independent dimensions of hyperactivity and aggression: a validation with playroom observational data. *J. Abnorm. Psychol.,* 91:183–198.

Pliszka, S. R. (1987), Tricyclic antidepressants in the treatment of children with attention deficit disorder. *J. Am. Acad. Child Adolesc. Psychiatry,* 26:127–132.

Sergeant, J. A. & Scholten, C. A. (1983), A stages of information approach to hyperactivity. *J. Child Psychol. Psychiatry,* 24:49–60.

Strauss, C. C., Lease, C. A., Last, C. G. & Francis, G. (1988), Overanxious disorder: an examination of developmental differences. *J. Abnorm. Child Psychol.,* 16:433–443.

Sternberg, S. (1969), Memory scanning: mental processes revealed by reaction time experiments. *American Scientist,* 57:421–457.

Swanson, J. M. & Cantwell, D. P. (1986), *Computerized assessment of children: cognitive tests, questionnaires and interviews.* Paper presented at the annual meeting of the American Academy of Child and Adolescent Psychiatry, Los Angeles, California.

Taylor, E., Schachar, R., Thorley, G., Wieselberg, H. M., Everitt, B. & Rutter, M. (1987), Which boys respond to stimulant medication? A controlled trial of methylphenidate in boys with disruptive behavior. *Psychol. Med.,* 17:121–143.

van der Meere, J. & Sergeant, J. (1987), A divided attention experiment with pervasively hyperactive children. *J. Abnorm. Child Psychol.,* 15:379–392.

——(1988), Focused attention in pervasively hyperactive children. *J. Abnorm. Child Psychol.,* 16:627–639.

Werry, J. S., Elkind, G. S. & Reeves, J. C. (1987), Attention deficit, conduct, oppositional, and anxiety disorders in children: III. laboratory differences. *J. Abnorm. Child Psychol.,* 15:409–428.

Zahn, T. P., Abate, F., Little, B. C. & Wender, P. H. (1975), Minimal brain dysfunction, stimulant drugs and autonomic nervous system activity, *Arch. Gen. Psychiatry,* 32:381–387.

25

Treatment of Obsessive-Compulsive Disorder With Clomipramine and Desipramine in Children and Adolescents: A Double-Blind Crossover Comparison

Henrietta L. Leonard, Susan E. Swedo, Judith L. Rapoport, Elisabeth V. Koby, Marge C. Lenane, Deborah L. Cheslow, and Susan D. Hamburger

National Institute of Mental Health, Bethesda, Maryland

Forty-eight children and adolescents with severe primary obsessive-compulsive disorder completed a 10-week double-blind crossover trial of clomipramine hydrochloride (mean dose [±SD], 150±53 mg/d) and desipramine hydrochloride (mean dose [±SD], 153±55 mg/d). Clomipramine was clearly superior to desipramine in significantly reducing obsessive-compulsive symptoms. Age at onset, duration and severity of illness, type of symptom, and plasma drug concentrations did not predict clinical response to clomipramine. Sixty-four percent of patients who received clomipramine as their first active treatment showed at least some sign of relapse during desipramine treatment. We further document the specificity of the antiobsessional effect of clomipramine and the need for maintenance treatment.

The considerable recent interest in obsessive-compulsive disorder (OCD) was prompted by the recognition that this is a common condition estimated to occur in 1% to 3% of the general population[1] and by the demonstration that the tricyclic antidepressant clomipramine hydrochloride is effective in treating this disorder.[2]

Reprinted with permission from *Archives of General Psychiatry*, 1989, Vol. 46, 1088–1092. Copyright © 1989 by the American Medical Association.

This study was supported in part by the Department of Health and Human Services, Public Health Service, Rockville, Md, National Research Service Award F35-MH09411-01.

The authors thank Nina Schooler, PhD, for helpful advice on design and statistical analysis.

Flament et al[3,4] have documented the efficacy of clomipramine for a group of 19 adolescents with severe primary OCD. However, that study, a placebo-controlled double-blind crossover trial, did not address the efficacy of clomipramine relative to that of another tricyclic antidepressant. There are several reasons for asking such a question. First, a crossover comparison between clomipramine and placebo, such as the Flament et al studies, was not in most cases truly "blind" because the anticholinergic side effects differentiated the active treatment phase. Most patients did particularly badly during the placebo phase when it was given second during the Flament et al studies, leaving open the possibility that a drug discrimination had been taught to the study patients who recognized that they were receiving placebo and experienced relapse. Second, the use of a comparison antidepressant addresses the question of what component of the antiobsessional response might be mediated by a nonspecific antidepressant or anxiolytic effect.

Several clinical treatment trials have utilized both a selective serotonin (5-hydroxytryptamine [5-HT]) reuptake blocker and another antidepressant for OCD.[2,5-8] However, these studies either did not demonstrate a significant difference between active treatments, had small sample size, lacked a placebo phase, and/or used comparison drugs with different side effect profiles.

Our study was a double-blind treatment trial crossover comparison of clomipramine and the tricyclic antidepressant desipramine hydrochloride, known to lack clomipramine's selective potency in blockade of serotonin reuptake,[9] in a sample of children and adolescents with severe primary OCD. The larger sample size and crossover design provided greater power for comparison of the two treatments, and more satisfactory blinding of the nonclomipramine phase.

Our study addressed the following two questions: (1) did clomipramine and desipramine differ significantly in their antiobsessional effects, and (2) if the two active drugs did differ, what was the rate of relapse on desipramine for those subjects receiving clomipramine as their first active treatment?

SUBJECTS AND METHODS

Subjects

Children and adolescents aged 6 to 18 years with severe primary OCD were obtained through self-referral and health care professionals. Subjects were screened by at least two psychiatrists at the Clinical Center of the National Institutes of Health, Bethesda, Md.

Inclusion criteria were rituals and/or repetitive thoughts deemed unreasonable by the patient that were experienced as distressful and causing significant interference at home, school, or with interpersonal functioning, in the absence of another mental disorder (such as Tourette's syndrome), schizophrenia, or organic mental disorder. In addition to these *DSM-III* criteria,[10] symptoms had to be present for at least 1 year. Applicants were excluded when there was any evidence of mental retardation (defined by a full-scale IQ below 70), thought disorder or delusional system, neurologic damage, primary affective disorder, or primary eating disorder. Other reasons for exclusion included symptoms that were too mild at the time of evaluation or uncooperativeness with study procedures. Secondary depression, defined by affective symptoms whose onset was subsequent to that of the obsessional illness, was not an exclusion criterion nor was a history of depression. At admission, all subjects underwent a full psychiatric and medical evaluation, and families were interviewed for historical data, including a detailed developmental history. All patients and their first-degree relatives were interviewed using structured psychiatric interviews, the Schedule for Affective Disorders and Schizophrenia[11] for family members 18 years and older, and the Diagnostic Interview for Children and Adolescents[12,13] for children over age 6 years.

Fifty children (32 boys and 18 girls) were accepted into the study and completed the initial baseline inpatient evaluation week. One child's condition improved spontaneously and did not enter the drug trial.

The study sample, therefore, consisted of 49 patients (31 boys and 18 girls), and values are reported as means $\pm$SDs. Mean age of the patient was 13.86 ± 2.87 years (range, 7 to 19 years). The mean full-scale IQ was 107.08 ± 13.07 (range, 71 to 135). The age of onset ranged from 5 to 16 years (10.23 ± 5.8 years), and the duration of illness ranged from 1 to 10 years (3.63 ± 2.74 years).

Only 12 of the children had not received any prior treatment. Thirteen had been hospitalized, 37 had had psychotherapy, and 3 had been treated with behavioral therapy. Twenty-four had had trials of at least one drug: 19 had taken an antidepressant: imipramine hydrochloride, 14; desipramine hydrochloride, 3; amitriptyline hydrochloride, 5, trazodone hydrochloride, 1; 8 had taken a neuroleptic; haloperidol, 2; trifluoperazine hydrochloride, 3; thiothixene, 2; thioridazine hydrochloride, 3; chlorpromazine hydrochloride, 2; perphenazine, 1; and 4 had taken an anxiolytic; alprazolam, 3; hydroxyzine hydrochloride, 1; and lorazepam, 1. Other agents used in trials were methylphenidate hydrochloride, 1; lithium carbonate, 1; clonidine, 1; and carbamazepine, 1. Drug combinations had been frequent. All medications were discontinued at least 2 weeks before admission; there was a 3-week minimum drug-free period for antidepressants and 6 weeks for antipsychotics.

Procedure

All patients were evaluated in a baseline 1-week inpatient assessment on an open pediatric ward. Structured psychiatric interview,[12,13] medical and developmental examination, and psychometric testing were carried out. Laboratory measures included complete blood cell count, thyroid functions, and liver chemistries, platelet monoamine oxidase and serotonin (5-HT); an electroencephalogram, a cerebral computed tomographic scan, and lumbar puncture for cerebrospinal fluid monoamines and metabolites also were obtained. Neuropsychological tests administered included Money's Road Map of direction sense[14] and Milner's stylus maze.[15] Psychophysiological measures of arousal and reaction time included spontaneous electrodermal fluctuations, heart rate, and skin conductance level.[16]

The drug trial was conducted on an outpatient basis for all subjects who were seen weekly for the 12-week study. During the first 2-week single-blind placebo phase, any subject with greater than 20% improvement on the Global OCD Scale would not be included in the active treatment trial. The study design is shown in Figure 1.

Active treatments then consisted of two consecutive 5-week treatment periods (labeled phase A and phase B, respectively) with randomized double-blind administration of clomipramine, or desipramine in doses targeting 3 mg/kg as tolerated. Clomipramine, desipramine, and placebo were supplied in 25-mg or 50-mg identical capsules and were administered on a fixed schedule: the dosage on the first day was 25 mg (for children weighing 25 kg or less) or 50 mg (for those weighing over 25kg) and increased by one capsule each week. The maximum dosage did not exceed 250 mg/d or 5 mg/kg. At the end of phase A, the dosage was tapered during the first week of phase B, and the phase B medication was increased concurrently. No other psychotropic drugs were administered.

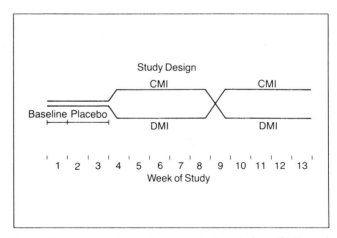

Figure 1. Design of clomipramine hydrochloride (CMI) and desipramine hydrochloride (DMI) crossover study for obsessive-compulsive children and adolescents.

Children receiving ongoing treatment with private psychotherapists were allowed to continue, but behavior modification was not a concurrent treatment during the study. The study was approved by the National Institute of Health Research Review Committee, Bethesda, Md, and each child and his parents gave ascent/informed consent for the investigation.

Clinical Assessment

Subjects and their families were seen weekly for behavioral ratings of depression, obsessive-compulsive symptomatology, and side effects. Behavioral ratings, described previously,[3,4] assessed obsessions (both self-rated and observed), depression, anxiety, global functioning, and side effects. Rating scales included the Leyton Obsessional Inventory-Child Version,[17] Obsessive-Compulsive Rating, Comprehensive Psychopathological Rating Scale,[18] National Institute of Mental Health (NIMH) Global Scales,[19] Brief Psychiatric Rating Scales,[20] and the Hamilton Depression Rating Scale.[21] Side effects were rated using the Subjective Treatment Emergent Symptoms Scale,[22] a checklist of 23 physical symptoms, rated none (0), slight (1), or much (2), and all of the clinical ratings were completed by a psychiatrist who was blind to the treatment condition.

At the end of the fifth week of each treatment phase, 12 hours after the administration of the previous dose of drug, blood was obtained for routine hematology and chemistry, platelet 5-HT, and plasma clomipramine, desmethylclomipramine, and desipramine measurements. Electrocardiography was repeated at the end of each treatment phase.

Data Analysis

Analysis of covariance, using baseline measures as the covariate, was utilized to examine differences between drug treatments of all clinical measures. A BMDP ANCOVA program[23] was used, with Bonferroni post hoc comparisons where appropriate. Side effects were examined for drug treatments and between drug and placebo using a repeated measures analysis of variance procedure (Statistical Analysis System)[24] with Bonferroni post hoc comparisons. An attempt was made to predict which factors might predict a positive response to clomipramine, using a Statistical Analysis System stepwise regression procedure.

Finally, a survival analysis[25] was utilized to calculate the cumulative proportion of subjects who remained well, as defined by the NIMH OCD Rating Scale, from the time of their last week receiving clomipramine (phase A—week 5) through the 5 weeks of desipramine treatment (phase B), for subjects who received clomipramine as their first active treatment (phase A).

TABLE 1
Clinical Ratings for Children and Adolescents With Severe Primary Obsessive-Compulsive Disorder (OCD) During Baseline, Placebo, Desipramine Hydrochloride, and Clomipramine Hydrochloride Treatment (N = 48)

Measure*	Baseline (Mean ± SD)	Placebo, wk 2	Mean ± SD		Drug†		Drug × Order†	
			Desipramine Hydrochloride, wk 5	Clomipramine Hydrochloride, wk 5	F	P	F	P
NIMH Obsessive-Compulsive Scale	8.5 ± 1.3	8.6 ± 1.5	8.0 ± 2.0	6.3 ± 2.3	16.62	.0002	24.60	.00001
Ward OCD Rating	14.5 ± 2.6	14.7 ± 2.5	13.6 ± 3.0	11.4 ± 3.6	21.16	.00001	13.50	.0007
CPRS-Obsessive-Compulsive Subscale	10.3 ± 3.4	9.7 ± 4.1	8.1 ± 4.5	6.9 ± 4.7	10.34	.003	8.41	.006
Insel	29.7 ± 8.1	29.9 ± 7.4	26.2 ± 10.4	20.2 ± 10.7	10.06	.004	26.95	.00001
LOI-Child Version								
Symptom	20.9 ± 8.5	18.6 ± 9.1	14.9 ± 10.2	14.4 ± 10.3	1.10	NS	...	...
Resistance	34.4 ± 20.3	31.7 ± 24.3	25.3 ± 24.6	24.7 ± 26.2	0.55	NS	...	...
Interference	35.9 ± 23.3	32.0 ± 26.5	26.4 ± 27.5	25.3 ± 28.5	0.86	NS	...	...
Hamilton Depression	7.5 ± 4.5	6.7 ± 5.2	6.6 ± 6.6	5.2 ± 4.9	8.47	.006	.88	NS
NIMH Depression	4.7 ± 2.0	4.6 ± 2.0	4.2 ± 2.6	3.0 ± 1.8	24.10	.00001	6.60	.01
NIMH Anxiety	5.8 ± 2.0	5.8 ± 2.3	5.0 ± 2.3	4.5 ± 2.1	3.31	NS	...	...
Global Functioning	7.6 ± 1.7	7.7 ± 1.7	7.0 ± 2.2	5.7 ± 2.4	19.34	.001	24.46	.00001

*NIMH indicates National Institute of Mental Health; CPRS, Comprehensive Psychopathological Rating Scale; and LOI, Leyton Obsessional Inventory; and NS, not significant.

†Analysis of covariance, clomipramine vs desipramine.

RESULTS

Of the 49 children who entered the treatment study, no subject's condition improved while being given placebo to a degree that they were dropped from treatment. Four subjects did not complete the trial. One boy discontinued in the second week of phase A (clomipramine) because he could not tolerate even a 25-mg dose; his data were not included. Three subjects left the study at week 3 of phase B and their final scores were used. Discontinuation was due to psychosis and depression requiring hospitalization (one case each) and noncompliance (one case).

For the 48 subjects whose data are reported for the treatment trial, the mean (±SD) dose of clomipramine hydrochloride at week 5 of treatment was 150±53 mg/d (3.01±0.73 mg/kg per day) and 153±55 mg/d (3.07±0.72 mg/kg per day) for desipramine hydrochloride, with a range of 50 to 250 mg/d for each drug.

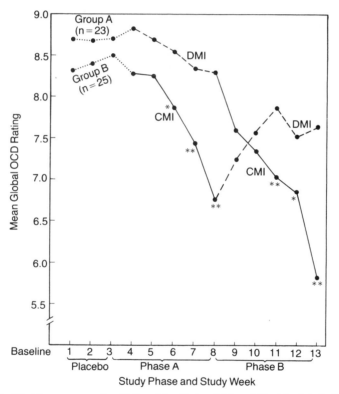

Figure 2. Weekly scores on the National Institute of Mental Health global obsessive-compulsive disorder (OCD) rating scale during placebo, desipramine hydrochloride (DMI), and clomipramine hydrochloride (CMI) treatment periods. Single asterisk indicates $P < .05$ by Bonferroni t statistic; double asterisk, $P < .01$ by Bonferroni t statistic.

Mean ($\pm$SD) plasma levels of clomipramine and its metabolite (desmethylclomipramine) at week 5 of treatment were 119$\pm$67 ng/mL (range, 13 to 325 ng/mL) and 278$\pm$154 ng/mL (range 44 to 639 ng/mL), respectively. Concentrations of the desmethyl metabolite were 2.3 times greater than those of clomipramine, with the correlation between the parent compound and its primary metabolite being .51. Mean ($\pm$SD) plasma levels of desipramine at week 5 of treatment were 182.73$\pm$160.64 ng/mL) range, 32 to 850 ng/mL).

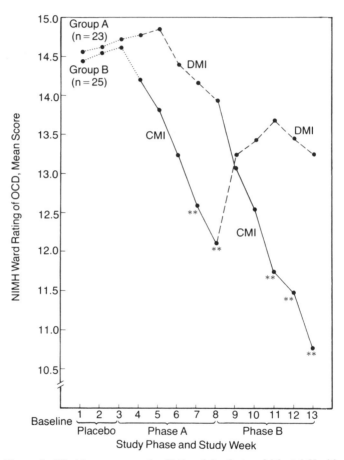

Figure 3. Weekly scores on the National Institute of Mental Health (NIMH) ward obsessive-compulsive disorder (OCD) rating during placebo, desipramine hydrochloride (DMI), and clomipramine hydrochloride (CMI) treatment periods. Asterisk indicates $P < .01$ by Bonferroni t statistic.

Clinical Response

Clomipramine but not desipramine produced a striking decrease in obsessive-compulsive ratings and in depression ratings as measured on the Hamilton NIMH Depression scales. Mean scores for baseline placebo, clomipramine, and desipramine treatments are given in Table 1 and Figures 2 and 3.

As shown, there is little benefit from placebo over baseline and a clear superiority of clomipramine over desipramine on most OCD rating scale measures. There is also a significant effect of drug order on these same rating scales (evident on inspection of Figures 1 and 2) shown in Table 1. When desipramine is given after clomipramine, subjects experienced relapse at a rate similar to that for placebo in our previous study.[3]

Figure 4 provides a graphic representation of the survival analysis, that is, the cumulative proportion of subjects (who received clomipramine as their first active medication in phase A) who did not have a relapse in the 5 weeks between their last dose of clomipramine (end of phase A) and the end of their phase B desipramine treatment (36%). As shown, 64% of the patients who were crossed over to

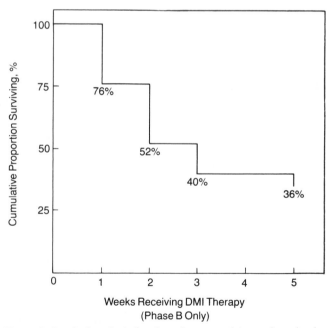

Figure 4. Survival analysis for obsessive-compulsive patients in phase B who received clomipramine hydrochloride as their first active treatment (phase A) and then were crossed over to desipramine hydrochloride (DMI) as their second active treatment (phase B).

desipramine showed some sign of relapse as defined by at least a one-point worsening on the NIMH Global OCD Scale by the fifth week receiving desipramine. A one-point worsening on the NIMH Global OCD Scale represented a noticeable increase in symptoms and was clinically meaningful.

As they experienced relapse, patients became more dysphoric, and as Table 1 shows, the Hamilton depression score was significantly higher for patients receiving desipramine than for those receiving clomipramine.

Side Effects

Side effects at the fifth treatment week on clomipramine and desipramine are shown in Table 2. The side effects of the two medications were similar except that tremor was greater with clomipramine than with desipramine and more patients experienced "other" side effects while receiving clomipramine, including chest pain, hot flashes, heartburn, rash, and acne. There tended to be a higher rate of sweating and dizziness while receiving clomipramine than desipramine although this was not statistically significant.

Predictors of Response

A stepwise regression analysis was carried out in an attempt to predict clinical response to clomipramine, as measured by the NIMH OCD Scale. Drug order was forced into the regression model first ($R^2 = 6\%$), followed by other selected variables, including sex, index and onset age, duration, severity, type of symptom, family history of OCD, neuropsychological and psychophysiological variables, cerebrospinal fluid monoamines and metabolites, and plasma drug concentrations. There was little significant prediction; skin conductance level and errors on the street map (toward direction) were the only variables that predicted response, accounting for 10% and 5% of the variance, respectively. In combination, including drug order, they accounted for 21% of the variance. (Lower skin conductance level and fewer map errors predicted, although weakly, a better response to clomipramine.) Neither plasma clomipramine nor desmethylclomipramine predicted clinical response to clomipramine.

COMMENT

Our study shows unequivocal superiority of clomipramine in comparison with another tricyclic antidepressant for the treatment of OCD. Most dramatic is the reversal of beneficial effect for the group receiving clomipramine first, even with maintenance of desipramine. Because both drugs were given in virtually identical doses, and because desipramine is an effective antidepressant, our study further

TABLE 2
Side Effects of Obsessive-Compulsive Children and Adolescents
During Clomipramine-Desipramine Hydrochloride Crossover
Study (N = 45)

Side Effect	No. (%) of Subjects			
	Baseline	Placebo	Desipramine Hydrochloride, wk 5	Clomipramine Hydrochloride, wk 5
Increased appetite	2 (4)	0 (0)	3 (7)	3 (7)
Poor appetite	7 (16)	2 (4)	6 (13)	6 (13)
Dry mouth	6 (13)	1 (2)	26*(58)	27* (60)
Increased salivation	1 (2)	1 (2)	0 (0)	1 (2)
Taste difference	0 (0)	0 (0)	0 (0)	1 (2)
Stiffness	5 (11)	0 (0)	1 (2)	2 (4)
Tremor	0 (0)	0 (0)	4 (9)	17*†(38)
Weakness	3 (7)	0 (0)	2 (4)	6‡ (13)
Tiredness	12 (27)	5 (11)	11 (24)	16‡ (36)
Headache	9 (20)	4 (9)	6 (13)	2 (4)
Itching	4 (9)	2 (4)	1 (2)	2 (4)
Constipation	3 (7)	2 (4)	5 (11)	8 (18)
Diarrhea	4 (9)	2 (4)	0 (0)	0 (0)
Nausea	2 (4)	1 (2)	1 (2)	2 (4)
Stomacheache	5 (11)	6 (13)	6 (13)	2 (4)
Urinary frequency	1 (2)	1 (2)	0 (0)	0 (0)
Difficulty urinating	0 (0)	0 (0)	0 (0)	2 (4)
Heart pounding	2 (0)	0 (0)	0 (0)	1 (2)
Dizziness	8 (18)	0 (0)	7 (16)	14* (31)
Blurry vision	4 (9)	2 (4)	1 (2)	4 (9)
Sweating	2 (4)	0 (0)	5 (11)	8* (18)
Difficulty sleeping	9 (20)	7 (16)	7 (16)	12 (27)
Other	0 (0)	1 (2)	1 (2)	7*†(16)

*P<.01, difference from placebo.
†P<.01, difference from desipramine.
‡P<.05, difference from placebo.

substantiates previous evidence that the drug's antiobsessional effect is independent of any nonspecific anxiolytic or antidepressant action. The higher Hamilton Depression scores while receiving desipramine than while receiving clomipramine supports our clinical impression that depression in OCD is most often secondary to impairment from OCD.

It is unlikely that desipramine is more beneficial than placebo for this population. Although our study utilized placebo only for an initial 2-week single-blind period, our prior clomipramine/placebo comparison using a similar patient population and design provides indirect placebo comparison data. In that earlier study, the slopes for the (minimal) improvement of patients receiving placebo in Phase A and for the deterioration of patients receiving placebo when given in phase B after clomipramine can virtually be superimposed on those for improvement in phase A with desipramine or deterioration in phase B of desipramine in the present study. Thus, an adverse drug desipramine/clomipramine interaction or an adverse effect of desipramine on OCD itself is unlikely.

Nineteen patients (38%) of the sample had not responded to a previous trial of a tricyclic antidepressant before entering the trial, which may have negatively biased the group's response to desipramine. However, we found no evidence that those patients with prior tricyclic drug treatment were more likely to respond differentially to clomipramine.

The deterioration rates found in this study need to be interpreted with caution with respect to clinical practice. The subjects had been given clomipramine for only 5 weeks, and it is possible that a longer treatment period would prevent or lessen later deterioration, and conversely that deterioration would have been greater if desipramine maintenance had been extended. Our clinical data suggest in fact that with a longer drug-free period, the incidence and degree of relapse are considerably greater. A double-blind maintenance/discontinuation study is currently in progress with subjects who have been receiving clomipramine from several months to several years to address this question systematically.

The selective efficacy of clomipramine and other serotonin reuptake blockers is of considerable practical and theoretical importance. Practically, because OCD is 20 to 60 times more common than previously believed,[1] a large number of patients are expected to benefit from these new treatments. Theoretically, the selective efficacy of drug treatment for complex behaviors linked by thoughts and behavioral routines that deal with cleanliness, danger, doubt, and guilt, supports the concept of preprogrammed behaviors most probably developed over evolutionary time at a level of complexity previously unimaginable in humans.[26]

REFERENCES

1. Karno M, Golding JM, Sorenson SB, Burnam MA. The epidemiology of obsessive-compulsive disorder in five US communities. *Arch Gen Psychiatry.* 1988;45:1094–1099.

2. Thoren P, Asberg M, Cronholm B, Jornestedt L, Traksman L. Clomipramine treatment of obsessive-compulsive disorder, I: a controlled clinical trial. *Arch Gen Psychiatry.* 1980;37:1281–1285.

3. Flament M, Rapoport JL, Berg C, Sceery W, Kilts C, Mellstrom B, Linnoila M. Clomipramine treatment of childhood obsessive-compulsive disorder. *Arch Gen Psychiatry.* 1985;42:977–983.

4. Flament M, Rapoport J, Murphy D, Berg CJ, Lake R. Biochemical changes during clomipramine treatment of childhood obsessive-compulsive disorder. *Arch Gen Psychiatry.* 1987;44:219–225.

5. Ananth J, Pecknold J, Van Den Steen N, Engelsmann F. Double-blind comparative study of clomipramine and amitryptyline in obsessive neurosis. *Prog Neuropsychopharmacol Biol Psychiatry.* 1981;5:257–262.

6. Insel TR, Murphy DL, Cohen RM, Alterman I, Kilts C. Linnoila M. Obsessive compulsive disorder: a double-blind trial of clomipramine and clorgyline. *Arch Gen Psychiatry.* 1983;40:605–612.

7. Insel T, Mueller E, Alterman I, Linnoila M. Murphy DL. Obsessive compulsive disorder and serotonin: is there a connection? *Biol Psychiatry.* 1985;20:1174–1188.

8. Volvavka J, Neziroglu F, Yaryura-Tobias J. Clomipramine and imipramine in obsessive-compulsive disorder. *Psychiatry Res.* 1985;14:83–91.

9. Ross SB, Renyi AL. Tricyclic antidepressant agents: comparison of the inhibition of the uptake of ^{3}H-nonadrenaline and ^{14}C-5-hydroxy-tryptamine in slices and crude synaptosome preparations of midbrain-hypothalamus region of the rat brain. *Acta Pharmacol Toxicol.* 1975;36:382–394.

10. American Psychiatric Association, Committee on Nomenclature and Statistics: *Diagnostic and Statistical Manual of Mental Disorders.* 3rd ed. Washington, DC: American Psychiatric Association; 1980.

11. Spitzer R, Endicott J. *Schedule for Affective Disorders and Schizophrenia.* 3rd ed. New York, NY: Biometrics Research Division, New York State Psychiatric Institute; 1978.

12. Herjanic B, Campbell JW: Differentiating psychiatrically disturbed children on the basis of a structured interview. *J Abnorm Child Psychol.* 1977;5:127–135.

13. Welner Z, Reich W, Herjanic B, Jung KG, Amado H. Reliability, validity, and parent-child agreement studies of the diagnostic interview for children and adolescents (DICA). *J Am Acad Child Adol Psychiatry.* 1987;26:649–653.

14. Money J, Alexander D, Walker HT. *A Standardized Road Map Test of Direction Sense.* Baltimore, Md: Johns Hopkins University Press; 1965.

15. Milner B. Visually guided maze learning in man: effects of bilateral hippocampal, bilateral frontal and unilateral cerebral lesions. *Neuropsychologia.* 1965;3:317–338.

16. Zahn TP, Rapoport JL. Acute autonomic nervous system effects of caffeine in prepubertal boys. *Psychopharmacology.* 1987;91:40–44.
17. Berg CJ, Rapoport JL, Flament MF. The Leyton obsessional inventory—child version. *J Am Acad Child Psychiatry.* 1986:25:84–91.
18. Asberg M, Montgomery SA, Perris C, Schalling D, Sedvall G. A comprehensive psychopathological rating scale. *Acta Psychiatr Scand.* 1978;271:5–27.
19. Murphy DL, Pickar D, Alterman IS. Methods for the quantitative assessment of depressive and manic behavior. In: Burdock EL, Sudilovsky A, Gershon S, eds. *The Behavior of Psychiatric Patients.* New York, NY: Marcel Dekker Inc; 1982:355–392.
20. Overall JE, Gorham DR. The Brief Psychiatric Rating Scale. *Psychol Rep.* 1962;10:799–812.
21. Hamilton M. Development of a rating scale for primary depressive illness. *Br J Soc Psychol.* 1967;6:278–296.
22. Campbell M, Palij M. Measurement of side effects including tardive dyskinesia. *Psychopharmacol Bull.* 1985;21:1063–1082.
23. BDMP, Statistical Software Manual. Berkeley: University of California Press; 1985.
24. *SAS User's Guide: Statistics.* 5th ed. Cary, NC: SAS Institute Inc; 1985.
25. Mausner JS, Kramer S. *Epidemiology: An Introductory Text.* Philadelphia, Pa: WB Sauders Co; 1985.
26. Bolles RC. Species typical response predispositions. In: Marler P, Terrance H, eds. *The Biology of Learning.* New York, NY: Springer-Verlag; 1984:425–436.

26

A Double-Blind Placebo Controlled Study of Desipramine in the Treatment of ADD: I. Efficacy

Joseph Biederman

Massachusetts General Hospital and Harvard Medical School, Boston

Ross J. Baldessarini

Harvard Medical School, Boston, and McLean Hospital, Belmont, Massachusetts

Virginia Wright and Debra Knee

Massachusetts General Hospital, Boston

Jerold S. Harmatz

Tufts University of Medicine and New England Medical Center, Boston

The tricyclic antidepressant drug desipramine (DMI) was evaluated in the treatment of young patients with attention deficit disorder with hyperactivity (ADDH) in an unselected sample of 62 clinically referred patients, 43 (69%) of whom previously responded poorly to psychostimulant treatment. The 42 children and 20 adolescents were assigned randomly to receive DMI (N = 31) or placebo (N = 31) for up to 6 weeks in a parallel groups, double-blind study. Clinically and statistically significant differences in behavioral improvement were found for DMI over placebo, at an average (± SEM) maximal daily dose of 4.6 ± 0.2 mg/kg; 68% of DMI-treated patients were considered very much or

Reprinted with permission from *Journal of the American Academy of Child and Adolescent Psychiatry,* 1989, Vol. 28, No. 5, 777–784. Copyright © 1989 by the American Academy of Child and Adolescent Psychiatry.

This work was supported in part by grants from Merrell-Dow Pharmaceutical Company and the Charlupski Foundation (to J.B.), as well as USPHS (NIMH) award and grants MH-31154, MH-36224, and MH-47370 (R.J.B.).

The authors thank Peter Rosenberger, M.D., David Gastfriend, M.D., and Kate Keenan for their help with this project, and Michael Jellinek, M.D. for encouragement.

much improved, compared with only 10% of placebo patients (p
<0.001). DMI was well tolerated, even at the relatively high doses
used. These findings suggest that DMI can be an effective treatment in
the management of pediatric patients with ADDH, including patients
who failed to respond to stimulants. Key Words: attention deficit disor-
der, desipramine.

Stimulants have been used widely in the treatment of attention deficit disorder with hyperactivity (ADDH). Yet, as many as 30% of children so treated do not improve (Barkley, 1977; Biederman and Jellinek, 1984). Because stimulants are short-acting drugs, their use is complicated by the need to take medicine in school and by a sometimes troublesome reemergence of symptoms on weekends and in the evening hours at home (Porrino et al., 1983). In addition, insomnia, dysphoric mood, tics, and some slowing of growth during development may occur with such treatment (Gittelman, 1980). Furthermore, although the ADDH syndrome and associated psychiatric symptoms can persist into adolescence and adulthood in at least 30% to 50% of patients who manifest ADDH as children (Gittelman et al., 1985; Weiss et al., 1985), there is little information regarding appropriate pharmacotherapy in the older age groups despite the increasingly frequent recognition of such patients (Varley, 1985). Concerns about treating adolescents with stimulant medication include at least the hypothetical risk of abuse and dependence by the patient or his associates (Goyer et al., 1982), and the common dislike by adolescents of the subjective effects of stimulant medication (Sleator et al., 1982).

These problems encourage the search for effective and safe alternatives to stimulant drugs in the treatment of ADDH. Tricyclic antidepressants (TCAs), mainly imipramine, have been proposed as an alternative treatment for this disorder (Gross, 1973; Huessy and Wright, 1970; Krakowski, 1965; Kupietz and Balka, 1976; Watter and Dreyfus, 1973; Zametkin and Rapoport, 1983). Possible advantages of TCAs over stimulants include a longer duration of action and the feasibility of once-daily dosing without symptom-rebound or insomnia, greater flexibility in dosage, the readily available option of monitoring plasma drug-levels (Preskorn et al., 1983), and minimal risk of abuse or dependence (Gittelman, 1980; Rapoport and Mikkelsen, 1978). Initial open trials (Gross, 1973; Huessy and Wright, 1970; Krakowski, 1965; Kupietz and Balka, 1976; Watter and Dreyfus, 1973), were followed by controlled studies (Greenberg et al., 1975; Rapoport et al., 1974; Waizer et al., 1974; Werry, 1980; Winsberg et al., 1972; Yepes et al., 1977) that generally showed TCAs to be superior to a placebo, although not always as effective as methylphenidate.

Desipramine (DMI) has not been well studied in pediatric populations until recently. Although similar to its precursor imipramine, DMI has relatively high selectivity against neuronal uptake of norepinephrine and, like other TCAs, appears eventually to enhance functional availability of norepinephrine and its activity at central alpha-1 adrenergic receptors (Baldessarini, 1985). Compared with other TCAs, DMI has relatively low affinity at muscarinic and histaminergic receptors and only moderate affinity at alpha-1 adrenergic receptors, and it is very weak against alpha-2, beta-adrenergic, and dopaminergic receptors (Baldessarini, 1985). Because of its pharmacologic properties, DMI may be associated with somewhat lesser risks of adverse effects than the tertiary-amine TCAs such as amitriptyline, clomipramine, doxepin, and imipramine.

Several open (Biederman et al., 1986; Gastfriend et al., 1984, 1985) and controlled (Donnelly et al., 1986; Garfinkel et al., 1983) studies have investigated the efficacy and toxicity of DMI in children with ADDH. In a double-blind, placebo-controlled, crossover study of 3 weeks duration for each phase, Garfinkel et al. (1983) compared the effects of methylphenidate, clomipramine, DMI, and placebo in 12 prepubertal boys with ADDH using daily doses of the TCAs up to 3.5 mg/kg. DMI and clomipramine were more beneficial than placebo, but somewhat less so than methylphenidate, in improving attentional and behavioral symptoms of ADDH; there was no improvement in cognitive performance with either of the TCA treatments. There were no important adverse effects and only mild increases in pulse rate and diastolic blood pressure were associated with all active drugs. Donnelly et al. (1986) studied 29 boys aged 6 to 12 years with ADDH in a parallel groups, double-blind, placebo-controlled study: 17 received DMI (mean daily dose, 3.4 mg/kg) and 12 received placebo for 14 days. Behavioral improvement with DMI was detected as early as day 3 and was sustained over the 2 weeks of the study. There were no important adverse effects, and only mild increases in pulse rate and diastolic blood pressure, with DMI treatment.

The authors have also reported favorable results in open, dose ranging, long-term trials of DMI in an unselected group of 12 adolescents (Gastfriend et al., 1984, 1985) and 18 children (Biederman et al., 1986) with ADDH, using daily doses of up to 5 mg/kg that were continued for up to 1 year. In these studies, 73% of the 30 patients had received pharmacologic treatments previously with an inadequate response or intolerable adverse effects but, after a mean period of 27 weeks (range 4-52 weeks) of follow-up, 80% of the patients were considered moderately or markedly improved on DMI. Adverse effects were mild, most appeared in the first 4 weeks of treatment, and were alleviated by dose reduction. Because of remaining uncertainties about the safety of TCAs in children, the authors also evaluated systematically the short- (4 to 12 weeks) and long- (13 to 52 weeks) term effects of DMI treatment on the cardiovascular system (Biederman et al., 1985) but found no symptomatic cardiovascular effects and only minor ECG changes associated with DMI treatment in daily oral doses as high as 5 mg/kg. Based on these preliminary studies and clinical experience with DMI, it was hypothesized that DMI at daily doses up to 5 mg/kg can be a safe and effective treatment for children and adolescents with ADDH. The present study reports the effects of DMI in a prospective, double-blind, placebo-controlled study of a total of 62 children and adolescents with ADDH. This is one of the largest experimental therapeutic trials of ADDH and the largest controlled trial of DMI in the pediatric population.

METHOD

Patients were drawn from consecutive outpatient referrals to the Pediatric Psychopharmacology Unit and Child Psychiatry Service of the Massachusetts General Hospital, Boston. All but two patients initially considered for the study ($N = 73$) met clinical criteria for *DMS-III* ADDH, manifested symptoms in at least two of three settings (home, school, clinic), and attained a score of 15 or more (out of 30) on the Conners Abbreviated Questionnaire by parent or teacher (see Guy, 1976); two children, aged 7 and 15 years, met clinical criteria for ADD without hyperactivity. The clinical diagnosis was confirmed in each case by using the module on attention deficit disorder from the Diagnostic Interview for Children and Adolescents, Parent Version (DICA-P) (Herjanic and Reich, 1982; Orvaschel, 1985). No patient needed to be excluded by having mental retardation (full scale IQ < 70), autism, psychosis, or another medical or neurological disorder or by abnormal results of psychiatric and medical evaluations given, including routine laboratory tests and initial ECG. Eleven patients failed to complete the protocol. The 62 subjects completing at least 3 weeks of the protocol ranged in age from 6 to 17 years; 42 were younger than 12 years, and 20 were 12 or older. All drugs were discontinued for at least 1 week before entering the protocol.

The trial was designed as a 6-week, double-blind, parallel groups, placebo-controlled protocol. Assenting patients were accepted into the study after their parents provided written informed consent under conditions approved by the hospital's Institutional Review Board. Patients were assigned randomly by a computer generated list to receive desipramine hydrochloride (DMI) ($N = 31$) or an equivalent amount of placebo ($N = 31$) in identical-appearing tablets. The dose was to be increased to the nearest convenient number of tablets to yield a dose ≥ 5.0 mg/kg by week 3 and resulted in a daily dose of DMI (or the equivalent amount of placebo) of ≤ 5.6 mg/kg given in two portions daily. However, in 22/31 DMI (as well as 16/31 placebo) treated patients, the maximal dose had to be lowered or increased more slowly due to apparent adverse effects, but no further increments were made after week 5. Compliance with treatment was monitored by weekly pill counts. No other psychotropic agents or formal psychological or behavioral therapy were administered during the study. At the end of the study, placebo-treated patients who did not improve were offered an open trial of DMI and all study procedures were repeated for another 6 weeks. In addition, patients who responded to DMI could continue its use under clinical treatment conditions.

After the final clinical ratings were obtained under double-blind conditions, the treatment code was opened to facilitate final laboratory assessments as well as follow-up dispositions. To reduce costs, only DMI-treated patients had end-of-treatment blood and ECG testing. Blood was drawn by antecubital venepuncture at 12 hours after last prior dose of DMI, after a minimum of 1 week on a stable drug regimen, for assay of the approximately steady-state serum level of DMI, as well as liver function tests and a complete blood count. DMI was separated by high performance liquid chromatography (HPLC) and detected with dual wave-length ultraviolet spectrometry sensitive to 20 ng/ml; intra- and interassay coefficients of variation (SD/mean) were <3% and <5%, respectively. In addition to the baseline ECGs given to all subjects, the DMI-treated patients also had an end-of-treatment ECG at the same time as the blood studies. Laboratory tests and ECGs were performed by the clinical laboratories of Massachusetts General Hospital. Laboratory personnel were unaware of the patients' clinical status or response to treatment. DMI plasma levels and cardiovascular findings are reported separately (see Biederman et al., 1989).

Response to treatment was assessed using the Conners Abbreviated Parent and Teacher Questionnaires (10 items, maximum score = 30) (Guy, 1976) completed by parents (weekly) and teachers (pre- and end-of-treatment); and physician-rated Clinical Global Impression (CGI) Scale (CGI, 1985) (weekly), which includes scales rating of Global Severity (1 = not ill, to 7 = extremely ill) and Global Improvement (GI, 1 = very much improved, to 7 = very much worse), and an Efficacy Index (1 = markedly improved with no side effects, to 16 = worse with marked side effects). The Continuous Performance Task (CPT) (Conners, 1985) and Paired Associated Learning Task (PALT) Swanson et al., 1979; Swanson, 1985) were administered by a trained research assistant as laboratory measurements of cognition before and at the end of treatment. The Children's Depression Inventory (CDI) (Kovacs, 1985) (maximum score = 54) was completed independently by each subject and mother before and at the end of treatment to evaluate depressive symptoms. Adverse effects during treatment were assessed systematically at each weekly clinical contact with the physician-rated Subjective Treatment-Emergent Symptoms Scale (STESS, 1985), which records reported and observed new symptoms. In addition, sitting and standing pulse and blood pressures were recorded by the supervising research physician at each visit.

Of the 73 patients screened, 62 (85%, 31 in each treatment condition) completed at least 3 weeks of the study protocol to provide usable data. The 11 patients (15%) who terminated prematurely (before week 3) were not included in the data analysis: four never started the protocol for administrative reasons; one was dropped after a pharmacy error was discovered in which placebo was given in week 1 and DMI in week 2; five had incomplete data collections; and one patient developed a rash during the first week on DMI and was discontinued. Eight placebo and one DMI patient were terminated prematurely between weeks 3 and 6 due to a deteriorating clinical course but were included in the data analysis (end-of-treatment ratings). The final data base thus involved 62 patients; 31 received DMI and 31 placebo. Differences between clinical effects associated with DMI and placebo were expressed as percent change scores on outcome measures calculated for each subject ([end-baseline]/baseline) × 100. Treatments were contrasted by application of independent Student's *t*-tests to each dimension for continuous data and by Yates-corrected chi-square analyses for categorical data. All analyses were two-tailed, and statistical significance was defined conservatively at the *1% level*; all data are reported as mean ± SEM unless otherwise stated. Because of the large number of patients (43/62 = 69%) included who by chance had received prior treatment with a stimulant without adequate benefit or with intolerable adverse effects, differences between DMI and placebo were reexamined by repeating all study analyses for this subsample with a prior history of treatment refractoriness.

RESULTS

Placebo and DMI treatment groups were similar in socioeconomic status (respectively, SES = 3.1 ± 0.2 vs. 3.3 ± 0.2, NS), full scale IQ (99.6 ± 2.8 vs. 103.3 ± 2.7, NS) male to female ratio (29/2 each), children to adolescents ratio (19/12 vs. 23/9, NS), and all but four patients (2 in each group) were Caucasian. Patients in the placebo and DMI groups ($N = 31$ each) also had similar clinical characteristics at baseline as expressed by the presence of comorbid psychiatric disorders, including learning difficulties (74.2% vs. 77.4%, NS), conduct disorder (35.5% vs. 38.7%, NS), and oppositional disorder (45.2% vs. 51.6%, NS). The groups also were closely similar in baseline ratings pertaining to ADDH by clinicians, parents, and teachers (Table 1), and in cognitive measures (PALT % errors = 57.6% ± 4.2% vs. 59.5% ± 2.9%, $t = 0.4$, $df = 48$, NS; CPT errors of commission = 24.8 ± 6.7 vs. 33.7 ± 10.1, $t = 0.7$, $df = 53$, NS; CPT errors of omission = 13.4 ± 3.1 vs. 14.2 ± 2.8, $t = 0.2$, $df = 53$, NS, each for placebo and DMI, respectively). By chance, the previously treatment-refractory patients were somewhat unevenly distributed between the two treatment groups (DMI group, 18 [58%] vs. placebo group, 25 [81%]; $\chi^2 = 2.7$, $df = 1$, $N = 62$, $p = 0.10$).

Daily doses (mg/kg) were similar for placebo and DMI treatment groups throughout the 6 weeks of the study (*week 1* = 1.6 ± 0.1 vs. 1.8 ± 0.1; *week 2* = 3.0 ± 0.2 vs. 3.0 ± 0.2; *week 3* = 4.2 ± 0.3 vs. 4.0 ± 0.2; *week 4* = 4.5 ± 0.2 vs. 4.3 ± 0.2; *week 5* = 4.7 ± 0.1 vs. 4.6 ± 0.1; *week 6* = 4.8 ± 0.1 vs. 4.6 ± 0.2). Because of occasional missing data and early dropouts, weekly ratings for weeks *1 + 2 + 3 + 4 + 5 + 6*, were combined to represent each 2-week period. While no significant differences in clinical efficacy between DMI and placebo were observed by weeks 1 + 2 at average daily doses of placebo and DMI of 2.4 ± 0.2 and 2.3 ± 0.2 mg/kg, respectively, differences were detected by weeks 3 + 4 (at average daily

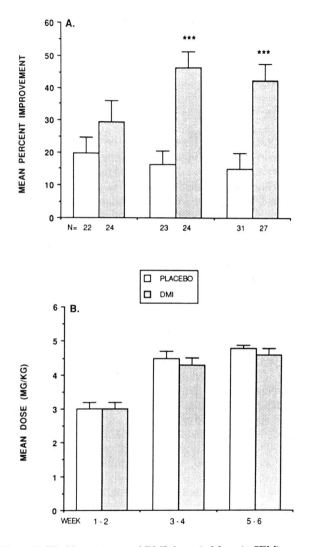

Figure 1. Weekly outcome and DMI dose. *A*, Mean (±SEM) percent change in Conners Abbreviated Parent Questionnaire scores and mean weight corrected daily doses (mg/kg). *B*, vs. duration of treatment by week period with DMI-(*solid bars*) and placebo-treated patients (*open bars*). By unpaired *t*-test (two-tailed) DMI vs. placebo, ** *p* <0.001;*** *p* <0.0001.

doses of 4.2 ± 0.2 and 4.4 ± 0.2 mg/kg) on Global Clinical Severity ratings (23.4% vs. 9.2% improvement, $t = 2.3$, $df = 41$, $p = 0.03$, trend) and Abbreviated Conners Parent Questionnaire scores 43.0% vs. 14.7% improvement, $t = 4.0$, $df = 40$, $p = 0.001$). This selective improvement on DMI was maintained by the end of the trial (weeks 5 + 6, 33.8% ± 3.4% vs. 9.1% ± 4.1%, $t = 4.7$, $df = 56$, $p = 0.0001$ and 42.1% ± 5.1% vs. 14.1% ± 4.9%, $t = 3.9$, $df = 56$, $p = 0.0003$ for Global Clinical Severity and Abbreviated Parent Conners Questionnaire, respectively) (Figure 1).

End point analysis (weeks 3 to 6) showed that 21/31 DMI subjects (68%) were considered *very much* (Clinical Global Improvement [CGI] score = 1) *or much* (CGI = 2) improved compared with only 3/31 (10%) of placebo subjects $\chi^2 = 22.0$, $df = 1$, $p = 0.0001$). DMI patients showed significantly more improvement than placebo patients in clinician's ratings, parent's ratings, and teacher's ratings (Table 1). In addition, DMI patients showed substantially more improvement in depressive symptoms as expressed in parental reporting, although this trend was not statistically significant at the 1% criterion (CDI-Parent mean [±SEM] percent change = 30.2% ± 9.4% vs. -2.4% ± 12.7%, $t = 2.0$, $df = 51$, $p = 0.05$, trend). Cognitive measures did not change significantly in either the DMI or placebo group (mean percent change for DMI vs. placebo, respectively: PALT = 14.0% ± 8.2% vs. 8.2% ± 7.5%, $t = 0.5$, $df = 47$, NS; CPT errors of commission = 13.8 ± 2.8 vs. 12.4 ± 3.0, $t = 0.3$, $df = 53$, NS; CPT errors of omission, 14.6 ± 2.7 vs. 16.6 ± 4.5, $t = -0.4$, $df = 53$, NS). Because there were relatively few adolescents in this study ($N = 20$: 8 given DMI, and 12 given placebo), statistical comparison of children and adolescents is not appropriate. Nevertheless, the patterns of mean changes in ADDH-related clinical outcome measures for the adolescents resembled those of the children (Table 1; Figure 2).

The appreciably higher (but statistically not significant) proportion of subjects previously unresponsive to stimulant treatment assigned, by chance, to the placebo group (25/31) than the DMI-treated group (18/31) raised concerns that the findings might be biased by this unequal distribution of possibly more difficult cases so as to favor DMI and disfavor placebo. Accordingly, the data for all 18 treatment-resistant subjects given DMI were reanalyzed and compared to the first 18 treatment-resistant subjects given placebo. This secondary analysis replicated the findings for the entire sample (at similar levels of statistical significance) concerning differences in improvement scores between DMI and placebo (overall rate of improvement [Global Improvement ≤2] = 0/18 vs. 13/18, $\chi^2 = 20.3$, $df = 1$, $p = 0.0001$) (Table 1 and Figure 2). A similar analysis was carried out to evaluate the effects of depressive symptoms on clinical outcome by stratifying subjects into two groups by the baseline scores on the CDI-Parent version below ("low") or above ("high") the median score of 17. No significant differences in outcome measures between DMI and placebo were detected in subjects with relatively high vs. low depressive scores.

TABLE 1
Clinical Characteristics of Sample at Baseline and End-Point Analysis of Improvement (Percent Change)

| | Baseline | | | | End of Treatment | | | |
| | Placebo | | DMI | | Placebo | | DMI | |
	Mean	±SEM	Mean	±SEM	% Change	±SEM	% Change	±SEM
Overall								
Clinician's Global Severity[a]	5.1	±0.1	5.2	±0.1	8.0	±3.8	33.8	±3.4***
Conners Questionnaire-Parent[b]	22.8	±0.8	21.8	±0.7	11.4	±5.1	42.1	±4.5**
Conners Questionnaire-Teacher[b]	17.3	±1.3	18.5	±1.2	12.6	±8.0	36.4	±4.9**
Children's Depression Inventory[c]	18.3	±1.3	16.1	±1.4	−2.4	±12.7	30.2	±9.4†
Adolescents[d]								
Clinician's Global Severity	4.9	±0.2	5.1	±0.3	7.1	±6.6	32.3	±6.0
Conners Questionnaire-Parent	23.1	±1.5	20.2	±0.8	23.9	±8.5	45.1	±8.9
Conners Questionnaire-Teacher	19.1	±2.1	13.7	±3.2	20.7	±11.4	27.7	±10.8
Children's Depression Inventory	17.5	±1.3	15.4	±3.6	14.7	±6.7	46.7	±20.1
Prior Treatment Refractory[e]								
Clinician's Global Severity	5.3	±0.1	5.1	±0.2	7.4	±3.8	34.2	±4.1***
Conners Questionnaire-Parent	23.4	±1.0	21.9	±0.9	6.9	±4.8	41.0	±5.6***
Conners Questionnaire-Teacher	18.4	±1.4	19.6	±1.7	10.0	±7.7	37.8	±5.4*
Children's Depression Inventory	19.5	±1.6	17.4	±2.0	−24.8	±18.8	19.5	±13.1

Note: by unpaired *t*-test (two-tailed); alpha = 1%; † $p < 0.05$ (strong trend); * $p < 0.01$; ** $p < 0.001$; *** $p < 0.0001$.

[a] Physician-rated Global Severity (1 = not ill, 7 = extremely ill); $N = 62$.

[b] Conners Abbreviated Parent and Teacher Questionnaires (10 items, maximum score = 30); $N = 59$.

[c] Children's Depression Inventory (CDI, maximum score = 54), completed by mother; $N = 57$.

[d] Since the number of participating adolescents was too small, no statistical tests were performed; data are presented for comparison purposes.

[e] Patients with a prior history of failure to at least one stimulant trial.

Overall, DMI treatment was well tolerated at the relatively high doses given. Adverse effects generally were mild and only slightly more common in association with DMI than with placebo treatment (risk of any adverse effect = 80.6% vs. 48.4% for DMI vs. placebo; $\chi^2 = 5.7$, $df = 1$, $p = 0.02$, strong trend). However, no significant differences were found in the rate of individual adverse effects between the DMI and placebo groups. Commonly reported adverse effects for DMI and placebo were dry mouth (32.3% vs. 19.4%), decreased appetite (29.0% vs. 12.9%), headaches (29.0% vs. 9.7%), abdominal discomfort (25.8% vs. 19.4%), tiredness (25.8% vs. 12.9%), dizziness (22.6% vs. 9.7%), and trouble sleeping (22.6% vs. 6.5%). No patient developed a serious complication. Only one female patient (not included in data analysis) was dropped for a side effect (rash); she was

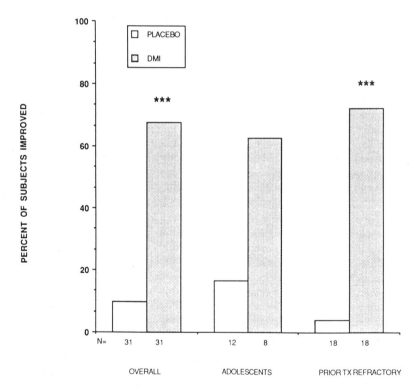

Figure 2. Rate of improvement in subgroups. Percentage of subjects improved (Clinical Global Improvement, CGI = 1 or 2) for DMI- (*solid bars*) and placebo-treated patients (*open bars*) for the entire sample, for adolescents (12 to 17 years), and for those with a prior history of failure to at least one stimulant trial. By chi-square (two-tailed) DMI vs. placebo *** $p < 0.0001$.

later treated again with DMI without recurrence of the rash (Biederman et al., 1988). Only two DMI subjects (6.5%) sustained a loss > 5% of initial weight, compared with 0% in the placebo group $\chi^2 = 0.52$, $df = 1$, NS).

Of the 28 (of 31) unimproved placebo patients, 27 (96%) consented to an open-label, 6-week, cross-over follow-up trial of DMI using a similar protocol to that of the double-blind phase and all but one showed clinical benefit without clinically significant adverse effects. Overall, 26 (96%) of patients were considered very much (Clinical Global Improvement [CGI] = 1) or much (CGI = 2) improved. The magnitude of improvement (mean ± SEM) on ratings by clinician (Global Severity = 2.9 ± 0.1), by parents (Abbreviated Conners = 56.0% ± 5.3%) and by teachers (Abbreviated Conners = 43% ± 7.1%) on ratings of ADD symptoms, as well as parents' ratings of depression scores (CDI-Parent = 45.8% ± 8.5%) was similar to that observed in DMI-treated patients under double-blind conditions.

DISCUSSION

In a 6-week, randomized, placebo-controlled trial of children and adolescents with ADDH, treatment with the TCA drug DMI at an average oral daily dose of 4.6 mg/kg was consistently more effective than a placebo. Overall, the response rate of DMI-treated patients (68%) was much higher than that of placebo-treated cases (10%). DMI patients showed statistically significant improvement in characteristic symptoms of ADDH as reported by parents and teachers as well as by physician's ratings, with a clinically meaningful end-point percent improvement from baseline scores on the order of 42%, 36%, and 34%, respectively.

It should be emphasized that this study, by chance, included a high (43/62 = 69%) and unequally distributed proportion (42% assigned to DMI and 58% to placebo) of cases of prior failure rate on at least one trial of a psychostimulant. This sampling pattern may have introduced a positive bias to DMI and a negative bias to the placebo response, both tending to favor DMI, and may limit the generalizability of these findings to largely treatment-refractory patients. However, secondary analysis of response measures for a sample selected to provide equal numbers of treatment-resistant cases treated with DMI or placebo ($N = 18$ cases in each group) yielded very similar results to those reported for the complete study sample ($N = 31$ per group) (Table 1, Figure 2). Nevertheless, in future studies, it may be appropriate to stratify subjects by prior history of treatment refractoriness. Avoidance of refractory patients altogether may be less feasible. Thus, many families of previously untreated children refused to participate in this study of a novel treatment for ADDH, and opted instead for conventional treatments. Others could appreciate the potential benefits of the proposed treatment but still refused to participate in a study with a 50% risk of assignment to placebo treatment for 6 weeks. This experience highlights the difficulty in recruiting subjects for pharmacological trials in a disorder for which effective treatments are widely available.

Even though the present study could not fully evaluate the impact of DMI treatment of ADDH at specific ages due to the relatively small numbers of patients at each year of age, and the limited number of adolescents included (8 adolescents given DMI and 12 given placebo), the findings for the adolescents yielded similar results to those reported for the complete study sample (Table 1, Figure 2), suggesting that DMI may also be effective in older patients. These results are consistent with an earlier open study at the Center that also found beneficial effects of DMI in adolescents with ADDH (Gastfriend et al., 1984, 1985). Although data are limited, the available literature suggests that stimulants too—particularly methylphenidate—may be effective in the treatment of adolescents with ADDH (Klorman et al., 1987; Varley, 1985) although stimulants may be less than ideal agents for this age group, as discussed in the Introduction. The search for appropriate alternative treatments for ADDH, particularly for adolescents and adults, has recently received renewed impetus since it is now evident that about 20% to 30% of children respond unsatisfactorily to stimulants and that in about 50% of cases of ADDH diagnosed in childhood, symptoms persist into adolescence and at least early adulthood (Gittelman et al., 1985; Weiss et al., 1985). The possible efficacy of DMI in the treatment of older cases of ADDH awaits confirmation in other studies with larger numbers of adolescent as well as adequate trials in adult patients.

The present study required 3 to 4 weeks to reach a significant drug versus placebo difference in benefits (Figure 1). This slow response, even to a maximum daily dose of DMI, appears to be inconsistent with previous reports of a more rapid response to imipramine (Greenberg et al., 1975; Rapoport et al., 1974; Waizer et al., 1974; Werry, 1980; Winsberg et al., 1972; Yepes et al., 1977) or DMI (Donnelly et al., 1986; Garfinkel et al, 1983) in ADDH. For instance, Donnelly et al. (1986) detected beneficial behavioral effects with DMI by day 3 (when the mean daily dose was 1.8 mg/kg), and these were sustained for the 2-week duration of the study at an average daily dose of 3.4 mg/kg. The design of the present study, requiring 3 weeks to reach daily doses in the 4.0 to 5.0 mg/kg range for reasons of safety, may account for the relative delay in observed response.

A relatively high target daily dose of DMI in the 4 to 5 mg/kg range was chosen based on inconsistent results reported with DMI at lower daily doses averaging 3.5 mg/kg (Donnelly et al., 1986; Garfinkel et al., 1983) and based on the authors' experience in preliminary open studies (Biederman et al., 1986; Gastfriend et al., 1984, 1985). This latter experience suggested that clinical benefits of DMI may be greater and more sustained (up to 12 months) (Biederman et al., 1986; Gastfriend et al., 1984, 1985) at daily doses higher than those of 2.5 to 3.5 mg/kg typical of earlier studies of TCAs in children (Biederman and Jellinek, 1984; Gittelman, 1980; Rapoport and Mikkelsen, 1978). In both the authors' previously reported open trials

(73%) (Biederman et al., 1986; Gastfriend et al., 1984, 1985) and the present controlled study (69%), most patients (71%) were previously refractory to, or had troublesome side effects on, stimulant therapy. Accordingly, it is possible that a requirement of relatively high doses of DMI may be selective for the treatment of stimulant-refractory ADDH patients. Thus, whether lower doses might be effective for newly treated or stimulant-responsive patients is not known and requires further investigation before broad clinical guidelines for the use of DMI in ADDH can be adequately specified. For the present time, in clinical practice, it is suggested that TCA treatment be individualized by slowly increasing doses, aiming to use the lowest effective dose, and be guided in children by clinical response, adverse effects, serum drug assays, and ECG monitoring (see Biederman et al., 1989).

Although this 6-week study was longer than the two previously reported DMI studies (Donnelly et al., 1986; Garfinkel et al., 1983), its findings provide evidence only for the *short-term* efficacy of DMI in the management of young patients with ADDH. It should be noted that Gittelman-Klein (1974), Rapoport et al. (1974), and Quinn and Rapoport (1975) have noted that *imipramine*, though indistinguishable from the stimulants during the initial phase of treatment, failed to have sustained clinical efficacy in a substantial proportion of children given relatively low doses (<3.0 mg/kg daily) of that tertiary-amine TCA. Moreover, Gittelman-Klein (1974) found in some cases that "over time, new difficulties appeared, such as temper outbursts, aggressiveness, and antagonistic behaviors." Other adverse effects of doses of *imipramine* in the 5 mg/kg dose range have included excitement, nightmares, insomnia, muscle pain, increased appetite, abdominal cramps, hiccups, bad taste, sweating, and flushed face, as well as a syndrome of forgetfulness and perplexity with marked irritability (Rapoport and Zametkin, 1980). We have not observed such effects with prolonged use of DMI in open, long-term trials at daily doses above 3.5 mg/kg, and only mild adverse effects but moderate to marked improvement in 80% of the 12 adolescents and 18 children with ADDH after a mean follow-up period of more than 6 months (27 weeks, range 4–52 weeks) (Biederman et al., 1986; Gastfriend et al., 1984, 1985). In the present study, DMI was well tolerated and there were no serious adverse effects. Only one patient was discontinued due to an apparent side effect (rash) but was later given DMI again without re-emergence of the rash. In addition, in contrast to the risk of treatment-emergent dysphoria (Gittelman, 1980; Pliska, 1987) reported in children treated with stimulants, DMI-treated patients showed a substantial *reduction* in depressive symptoms compared with placebo-treated patients. This outcome is consistent with previous reports (Garfinkel et al., 1983; Pliska, 1987; Staton et al., 1981), suggesting that TCAs may be effective in improving depressive symptoms in children with ADDH.

At the end of the present double-blind protocol, patients were given the option of an elective open-label but otherwise protocol-guided DMI follow-up treatment for placebo non-responders. Despite the inherent limitations in such uncontrolled experience, it is interesting that of 28 (out of 31) unimproved placebo patients, 27 elected to participate in the open label study, and 26 (96%) showed clinical benefit without clinically significant adverse effects.

In further contrast to reported results from other studies with tertiary-amine TCAs (imipramine or amitriptyline) (Ross et al., 1984; Watter and Dreyfus, 1973; Winsberg et al., 1972), DMI treatment was not associated with significantly improved (or worsened) performance on short-term laboratory measures of cognition in the present study. This observation is consistent with other studies of DMI that examined cognitive variables in children with ADDH (Donnelly et al., 1986; Garfinkel et al., 1983) and in normal adults (Sprague and Sleator, 1977) and suggests that brief DMI treatment may affect behavior more than cognition or that measurable cognitive effects may require long-term assessment, perhaps under more academically realistic conditions (as by following grades and scholastic achievement rest scores). More work needs to be done to evaluate positive or negative cognitive effects of prolonged drug treatment of ADDH patients with TCAs as well as with stimulants (Puig-Antich et al., 1987).

Additional results from this study, reported separately (see Biederman et al., 1989), indicate that DMI treatment led to *asymptomatic* and generally small, but sometimes statistically significant, effects in diastolic blood pressure, heart rate, and ECG cardiac conduction times (all increased). These cardiovascular changes were associated weakly with steady-state DMI serum concentrations above the median (152 ng/ml). Although the clinical significance of these findings is unknown, the conduction defects encountered may be dangerous and indicate that prudent practice includes routine ECG monitoring when doses of TCAs above 3.5 mg/kg are used, as was recommended previously (Hayes et al., 1975). Since dose was not significantly associated with serum levels of DMI, but serum levels above 150 ng/ml were associated with somewhat greater risk of reduced efficiency of cardiac conduction, monitoring of DMI serum levels as well as ECG during treatment are wise components of TCA therapy of children and adolescents so as to optimize the probability of beneficial response and reduce the risk of cardiovascular toxicity.

The pharmacological mechanism of action of DMI in ADDH remains unknown. Donnelly et al. (1986) found that DMI treatment decreased both plasma norepinephrine levels and urinary excretion of its metabolite MHPG in children with ADDH. Since DMI has a powerful and selective inhibitory effect on the neuronal uptake of norepinephrine and alters its metabolism and effects on adrenergic receptors in the mammalian brain, these findings may suggest that the somewhat delayed anti-ADDH effects of DMI, like its antidepressant effects, may be related to the drug's actions on this central neurotransmitter system by actions partly shared with those of stimulants (Baldessarini, 1985).

In conclusion, the present controlled study adds to clinical experience and other relatively short-term trials indicating that DMI may be an effective and well-tolerated treatment for many children with ADDH, including those who have failed to respond to stimulants and perhaps, for those for whom a long-acting medicine is preferable, or for those with associated depressive symptoms. Additional studies are needed to test the impression that DMI may be useful in the treatment of adolescent or adult patients with a childhood history of ADDH and to evaluate whether daily doses of 4 to 5 mg/kg are also needed in medication-naive or stimulant-responsive patients. TCA therapy in children and adolescents, especially when daily doses above 3.5 mg/kg are employed, requires optimization clinically and by assay of serum drug levels and ECG.

REFERENCES

Baldessarini, R. J. (1985), *Chemotherapy in Psychiatry.* Cambridge, MA: Harvard University Press, pp. 130–234.

Barkley, R. A. (1977), A review of stimulant drug research with hyperactive children. *J. Child Psychol. Psychiatry,* 18:137–165.

Biederman, J., Baldessarini, R. J., Wright, V. et al. (1989), A double-blind placebo controlled study of desipramine in the treatment of ADD: II. Serum drug levels and cardiovascular findings. *J. Am. Acad. Child Adolesc. Psychiatry,* 28(5).

———Gastfriend, D. R., Jellinek, M. S. et al. (1985), Cardiovascular effects of desipramine in children and adolescents with attention deficit disorder. *J. Pediatrics,* 106:1017–1020.

——— ——— ———(1986), Desipramine in the treatment of children with attention deficit disorder. *J. Clin. Psychopharmacol,* 6:359–363.

———Gonzalez, E., Bronstein, B. et al. (1988), Desipramine and cutaneous reactions in pediatric outpatients. *J. Clin. Psychiatry,* 49:178–183.

———Jellinek, M. S. (1984), Psychopharmacology in children. *N. Engl. J. Med.,* 310:968–972.

CGI (Clinical Global Impression) Scale-NIMH (1985), *Psychopharmacol. Bull.* 21:839–844.

Conners, C. (1985), The computerized continuous performance test. *Psychopharmacol. Bull.,* 21:891–892.

Donnelly, M., Zametkin, A. J., Rapoport, J. E. et al. (1986), Treatment of childhood hyperactivity with desipramine: plasma drug concentration, cardiovascular effects, plasma and urinary catecholamine levels, and clinical response. *Clin. Pharmacol. Ther.,* 39:72–81.

Garfinkel, B. D., Wender, P. H. & Sloman, L. (1983), Tricyclic antidepressants and methylphenidate treatment of attention deficit disorder in children. *J. Am. Acad. Child Psychiatry,* 2:343–348.

Gastfriend, D. R., Biederman, J. & Jellinek, M. S. (1984), Desipramine in the treatment of adolescents with attention deficit disorder. *Am. J. Psychiatry,* 141:906–908.

——— ——— ———(1985), Desipramine in the treatment of attention deficit disorder in adolescents. *Psychopharmacol. Bull,* 21:144–145.

Gittelman, R. (1980), Childhood disorders. In: *Drug Treatment of Adult and Childhood*

Psychiatric Disorders, ed. D. Klein, F. Quitkin, A. Rifkin & R. Gittelman. Baltimore, Williams & Wilkins, pp. 576–756.

——Mannuzza, S., Shenker, R. et al. (1985), Hyperactive boys almost grown up. *Arch. Gen. Psychiatry,* 42:937–947.

Gittelman-Klein, R. (1974), Pilot clinical trial of imipramine in hyperkinetic children. In: *Clinical Uses of Stimulant Drugs in Children,* ed. C. K. Conners. The Hague, Netherlands: Excerpta Medica. Foundation, pp. 192–201.

Goyer, P. F., Davis, G. C. & Rapoport, J. S. (1982), Abuse of prescribed stimulant medication by a 13 year old hyperactive boy. *J. Am. Acad. Child Psychiatry,* 18:1170–1175.

Greenberg, L., Yellin, A., Spring, C. et al. (1975), Clinical effects of imipramine and methylphenidate in hyperactive children. *International Journal of Mental Health,* 4:144–156.

Gross, M. D. (1973), Imipramine in the treatment of minimal brain dysfunction in children. *Psychosomatics,* 14:283–285.

Guy, W. (ed.) (1976), *ECDEU Assessment Manual for Psychopharmacology, Revised* (NIMH Publication No. [ADM] 76–338). Washington, DC: U.S. Government Printing Office.

Hayes, T. A., Panitch, M. L. & Barker, E. (1975), Imipramine dosage in children: a comment on imipramine and electrocardiographic abnormalities in hyperactive children. *Am. J. Psychiatry,* 132:545–547.

Herjanic, B. & Reich, W. (1982), Development of a structured psychiatric interview for children: agreement between child and parent on individual symptoms. *J. Abnorm. Child Psychol.,* 10:307–324.

Huessy, H. R. & Wright, A. L. (1970), The use of imipramine in children's behavior disorders. *Acta Paedopsychiatrie,* 37:194–199.

Korman, R., Coons, H. W. & Borgstedt, A. D. (1987), Effects of methylphenidate on adolescents with a childhood history of attention deficit disorder: I. Clinical findings. *J. Am. Acad. Child Adolesc. Psychiatry,* 26:363–367.

Kovacs, M. (1985), CDI (The Children's Depression Inventory). *Psychopharmacol. Bull.,* 21:995–1000.

Krakowski, A. J. (1965), Amitriptyline in the treatment of hyperkinetic behavior syndrome in children. *Psychosomatics,* 6:355–360.

Kupietz, S. & Balka, E. (1976), Alterations in vigilance performance of children receiving amitriptyline and methylphenidate pharmacology. *Psychopharmacology,* 50:29–33.

Orvaschel, H. (1985), Psychiatric interviews suitable for use in research with children and adolescents. *Psychopharmacol. Bull.,* 21:737–748.

Pliska, R. (1987), Tricyclic antidepressants in the treatment of children with attention deficit disorder. *J. Am. Acad. Child Psychiatry,* 26:127–132.

Porrino, L., Rapoport, J., Behar, D. et al. (1983), A naturalistic assessment of motor activity of hyperactive boys. II. Stimulant drug effects. *Arch. Gen. Psychiatry,* 30:789–793.

Preskorn, S. H., Weller, E. B., Weller, R. A. et al. (1983), Plasma levels of imipramine and adverse effects in children. *Am. J. Psychiatry,* 140:1332–1335.

Puig-Antich, J., Perel, J. M., Lupatkin, W. et al. (1987)., Imipramine in prepubertal major depressive disorder. *Arch. Gen. Psychiatry*, 4:81–89.

Quinn, P. O. & Rapoport, J. L. (1975), One-year-follow-up of hyperactive boys treated with imipramine or methylphenidate. *Am. J. Psychiatry*, 10:387–390.

Rapoport, J. L. & Mikkelsen, E. J. (1978), Antidepressants. In: *Pediatric Psychopharmacology*, ed. J. D. Werry. New York: Brunner/Mazel, pp. 208–233.

———Quinn, P., Bradbard, G. et al. (1974), Imipramine and methylphenidate treatment of hyperactive boys: a double-blind comparison. *Arch. Gen. Psychiatry*, 30:789–793.

———Zametkin, A. (1980), Attention deficit disorder. *Psychiat. Clin. North Am.*, 3:425–442.

Ross, R. J., Smallberg, G. & Weingartner, H. (1984), The effects of DMI on cognitive function in healthy subjects. *Psychiatry Res.* 12:89–97.

Sleator, E. K., Ullman, R. K. & von Neumann, A. (1982), How do hyperactive children feel about taking stimulants and will they tell the doctor? *Clin. Pediatrics*, 21:474–479.

Sprague, R. L. & Sleator, E. K. (1977), Methylphenidate in hyperkinetic children: differences in dose effects on learning and social behavior. *Science*, 198:1274–1276.

Staton, R. D., Wilson H. & Brumback, R. A. (1981), Cognitive improvement associated with tricyclic antidepressant treatment of childhood major depressive illness. *Percept. Mot. Skills*, 53:219–2324.

STESS (Subjective Treatment Emergent Symptom Scale)-NIMH (1985), *Psychopharmacol. Bull.*, 21:1073–1076.

Swanson, J. M. (1985), Measures of cognitive functioning appropriate for use in pediatric psychopharmacology research studies. *Psychopharmacol. Bull.*, 21:887–890.

——— Barlow, A. & Kinsbourne, M. (1979), Task specificity of responses to stimulant drugs in laboratory tests. *International Journal of Mental Health*, 8:67–82.

Varley, C. K. (1985), A review of studies of drug treatment efficacy with attention deficit disorder with hyperactivity in adolescents. *Psychopharmacol. Bull.*, 21:216–221.

Waizer, J., Hoffman, S. P., Polizos, P. et al. (1974), Outpatient treatment of hyperactive school children with imipramine. *Am J. Psychiatry*, 131:587–591.

Watter, N. & Dreyfuss, F. E. (1973), Modifications of hyperkinetic behavior by nortriptyline. *Virginia Medicine*, 100:123–126.

Weiss, G., Hechtman, L., Milroy, T. et al. (1985), Psychiatric status of hyperactive adults: a controlled prospective 15-year follow-up of 63 hyperactive children. *J. Am. Acad. Child Psychiatry*, 24:211–220.

Werry, J. (1980), Imipramine and methylphenidate in hyperactive children. *J. Child Psychol. Psychiatry*, 21:27–35.

Winsberg, B. G., Bialer, I., Kupietz, S. et al. (1972), Effects of imipramine and dextroamphetamine on behavior of neuropsychiatrically impaired children. *Am. J. Psychiatry*, 128: 1425–1431.

Yepes, L. E., Balka, E. B., Winsberg, B. G. et al. (1977), Amitriptyline and methylphenidate treatment of behaviorally disordered children. *J. Child Psychol. Psychiatry*, 18:39–52.

Zametkin, A. & Rapoport, J. L. (1983), Tricyclic antidepressants and children. In: *Drugs in Psychiatry, Vol. I. Antidepressants*, ed. G. D. Burrows, T. R. Norman & B. Davies. Amsterdam: Elsevier, pp. 129–147.

Part VI

PSYCHOSOCIAL ISSUES

The papers in this section address a range of issues that are at the interface between clinical practice and social policy. The paper by Bailey succeeds admirably in its goals of updating child and adolescent psychiatrists on the current status of substance abuse among youth, in delineating areas of needed research and in encouraging practitioners to become more active in the prevention, diagnosis, and treatment of these conditions. A glossary of definitions is provided to guide the reader through Bailey's lucid and succinct consideration of the epidemiology, etiology, diagnosis, and treatment of substance abuse. Clearly stated conclusions emphasize the magnitude of the problem and the fact that treatment remains variable with no clear guidelines regarding what works best or how to measure outcome. His call for the active participation of child and adolescent psychiatrists in preventative, educative, consultative, and collaborative efforts with others in the field is an important message to the profession.

That adolescent suicide is a serious public problem is unquestioned. Brent, Kerr, Goldstein, Bozigar, Wartella, and Allen have utilized an unfortunate "experiment in nature" to expand our understanding of the relationship between exposure to suicide in susceptible adolescents and the subsequent development of suicidal behavior. The data upon which their paper is based were collected when mental health professionals were asked to provide services for students at a high school after two students had committed suicide within four days. Interviews were conducted with parents, teachers, and friends of the victims to reconstruct the events leading up to the suicides, and students through to be at high risk (110 in all) were referred for mental health screening. In addition, referrals to pediatric emergency facilities and community clinics were monitored to learn if students and their families were seeking psychiatric treatment independent of screening efforts, which led to the identification of an additional 14 at-risk students. During an 18-day period, in addition to the two suicides, seven students attempted suicide, and 23 others manifested suicidal ideation. Compared with expected rates, the frequency of both completed and attempted suicide were markedly elevated. The characteristics of students who became suicidal are similar to those reported in other studies in that they were more likely than their nonsuicidal counterparts to be currently depressed and to have had past episodes of depression and suicidality. Close friends of victims manifested suicidality at a lower psychopathological threshold than those who were less close to the victims. The data are convincing with regard to the need for the rapid initiation of on-site screening of students at risk for suicidality subsequent to exposure, by trained clinicians who have access to appropriate referral sources. However, to limit the possibility that the continued presence of mental health workers provokes an exacerbation of the epidemic, the authors urge that they be withdrawn as soon as the demand for services subsides.

In the next paper, Lewis, Lovely, Yeager, and Femina focus attention on another issue of major social and clinical importance. The paper is another in Lewis' series of studies of violent youth. Follow-up data on 95 formally incarcerated delinquents obtained from adult FBI and police records are reported. The application of sophisticated data analytic techniques has permitted the more precise specification of the association between childhood and adult aggression. Although nearly all very violent adults appear to have been violent as juveniles, many violent juveniles do not become violent adults.

The data suggest that there are combinations of intrinsic vulnerabilities and environmental stressors indentifiable in adolescence, if not before, that help explain which delinquents will go on to commit violent crimes as adults. Delinquent children with combinations of psychiatric, neurological, and cognitive vulnerabilities appear to be at somewhat greater risk of continuing violence than their more intact counterparts. In addition, delinquent children who have been brutally abused and/or have been raised in extraordinarily violent homes are at greater risk for ongoing violence than those whose home environments have been more benign. Within this sample of delinquents, a constellation of interacting clinical and environmental variables is a far better predictor of future violent behavior than is early aggression alone. The findings represent a significant contribution to the literature on conduct disorder, pointing the way toward the more precise delineation of intervention strategies and underscoring the importance of adequate neuropsychiatric assessment of conduct disordered children and youth.

Yet another interface issue is that of the sexual abuse of children. The widespread documented incidence of child sexual abuse and the incontrovertible evidence of the harm it causes victims has led to a nationwide explosion of programs to prevent its occurrence. Repucci and Haugaard provide a thoughtful review of the status of sexual abuse prevention problems that addresses the complexity of teaching children of different ages about how to recognize abuse and how to be self-protective. They conclude that most evaluations of preventative programs suffer from basic design problems and present few results indicative of either primary prevention or detection. Without more thorough evaluations of ongoing programs, the authors suggest that we cannot conclude with confidence that they are effective, nor can we be sure that they are causing more good than harm. Programs may adversely affect a child's positive relationships with meaningful people or cause undue worry or fear, at least in the short run. Moreover, sexual abuse prevention programs may increase the risk for some children if adults assume that competence to deal with the problem has been effectively taught and, as a result, are less vigilant. The importance of these questions is clear. As the authors indicate, unless prevention programs contain a meaningful evaluation component, they may make adults feel better but without really protecting children.

Krener and Miller add to the growing literature on the social consequences and psychiatric implications of HIV infection by presenting five clinical situations involving children and adolescents exposed to human immunodeficiency virus. The vignettes that were chosen to illustrate the psychosocial spectrum of the disease include accounts of an at-risk gay youth, an infant with AIDS, an HIV positive hemophiliac adolescent, and an HIV positive prostitute. An example of a consultation to a community health center regarding AIDS education for drug-abusing adolescents is also provided. The authors describe the particular problems faced by psychiatrists as they apply their skills in individual and family therapy, neuropsychological assessment, and psychopharmacological management to an increasing number of AIDS-related problems. As the authors point out, the psychiatric profession has a history of valuable contributions to the understanding of patient-physician relationships. Expanding that understanding to the ethical sociological, neuropsychiatric, and human impact of the HIV epidemic is the next challenge. The clinical interventions described in this paper provide an exemplary model.

27

Current Perspectives on Substance Abuse in Youth

George W. Bailey

*Childrens Hospital National Medical Center and George
Washington School of Medicine*

The literature on substance abuse in youth is reviewed and current terminology is defined. Perspectives are presented on epidemiology, etiology, diagnosis and differential diagnosis, prevention, treatment, outcome, associated problems, issues of interface with other professionals, and directions for future research. Substance abuse in children and adolescents is a major public health problem. The definitive cause is unknown; there is a progression from legal to illegal drugs. Prevention methods are most effectively aimed at stopping initial use, and treatment remains variable. Child and adolescent psychiatrists are encouraged to become more involved in the problem. Key Words: child, adolescent, substance abuse, child and adolescent psychiatrist.

This paper is a selective review of the literature on substance abuse in children and adolescents and has a threefold purpose: first, to update child and adolescent psychiatrists on the current status of substance abuse in youth; second, to delineate areas of needed research; third, to encourage child and adolescent psychiatrists to become more active in prevention, diagnosis, treatment, research, and issues of interfacing with others already active in this field.

Reprinted with permission from *Journal of the American Academy of Child and Adolescent Psychiatry,* 1989, Vol. 28, No. 2, 151–162. Copyright © 1989 by the American Academy of Child and Adolescent Psychiatry.

SPECIAL CONSIDERATIONS ON YOUTHFUL SUBSTANCE ABUSE

Integrating the literature quickly establishes two important issues. The first is that most of the current substance abuse information and research comes from adult (generally male) alcohol studies; little is known about the applicability of an alcohol treatment model to other drugs of abuse; and even less is known about the comparability of substance abuse in youth and adults (Blum, 1987). These are important when attempting to understand, interpret, extrapolate and generalize data in terms of child and adolescent issues.

The second is the ambiguity of definitional terms. There seem to be as many definitions of substance abuse as there are treatment programs. In reviewing much of the literature, one is often left with a sense that words are subjectively defined to mean what the writer wants them to mean.

One definition has gained considerable acceptance and there is a growing consensus in the field that all compulsive abuse of mind-altering substances is part of a single biopsychosocial disease called *chemical dependency* (Wheeler and Malmquist, 1987). This generic term replaced the older more pejorative term *addiction* and describes the compulsive use of chemicals and the inability to resist the impulse to use them despite negative consequences in major areas of one's life.

Subjective use of terminology causes ambiguity and confusion and delineates the need for standardization of substance abuse terminology. Major definitional issues remain about what constitutes alcohol and drug abuse, misuse, and abuse during the teen and younger years. Appendix 1 is a compilation of generally accepted definitions and terminology now used in the substance abuse field.

EPIDEMIOLOGICAL CONSIDERATIONS

The use of illicit substances in the United States blossomed in the late 1960s and early 1970s among the mainstream of American youth, making almost normative certain behaviors previously considered quite deviant and found only among small and marginal groups of the population (Johnston et al., 1987). It began with college students and spread rapidly up and down the age spectrum. While the spread to older ages was less dramatic, the downward drift, first to adolescents and more recently to preadolescents has been very dramatic (Miller, 1983).

It is important that child and adolescent psychiatrists be current and familiar with drugs of abuse in their area, the patterns of use, the "street names," and the clinical presentation in relation to psychiatric symptomatology.

There are five general categories of legal substances of abuse: alcohol, nicotine, psychoactive medications, over-the-counter medications, and inhalants. Alcohol includes beer, wine ("coolers" are particularly popular) (Johnson, 1988), and hard liquor; nicotine includes cigarettes and smokeless tobacco (snuff and chewing tobacco) (Connolly et al., 1986).

The psychoactive medications are generally prescribed by physicians, including psychiatrists, and constitute a significant source of abusable drugs (Roush et al., 1980). This general category includes stimulants, sedatives, hypnotics, narcotic and nonnarcotic analgesics, and antimuscarinics (benztropine, trihexyphenidyl) (Dilsaver, 1986). Johnston et al. (1987) report preliminary data suggesting that children who received psychoactive drugs from physicians before taking them on their own show greater rates of illicit drug use than children who were never prescribed such agents.

Over-the-counter medications (OTCs) include cough, cold, sleep, and weight reduction aids containing phenylpropanolamine, ephedrine, pseudoephedrine, caffeine, amphetamine substitutes, and atropine compounds (Pentel, 1984).

The last group of legal drugs are the inhalants. These are cheap, readily available, easily attained, and found in almost every household. They are often the first mind-altering substance used by younger children who, as adolescents, tend to abandon them after a year or two as they advance to other substances (McHugh, 1987). These include toluene (glues, adhesives, acrylic paint, paint thinners, and automotive products); halogenated hydrocarbons (solvents, degreasers, typewriter correction fluids, spot removers, and freon); nitrous oxide (propellant for whipped cream and power boosters for automobiles and motorcycles), and aliphatic nitrites, commonly called "poppers" or "snappers" (amyl, *n*-butyl, and isobutyl nitrite).

Illegal drugs include marijuana; cocaine/"crack"; hallucinogens such as lysergic acid diethylamide (LSD), mescaline, psilocybin ("magic mushrooms"), and phencylidine (PCP); opioids; and heroin.

Synthetic compounds created by underground chemists and designed to mimic scheduled psychoactive drugs are a new source of drugs of abuse (Petersen, 1987). According to Ruttenber (1985) these illegal analogs, often glamorized as "designer drugs," generate concern because of their impending epidemic use.

The National Institute on Drug Abuse (NIDA) sponsors two major sources of epidemiologic data. They are the Monitoring the Future Survey, a yearly survey of public and private high school seniors; and the National Household Survey on Drug Abuse, a periodic survey of representative households in the continental United States (see NIDA, 1985). Both surveys are from the general population and are considered to be reliable indicators for substance abuse among the "normal" population.

Highlights from the 1987 Monitoring the Future Survey (Johnston et al., 1988) suggest initial optimism. For example, in 1987 there was continuing decline in the use of marijuana, stimulants, sedatives, and methaqualone. There was also a substantial decline in cocaine use for the first time in eight years.

Less optimistically, despite the apparent decline of cocaine use, there is still serious concern about the "crack epidemic." There was also little change in the use of

LSD, heroin, and opioids, and evidence of a continuing gradual increase in the use of inhalants.

The least optimistic data concerned the two most common legal drugs of abuse. Despite a decline in alcohol use in the three preceding years, there was no further decline in 1987 and, as in every year since 1984, there was no significant reduction in cigarette smoking. This is a matter of grave concern because cigarettes alone will cost the lives of more young people than all the other drugs combined (Johnston et al., 1988).

Most young people experiment with alcohol and drugs and some use them regularly for a period of time, yet the majority will not develop serious problems or significant negative consequences in their life. Data suggest that most adolescents "mature out" of substance abuse (Kandel and Logan, 1984). Wheeler and Malmquist (1987) report that only an estimated 6 to 10% of adolescents meet the criteria for chemical dependency. They do not specify, however, if they mean all adolescents or only those in treatment facilities.

There is no definitive way to detect who will progress into chemical dependency and who will not.

Substance abuse is best viewed as a continuum with *nonusers* (Appendix 1) at one end and *compulsive users* (Appendix 1) at the other. Between the two extremes is a large spectrum of youths who experience alcohol and drug use in several different ways. Generally, they are seen as either *experimental users* (Appendix 1) or *casual users* (Appendix 1).

One of the most influential attempts to describe the patterns of substance abuse is the concept of "stages" (Kandel, 1975; Macdonald, 1984; DuPont, 1987). Kandel posits there is a developmental process in which adolescents became initiated into substance abuse through a sequence of stages with each prior drug stage acting as a potential gateway to the next stage (Kandel et al., 1987a, b).

She proposes that adolescents progress from legal to illegal and from less to more serious drugs. The stages begin with the legal drugs and include (a) no use of any drug, (b) use of beer or wine, and (c) use of cigarettes and hard liquor. At this point the use of illegal drugs begins with (d) marijuana and (e) other illicit drugs such as cocaine/"crack," hallucinogens, heroin, and opioids. According to Kandel, drugs begun in earlier stages are "carried over" and continued in the next stage as new drugs are added to the substance abuser's repertoire.

More recently Donovan and Jessor (1983) suggested that *problem drinking* (Appendix 1) is a stage that exists after marijuana use and before heroin and cocaine.

Voss and Clayton (1987) report that an overwhelming majority of young people follow this consistent and predictable pattern of progression regardless of variable differences in gender, ethnicity, size of community, or region of the country.

Inherent in this stage concept is the notion of "gateway drugs," i.e., the ones used first. Alcohol and tobacco products are the primary gateway drugs. Causal relationships remain undetermined; however, data show that cigarette and alcohol use relate strongly to use of illicit drugs such as marijuana and cocaine (Voss and Clayton, 1987).

The continuation of drugs from one stage to another had produced an important characteristic of substance abuse in children and adolescents: multiple drug use. Multiple drug use is the rule, not the exception, for the overwhelming majority of substance-using adolescents (Clayton, 1986), and this phenomenon complicates several aspects of diagnosis, treatment, prognosis, and research. First, drugs added together produce different effects than single drugs and produce a mixed symptom pattern. Second, many illicit drugs are altered by contaminants, adulterants, diluents, and haphazard quality control, which significantly adds to their morbidity. Third, multiple drug use confounds research studies designed for one specific drug.

According to Clayton (1986), the most common reason for using drugs in combination is to enhance the effects of one drug with another (e.g., alcohol heightens the "mellowing out" effect of marijuana). In addition, multiple drugs are used to counteract the effects of one drug with another (e.g., a benzodiazepine ameliorates the "wired" effect of amphetamines); when a substitute is needed for an unavailable preferred drug (use of propoxyphene until codeine can be obtained); and to conform to what others in the peer group are doing (e.g., the prevalence of alcohol plus marijuana is so high in certain groups of substance abusing adolescents that it becomes the norm).

There is an understandable tendency in the drug and alcohol fields to be substance specific. Multiple drug use, however, must be recognized and dealt with realistically (Clayton, 1986). Diagnostic instruments such as the Users Manual for adolescent substance abuse (forthcoming from NIDA) and those of Winters and Henley (see below) are helpful to identify multiple drug users for epidemiological, diagnostic, and treatment purposes.

An important epidemiological task is the identification of children and adolescents at risk for serious substance abuse. For example, the Comprehensive Drug Abuse Treatment, Rehabilitation, and Treatment Act of 1986 identified nine categories of youth presumed to be at risk: children of substance abusers; victims of physical, sexual or psychological abuse; school dropouts; pregnant teenagers; economically disadvantaged youth; delinquent youth; youth with mental health problems; suicidal youth; and disabled youth (Kumpfer, 1987).

Unquestionably, the most vulnerable child is the child of an alcoholic or other substance abuser. There are an estimated 7 million children below the age of 18 who are the children of alcoholics (Russell et al., 1985) and many more with parents who abuse other substances. Children of alcoholics are significantly more likely to become alcoholic (Goodwin, 1985; Shuckit, 1985) and more likely to marry a substance abuser (Woititz, 1983). In addition, Bennett et al. (1988) found cognitive, behavioral, and emotional difficulties in school age children with alcoholic parents.

Despite impressive work in the epidemiology of substance abuse, the question of correlation and applicability of child, adolescent, and adult issues remains unanswered.

ETIOLOGICAL CONSIDERATIONS

The cause of substance abuse in children and adolescents is unknown. Children use drugs for a host of reasons (Morrison and Smith, 1987). For example, they are readily available; they are a quick, easy, and cheap way to feel good; they are a means of gaining acceptance in peer relationships; they help modify unpleasant feelings, reduce disturbing emotions, relieve tension and stress, alleviate depression, and help cope with life pressures.

These are insufficient reasons to adequately explain the etiologic phenomena. There is almost universal agreement that no solitary cause or specific reason accounts for all types of drug use or applies to all types of drug abusers (Newcomb et al., 1986).

The extreme, chemical dependency, is now seen by most substance abuse experts as a "final common pathway" determined by a multitude of factors including genetic vulnerability, environmental stressors, social pressures, psychiatric problems and individual personality characteristics (Newcomb et al., 1986). Substance abuse is an excellent example of a condition reflecting a biopsychosocial determination.

A. Biological

Genetic studies are particularly promising. In addition to their own work, several authors (e.g., Schuckit, 1983; Goodwin, 1985) cite twin, family, and adoption studies that show strong genetic contribution to substance abuse in children and adolescents.

A family history is very important in assessing a child or adolescent for substance abuse. A three generational genogram verified by as many family members as possible will significantly increase the yield of important information for the clinician (Baker et al., 1987).

B. Psychological

Psychological factors are less clearly understood. Often, behavioral traits associated with adolescent alcohol and drug use such as rebelliousness, poor school performance, delinquency, and criminal activity (Kandel, 1982), and personality traits such as low self-esteem, anxiety, depression, and lack of self-control predate the onset of drug use (Carroll, 1981; Kandel, 1981).

Although not universally accepted, the search for an "addictive personality" (Vaillant, 1980) continues. A longitudinal study of children who later become adult problem drinkers (McCord, 1972) and a more recent study by Hartocollis (1982) support the hypothesis that certain personality traits and defense configurations are well entrenched before the development of alcoholism.

C. Social

Many studies address social factors contributing to substance abuse. For example, Botvin (1986) suggests that several psychosocial factors (social, cognitive, attitudinal, personality, and developmental) may play a role in the initiation of substance abuse. The association is not pure, however. Botvin concludes that although these appear to be primarily responsible for initiating substance abuse, pharmacological factors become increasingly important in reinforcing and maintaining regular patterns of use.

Semlitz and Gold (1986) summarized the more important social antecedents of substance abuse. These include parental and peer drug use and their approval of such use; the adolescent's own beliefs and norms about drug use and its harmfulness; a predisposition toward nonconformity, rebellion and independence; low academic performance and motivation; and engaging in "problem behaviors" reflecting deviance from appropriate adolescent activities.

In addition, Newcomb et al. (1986) cite several references suggesting that maternal drug use, low self-esteem, depression, psychological distress, poor relationships with parents, low sense of social responsibility, and lack of religious commitment are all important social determinants.

The literature reflects a consensus that attitudes and practices regarding the use of alcohol and possibly other drugs come first from parents and then from peers (Hartocollis, 1982).

Environmental substance use patterns are powerful predictors of problems in children and adolescents (Harford and Grant, 1987). For example, parents of adolescents who use illicit drugs are more likely to be illicit drug users themselves (Kandel, 1974).

Social contexts outside the home are also important variables. Where, and with whom, young people use substances and the meaning and structure of drinking situations play critical roles in initiation and maintenance of substance abuse (Harford and Grant, 1987).

The disease concept of alcoholism is almost universally accepted within the medical and alcoholism treatment communities. Chemical dependency is conceptualized in much the same way by many in the addictions field (e.g., Macdonald and Newton,

1981). One danger of dogmatic acceptance that all substance abuse and chemical dependency is secondary to a disease is that it circumvents the necessity of thorough, individualized assessment and treatment. This has been one criticism of treatment programs run by nonphysicians (Peele, 1987).

Despite work on multidimensional models of alcoholism, clinically we are still a long way from consensus on what constitutes alcohol abuse and alcoholism (Blum, 1987) in adults and even further in children and adolescents.

DIAGNOSIS

DSM-III-R does not distinguish between childhood, adolescent, and adult substance abuse and is of limited value for making the diagnosis in children and adolescents.

Halikas et al. (1984) modified the adult criteria in *DSM-III* and applied them to a select population of juvenile offenders. While reporting promising preliminary data, the group cautioned against generalization and identified the need for additional study.

Diagnosing substance abuse rests on the realization that all children and adolescents are at risk but some considerably more than others. Making the diagnosis of alcohol and drug abuse must be part of a comprehensive diagnostic approach. As noted earlier, the NIDA Users Manual will provide important diagnostic tools. Meanwhile, Farrow and Deisher (1988) offer a practical guide to the office assessment of adolescent substance abuse.

Sources of diagnostic information include the following.

A. History and Mental Status Examination

Anglin (1987) and Farrow and Deisher (1988) provide excellent reviews on the important issues of history taking and interviewing guidelines. Information obtained from the child or adolescent needs verification by parents, teachers, referral sources, and others involved.

B. Physical Examination

Clinical medicine plays an important role in the detection and management of youthful substance abuse (MacKenzie et al., 1987) and the physical examination is an integral part of the diagnostic process. For those who choose not to do their own physical and neurological examinations, other colleagues may be helpful consultants for this critical aspect of the comprehensive assessment.

C. Self-Report

A major concern with self-report measures is the possibility of underreporting. One effort to increase their accuracy is the use of a bogus pipeline. This is a method of telling subjects their self-reports will be verified by the researchers with a biological test (e.g., saliva analysis) when no verification actually occurs. Two studies (Werch et al., 1987; Campanelli et al., 1987) that investigated this method met with mixed success in assessing adolescent cigarette smoking and neither was able to show its efficacy, or recommend its use.

Barnea et al.'s (1987) review of the literature, and their own longitudinal adolescent study using self-report techniques, showed a high rate of reliability in self-reporting of substance abuse both cross-sectionally and longitudinally.

Other clinical studies also report favorable use of self-report questionnaires. Silver et al. (1987), for example, examined the relationship between a self-report questionnaire for marijuana use and urine screens in adolescents and demonstrated good concordance between the subject's admission of use and a positive urine.

D. Structured Interview and Standardized Tests

Identification of "negative consequences" can be done by use of structured questionnaires or a directed interview (Farrow and Deisher, 1988). Significant work in this area has occurred with adult substance abusers. Examples include the Michigan Alcoholism Screening Test (MAST) (Selzer, 1971); the MacAndrews Alcoholism Scales (MAC) (MacAndrews,) 1965); and the Addiction Severity Index (ASI) (McLellan et al., 1980).

Preliminary studies have investigated use of such tests in adolescents and young adults. For example, Rathus et al. (1980) studied the MAC on adolescents. They found evidence that the MAC may identify a psychological tendency toward substance dependence. It did not, however, confirm the existence of substance abuse; nor did it quantify or analyze the type or nature of such dependence.

MacAndrews (1986) also developed another Minnesota Multiphasic Personality Inventory (MMPI) derived scale, the Substance Abuse Proclivity Scale (SAP Scale). He was able to identify a subgroup of adolescent males who used substances in such a manner that treatment was required and thereby demonstrated that predisposition was measurable psychometrically.

The Michigan Alcoholism Screening Test (MAST), is a well-accepted adult assessment instrument. Favazza and Cannell (1977) and Silber et al. (1985) used it with college students and found it effective. More recently, Anderson (1987) used a computerized version of the MAST on a college population. The participants found the test to be acceptable and believed that it accurately represented their drinking habits.

The CAGE, originated by Ewing and Rouse in 1970 and later validated by Mayfield et al. (1974) and Beresford et al. (1982) is generally accepted by clinicians in the field. It is a clinician-administered face-to-face interview consisting of four questions (see Appendix 2). While there are no studies to date using the CAGE test in children or adolescents, it is easily administered, less intimidating than more structured assessment instruments, and an easy addition to any physician's assessment repertoire.

The Chemical Dependence Adolescent Assessment Project developed a multi-dimensional questionnaire, the Personal Experience Inventory (Winters and Henley, 1988), consisting of three distinct instruments for the assessment of adolescent substance abuse. These include a self-report chemical abuse problem severity inventory; a self-report inventory of personal, family, and social factors that predispose, perpetuate, or accompany adolescent chemical involvement; and a structured interview organized around the *DSM-III-R* diagnostic criteria for psychoactive use disorders.

The Children of Alcoholics Screening Test (CAST) is a reliable and valid instrument to identify children of alcoholics (Jones, 1983). Use of the CAST on an inpatient psychiatry service for latency-aged children indicates significant accuracy in identifying these youngsters despite a reported negative family history for alcohol abuse (personal experience; Bailey, in prep).

E. Laboratory Diagnosis

Schuckit (1988) reviewed laboratory methods for enhancing diagnostic accuracy of alcoholism in adults and Chan et al. (1987) did the same for late adolescents and young adults. Both concluded that preliminary studies are promising.

Farrow et al. (1987) concluded that there are no definitive screening tests for alcoholism and drug abuse in pediatric and adolescent populations. However, they support the hypothesis (Abramovicz, 1985) that young substance abusers may exhibit acute, usually time-limited complications but appear well in intervening periods despite continual substance ingestion.

F. Drug Screening

The use of toxicology screens for detection of substance use and abuse is controversial. There are several excellent reviews regarding general information (Stewart, 1982; Schwartz and Hawks, 1985; MacKenzie et al., 1987); moral, ethical, philosophical and legal considerations (King, 1987; Silber, 1987; Goldsmith, 1988); and the concordance of toxicological screens with clinical and historical data (Silver et al., 1987).

Child and adolescent psychiatrists have two responsibilities in this area: (a) to have a general knowledge of common laboratory methods of toxicological analysis, including the advantages and disadvantages of each; and (b) to know how to order, understand, and interpret these findings to patients, their families, and consultees.

A negative screen does not necessarily mean that drug use is absent; nor does a positive screen necessarily mean that drugs are the cause of the immediate symptoms or that the person was under the influence at the time of the test (Stewart, 1982). Any presumptive positive screen requires confirmation by a well-documented reference procedure such as gas chromatography/mass spectrometry (Stewart, 1982).

Drug interference by other pharmacologically active agents may interfere with drug screening. This is particularly important with multiple drug users (Stewart, 1982). MacKenzie et al. (1987) reviewed the important issues of false negative and false positives results.

A positive test drug screen is only one step in an otherwise critical process. Appropriate utilization of the screening results must be integrated into a comprehensive clinical assessment and cogent presentation to the child or adolescent and his/her family. The interpretation of this important data by nonmedical personnel is an area for significant concern. Interpretation of positive drug screens requires that the clinician be knowledgeable about medicine, pharmacology, drug kinetics, and drug effects (Goldsmith, 1988).

Gold and Dackis (1986) enumerated absolute indications for urine testing. They include all adolescents with psychiatric symptoms; high risk adolescents (runaways, delinquents, etc.); adolescents with mental status or performance changes; acute-onset behavior states; adolescents with recurrent respiratory ailments, recurrent accidents or unexplained somatic symptoms and for monitoring abstinence.

DIFFERENTIAL AND DUAL DIAGNOSIS

Macdonald (1984) points out that adolescent substance abuse is probably the most commonly missed pediatric diagnosis. Child and adolescent psychiatrists are well suited to the challenge of both differential and *dual diagnosis* (Appendix 1).

Substance abuse may be a manifestation of psychopathology, an effect of psychopathology or unrelated to psychopathology. An essential issue is to determine which one or which combinations may be operating in a particular child or adolescent (Carter and Robson, 1987).

The differential diagnosis in assessment of physical emotional, behavioral, academic and social problems in children and adolescents should include consideration of substance abuse by the patients and/or by their parents. These ubiquitous difficulties are often clues that alert the informed clinician.

Several studies indicate an association between substance abuse and unipolar depression (Kashani et al., 1985; Deykin et al., 1987); bipolar disorder (Famuiaro et al., 1985); antisocial behavior (e.g., Robins, 1978; Cantwell, 1978; Clayton, 1986);

attention-deficit hyperactivity disorder (e.g., Gittelman et al, 1985); borderline personality disorder (Loranger and Tullis, 1985); and suicide (Fowler et al., 1986; Rich et al., 1988).

Other researchers have examined the issue of dual diagnosis (co-morbidity) of substance abuse and additional psychiatric conditions (e.g., Groves et al., 1986; Lavik and Onstad, 1986).

Children and adolescents whose parents are alcohol and drug abusers are at increased risk for development of psychiatric disorders. Associated disorders include attention deficit disorder, conduct disorders, learning disorders, anxiety disorders, affective disorders, eating disorders, personality disorders, and psychosis (Russell et al., 1985).

ASSOCIATED PROBLEMS

There are issues associated with child and adolescent substance abuse that are emerging as significant problems but have not yet been seriously studied.

Acquired immunodeficiency syndrome (AIDS), AIDS-related complex (ARC), and seropositivity with the human immunodeficiency virus (HIV) have become major public health issues and their association with substance abuse is well established (e.g., Petersen, 1987). Clearly, practices within the drug-using subculture have an impact on the spread of AIDS within the community (Petersen, 1987) and this association has far-reaching ramifications for the fields of substance abuse prevention, diagnosis, and treatment.

Although the primary spread in substance abusers is by intravenous (IV) drug taking, one cannot discount the importance of adolescent sexual activity, both heterosexual and homosexual. The effect is that more HIV-infected persons are entering substance abuse treatment programs (Drucker, 1986). In fact, many of them learn of their HIV status as part of a substance abuse assessment.

Bakti (1988) reviewed the impact of the AIDS spectrum on substance abuse treatment and determined a unique set of circumstances. AIDS-related issues that complicate usual substance abuse treatment include increased difficulty maintaining abstinence from drugs; measures to protect the patient's health and the health of others by preventing viral spread; severe medical and psychiatric problems that may overshadow the importance of substance abuse as the main focus of treatment; and limitations of the usual clinical practice of orienting treatment toward the future.

The issue of confidentiality takes on new perspectives when dealing with the AIDS-substance abuse combination. Child and adolescent psychiatrists should have an understanding of the more important legal matters such as confidentiality and disclosure (Pascal, 1987).

Perinatal substance abuse has become an increasingly important area of concern and research because of mounting evidence of the association between substance abuse and infant morbidity and mortality (Petersen, 1987). The most studied and reported relationship between substance abuse and the effect on the developing organism has dealt with the fetal alcohol syndrome (FAS). This complication of alcohol abuse occurs in 1 out of 5,000 births and is the leading preventable cause of mental retardation (NIDA, 1987).

The full fetal alcohol syndrome includes a triad of growth retardation, central nervous system dysfunction and craniofacial dysmorphology. This syndrome is actually a spectrum of symptoms with the full triad representing one extreme. Lesser degrees or partial conditions are termed *fetal alcohol effects* (Streissguth et al., 1980; Little et al., 1982) with the penetrance related to the timing and amount of alcohol consumed by the mother (Rosett et al., 1983).

The syndrome is generally recognized in the neonatal period; however, Larson and Bohlin (1987) report the clinical picture might not be recognized until preschool age when the characteristic physical features become more evident or later when additional behavioral symptoms such as inattention, distractability, and hyperactivity are present.

Petersen (1987) cites recent research that the symptoms usually attributed to FAS are also found when the pregnant mother is a marijuana user. Clinical differentiation between the two may be difficult because pregnant adolescent females are more likely to abuse alcohol and drugs simultaneously.

The fetal effects of cocaine (Chasnoff et al., 1986, 1987) and other substances of abuse have also been studied. Sonderegger (1986) provided an overview of some of the more important ones and, in addition, reviewed important legal issues inherent in this problem.

Substance abuse is a potent causative factor in perinatal morbidity and mortality among adolescents, yet the pregnant adolescent is absent in most substance-use research (Pletch, 1988). Pletch warns that it is unwise to generalize the results of substance use research from nonpregnant to pregnant adolescents or the results of teratological research from adults to adolescents.

PREVENTION

Major emphasis in this area is directed at preventing the initiation of drug and alcohol use. Two early efforts at prevention, "affective education" (Goodstadt, 1978) and "affective-humanistic education" (Swisher, 1979), proved generally ineffective at changing actual substance use (Petersen, 1987; DuPont, 1987). In addition, the abstinence of "Just Say No" model shows only minimal effectiveness (Botvin, 1984).

Recent reviews (Botvin and Wills, 1985; Flay, 1985) indicate the most promising current preventive approaches focus primarily on psychosocial factors that promote initiation of substance use. The better results come from programs aimed at cigarette smoking; however, the efficacy beyond two years has not been demonstrated (Petersen, 1987).

There are two general approaches. The social influences approach, based primarily on the work of Evans et al. (1978), focuses on influences that promote substance use (parental, peer, media pressures) and teaches specific coping skills to resist these pressures.

Others have elaborated on this model and used peer leaders, public commitments, role playing and social reinforcement techniques (e.g., Botvin and Eng, 1982; Hurd et al., 1980). Their studies showed reduction in the onset of cigarette smoking; however, the reduction was greatest shortly after the program ended and tended to diminish over time (Petersen, 1987).

The second approach, based jointly on Bandura's social learning theory (1977) and Jessor and Jessor's problem behavior theories (1977) is called personal and social skills training. Building on the same principles as the social influence model, this approach also includes acquisition of more general personal and social skills. The content of programs varies considerably, yet all programs encompass two or more of the following: problem-solving and decision-making skills; cognitive skills for resisting social pressures; self-control and self-esteem enhancement skills; learning nondrug using coping alternatives; enhancement of interpersonal skills; and assertiveness training. These are taught through instruction, demonstration, reinforcement, behavioral rehearsal and "homework" assignments.

All follow-up studies up to one year report significant efficacy of the personal and social skills training (Petersen, 1987). Botvin (1986) reported that the combination of personal-social skills training and social influence techniques produced the best results.

Botvin also noted there is only limited evidence about the effects of prevention strategies on substance use other than cigarette smoking. Preliminary studies using personal-social skills training, however, show significant reduction in both marijuana and excessive drinking.

Although promising, there are significant limitations to both approaches. The focus is primarily on cigarette smoking; there are no firm conclusions about which program components are the most or least important; follow-up has been 2 years or less; and studies are restricted primarily to white, middle-class populations.

Other preventive programs have not been subject to scientific scrutiny, but there are anecdotal reports of their success (Petersen, 1987). These programs include student-initiated programs such as Students Against Drunk Driving (SADD) and various parent movements. The latter, sometimes called "grassroot programs," involve community-based programs organized and implemented by parents (e.g., Mothers Against Drunk Driving [MADD]). Manatt has written a detailed description of the parents' movement (1983).

According to Petersen (1987), research on the prevention of substance abuse remains in its infancy with virtually all studies to date having serious deficiencies and limitations in their general applicability.

TREATMENT

There is no definitive treatment for either substance misuse or chemical dependency, yet there are multiple treatment philosophies and modalities. Finding the most appropriate treatment for a specific child or adolescent is a difficult task. A recent publication from NIDA entitled Adolescent Drug Abuse: Analysis of Treatment Research, addresses the issue (Rahdert and Grabowski, 1988).

Means to effectively divide substance-abusing patients into homogeneous subgroups with common treatment problems would allow for better and more cost-effective treatment. McLellan et al. (1985) developed the Addiction Severity Index to achieve such a patient-treatment match. Although it has proved reliable in adult substance abusers, it has not yet been tested on children or adolescents.

Until more effective means of selecting treatment approaches become available, practitioners must select from the programs available in their area. For the purposes of organization, these fall into four general categories: outpatient, inpatient, aftercare, and residential/therapeutic communities.

Most treatment programs share general features such as abstinence from substances of abuse, group therapy with other substance abusers, adjunctive use of self-help groups such as Alcoholic Anonymous (AA) and Narcotics Anonymous (NA) and the philosophy that the problem is "arrested" rather than cured (Hoffman et al., 1987).

A. Outpatient

Most youthful substance abusers are treated as outpatients; however, there are inherent difficulties in doing so. Examples include *denial* (see Appendix 1) of the problem by the youth and/or the family, basic adolescent mistrust of adult intrusiveness, continued association with substance-abusing peer groups, unwillingness to abstain, and lack of self-motivation. Such difficulties make confrontation of the problem difficult on an outpatient basis (Wheeler and Malmquist, 1987).

Many practitioners believe there is no effective outpatient treatment for adolescent chemical dependency (Wheeler and Malmquist, 1987), while others disagree. Semlitz and Gold (1986), for example, have outlined clinical criteria for outpatient treatment. These include the absence of acute medical or psychiatric problems, absence of chronic medical problems precluding outpatient treatment, willingness to abstain from all mood-altering drugs, cooperation with random urine screening, previously successful outpatient treatment, family interest and involvement in the treatment process, and self-motivation for treatment.

Outpatient treatment is a generic mixture of resources available in a particular community. Community-based resources include hotlines; drug and alcohol counseling and information centers; specialized staffs in emergency rooms; half-way houses; educational, occupational, and vocational services; social and legal services; self-help groups and community mental health centers. These services are generally available to meet the needs of children, adolescents and families with varying degrees of substance-related problems and often are the major resources for those with limited financial means or health insurance.

Wheeler and Malmquist (1987) characterized the more structured types of outpatient care into substance abuse counseling (intended to limit progression of substance use); aftercare (designed to support those returning from an inpatient stay); day treatment (an alternative to inpatient or residential treatment for selected adolescents); and family programming (intended to educate and support the family members of a chemically dependent adolescent).

Halfway houses, which are not primary treatment facilities, are available in most larger communities. They are structured settings from which the recovering adolescent may reenter the community while not immediately returning to the home environment. Participants generally receive additional treatment and support outside the halfway house at community facilities.

B. Inpatient

The Minnesota Model has been very influential in setting the standards for most inpatient treatment programs (Wheeler and Malmquist, 1987). This model (a) provides a structured, time-limited inpatient stay (generally less than 2 months); (b) bases its treatment philosophy on the disease concept of chemical dependency; and (c) stresses an ongoing commitment to an AA-like 12-step recovery program.

The issue of *detoxification* is an important and often misunderstood concept in relation to inpatient treatment programs. By strict definition (see Appendix 1), less than 5% of those entering an inpatient treatment program require specific medical detoxification (CATOR, 1986).

The services include a comprehensive diagnostic assessment and psychosocial and academic evaluations, and an active family involvement in the treatment process is required. Considerable emphasis is placed on educating the youth and the family about chemical dependency with the goal of exploring and developing alternatives to chemical use.

Psychotherapeutic interventions consist of individual (especially if there are concomitant psychiatric conditions), group (social skills and assertiveness training, leisure activity planning), and family therapy and attendance at AA/NA meetings. Academic and vocational interventions are also important.

The staff is multidisciplinary and typically consists of psychiatrists, pediatricians or adolescent specialists, psychologist, chemical dependency counselors, nurses, teachers, and occupational-recreational therapists. Legal consultation is often available also.

C. Aftercare

All inpatient programs recognize the need for follow-up or aftercare. This may involve intensive, partial day-programs, weekly aftercare meetings, or both. Aftercare is critical regardless of the form it takes because the adolescent faces the greatest temptations in maintaining abstinence once returned to the home environment (Wheeler and Malmquist, 1987).

Sobriety is maintained through continuation in a self-help group (AA/NA). "Ninety meetings in ninety days" is a common expectation of chemically-dependent adolescents when they leave an inpatient program.

D. Residential/Therapeutic Community

Residential treatment is generally indicated for substance abusing youth with additional psychiatric, behavioral (generally antisocial), social, or family problems and who have been unsuccessful following an inpatient stay (Wheeler and Malmquist, 1987).

The therapeutic community is a highly structured, nonpermissive, drug-free residential setting. The intensive daily routine involves encounter groups (typically highly confrontational), individual counseling, tutorial learning sessions, remedial and formal education, daily chores, and open, frank communications directed at acceptance of one's responsibility within the community. There is also a strong emphasis on AA/NA components. The staff is primarily paraprofessionals who generally are graduates from the program and in their own recovery process.

The length of stay varies from 6 months to up to 2 years. Some therapeutic communities (e.g., Straight, Inc.) initially use a "swap" program where enrollees are sent to each other's home or the homes of "foster parents."

OUTCOME

The untreated use of alcohol and drugs by children and adolescents has several possible outcomes. Some experiment and stop, others continue to use casually without significant consequences, some progress to chemical dependency, and some die. Several authors review various aspects of outcome (e.g., Holmberg, 1985; Kandel et al., 1986; Friedman and Glickman, 1987).

Most outcome studies examine response to treatment; however, attempting to integrate the literature on the matter is baffling. There are many methodological considerations in evaluating treatment outcome. There is little agreement on what constitutes successful treatment outcome (e.g., abstinence vs. successful life function vs. controlled use) or how to measure it (e.g., treatment effect vs. "maturing out" effects). There is also weak correlation between short-term and long-term treatment outcome. For example, McLellan et al. (1982) report short-term treatment efficacy in adolescents but far from compelling evidence for long-term efficacy.

Hoffman et al. (1987) identified six difficulties that need addressing before adequate assessment of treatment efficacy can be accomplished. These are (1) differences in perspectives and definitions of substance-related problems by referral sources, (2) differential characteristics of patient populations, (3) differential characteristics of treatment programs, (4) lack of categorization of patient-treatment match, (5) lack of measurement of an adolescent's individualized treatment response and (6) failure to identify and use appropriate outcome variables.

Relapse (Appendix 1) is an important feature of chemical dependency; however, it is poorly understood or researched. In a recent review, Saunders and Allsop (1987) were unable to reach consensus on how to define relapse and pointed to the need for further research on this important issue.

Despite multiple unknowns regarding treatment outcome, child and adolescent psychiatrists will invariably be asked to evaluate and interpret the claims and reported treatment successes of programs in their area and to help patients and their families to choose the best available treatment program.

ISSUES OF INTERFACE

The child and adolescent psychiatrist is in a unique position to work with others who treat youthful substance abusers and their families. Besides providing direct service and expertise, he or she can interface in four major areas: education, prevention, consultation, and collaboration.

Education efforts may involve several levels: patients and their families; psychiatric (adult and child) and nonpsychiatric physicians at the trainee level and later (through continuing medical education); other mental health professionals; community resources such as schools, self-help groups, employee assistance programs, the media, the religious community, the juvenile justice system, social agencies; and, especially, the general public.

In the area of prevention, the child and adolescent psychiatrist can provide consultation and liaison services to all the above and to the community at large. He or she can help these groups to identify risk factors for vulnerable children, adolescents and families. These risk factors include being the child of a substance abusing parent, genetic and environmental factors, and personality factors such as impaired peer relations, social isolation, and low self-esteem.

A very important liaison service the child and adolescent psychiatrist can offer these youths, their families, and the professionals who work with them is an understanding of the critical dynamic of *enabling* (Wegscheider, 1981) (see Appendix 1). Identification and understanding of this enabling process can have a profound effect on disrupting the perpetuation of substance abuse.

As a consultant, the child and adolescent psychiatrist can provide a comprehensive medical, developmental, psychosocial, and psychiatric assessment. Accurate diagnosis is particularly important to determine whether the substance abuse complicates other psychiatric conditions. If so, it will require the skills and expertise of a child and adolescent psychiatrist to determine which diagnosis is primary and whether the substances may have precipitated, masked or ameliorated symptomatology.

In any child or adolescent with coexisting psychiatric conditions, the psychiatrist should have continued involvement. This will include neuropsychiatric evaluation in the form of mental status examination, ongoing assessment and management of serious psychiatric complications such as suicidal and homicidal risk, and the need for psychopharmacological and psychotherapeutic intervention.

The child and adolescent psychiatrist should also play a major role in setting standards of care as well as developing and supporting comprehensive quality assurance. He or she should be knowledgeable about available treatment facilities and resources in order to make referral to appropriate facilities for services individualized to the specific needs of the child and adolescent.

FUTURE DIRECTIONS

Basic psychiatric research is needed in the pathogenesis, prevention, diagnosis, and treatment of substance abuse in children and adolescents. Clarification and delineation of standardized terminology and appropriate diagnostic criteria specific for children and adolescents are of particular importance. Research in treatment efficacy and evaluation of treatment outcome are also crucial.

CONCLUSIONS

Substance abuse in children and adolescents is a major public health problem that continues to pervade our society at an alarming rate without significant signs of abating. It involves two groups of children and adolescents: those who abuse alcohol and drugs and those whose parents abuse alcohol and drugs.

The definitive cause of youthful substance abuse is unknown, but considerable data indicate it is a multidimensional disorder with a biopsychosocial determination.

The majority of children and adolescents who use alcohol and drugs do not become chemically dependent, but we do not, as yet, know why. In those who do, the predisposition is determined by multiple factors.

There is a definite progression from legal to illegal drugs, and drugs begun in one stage are generally continued in the next. Early onset of alcohol and drug abuse correlate strongly with significant later difficulties.

Prevention methods are most effectively aimed at stopping initial use, and there are promising techniques under study.

Treatment remains variable with no clear guidelines regarding what works best or how to measure outcome.

Areas of interface with those who assess and treat these youths are very important and worthy of every child and adolescent psychiatrist's attention and efforts. The major areas of interface include prevention, education, consultation, and collaboration.

More studies on substance abuse in children and adolescents are needed. More studies on the effect of having a substance-abusing parent are needed. They should be done by those who are comprehensively trained to develop, conduct, and interpret them. The child and adolescent psychiatrist is in a unique position to accomplish this.

APPENDIX 1

Substance Abuse Definitions

The following are definitions commonly used in published studies on substance abuse. Sources are quoted when possible; otherwise, definitions are part of the generally accepted language in the field and have no readily identified source.

Abstinence: (medical definition) any psychologically or physiologically significant period during which the self-administration of the agent in question ceases.

Binge drinking/substance abusing: the periodic use of alcohol and drugs (typically weekends), often to the point of significant intoxication. Although episodic, it carries the risk and liability of chemical dependency in a predisposed person.

Blackout: a chemically-induced form of amnesia that occurs with regular or heavy use of alcohol or other mind-altering drugs. Generally accepted as a sign of chemical dependency.

Casual user: a user involved in alcohol and drug use who makes a continuing conscious effort never to lose control over the occasional use (cited in Petersen, 1987).

Chemical dependency: the compulsive use of chemicals and the inability to resist the impulse to use them despite negative consequences in the major areas of one's life.

Compulsive drug user: one who has lost control over the use of alcohol and drugs and whose life revolves around obtaining, maintaining, and using a supply of alcohol and drugs (cited in Petersen, 1987).

Current use: use of alcohol or drugs in the past 30 days (NIDA).

Denial: the process secondary to and specific to substance abuse whereby the user is unable to perceive him/her-self, others, or circumstances as they really are. It functions to alter one's perception of reality, repress the painful consequences that occur, and allow the substance abuse and disease process to progress. This phenomenon of addictive disease must be clearly differentiated from the traditional psychiatric defense mechanism of denial (Morrison and Smith, 1987).

Detoxification: generically means withdrawing the drug upon which the person is dependent (cited in Petersen, 1987). It has a specific medical meaning, however. This is a process by which a person who is physically and psychologically dependent on a drug is withdrawn from that drug by (a) gradually decreasing (tapering) the dosage of the drug, or (b) substitution of another drug that is more easily discontinued (Wilford, 1981).

Drug of abuse: any substance, taken through any route of administration, that alters the mood, level of perception, or brain function (Schuckit, 1984).

Drug abuse: there is no universally accepted definition.

   a. A physical or psychic state resulting from the interaction of a person and a drug characterized by behavioral and other responses that always include a compulsive desire or need to use the drug on a continuous basis in order to experience its effect and/or avoid the discomfort of its absence (World Health Organization, 1964).

   b. Use of a mind-altering substance in a way that differs from generally approved medical or social practices (Johnston et al., 1981).

   c. Continued use of a substance despite negative consequences caused by its use.

Dual diagnosis: the coexistence or co-morbidity of substance abuse and other psychiatric disorders.

D.U.I.: (driving under the influence) driving after the use of a mind-altering substance and while the effects of the substance are still present. Many teens do this, yet do not take it as seriously as D.W.I. (driving while intoxicated).

Enabling: process whereby people involved with the chemically dependent person consciously or unconsciously allow him/her to continue the substance use and prevent him/her from having to face and deal with the consequences of the substance use (Wegscheider, 1981).

Euphoric recall: a process secondary to denial in which the substance abuser remembers only the good aspects of substance use.

Experimental user: a user motivated by peer and social pressures and/or a need for new experiences or heightened stimulation to "try anything at least once." Usually use alcohol or drugs once or twice with no intention of going beyond the experimental level (cited in Petersen, 1987).

Heavy drinking: drinking of five or more drinks in a row on at least one occasion in the previous two weeks (NIDA).

Intervention: a therapeutic maneuver designed to break through the denial of a chemically dependent person. The goal is to have them accept treatment now rather than "hit bottom." Important persons in their life confront the user with specific examples of how substance abuse has interfered with their life and the lives of others. Each person states consequences they will enact if the chemically dependent person does not accept treatment. This is a risky maneuver and is best handled by persons trained to use it appropriately.

Non-user: a person who has never used drugs inappropriately (cited in Petersen, 1987).

Physical dependence: condition in which the body has physiologically adapted to the chronic use of a substance with the development of physical symptoms when the drug is stopped or withdrawn (Schuckit, 1984).

Problem drinking: being drunk six or more times in the last year and/or negative consequences in two of five areas of life (home, school, friends, legal, driving while intoxicated) (NIDA).

Psychological dependence: a subjective term that is difficult to quantify, centering on the user's needing the drug in order to reach a maximal level of functioning or feeling of well-being (Schuckit, 1984).

Regular user: one who uses weekly or more often.

Relapse: (medical definition) the return of a disease after its apparent cessation (Taylor, 1988). The chemical dependency field has not settled on a standard definition. Most commonly used definitions include:

a. return to pretreatment levels of morbidity (Armour et al., 1978);
b. any drug use after initiating a period of abstention (Oxford and Edwards, 1977).

Recidivism (repetition of an offense or crime) is no longer used in chemical dependency field to describe relapses.

Tolerance: a condition in which there is a need for higher and higher doses of a substance in order to achieve the same effect (Schuckit, 1984).

Withdrawal: a condition marked by the appearance of psychologic symptoms when a drug is reduced or stopped quickly (Schuckit, 1984).

APPENDIX 2

The CAGE Test

Essential features of the test (Ewing and Rouse, 1970; Ewing 1984):

    C: cut down
    A: annoyed
    G: guilty
    E: eye-opener

Exact wording of the original questions:

1. Have you ever felt you ought to *C*ut down on your drinking?
2. Have people *A*nnoyed you by criticizing your drinking?
3. Have you ever felt bad or *G*uilty about your drinking?
4. Have you ever had a drink first thing in the morning to steady your nerves or get rid of a hangover? (*E*ye-opener)

The physician in clinical practice can paraphrase the four questions to suit the occasion without significantly altering their validity, provided that the clinician specifically focuses on Cutting down, Annoyance by criticism, Guilty feelings, and Eye-openers (Ewing, 1984).

Scoring:

    a. Two or more affirmative replies are the most discriminating in clinical populations (Mayfield et al., 1974).
    b. According to originators, even one affirmative reply calls for further inquiry (Ewing and Rouse, 1970).

REFERENCES

Abramovicz, M. (ed.) (1985), Acute drug abuse reactions. *Medical Letters,* 27:77–80.

Anderson, J. L. (1987), Computerized MAST for college health service. *J. Am. Coll. Health,* 36:83–88.

Anglin, T. A. (1987), Interviewing guidelines for the clinical evaluation of adolescent substance abuse. *Pediatr. Clin. North Amer.,* 34:381–398.

Armour, D., Polich, J. & Stambul, H. (1978), Alcoholism and treatment. New York: Wiley.

Baker, N. J., Berry, S. & Adler, L. (1987), Family diagnoses missed on a clinical inpatient service. *Am. J. Psychiatry,* 144:630–632.

Batki, S. L. (9188), Psychiatric aspects of treatment of IV drug abusers with AIDS. *Hosp. Community Psychiatry,* 39:439–441.

Bandura, A. (1977), *Social Learning Theory.* Englewood Cliffs, NJ: Prentice-Hall.

Barnea, Z., Rahau, G., & Teichman, M. (1987), The reliability and consistency of self-reports on substance use in a longitudinal study. *Br. J. Addict.,* 82:891–898.

Bennett, L. A., Wolin, S. J. & Reiss, D. (1988), Cognitive, behavioral, and emotional problems among school-age children of alcoholic parents. *Am. J. Psychiatry,* 145:185–190.

Beresford, T., Low, D., Hall, R., Adduci, R. & Groggans, (1982), Alcoholism assessment on an orthopedic surgery service. *J. Bone Joint Surg.,* 64:730–773.

Blum, R. W. (1987), Adolescent substance abuse. *Pediatr. Clin, North Am.,*34:523–537.

Botvin, G. (1984), Prevention Research in Drug Abuse and Drug Abuse Research. Rockville, MD: National Institute on Drug Abuse, pp. 39–40.

Botvin, G. J. & Eng. A. (1982), The efficacy of a multi-component approach to the prevention of cigarette smoking. *Prev. Med.,* 11:199–211.

——Wills, T. A. (1985), Personal and social skills training: cognitive-behavioral approaches to substance abuse prevention. In: *Prevention Research: Deterring Drug Abuse in Children and Adolescents,* eds. C. Bell & Battles, Rockville, MD: National Institute on Drug Abuse.

——(1986), Substance abuse prevention research. *J. School Health,* 56:369–374.

Campanelli, P. C., Dielman, T. E. & Shopey, J. T. (1987), Validity of adolescents self-report of alcohol use and misuse using a bogus pipeline procedure. *Adolescence,* 22:7–22.

Cantwell, D. P. (1978), Hyperactivity and antisocial behavior. *J. Am. Acad. Child Psychiatry,* 17:252–262.

Carroll, J. K. (1981), Perspectives on marijuana use and abuse and recommendations for preventing abuse. *Am. J. Drug Alcohol Abuse,* 8:259–282.

Carter, Y. H. & Robson, W. J. (1987), Drug misuse in adolescence. *Arch. Emerg. Med.,* 4:17–24.

CATOR (1986), *Chemical Abuse/Addiction Treatment Outcome Registry.* St. Paul, MN: CATOR.

Chan, A. W. K., Welte, J. W. & Whitney, R. B. (1987), Identification of alcoholism in young adults by blood chemistries. *Alcohol,* 4:175–179.

Chasnoff, I. J., Burns, W. J., Schnoll, S. H. & Burns, K. A. (1986), Effects of cocaine on pregnancy outcome. *Natl. Inst. Drug Abuse Res. Monogr. Ser.,* 67:335–41.

——Burns, K. A. & Burns, W. J. (1987), Cocaine use during pregnancy. *Neurotoxicol. Teratol.,* 157:686–90.

Clayton, R. R. (1986), Multiple drug use. *Recent Dev. Alcohol.,* 4:7–38.

Connolly, G. N., Winn, D. M., Hecht, S. S., Henningfield, J. E., Walker, B. & Hoffman, D. (1986), The re-emergence of smokeless tobacco. *N. Engl. J. Med.,* 314:1020–1027.

Deykin, E. Y., Levy, J. C. & Wells, V. (1987), Adolescent depression, alcohol, and drug abuse. *Am. J. Public Health,* 77:178–182.

Dilsaver, S. C. (1986), Antimuscarinic agents as substances of abuse. *J. Clin, Psychopharmacol.,* 8:14–22.

Donovan, J. E. & Jessor, R. (1983), Problem drinking and the dimension of involvement with drugs: a Guttman scalogram analysis. *Am. J. Public Health,* 73:468–472.

Drucker, E. (1986), AIDS and addiction in New York City. *Am. J. Drug Alcohol Abuse,* 12:165–181.

DuPont, R. L. (1987), Prevention of adolescent chemical dependency. *Pediatr. Clin. North Am.,* 34:495–505.

Evans, R. I., Rozelle, R. M., Mittlemark, M. B., Hansen, W. B., Bane, A. L. & Havis, J. (1978), Deterring the onset of smoking in children. *Journal of Applied Social Psychology,* 8:126–135.

Ewing, J. A. & Rouse, B. A. (1970), *Identifying the hidden alcoholic.* Paper presented at the 29th International Congress on Alcohol and Drug Dependence, Sydney, Australia.

———(1984), Detecting alcoholism. The CAGE questionnaire. *JAMA,* 252:1905–1907.

Famularo, R., Stone, K. & Popper, C. (1985), Preadolescent alcohol abuse and dependence. *Am. J. Psychiatry,* 140:1187–1189.

Farrow, J. A., Rees, J. M. & Worthington-Robert, B. S. (1987), and marijuana abusers. *Pediatrics,* 79:218–223.

———Deisher, R. (1988), A practical guide to the office assessment of adolescent substance abuse, *Pediatr. Ann.,* 15:675–684.

Favazza, A. R. & Cannell, B. (1977), Screening for alcoholism among college students. *Am. J. Psychiatry,* 134:1414–1416.

Flay, B. R. (1985), Psychosocial approaches to smoking prevention. *Health Psychol.,* 4:449–488.

Fowler, R. C., Rich, C. L. & Young, D. (1986), San Diego suicide study. II. Substance abuse in young cases. *Arch. Gen. Psychiatry,* 43:962–965.

Friedman, A. S. & Glickman, N. W. (1987), Effects of psychiatric symptomatology on treatment outcome for adolescent male drug abusers. *J. Nerv. Ment. Dis.,* 175:425–430.

Gittelman, R., Mannuzza, S., Shenker, R. & Bonagura, N. (1985), Hyperactive boys almost grown up. I. *Arch. Gen. Psychiatry,* 42:937–947.

Gold, M. S. & Drakis, G. A. (1986), Role of the laboratory in the evaluation of suspected drug abuse. *J. Clin. Psychiatry,* 47:17–23.

Goldsmith, M. F. (1988), Drug testing upheld, decried: physicians asked to decide. *JAMA,* 259:2341-2342.

Goodstadt, M. S. (1978), Alcohol and drug education. *Health Education Monographs,* 6:263–279.

Goodwin, D. W. (1985), Alcoholism and genetics. *Arch. Gen. Psychiatry,* 42:171–174.

Groves, J. B., Batey, S. R. & Wright, H. H. (1986), Psychoactive drug use among adolescents with psychiatric disorders. *Am J. Hosp. Pharm.,* 43:1714–1718.

Halikas, J. A., Lyttle, M. D., Morse, C. L. & Hoffman, R. G. (1984), Proposed criteria for the diagnosis of alcohol abuse in adolescents. *Compr. Psychiatry,* 25:581–585.

Harford, T. C. & Grant, B. F. (1987), Psychosocial factors in adolescent drinking contexts. *J. Stud. Alcohol,* 48:551–557.

Hartocollis, P. C. (1982), Personality characteristics in adolescent problem drinkers. *J. Am. Acad. Child Psychiatry,* 21:348–353.

Hoffman, N. G., Sonis, W. A. & Halikas, J. A. (1987), Issues in the evaluation of chemical dependency treatment programs for adolescents. *Pediatr. Clin. North Am.,* 34:449–459.

Holmberg, M. B. (1985), Longitudinal studies of drug abuse in a fifteen-year-old population. *Acta Psychiatr. Scand.,* 71:80–91.

Hurd, P. D., Johnson, C. A. & Pechacek, T. (1980), Prevention of cigarette smoking in seventh grade students. *J. Behav. Med.,* 3:15–28.

Jessor, R. & Jessor, S. L. (1977), *Problem Behavior and Psychological Development: A Longitudinal Study of Youth.* New York: Academic Press.

Johnson, E. M. (1988), Wine coolers: they're not a "soft" drink. In: *Schools Without Drugs. The Challenge,* Vol. 2, Issue 5. Washington, DC: U.S. Department of Education.

Johnston, L. D., Bachman, J. G. & O'Malley, P. M. (1981), Drugs and the nation's high school students. In: *Drug Abuse in the Modern World,* ed. G. G. Nahas & H. C. Frick. New York: Pergamon.

—— O'Malley, P. M. & Bachman, J. G. (1987), Psychotherapeutic, licit, and illicit use of drugs among adolescents. *J. Adolesc. Health Care,* 8:36–51.

—— —— —— (1988), *Illicit Drug Use, Smoking, and Drinking by America's High School Students, College Students, and Young Adults. 1975–1987.* Rockville, MD: National Institute on Drug Abuse.

Jones, J. W. (1983), *The Children of Alcoholics Screening Test.* Chicago, IL: Camelot Unlimited.

Kandel, D. B. (1974), Inter- and intragenerational influences in adolescent marijuana use. *Journal of Social Issues,* 30:107–135.

—— (1975), Stages in adolescent involvement in drug use. *Science,* 190:912–914.

—— Kessler, R. & Margulies, R. (1978a), Antecedents of adolescent initiation into stages of drug abuse. *Journal of Youth Adolescence* 7:13–40.

—— —— —— (1978b), Adolescent initiation into stages of drug use. In: *Longitudinal Research on Drug Use,* ed. D. B. Kandel. Washington, DC: Hemisphere-Wiley, pp. 75–100.

—— (1981), *Frequent marijuana use: correlates, possible effects, and reasons for using and quitting.* Paper presented at American Counsel on Marijuana Conference, "Treating the Marijuana Dependent Person," Bethesda, Md.

—— (1982). Epidemiological and psychosocial perspectives on adolescent drug use. *J. Am. Acad. Child Psychiatry,* 21:328–347.

—— Logan, J. A. (1984), Patterns of drug use from adolescence to young adulthood: I. Periods of risk for initiation, continued use, and discontinuation. *Am. J. Public Health,* 74:660–666.

—— Davies, M. A., Karus, D. & Yamaguchi, K. (1986), The consequences in young adulthood of adolescent drug involvement. *Arch. Gen. Psychiatry,* 43:746–754.

Kashani, J. H., Keller, M. B., Solomon, N., Reid, J. C. & Mazzola, D. (1985), Double depression in adolescent substance abusers. *J. Affective Disord.,* 8:153–157.

King, N. M. P. (1987), Moral and legal issues in screening for drug use in adolescents. *J. Pediatr.,* 111:249–250.

Kumpfer, K. L. (1987), *Prevention of drug abuse. A critical review of risk factors and prevention strategies.* Paper prepared for the American Academy Child and Adolescent Psychiatry's Project Prevention: An Intervention Initiative.

Larson, G. & Bohlin, A. B. (1987), Fetal alcohol syndrome and preventive strategies. *Pediatrician,* 14:51–56.

Lavik, N. J. & Onstad, S. (1986), Drug use and psychiatric symptoms. *Acta Psychiatr. Scand.*, 73:437–440.

Little, R. E. Graham, J. M. & Samson, H. H. (1982), Fetal alcohol effects in humans and animals. *Adv. Alcohol Subst. Abuse*, 1:103–125.

Loranger, A. W. & Tullis, E. H. (1985), Family history of alcoholism in borderline disorders. *Arch. Gen. Psychiatry*, 42:153–157.

MacAndrews, C. (1965), The differentiation of male alcoholic outpatients from non-alcoholic psychiatric patients by means of the MMPI. *Quarterly Journal of Study of Alcohol*, 26:238–246.

_____(1986), Toward the psychometric detection of substance misuse in young men: The SAP Scale. *J. Study Alcohol*, 47:161–166.

Macdonald, D. I. & Newton, M. (1981), The clinical syndrome of adolescent drug abuse. *Adv. Pediatr.*, 28:1–25.

_____(1984), Drugs, drinking and adolescents. *Am. J. Dis. Child.*, 138:117–125.

MacKenzie, R. G., Cheng, M. & Haftel, A. J. (1987), The clinical utility and evaluation of drug screening techniques. *Pediatr. Clin. North Am.*, 34:423–438.

Manatt, M. (1983), *Parents, Peers, and Pot II* [DHHS Pub. No. 83–1290]. Washington, DC: U.S. Govt. Printing Office.

Mayfield, D. G., McLeod, G. & Gall, P. (1974), The CAGE questionnaire: validation of a new alcoholism screening instrument. *Am. J. Psychiatry*, 131:1121–1123.

McCord, J. (1972), Etiological factors in alcoholism. *Quarterly Journal of Study of Alcohol*, 33:1020–1027.

McHugh, M. J. (1987), The abuse of volatile substances. *Pediatr. Clin. North Am.*, 34:333–340.

McLellan, T. A., Luborsky, L., Woody, G. E. & O'Brien, C. P. (1980), An improved diagnostic evaluation instrument for substance abuse patients. *J. Nerv. Ment. Dis.*, 168:26–33.

McLellan, A. T., Luborsky, L., O'Brien, C. et al. (1982), Is treatment for substance abuse effective? *JAMA*, 247:1423–1428.

_____Luborsky, L., Cacciola, J. et al. (1985), New data from the Addiction Severity Index. *J. Nerv. Ment. Dis.*, 173:412–423.

Miller, J. (1983), *National Survey on Drug Abuse: Main Findings, 1982* [DHHS Pub. No. 83–1263]. Washington, DC: U.S. Govt. Printing Office.

Morrison, M. M. & Smith, Q. T. (1987), Psychiatric issues of adolescent chemical dependence. *Pediatr. Clin. North Am.*, 34:461–480.

National Institute on Drug Abuse (1985), *National Household Survey on Drug Abuse.* Rockville, MD: Author.

Newcomb, M. D., Maddahian, E. & Bentler, P. M. (1986), Risk factors for drug use among adolescents. *Am. J. Public Health*, 76:525–531.

Oxford, J. & Edwards, J. (1977), *Alcoholism.* Oxford University Press. Pascal, C. B. (1987), Selected legal issues about AIDS for drug abuse treatment programs. *J. Psychoactive Drugs*, 19:1–12.

Peele, S. (1987), What can we expect from treatment of adolescent drug and alcohol abuse. *Pediatrician*, 14:62–69.

Pentel, P. (1984), Toxicity of over-the-counter stimulants. *JAMA,* 252:1898–1903.

Petersen, R. C. (ed.) (1987), *Drug Abuse and Drug Abuse Research. The Second Triennial Report to Congress.* Rockville, MD: National Institute on Drug Abuse.

Pletch, P. K. (1988), Substance use and health activities of pregnant adolescents. *J. Adolesc. Health Care,* 9:38–45.

Rathus, S. A., Cox, J. A. & Ortins, J. B. (1980), The MacAndrews Scales as a measure of substance abuse and delinquency among adolescents. *J. Clin. Psychol.,* 36:579–583.

Rahdert, E. R. & Grabowski, J. (eds.) (1988), *Adolescent Drug Abuse: Analyses of Treatment Research* [National Institute on Drug Abuse Research Monograph #77]. Rockville, MD: National Institute on Drug Abuse.

Rich, C. L., Fowler, R. C., Fogarty, L. A. & Young, D. (1988), San Diego suicide study. III. Relationships between diagnosis and stressors. *Arch. Gen. Psychiatry,* 45:589–592.

Robins, L. N. (1978), Sturdy childhood predictors of adult antisocial behavior. *Psychol. Med.,* 8:611–622.

Rosett, H. L., Weiner, L., Lee, A., Zuckerman, B., Dooling, E. & Oppenheimer, E. (1983), Patterns of alcohol consumption and fetal development. *Obstet. Gynecol.,* 61:539–546.

Roush, G. C., Thompson, W. D. & Berberian, R. M. (1980), Psychoactive medicinal and nonmedicinal drug use among high school students. *Pediatrics,* 66:709–715.

Russell, M., Henderson, C. & Blume, S. B. (1985), *Children of Alcoholics. A Review of the Literature.* New York: Children of Alcoholics Foundation, Inc.

Ruttenber, J. (1985), Designer Drugs. In: *Patterns and Trends in Drug Abuse: A National and International Perspective,* ed. N. J. Kozel. Rockville, MD: National Institute on Drug Abuse.

Saunders, B. & Allsop, S. (1987), Relapse: a psychological perspective. *Br. J. Addict.,* 82:417–429.

Schuckit, M. A. (1983), Alcoholic men with no alcoholic first-degree relative. *Am. J. Psychiatry,* 140:439–443.

——(1984), *Drug and Alcohol Abuse: A Clinical Guide to Diagnosis and Treatment.* New York: Plenum.

——(1985), Genetics and the risk for alcoholism. *JAMA,* 254:2614–2617.

——(1986), Genetic and clinical implications of alcoholism and affective disorder. *Am. J. Psychiatry,* 143:140–147.

——(1988), Alcoholism: methods for better diagnosis. *Psychiatric Times,* V(6):1,15–17.

Schwartz, R. H. & Hawks, R. L. (1985), Laboratory detection of marijuana use. *JAMA,* 254:788–792.

Selzer, M. L. (1971), The Michigan Alcoholism Screening Test: the quest for a new diagnostic instrument. *Am. J. Psychiatry,* 127:1653–1658.

Semlitz, L. & Gold, M. S. (1986), Adolescent drug abuse. *Psychiatr. Clin. North Am.,* 9:455–473.

Silber, T. J., Capon, M. & Kuperschmidt, I. (1985), Administration of the Michigan Alcoholism Screening Test (MAST) at a student health service. *J. Am. Coll. Health,* 33:229–233.

——(1987), Adolescent marijuana use: screening and ethics. *Adolescence,* XXII.

_____Getson, P., Ridley, S., Iosefsohn, M. & Hicks, J. (1987), Adolescent marijuana use: concordance between questionnaire and immunoassay for cannabinoid metabolites. *J. Pediatr.,* 111:229–302.

Sonderegger, T. B. (1986), Overview of perinatal substance abuse. *Neurobehav. Toxicol. Teratol.,* 8:325–327.

Stewart, D. C. (1982), The use of the clinical laboratory in the diagnosis and treatment of substance abuse. *Pediatr. Ann.,* 11:669–682.

Streissguth, A. P., Landesman-Dwyer, S., Martin, J. C. et al (1980), Teratogenic effects of alcohol in humans and laboratory animals. *Science,* 209:353–361.

Swisher, J. D. (1979), Prevention issues. In: *Handbook on Drug Abuse,* ed. R. L. Dupont, Goldstein, A. & O'Donnell, J. Washington, DC: National Institute on Drug Abuse, pp. 423–435.

Taylor, E. J. (ed.) (1988), *Dorland's Illustrated Medical Dictionary,* 27th ed. Philadelphia, PA: W. B. Saunders.

Vaillant, G. E. (1980), Natural history of male psychological health: VIII. Antecedents of alcoholism and "orality." *Am. J. Psychiatry,* 137:181–186.

Voss, H. L. & Clayton, R. R. (1987), Stages in involvement with drugs. *Pediatrician,* 14:25–31.

Wegscheider, S. (1981), *Another Choice. Hopes and Health for the Alcoholic Family.* Palo Alto, CA: Science and Behavior Books, Inc.

Werch, C. E., Gorman, D. R., Marty, P. J., Forbes, J. & Brown, B. (1987), Effects of the bogus pipeline on enhancing validity of self-reported adolescent drug use measures. *J. Sch. Health,* 57:232–236.

Wheeler, K. & Malmquist, J. (1987), Treatment approaches in adolescent chemical dependency. *Pediatr. Clin. North Am.,* 34:437–447.

WHO Expert Committee on Addiction-Producing Drugs. (1964), 13th Report publication 273, World Health Organization Technical Report Series, Geneva.

Wilford, B. B. (1981), *Drug Abuse. A Guide for the Primary Care Physician.* Chicago, IL: American Medical Association.

Winters, K. & Henley, G. (1988), *The Personal Experience Inventory.* Los Angeles, CA: Western Psychological Services.

Woititz, J. G. (1983), *Adult Children of Alcoholics.* Pompano Beach, FL: Health Communications, Inc.

28

An Outbreak of Suicide and Suicidal Behavior in a High School

David A. Brent

Western Psychiatric Institute and Clinic, Pittsburgh

Mary Margaret Kerr

Pittsburgh Board of Education

Charles Goldstein

Brookside Hospital, Nashua, New Hampshire

James Bozigar, Mary Wartella, and Marjorie J. Allan

Western Psychiatric Institute and Clinic, Pittsburgh

In a high school of 1,496 students, two students committed suicide within 4 days. During an 18-day period that included the two suicides, seven students attempted suicide and an additional 23 manifested suicidal ideation. Compared to expected rates, the rates of both completed and attempted suicide were markedly elevated. Seventy-five percent of the members of the cluster had at least one major psychiatric disorder antedating their exposure. One hundred ten students thought to be at high risk were psychiatrically screened on site. Within this group, students who became suicidal after exposure were more likely than their nonsuicidal counterparts to be currently depressed and to have had past episodes of depression and suicidality. Close friends of the victims manifested suicidality at a lower psychopathological threshold than those who were less close to the victims. Students who are friends of a victim

Reprinted with permission from *Journal of the American Academy of Child and Adolescent Psychiatry.* 1989, Vol. 28, No. 6, 918–924. Copyright © 1989 by the American Academy of Child and Adolescent Psychiatry.

This work was supported by a Clinical Investigator Award from NIMH 1K08 MH00581-01 (D.A.B.), the William T. Grant Foundation Grants, 8601063-86 (D.A.B.), and 53586 (M.M.K.), and appropriation from the Commonwealth of Pennsylvania. The support of school personnel, the involved school board, and the staff of the catchment area community mental health center were essential to this work. Finally, we would like to thank Dr. Madelyn Gould, who made very helpful editorial comments.

or who have a history of affective disorder and/or previous suicidality
should be screened for suicidality after exposure. Key Words: suicide,
cluster, epidemic, school, risk factor.

The epidemic rise in adolescent suicide over the past three decades has resulted in increased investigatory efforts into this serious public health problem (Shaffer and Fisher, 1981; Shaffer et al., 1988). Among the putative risk factors that the U.S. Public Health Service has targeted as worthy of further scrutiny is the relationship between exposure to suicide in susceptible adolescents and the subsequent development of suicidal behavior (Davidson and Gould, 1988). The view that an adolescent suicide may trigger a cluster of subsequent suicides among the contacts of the victim (often termed the "contagion" hypothesis) has elicited widespread concern among educational and mental health professionals. However, there have been few efforts to evaluate the range or extent of the effects of exposure to suicide, and little is known about what factors may predispose to suicidality in adolescents who are so exposed. Consequently, coherent and empirically based guidelines for a rational public health response to an adolescent suicide have been difficult to develop.

In this paper, the authors review the evidence supporting the "contagion" hypothesis and describe their clinical experience with students of a high school in which a cluster of suicidal behavior occurred. On the basis of this experience, policy and research recommendations regarding the deleterious effects of exposure to suicide are advanced.

There are several lines of research suggesting that exposure to suicide may increase the risk for suicide in those so exposed. First, within localized geographic areas, there have been reports of outbreaks of adolescent suicide and suicidal behavior far in excess of the expected frequency (i.e., suicide clusters) (Coleman, 1987; Gould et al., in press; Robbins and Conroy, 1983; Ward and Fox, 1977). Second, suicide and suicidal behavior are more common in the familial and nonfamilial networks of suicidal individuals (Harkavy-Friedman et al., 1987; Kety, 1986; Kreitman et al., 1970; Roy, 1983; Shafii et al., 1985; Smith and Crawford, 1986). Third, media publicity has been reported to be followed by an increase in the suicide rate of about 7–10%, regardless of whether such publicity is propagated by front page newspaper headlines, television news reports, or fictional docudramas (Gould and Shaffer, 1986; Gould et al., 1988; Phillips, 1974; Phillips and Carstensen, 1986; Schmidtke and Hafner, 1988; Shepherd and Barraclough, 1978). Moreover, the increase in the suicide rate following media publicity appears to be confined to the adolescents and young adult age groups (Phillips and Carstensen, 1988; Schmidtke and Hafner, 1988).

Anecdotal reports of suicide clusters indicate that such "cluster victims" show a high prevalence of known risk factors for suicide, including recent legal problems, family loss and disruption, depression, substance abuse, and personality disorder

(Ashton and Donnan, 1981; Dizmang et al., 1974; Robbins and Conroy, 1983; Ward and Fox, 1977). Some additional clues about specific risk factors for imitative suicides may be drawn from studies of nonsuicidal psychosocial epidemics of psychosomatic illness which demonstrate that histrionic personality traits, conduct disorder, and family disruption due to death or divorce characterize schoolchildren most likely to be affected by these epidemics (Helvie, 1968; Knight et al., 1965; Small and Nicholi, 1982). Therefore, it is likely that those adolescents most vulnerable to the effects of exposure to suicide are those with some preexisting psychiatric difficulties, social impairment, and family disruption.

In the present report, the authors describe the profile of adolescents who became suicidal subsequent to two suicides among their fellow students within a 4-day period. The following questions about risk factors for suicidality among high school students subsequent to exposure to a student suicide are addressed: (1) Did the outbreak of suicide and suicidal behavior described in this report constitute a statistically significant cluster? (2) What were the characteristics of those students involved in the cluster? (3) Among a sample of 110 students psychiatrically screened on site at the high school, how did suicidal and nonsuicidal students differ with respect to their relationship to the suicide victims, exposure to the suicide, and prior psychiatric vulnerability?

METHOD

Within a period of 4 days, two students in a high school of 1,496 pupils committed suicide. After the second of the two suicides, our program, Services for Teens at Risk, as well as other clinicians from Western Psychiatric Institute and Clinic (WPIC) and the community mental health center serving the catchment area including this high school, were called to provide services for students at the high school. Three steps were taken to ascertain and attenuate the impact of the suicides on the student body:

1. The parents, teachers, and friends of the suicide victims were interviewed to reconstruct the events of the suicides using the method of the "psychological autopsy" (Brent et al., 1988a, b). The information gathered from this process made it possible to counter various distortions about the circumstances of the two students' deaths (e.g., the deaths were really homicides, the suicide victims were well-adjusted, etc.) and to identify which students were closest to the victims, last saw the victims alive, and might have been exposed to the suicidal act.

2. Mental health professionals met with all the students in the high school in their homeroom classes. Students were referred for additional mental health screening if they: (a) requested additional psychological help, (b) were identified by another student as needing mental health services, (c) appeared visibly upset during the meeting, (d) were friends of one of the suicide victims, (e) had attended one of the funerals, and/or (f) were known to have had prior psychiatric problems. During the

3 weeks after the initial suicides and suicidal behavior, a total of 110 students thought to be at high risk for imitation were referred for mental health screening at the high school.

The screening interviews with the 110 students were conducted by experienced clinicians (master's or doctoral level) well trained in research diagnostic interviewing using standardized assessment format that included the following: (a) past and present suicidality; (b) past and current psychiatric treatment; (c) *DSM-III* symptoms and diagnosis for past and current substance abuse, conduct disorder, and major depression; (d) parental psychopathology; (e) relationship to the victim; and (f) funeral attendance. Although a formal semi-structured interview schedule was not followed, clinicians interviewed the students as to the presence or absence of psychiatric disorder by coverage of diagnostic criteria. Parental psychopathology was assessed by asking the adolescents about *DSM-III* symptoms of substance abuse, depression, antisocial disorder, and suicidality in their parents. In the majority of cases (88%), information obtained from the student was confirmed with a parental informant by a telephone interview. The relationship of the student to the suicide victims was defined as follows: (a) close relationship: the student and victim previously exchanged confidences on a regular basis, (b) friendship: the student engaged in social activities with the victim, (c) and acquaintanceship: the student merely knew the victim to say hello and exchange pleasantries. Closeness of relationship to the victim was verified by school faculty and other friends of the victims. All cases were presented to the senior author, and ambiguous or contradictory information was clarified by reinterviewing the child and/or parent.

3. Referrals to two pediatric emergency facilities, WPIC, and the catchment area community mental health center were monitored to learn if students and their families also sought psychiatric treatment independent of our screening efforts. An additional 14 students who either were seriously suicidal or attempted suicide were identified through this procedure. Ten of these were contacted and interviewed using the same format as the students who were screened in the mental health center. Information on the remaining four were obtained using secondary sources: for two, psychiatric hospital records were reviewed (both hospitalized at WPIC), and information for another two were obtained from interviews with parents and teachers.

In summary, a total of 32 students were identified who were involved in this suicidal cluster: (1) two suicide victims; (2) 16 suicidal students identified through mental health screening in the schools; and (3) 14 suicidal students who were found to have presented at one of two major pediatric emergency rooms, at WPIC, or at the catchment area mental health facility. It is likely that additional suicidal students were not identified, as the records of all treatment facilities in the region were not reviewed, and only 7% of the student body were systematically screened.

Data analysis. The rates of suicide and attempted suicide were compared with the expected rates by use of the Poisson statistic (Hays, 1981). Suicidal students were compared with those who were not by use of the chi-square statistic with Yates correction for continuity. The multivariate contribution of specific variables to suicidal outcome was tested through logistic regression, and the individual contributions of suicidal risk factors were expressed by use of odds ratios and 95% confidence intervals (Schlesselman, 1982). The interaction of relationship with the suicide victim, prior and current psychopathology, and suicidality was examined through the use of log-linear analyses (Bishop et al., 1975).

RESULTS

Description of the outbreak. The site of the cluster was a high school of 1,496 students in an urban, working-class neighborhood. A self-inflicted firearms death (ruled undetermined) of a 21-year-old ex-student preceded the cluster by 6 weeks (Case 00, see Table 1). The cluster began when, within a 7-day period, two students made suicide attempts, one made a suicidal gesture, and two students committed suicide, the first by firearms, the second by hanging. The first student suicide victim (Case 04) was a friend both of the 21-year-old ex-student suicide victim (Case 00), and attempter 01, an acquaintance of gesturer 02, and a close friend of attempter 03. The suicide of the second student (Case 05), an acquaintance of the first student suicide, 4 days later led to the authors' involvement in the high school. At this point in time (Day 07), the authors began screening efforts in the school and subsequent to Day 07, 19 students were identified as having suicidal ideation with a plan or having made a suicidal threat and five additional students made suicide attempts. In summary, within 4 days, two students committed suicide and within the 18 days including the first suicide, seven students attempted suicide and 23 manifested serious suicidal ideation.

Does this outbreak of suicidality represent a cluster? The two suicides in the high school of 1,496 students occurred within 4 days. Assuming a rate of 8.5 per 100,000 students per year (the national suicide rate among 15- to 19-year-olds reported by the CDC in 1980 [Center for Health Promotion and Education, 1985], one would expect to see 0.00139 suicides in this high school of 1,496 students in 4 days, so that the observed rate was 1,435 times of that expected. Using the Poisson distribution, the number of suicides that occurred in this high school within 4 days was markedly increased beyond chance ($p = 0.00001$).

Seven students made suicide attempts within 18 days. Assuming that the 12-month prevalence of suicide attempts among high school students is 4% (Smith and Crawford, 1986), one would expect to have observed 3.0 suicide attempts within 18 days, so that the observed rate was 2.3 times the expected rate, which, according to the Poisson statistic, is unlikely to have occurred due to chance alone ($p = 0.03$).

TABLE 1
Characteristics of the Cluster of Suicidal Students

Case	Day	Suicidality	Method	Age	Sex	Exposure	Relationship	Diagnosis*
00	–	Undetermined	Firearms	20	M	–	–	–
01	01	Attempt	Cutting	15	F	–	Friend	Bipolar, CD, ADD
02	02	Gesture	OD	15	F	None	Acquaintance	MDD, CD
03	02	Attempt	OD	16	M	Heard	Close friend	MDD
04	03	Completion	Firearms	16	M	Heard	Friend	SA, CD
05	07	Completion	Hanging	15	M	Heard	Acquaintance	MDD, SA
06	08	Threat	Jumping	12	M	Heard	Friend	MDD
07	08	Ideation	None	16	M	Heard	Acquaintance	MDD
08	09	Ideation	None	16	M	Heard	Acquaintance	MDD, SA
09	09	Ideation	None	14	F	Funeral	Best friend	Adj. dis.
10	09	Ideation	None	16	F	–	–	None
11	09	Ideation	None	17	F	Funeral	Friend	MDD
12	09	Ideation	None	15	F	–	–	MDD, CD, SA
13	09	Attempt	OD	17	F	–	–	MDD
14	10	Attempt	OD	15	F	Heard	Acquaintance	MDD
15	11	Ideation	Automobile	18	M	Heard	Acquaintance	MDD
16	12	Ideation	None	15	F	Heard	Close friend	MDD, CD
17	12	Ideation	OD	15	F	Funeral	Friend	MDD, CD
18	12	Threat	Cutting	13	F	Heard	Friend	MDD
19	12	Ideation	None	13	F	–	–	None
20	13	Attempt	OD	16	M	Funeral	Close friend	MDD, CD, SA
21	13	Ideation	None	18	M	–	–	None
22	13	Ideation	None	16	F	Funeral	Close friend	None
23	13	Ideation	Firearms	15	F	Heard	Close friend	Adj. dis., SA
24	13	Ideation	None	17	M	Funeral	Friend	MDD
25	14	Attempt	Hanging	16	F	–	Close friend	MDD
26	14	Ideation	–	17	M	Funeral	Best friend	Adj. dis.
27	14	Threat	–	16	F	Heard	Acquaintance	CD
28	14	Threat	–	15	F	Heard	Acquaintance	MDD
29	15	Threat	–	15	M	–	Acquaintance	Adj. dis.
30	16	Threat	Cutting	13	M	Heard	Acquaintance	CD
31	18	Attempt	OD	15	F	Heard	Friend	MDD
32	18	Gesture	OD	15	F	Funeral	Friend	Cyclothymia

* CD = conduct disorder; ADD = attention deficit disorder; MDD = major depressive disorder; SA = substance abuse; Adj. dis. = adjustment disorder.

Characteristics of those involved in the cluster. Of the 32 students involved in the cluster, 14 (43.8%) were male, all were white, and the median age was 15 (see Table 1). Two completed suicide, seven attempted suicide, two made suicidal gestures, five made suicidal threats, and 16 manifested serious suicide ideation. As noted above, the first three members of the cluster Cases 01–03, (two attempters and a gesturer) were a friend, close friend, and acquaintance of the first suicide victim (Case 04), respectively. Of the 28 cluster members who became suicidal after the first suicide, seven (25.0%) members of the cluster were close friends of one of the suicide victims, seven were friends (25.0%), nine (32.1%) were acquaintances, and in five cases the relationship was not ascertained (17.9%). Only nine of the 28 (32.1%) attended the funeral of one of the victims. The majority (75%) of the cluster members ($N = 32$) had at least one major psychiatric disorder that antedated the cluster: 20 (62.5%) had preexisting affective disorders, eight (25%) had conduct disorders, and five (15.6%) had substance abuse disorders (sum greater than 100.0% because some cluster victims had more than one diagnosis). Those who were close friends of one of the victims were much more likely to be classified as having an adjustment disorder or no psychiatric disorder than were friends or acquaintances (50.0% vs. 5.5%; Fisher's exact test, $p = 0.04$).

Characteristics of students screened in the high school. Of the 110 students screened in the high school, 98.1% were white (as compared to 77.2% of the student body ($\chi^2 = 26.52\ p < 0.0001$), 70.3% were female (as compared to 50% of the student body, $\chi^2 = 18.14$, $p < 0.0001$), and they had a similar grade distribution to the high school as a whole. Three fifths (60.9%) described themselves as a friend or close friend of one of the victims, and 57% (of the 93 screened for whom this information was available) reported having attended one or both of the funerals.

This group reported having had substantial past psychiatric difficulties: 19.3% had previous psychiatric treatment, 28.2% had had a previous history of depression, 19.1% reported conduct disturbances, 24.5% reported previous difficulties with substance abuse, and almost one-third (31.8%) had had previous suicidality. Almost one in eight (11.9%) had made a suicide attempt in the past. One-third of the students screened had at least one parent with a major psychiatric disorder.

Comparison of students with and without suicidality at the time of assessment. Sixteen of the 110 (14.5%) students screened showed suicidal ideation with intent to die or a concrete suicidal plan that had its onset *after* the exposure. The suicidal and nonsuicidal students were compared on the basis of demographics, funeral attendance, relationship with the suicide victims, and past and current psychopathology. The only significant contrast was that the suicidal students were more likely to come from the 10th grade ($\chi^2 = 10.20$, $df = 3$, $p = 0.03$, see Table 2), although posthoc pairwise contrasts were not significant.

Several past and current psychiatric conditions were associated with current suicidality (see Table 3). When compared to nonsuicidal students, the suicidal stu-

TABLE 2
Demographic, Relationship, and Exposure Characteristics of
Currently Suicidal Students Screened Subsequent to Exposure to
Suicide (%)

Demographic Relationship, and Exposure	Suicidal ($N = 16$)	Nonsuicidal ($N = 94$)	χ^2	df	p
Grade			10.20	3	0.03
9	13.3	19.6			
10	60.0	22.8			
11	6.7	28.3			
12	20.0	29.3			
Race (% white)	100.0	88.9	0.34	1	NS
Sex (% male)	31.2	29.8	0.01	1	NS
Relationship[a]			4.23	4	NS
Did not know	0.0	5.7			
Acquaintance	16.7	29.5			
Friend	33.3	17.1			
Close friend	41.7	44.3			
Best friend	8.3	3.4			
Exposure to suicide[b]			0.53	1	NS
(% attended funeral)	55.6	66.7			

[a] Due to missing data, for suicidal, $N = 12$, for nonsuicidal, $N = 88$.
[b] Due to missing data, for suicidal, $N = 15$, for nonsuicidal, $N = 93$.

TABLE 3
Psychiatric Characteristics of Current Suicidal Students Screened
Subsequent to Exposure to Suicide (%)

	Suicidal ($N = 16$)	Nonsuicidal ($N = 94$)	χ^2	df	p
Past psychiatric disorder					
Past psychiatric treatment	33.3	17.0	1.29	1	NS
Past suicidality	62.5	26.6	6.55	1	0.01
Past major depression	56.3	23.4	5.76	1	0.02
Past conduct disorder	25.0	18.1	0.09	1	NS
Past substance abuse	43.8	21.3	2.61	1	0.10
Current psychiatric disorder					
Major depression	68.8	20.2	13.89	1	0.0002
Conduct disorder	31.3	13.8	1.89	1	NS
Substance abuse	31.3	16.0	1.24	1	NS
Psychiatric disorder in at least one parent	43.8	30.9	1.01	1	NS
Disposition					
School follow-up	6.3	72.3	36.02	2	<0.0001
Outpatient	75.0	27.7			
Inpatient	18.7	0.0			

dents were more likely to have been suicidal in the past (62.5% vs. 26.6%, $\chi^2 =$ 6.55, $p = 0.01$), to have an episode of major depression in the past (56.3% vs. 23.4%; $\chi^2 = 5.76$, $p = 0.02$), or to be in the midst of a current major depression (68.8% vs. 20.2%, $\chi^2 = 13.89$, $p = 0.0002$). Suicidal students showed a nonsignificant tendency to be more likely than nonsuicidal students to have a past history of substance abuse (43.8% vs. 21.3%; $\chi^2 = 2.61$, $p–0.10$). Not surprisingly, many more of the suicidal than nonsuicidal students were referred for psychiatric treatment (93.7% vs. 27.7%, $\chi^2 = 28.51$, $p < 0.0001$). Logistic regression indicated that two of the above-noted screening items, current major depression (odds ration [O.R.] $= 2.6$, 95% confidence interval [C.I.] $= 1.4$ to 4.7) and past suicidality (O.R. $= 1.7$, 95% C.I. $= 1.1$ to 3.1) each contributed significantly to the classification of suicidal students. These two variables correctly classified 13 out of 16 of the suicidal students (81.3%).

The interaction of relationship to the victims, prior and current psychopathology, and current suicidality. Students who were close friends of the victims appeared to become suicidal at a lower psychopathological threshold than did students less close to the victims. For example, fewer than half of the suicidal close friends of the victims had a past or current affective disorder (3/7), whereas *all* of the suicidal students who were less close to the victims had a past or current affective disorder (7/7) (see Table 4, interaction of affective disorder $\times$ closeness of relationship $\times$ suicidality, log-likelihood $\chi^2 = 6.11$, $df = 1$, $p = 0.01$).

TABLE 4

Closeness of Relationship to the Victim, Affective Disorder, and Suicidality among the Students[a,b]

Best or Close Friend (F)	Past or Current Affective Disorder (A)	Current Suicidality (S)	
		No	Yes
No	No	36	0
	Yes	9	7
Yes	No	33	4
	Yes	8	3

[a] FAS interaction term, log-likelihood, $\chi^2 = 6.11$, $df = 1$, $p = 0.014$.

[b] Due to missing values, total N reduced from 110 to 100.

DISCUSSION

Summary

In the present study, the existence of a cluster of suicide and suicidal behavior unlikely to have occurred by chance alone has been documented. Moreover, the clinical characteristics of those individuals who were part of this cluster have been described. Students with current major depression and those with past problems with depression and suicidality were the most likely to become suicidal subsequent to exposure. Prior and current psychopathology appeared to predict suicidality following exposure to a greater degree than did the closeness of the relationship to the suicide victim or attendance at the funeral. However, those students who were close friends of the suicide victims appeared to have become suicidal at a lower threshold of psychopathology than did exposed students who were not as close to the victims. The relationship of these results to previous reports of suicidal clusters, the limitations of this study, and the implications of these findings for further clinical practice and research will be discussed.

Epidemics of suicidal behavior actually occur. This report adds to other descriptions of outbreaks of suicide and suicidal behavior in localized geographic areas (Coleman, 1987; Dizmang et al., 1974; Robbins and Conroy, 1983; Ward and Fox, 1977). It is probable that the prevalence of suicidal behavior following the student suicides have been underestimated, because all students were not screened in a systematic fashion and because the records of all treatment facilities where suicidal students might have presented were not reviewed. Despite this limitation, the authors were able to establish that the incidence of suicide and suicidal behavior in the area under observation was markedly elevated compared to national and local normative data (Brent et al., 1987; Center for Health Promotion and Education, 1985; Shaffer and Fisher, 1981), thereby supporting the view that suicidal contagion is a real phenomena among adolescents (Davidson and Gould, 1988).

Psychiatric vulnerability of cluster victims. The present finding that students who become suicidal subsequent to exposure were much more likely to have had prior and current psychiatric difficulties than exposed but nonsuicidal students is consistent with previous clinical descriptions of epidemic outbreaks of suicidal and nonsuicidal behavioral disturbances (Ashton and Donnan, 1981; Dizmang et al., 1974; Helvie, 1968; Knight et al., 1965; Robbins and Conroy, 1983; Small and Nicholi, 1982; Ward and Fox, 1977). Moreover, the contribution of affective disorder, both past and current, and past suicidality to the risk for current suicidality has been well established in both clinical and community samples (Brent et al., 1986; Brent, 1987; Crumley, 1979; Robbins and Alessi, 1985; Robins, 1989; Pfeffer et al., 1979, 1980, 1982, 1984; Velez and Cohen, 1988). Therefore, one may be justified in asking whether these students would have become suicidal regardless of their exposure.

The statistically significant increase in suicide attempts observed relative to those expected indicates that, at the least, the suicidal cases were "brought forward" by the exposure. The lack of pre-exposure baseline information on the rates of suicidal behavior in the high school makes it impossible to discern if these suicidal cases were, in fact, new cases. However, previous ecological studies on the impact of media publicity about suicide have suggested that publicity does increase the rate rather than merely bringing cases forward in time (Gould and Shaffer, 1986; Phillips, 1974; Phillips and Carstensen, 1986).

Exposure. Attendance at the funeral appears to play little role in the development of suicidality relative to psychopathology. This is not to say that the "dose" of exposure to the suicide is unimportant. In fact, studies on the impact of media publicity on suicide rates suggest a dose-response effect (Phillips, 1974; Phillips and Carstensen, 1986; Schmidtke and Hafner, 1988). The degree of exposure to suicide that has been reported to elicit psychopathology appears to be at the level of either discovering the body or witnessing the suicidal act (Rudestam, 1977). None of the students interviewed experienced an exposure of such an intensity.

Relationship to the victim. The apparently minor role that closeness to the victim played in the psychopathological response of exposed students may be attributable to the manner in which "closeness" was ascertained. This variable was assessed via a single question to the student, albeit one verified by parents and teachers. Another limitation with regard to the assessment of the potentially pathogenic role of exposure to suicidality is that only the relationship of the cluster students to the two suicide *victims* was assessed. It is possible that some of the cluster students were close friends with each other and that the propagation of this epidemic occurred through the vectors of these other relationships. Finally, the relationship to the suicide victim may not be a powerful predictor of suicidality in part because it is collinear with psychopathology (Shafii et al., 1988). The *high* prevalence of psychopathology among close friends of the suicide victims, combined with their tendency of these close friends to become suicidal at a *lower* psychopathological threshold than mere friends or acquaintances indicates that adolescents should be regarded as a high suicide risk following the suicide of a close friend.

Sampling. Before discussing the clinical and research implications of these findings, it is important to address another limitation of this study, the sampling frame for the subjects. For clinical and logistical reasons, students were screened on the basis of putative risk factors: funeral attendance, friendship with the victim, and prior and current psychiatric disorder (CDC, 1988). The impact of exposure to suicidality on the 93% of the students who were not screened is therefore unknown. It is also uncertain if the risk factors for suicidality obtained in a more representative sample of students would be similar to those obtained in the high-risk sample. However, the risk factors associated with suicidality in this sample have been previously reported in community studies (Pfeffer et al., 1982; Robins, 1989; Velez and

Cohen, 1988). Because the present sampling frame for screening tended to select students who were loaded with psychiatric risk factors for suicidality, the bias of this study would be toward *not* finding a relationship between these risk factors and suicidality. Therefore, it is likely that these findings with regard to risk factors for suicidality following exposure can be generalized to other settings, given their convergence with the results from other clinical and community samples.

Recommendations

Based upon this experience, the authors concur with the recommendations of the Council for Disease Control for screening students at risk for suicidality subsequent to exposure (CDC, 1988). The risk for suicidality appears to be greatest among those with psychiatric vulnerability antedating the exposure, particularly past or current affective disorder and past suicidality. Those who were close friends of the victims may also be at risk, even if they do not have current or past psychopathology. Screening exposed students for suicidality is best accomplished on-site in the school by trained clinicians who have access to both inpatient and outpatient referral sources.

The optimal length of time to maintain a clinical presence in the school is unknown, but by 3 weeks, most of the new-onset suicidal students within the crudely defined high-risk groups had been identified. The authors were concerned that by prolonging the presence of mental health workers in the school, exposure might be inadvertently exacerbated, thereby prolonging the suicidal epidemic. This is not an inconsequential consideration, as there has been at least one documented psychosocial epidemic in which the public health investigation appeared to provoke a recrudescence of psychosomatic symptomatology among the index population (Knight et al., 1965). Therefore, the presence of mental health workers on site in the school should be withdrawn as soon as the demand for such services subsides.

Further research is required to verify and extend these results by studying a representative sample of exposed and unexposed students prospectively subsequent to the suicide of a classmate. In this way, the time course of normative and pathological psychological responses to exposure to suicide can be detailed, and a more precise understanding of the mechanisms that predispose to suicidal contagion may be elucidated.

REFERENCES

Ashton, J. R., & Donnan, S. (1981), Suicide by burning as an epidemic phenomenon: an analysis of 82 deaths and inquests in England and Wales in 1978–1979. *Psychol. Med.,* 11:735–739.

Bishop, Y. M. M., Fienberg, S. E. & Holland, P. W. (1975), *Discrete Multivariate Analysis. Theory and Practice.* Cambridge, MA: The MIT Press.

Brent, D. A. (1987), Correlates of the medical lethality of suicide attempts among children and adolescents. *J. Am. Acad. Child Adolesc. Psychiatry*, 26:87–89.

_____Kalas, R., Edelbrock, C., Costello, A. J., Dulcan, M. K. & Conover, N. (1986), Psychopathology and its relationship to suicidal ideation in childhood and adolescents. *J. Am. Acad. Child Psychiatry*, 25:666–673.

_____Perper, J. & Allman, C. (1987), Alcohol, firearms, and suicide among youth: temporal trends in Allegheny County, Pennsylvania 1960–1983. *JAMA*, 257:3369–3372.

_____ _____Goldstein, C. E. et al. (1988a), Risk factors for adolescent suicide. *Arch. Gen. Psychiatry*, 45:581–588.

_____ _____Kolko, D. J. & Zelenak, J. P. (1988b), The psychological autopsy: methodologic considerations for the study of adolescent suicide. *J. Am. Acad. Child Psychiatry*, 27:362–366.

Centers for Disease Control (1988), CDC recommendations for a community plan for the prevention and containment of suicide clusters. *MMWR*, 37 (Suppl. no. S-6): 1–12.

Center for Health Promotion and Education (1985), *Suicide Surveillance 1970–1980.* Atlanta: U.S. Dept of Health and Human Services, Centers for Disease Control.

Coleman, L. (1987), *Suicide Clusters.* Boston: Faber & Faber, Inc.

Crumley, F. E. (1979), Adolescent suicide attempts. *JAMA*, 241:2404–2407.

Davidson, L. & Gould, M. S. (1988), Contagion as a risk factor for youth suicide. In: *United States Department of Health and Human Services: Report on the Secretary's Task Force on Youth Suicide, Vol 2; Risk Factors for Youth Suicide.* Washington, DC: U.S. Government Printing Office.

Dizmang, M., Watson, J., May, P. et al. (1974), Adolescent suicide at an Indian reserve. *Am J. Orthopsychiatry*, 44:43–49.

Gould, M. S. & Shaffer, D. (1986), The impact of suicide in television movies: evidence of imitation. *N. Engl. J. Med.*, 315:690–694.

_____Wallenstein, S. & Kleinman, M. (in press), *Time-space clustering of teen suicide. Am. J. Epidemiol.*

_____Shaffer, D. & Kleinman, M. (1988), The impact of suicide in television movies: replication and commentary. *Suicide Life Threat. Behav.*, 18:90–99.

Harkavy-Friedman, J. M., Asnis, G. M. & Boeck, M. (1987), Prevalence of specific suicidal behaviors in high school sample. *Am. J. Psychiatry*, 144:1203–1206.

Hays, W. L. (1968), *Statistics,* Ed. 3. New York: Holt Rinehard and Winston, Inc., pp. 435–437.

Helvie, C. O. (1968), An epidemic of hysteria in a high school. *J. Schl. Health*, 38:505–509.

Kety, S. S. (1986), Genetic factors in suicide. In: *Suicide,* ed. A. Roy. Baltimore: Williams & Wilkins, pp. 41–45.

Knight, J. A. Friedman, T. I. & Sulianti, J. (1965), Epidemic hysteria: a field study. *Am. J. Public Health*, 858–865.

Kreitman, N., Smith, P. & Tan, E. S. (1970), Attempted suicide as language: an empirical study. *Br. J. Psychiatry,* 116:464–473.

Pfeffer, C. R., Conte, H. R., Plutchik, R. & Jerrett, I. (1979), Suicidal behavior in latency-age children: an empirical study. *J. Am. Acad. Child Psychiatry,* 18:679–692.

―――― ―――― ――――et al. (1980), Suicidal behavior in latency-age children. *J. Am. Acad. Child Psychiatry,* 19:703–710.

Pfeffer, C. R., Solomon, G., Plutchik, R., Mizruchi, M. S. & Weiner, A. (1982), Suicidal behavior in latency-age psychiatric inpatients: a replication and cross-validation. *J. Am. Acad. Child Psychiatry,* 21:564–569.

――――Zuckerman, S., Plutchik, R. et al. (1984), Suicidal behavior in normal school children: a comparison with child psychiatric inpatients. *J. Am. Acad. Child Psychiatry,* 23:416–423.

Phillips, D. P. (1974), The influence of suggestion on suicide: substantive and theoretical implications of the Werther effect. *American Social Review,* 39:340–359.

――――Carstensen, L. L. (1986), Clustering of teenage suicides after television news stories about suicide. *N. Engl. J. Med.,* 315:685–689.

Robbins, D. & Conroy, R. (1983), A cluster of adolescent suicide: Is suicide contagious? *J. Adolesc. Health Care,* 364:253–255.

Robbins, D. R. & Alessi, N. E. (1985), Depressive symptoms and suicidal behavior in adolescents. *Am. J. Psychiatry,* 142:588–592.

Robins, L. N. (1989), *Alcohol, drug abuse and mental health administration.* Report of the Secretary's Task Force on Youth Suicide. Vol. 4: Strategies for the Prevention of Youth Suicide [DHHS Publ. No. (ADM) 89–1624]. Washington, DC: U.S. Government Printing Office, pp. 94–114.

Roy, A. (1983), Family history of suicide. *Arch. Gen. Psychiatry,* 40:971–974.

Rudestam, K. E. (1977), Physical and psychological responses to suicide in the family. *J. Consult. Clin. Psychol.,* 45:162–170.

Schlesselman, J. J. (1982), *Case-Control Studies: Design, Conduct Analysis.* New York: Oxford University Press.

Schmidtke, A. & Hafner H. (1988), The Werther effect after television films: new evidence for an old hypothesis. *Psychol. Med.,* 18:665–676.

Shaffer, D. & Fisher, P. (1981), The epidemiology of suicide in children and young adolescents. *J. Am. Acad. Child Psychiatry,* 20:545–561.

―――― ――――Garland, A. Gould, M., P. & Trautman, P. (1988), Preventing teenage suicide: a critical review. *J. Am. Acad. Child Adolesc. Psychiatry,* 27:675–687.

Shafii, M., Carrigan, S., Whittighill, J. R. & Derrick, A. (1985), Psychological autopsy of completed suicide in children and adolescents. *Am. J. Psychiatry,* 142:1061–1064.

――――Seltz-Lenarsky, J., Derrick, A. M. et al. (1988), Comorbidity of mental disorders in the post-mortem diagnosis of completed suicide in children and adolescents. *J. Affect. Disord.,* 227–233.

Shepherd, D. & Barraclough, B. M. (1978), Suicide reporting: information or entertainment? *Br. J. Psychiatry,* 132:283–287.

Small, G. W. & Nicholi, A. M., (1982), Mass hysteria among school children. *Arch. Gen. Psychiatry,* 39:721–724.

Smith, K. & Crawford, S. (1986), Suicidal behavior among "normal" high school students. *Suicide Life Threat. Behav.,* 16:313–325.

Velez, C. N. & Cohen, P. (1988), Suicidal behavior and ideation in a community sample of children: maternal and youth reports. *J. Am. Acad. Child Adolesc. Psychiatry,* 27:349–356.

Ward, J. A. & Fox, J. (1977), A suicide epidemic on an Indian reserve. *Canadian Psychiatric Association Journal,* 22:423–426.

29

Toward a Theory of the Genesis of Violence: A Follow-up Study of Delinquents

Dorothy Otnow Lewis
New York University School of Medicine

Richard Lovely
John Jay College of Criminal Justice, New York

Catherine Yeager and Donna Della Famina
New York University School of Medicine

The results of a follow-up study of 95 formerly incarcerated delinquents are reported. Adult F.B.I. and state police records were used. All but six of the subjects had adult criminal records. The average number of adult offenses was 11.58. Juvenile violence alone did not distinguish well between those who would and would not go on to adult violent crime. Seventy-seven percent of the more violent juveniles and 61% of the less violent juveniles committed adult aggressive offenses. The interaction of intrinsic vulnerabilities (cognitive, psychiatric, and neurological) and a history of abuse and/or family violence was a better predictor of adult violent crime. Key Words: delinquents, follow-up study, abuse, family violence, neurological impairment.

The causes of violence are poorly understood. It is well established that violence in childhood is associated with later violence (Monahan, 1981). As a variable, however, early aggression can only predict adult violence; it has no implications for understanding its causes, treatment, or prevention. While nearly all very violent adults appear to have been violent as juveniles, many violent juveniles do not become violent adults. How can one explain why some do and some do not? Are there more useful variables than early aggression that have implications for treat-

Reprinted with permission from *Journal of the American Academy of Child and Adolescent Psychiatry,* 1989, Vol. 28, No. 3, 4 31–436. Copyright © 1989 by the American Academy of Child and Adolescent Psychiatry.

ment and prevention? Are there combinations of intrinsic and environmental factors that distinguish between those aggressive children who are likely to continue their violent careers, and those who will not?

The purpose of this paper is twofold: (1) to report the results of a 7-year follow-up study of incarcerated juveniles; and (2) to test the hypothesis that a constellation of certain kinds of neuropsychiatric vulnerabilities, interacting with violent abusive family environments, predicts adult violence better than does early violence alone.

THE LITERATURE

Considering the magnitude of violent crime in the United States, there have been remarkably few follow-up studies of aggressive children and adolescents and even fewer studies that consider issues other than previous antisocial behaviors, for purposes of prediction. Lefkowitz et al. (1977) reported that aggression at 8 years of age was predictive of future aggression; Wolfgang et al. (1972, 1984) reported that the degree of early antisocial behavior and being black were predictive of ongoing criminality; and Robins (1966), in a study using records from a child guidance clinic, found that early antisocial behavior was associated with the adult diagnosis of sociopathic personality. Faretra's (1981) follow-up study of violent and suicidal adolescent psychiatric inpatients also reported a high prevalence of adult violent crime in former adolescent psychiatric inpatients. Finally, Loeber and Dishion (1983), after an extensive literature review, concluded that early conduct and academic problems and poor family discipline and supervision were the best predictors of delinquency.

Most of the studies cited above used data from police files, school records, and clinic or hospital records. These resources allow the study of large numbers of subjects but limit the kinds of variables to those that are readily available. Clinical data that are now recognized as essential for the evaluation of violent individuals (e.g., histories of CNS trauma, EEG results and psychomotor epileptic symptoms, evidence of cognitive impairment, histories of physical abuse, etc.) are not uniformly available in clinic or hospital records.

Studies of delinquent adolescents and criminal adults by the present authors and their colleagues (Lewis et al., 1976a, b, 1979, 1985, 1986, 1987, 1988) have consistently demonstrated associations among signs and symptoms of neuropsychiatric and cognitive impairment, upbringing in abusive, violent families, and aggressive behaviors in childhood and adolescence. Of special note was the finding that a constellation of neuropsychiatric vulnerabilities and abusive, violent families distinguished more aggressive nondelinquent subjects from their nonaggressive nondelinquent peers (Lewis et al., 1987). Thus, it would seem that a constellation of particular intrinsic vulnerabilities and specific kinds of family stressors is associated with aggressiveness in general and not simply with having been designated delinquent or criminal. The authors of this study wondered whether the same kinds of intrinsic and environmental disturbances associated with juvenile aggression were predictive of adult violence.

The current study, in addition to exploring the association between juvenile violence and adult criminality, examines data gathered from psychiatric, neurological, and psychological evaluations performed expressly for research purposes. It differs from the Robins (1966) and Faretra (1981) studies in two important ways: (1) it was based on clinical evaluations rather than record reviews, and (2) the study sample was composed entirely of incarcerated delinquents rather than hospitalized or child guidance center referred patients.

When this follow-up study was begun, the authors hypothesized that intrinsic vulnerabilities—psychiatric, neurological, or cognitive—when coupled with an upbringing in an abusive and/or violent household, would be associated with adult criminal violence. They further hypothesized that the effect of this combination of variables on violence would not simply be additive but would gain power by virtue of an interaction between the intrinsic and environmental components.

METHOD

Sample

This follow-up study is one of a series of reports on a group of incarcerated juveniles who were originally studied in the late 1970s (Lewis et al., 1979). The original sample consisted of 97 boys incarcerated at the only correctional school in Connecticut during an 18-month period in the late 1970s. The selection of subjects has been described (Lewis et al. 1979). Unfortunately, at the time, there was considerable local and national concern regarding studies of neuropsychiatric and intellectual factors, and it was impossible to recruit a comparison sample of demographically comparable nondelinquents. Thus, Lewis et al. were limited to studying incarcerated delinquents only. So that violent and relatively nonviolent juveniles could be compared, the sample was divided into 79 more-violent subjects, and 18 less-violent subjects, based on reliable ratings of violent behaviors (Lewis et al., 1979). Given the sample limitations, findings from this follow up study may not be able to be extrapolated to other juvenile populations.

Within the sample, 37% of the subjects were white, 41% were black, 21% were Hispanic, and 1% Oriental. The subjects' ages at the time of evaluation ranged from 12.4 years to 17.4 years (mean 15 years 3 months, median 15 years, 3 months). Ages at the time of follow-up ranged from 19.9 years to 25.2 years (mean 22.5 years, median 22.7 years). The overwhelming majority of the subjects were from classes IV and V according to the Hollingshead and Redlich criteria (Hollingshead and Redlich, 1958).

By the time of follow-up, six subjects had died. Of these, two died shortly after release from the correctional school. Since they had insufficient time to commit offenses as adults, their data were dropped from the follow-up study. Thus, the final number of subjects was 95, 77 very violent, and 18 less violent.

Psychiatric and Neurological Evaluation

The original psychiatric evaluation has been described (Lewis et al., 1979, 1987). To summarize briefly, it consisted of a lengthy semistructured interview that was devised because there was no existing diagnostic protocol for children or adolescents that dealt adequately with topics such as medical history, history of neuropsychiatric symptoms (e.g., lapses, memory impairment, metamorphopsias), qualities of temper, or histories of physical abuse and family violence, all topics essential to the workup of antisocial individuals. The instrument has since been tested on adolescent inpatients, and the data obtained from it in the areas mentioned above were found to be more comprehensive than those obtained after a 2-week period of routine psychiatric assessment on an adolescent inpatient teaching service.

In addition to obtaining historical information, a systematic mental status examination was conducted by both the neurologist and the psychiatrist. The criteria for determining the presence or absence of psychotic symptoms were clearly defined and have been described (Lewis et al., 1979, 1987).

Standard neurological examinations, which have been described (Lewis et al., 1979, 1987), were carried out be a senior neurologist. A brief test of reading grade level, including word recognition and paragraph comprehension, was also performed by the neurologist.

Neurological history, including a detailed history of CNS injury and psychomotor symptoms, was obtained by the neurologist as well as the psychiatrist.

In addition to the neurological examination, sleep deprived electroencephalograms were performed and were read by a senior neurologist at a local medical school.

Pychoeducational Testing

Psychological testing, consisting of the Weschler Intelligence Scale for Children (revised) (Weschler, 1974), the Bender-Gestalt Test (Bender, 1946), and the Rorschach Test (Rorschach, 1945), was performed.

Reading grade level was assessed as part of the correctional school's routine educational evaluation and has been described (Lewis et al., 1979). Reading level discrepancy was calculated by subtracting the subject's reading grade level score from his expected grade level for age and IQ.

Abuse and Family Violence

Certain other issues were covered both by the neurologist and the psychiatrist. For example, both tried to ascertain whether or not the child had been a victim of abuse or had witnessed extreme violence. Because issues of abuse are so important to this follow-up study, criteria for positive coding will be repeated here. A child was considered to have been a victim of abuse by his parents, guardian, or others if he had been punched, beaten with a stick, board, pipe, or belt buckle, or beaten with a belt or switch other than on the buttocks. He was also considered to have been abused if he had been deliberately cut, burned, or thrown down stairs or across a room. A child was considered not to have been abused if he was only struck with an open hand or beaten with the leather part of a belt or with a switch on the buttocks only. For purposes of this follow-up study, subjects were also categorized as abused if their parents had been referred to Protective Services for abuse or neglect. Family violence was considered to have occurred if parents or other close family members had assaulted each other physically or threatened each other with weapons.

Issues of Veracity

When dealing with information obtained from delinquents or criminals the issue of veracity is paramount. Because the majority of this sample of juveniles was born before the Battered Child Syndrome was reported (Kempe et al., 1962), and before mechanisms were standardized for reporting abuse, it was not always possible to verify juveniles' reports with official records of abuse. However, in addition to the clinicians' interviews with subjects, there was a wealth of data from other social service agencies, parent interviews, and hospital records, as well as from scars over subjects' faces and bodies, that tended to substantiate what children said. In fact, subsequent reviews of hospital records, and interviews years later with subjects themselves, indicated that in adolescence they tended to underreport their experiences of having been abused and of having witnessed family violence.

Categorization of Intrinsic Vulnerabilities.

Intrinsic vulnerabilities are defined here as impairments or dysfunctions that interfere with or limit the normal socialization of a child. From the authors' previous studies of the association of clinical signs and symptoms and juvenile violence, three general categories of such intrinsic vulnerabilities were identified: (1) episodic psychotic symptoms, (2) neurological/limbic dysfunction, (3) cognitive impairment.

Episodic psychotic symptoms. Subjects in this study were considered to have episodic psychotic symptoms if, at any time, they experienced paranoid ideation, or visual or auditory hallucinations as previously defined (Lewis et al., 1979), or if, during psychiatric interviews, they were loose, rambling, or illogical.

Neurological/limbic dysfunction. A subject was classified as having neurological or limbic dysfunction if he had three or more psychomotor symptoms, as previously defined (Lewis et al. 1987), or if he had a history of seizures or an abnormal EEG.

Cognitive impairment. The following measures of cognitive impairment were used: (1) a reading ability of 3 or more years below that expected for age and intelligence *and* (2) either an inability to subtract serial 7s or an inability to recall four digits backward. IQ alone was not used, because in the original study, it did not distinguish between more- and less-violent groups significantly. Furthermore, it was found that brain dysfunction rather than simply low intelligence is more closely associated with problems in judgment and impulse control. Although it would have been desirable to have had a more robust measure of cognitive impairment based on a standardized battery of neuropsychological tests such as the Halstead-Reitan Battery (Halstead and Reitan, 1979), funding limitations precluded obtaining such measures.

Thus, a continuous variable was created, Intrinsic Vulnerabilities, encompassing episodic psychotic symptoms, neurological/limbic dysfunction, and cognitive impairment (min. value = 0, max. value = 3).

Categorization of Environmental Stressors

For purposes of this study, environmental stressors were defined as having been physically abused, and/or having witnessed extreme violence between family members, both as defined above. Of the 95 subjects, 60% (N = 57) had both been abused and had witnessed extraordinary family violence. In addition 16 had indisputable evidence of abuse only and seven had similarly clear evidence of extreme family violence only. However, in these 23 cases, there was also material available suggesting the likelihood that both had occurred. Since, in this sample, the two experiences usually went together, it was decided to not distinguish between those who had been abused and those who had been exposed to violence. For this reason, the environmental variable *Abusive, Violent Family* was created to reflect either experience.

Measures of Adult Violence and Criminality

With proper respect for and assurances of confidentiality, the authors were able to obtain the following data regarding adult offenses: (1) number, nature, and timing of arrests according to state police records; (2) number, nature, and timing of arrests according to F.B.I. records; and (3) duration and timing of incarcerations. Thus, adult arrest data was exceptionally complete.

After the arrest data were obtained, the nature of the offenses was coded in two different ways. First, each offense was coded to reflect its severity according to the Connecticut State Penal Code. The penal code divides offenses into felonies and misdemeanors. Within each of these categories, the severity of the offense is classified as A, B, C, or D, in descending order of seriousness. For purposes of assessing adult violence, one of our outcome measures was numbers of A felonies plus numbers of B felonies. These felonies included murder, sexual assault, kidnapping, and robbery.

The alphabetical classification of offenses used by the police did not always reflect the aggressive nature of criminal acts, since lesser degrees of felonies and some misdemeanors are violent. Therefore, offenses were also coded in terms of the descriptive nature of the acts. Thus the following acts were grouped together as Aggressive Offenses: murder or attempted murder; kidnapping or unlawful restraint; sexual assault of any kind; nonsexual assault of any kind; robbery of any kind; and burglary with weapons or explosives or in which physical injury occurred (i.e., Burglary I). The category of Nonaggressive Offenses encompassed all other offenses such as stealing of any kind, including certain forms of burglary in which no physical harm occurred, and other lesser offenses such as breach of the peace in which no individual was injured.

Coding offenses in these two different ways allowed the data to be analyzed in more meaningful ways than would have been possible had simply felony and misdemeanor alphabetical classifications been used. Also, a subject's total number of offenses, regardless of their nature was recorded.

In addition, the numbers of prison days a subject was incarcerated was tabulated. By subtracting the numbers of days incarcerated from the numbers of days between discharge from juvenile corrections and follow-up, the number of offenses committed per year at liberty could be calculated.

A word should be said about the limitations of using recorded offenses only. Many violent acts never come to the attention of the police. Furthermore, the classification of an offense sometimes reflects plea bargaining. Thus, official records underestimate actual violence. On the other hand, they are objective.

FINDINGS

The follow-up data revealed a distressing picture. Of the 95 subjects, all but six had an adult criminal record. The average total number of adult offenses was 11.58 (median 9, range 0 to 64). Moreover, 48 of the 95 had committed at least one A or B felony (mean 1.46, range 0 to 11). Nine had been arrested for murder or attempted murder, 12 for sexual assault, nine for kidnapping or unlawful restraint, 58 for nonsexual assault, and 44 for robbery or Burglary I. In fact, 69 of the 95 subjects had committed one or more aggressive offenses, as categorized above. The average number of aggressive offenses was 3.52 (median 2, range 0 to 16). Over 80% of subjects had spent time in jail or prison. Time imprisoned ranged from 0 to 2,604 days ($\bar{X}$ = 745 days, median = 537 days).

Juvenile Violence vs. Adult Violence

To what extent did those who were aggressive as juveniles turn out to be violent adults? Of those who had been classified seriously violent as juveniles, 77% had an adult arrest record for aggressive offenses, but so did 61% of the subjects who were not classified seriously violent as juveniles. Thus, early violence per se did not distinguish well those who would become violent adults from those who would not. In fact, early violence alone misclassified 23% of the more violent juveniles and 61% of the less violent juveniles in terms of future adult violence.

Intrinsic Vulnerabilities, Family Stressors, and Violence

If intrinsic vulnerabilities and abusive, violent families contribute to the production of violence, then these variables might be expected to perform as better indicators of future violence than simply early violent behavior. The authors' concern, however, was not simply to predict adult violence, but also to take a step toward understanding the dynamics of the causes of violence.

Because of the relatively small number of subjects in relation to the number of variables and combinations thereof, it was not possible to study the relationship of isolated specific vulnerabilities to outcome. For example, almost all of the subjects who had only one intrinsic vulnerability (i.e., either episodic psychotic symptoms, or neurological/limbic dysfunction, or cognitive impairment), had also been abused or raised in violent homes. Similarly, only seven subjects had histories of abuse and/or family violence and no intrinsic vulnerabilities at all. However, the sample size did permit us to determine whether the numbers of intrinsic vulnerabilities and their interaction with violent abusive home environments were associated with increasing levels of adult violence. Therefore the data were analyzed in terms of the relationship to criminal outcome of numbers of intrinsic vulnerabilities with and without a history of abuse and/or family violence.

Subjects were divided into the following groups:

  I: Those with neither Intrinsic Vulnerabilities nor Abusive, Violent Families (*N* = 6)

 II: Those with Intrinsic Vulnerabilities only (*N* = 9)

III: Those with Abusive, Violent Families only (*N* = 7)

 IV: Those with one Intrinsic Vulnerability *and* Abusive, Violent Families (*N* = 17)

V: Those with two Intrinsic Vulnerabilities *and* Abusive, Violent Families (N = 34)

VI: Those with all three Intrinsic Vulnerabilities *and* Abusive, Violent Families (N = 22).

Tables 1 and 2 illustrate the relationship of adult criminal violence to Intrinsic Vulnerabilities and Abusive, Violent Families. As can be seen, subjects seem to fall into three different levels of criminality. Those few subjects with neither Intrinsic Vulnerabilities nor Abusive, Violent Families have extremely low rates of serious

TABLE 1

Numbers of A plus B Felonies, Aggressive Offenses, Total Offenses, and Days Incarcerated for Subjects in Categories I-VI

	Category[a]	Mean	Median
A plus B felonies	I	0.2	0.0
	II	0.7	0.0
	III	0.6	0.0
	IV	0.5	0.0
	V	1.8	1.0
	VI	2.7	1.5
Aggressive offenses	I	0.0	0.0
	II	2.1	2.0
	III	1.9	1.0
	IV	2.2	1.0
	V	4.4	3.5
	VI	5.4	4.0
Total numbers of offenses	I	2.2	2.5
	II	9.8	6.0
	III	11.9	10.0
	IV	10.2	3.0
	V	11.0	10.0
	VI	16.8	13.5
Numbers of days incarcerated	I	1.0	0.0
	II	337.7	13.0
	III	562.1	20.0
	IV	563.3	376.0
	V	750.8	604.0
	VI	1214.4	1123.0

[a] I—Neither Vulnerabilities nor Abusive, Violent Families; II—Intrinsic Vulnerabilities only; III—Abusive, Violent Families only; IV—One Vulnerability and Abusive, Violent Families; V—Two Vulnerabilities and Abusive, Violent Families; VI—Three Vulnerabilities and Abusive, Violent Families.

TABLE 2
Rates of A plus B Felonies, Aggressive Offenses, and Total
Offenses per Year at Liberty for Subjects in Categories I-VI

	Category[a]	Mean	Median
A plus B felonies	I	0.0	0.0
	II	0.2	0.0
	III	0.2	0.0
	IV	0.2	0.0
	V	0.7	0.2
	VI	2.5	0.5
Aggressive offenses	I	0.0	0.0
	II	0.5	0.3
	III	0.6	0.2
	IV	0.8	0.3
	V	2.6	0.8
	VI	4.6	1.2
Total offenses	I	0.4	0.5
	II	2.2	1.2
	III	3.5	1.7
	IV	3.0	0.9
	V	5.6	2.1
	VI	15.4	3.8

[a] See Table 1 for explanation of categories.

criminality, whatever the measure used, be it A plus B felonies, Aggressive Offenses, or Total Numbers of Offenses.

Of some surprise was the finding that subjects in group IV, with one Intrinsic Vulnerability and a history of Abusive Violent Families, had no more serious criminal records than did those in groups II and III with either Intrinsic Vulnerability or Abusive, Violent Families. The authors had thought originally that any vulnerability, coupled with abuse and/or family violence would be more detrimental than vulnerabilities alone or abuse alone. Of note, of the nine subjects in group II, with Intrinsic Vulnerabilities only, just one had a single vulnerability; the rest had two or three, suggesting fairly extensive impairment. These subjects with one to three Intrinsic Vulnerabilities were collapsed into one category because of their extremely small numbers. Thus, groups II, III and IV fell into a middle level of criminality, with more serious criminality than subjects in category I but several times less serious criminality than subjects in categories V and VI.

Most striking, and consistent with the hypothesis, were the high rates of criminality in subjects in groups V and VI. Severe neuropsychiatric and/or cognitive handicaps (2 or more kinds of intrinsic vulnerabilities) coupled with an upbringing in an abusive, violent household were associated with serious adult violent criminality.

Patterns of Vulnerabilities and Environmental Stressors in Murderers

Murder is the most serious of crimes. For this reason the authors looked specifically at the patterns of vulnerabilities and stressors in the nine subjects who, as adults, committed murder. Six of the nine had three vulnerabilities and a history of abuse and/or family violence. The remaining three had two vulnerabilities and a history of abuse and/or family violence. Thus all fell into the seriously impaired as well as abused categories.

Log-Linear Analysis

Central to the theoretical thrust of this study was to test whether intrinsic vulnerabilities and abuse had independent effects on criminal outcomes or whether they interacted to heighten the level of violence. Tables 1 and 2 reveal a pattern of sharp increases in the size of the outcome variable when the number of intrinsic vulnerabilities in conjunction with a history of abuse and/or family violence jumps from one to two and then from two to three. This is consistent with the hypothesis that there is an interactive effect between Intrinsic Vulnerabilities and Abusive, Violent Families. As a way to test this hypothesis, a log-linear analysis was conducted, using as an outcome variable ever having committed an aggressive offense as an adult (Variable name = AGGOFF). An index of vulnerabilities from 0 to 3 was used as an independent variable indicating the extent of intrinsic impairment (Variable name = VULS). Abusive, violent families were used as the independent variable indicating extreme environmental stress (Variable name = ABVIOL).

The goal of the log-linear analysis is to reproduce the actual profile of the sample by specifying a model comprised of the hypothesized interactions among the independent variables. As can be seen in Table 3, the distribution of subjects across the

TABLE 3

Log-Linear Models for 3-Way Cross Tabulation of Intrinsic
Vulnerabilities (VULS), Abuse, Violent Families (ABVIOL), and
Aggressive Offenses (AGGOFF)

Fitted Marginals/LogLinear Models (Outcome Variable = AGGOFF)	Likelihood Ratio	df	p Value
{VULS ABVIOL}	14.42	6	0.03
{VULS ABVIOL}{VULS AGGOFF}	10.81	5	0.06
{VULS ABVIOL}{ABVIOL AGGOFF}	12.31	5	0.03
{VULS ABVIOL}{ABVIOL AGGOFF}{VULS AGGOFF}	6.11	4	0.19[a]

[a] This interactive combination of variables did not differ significantly from the actual clinical data and, thus, supported the interactive hypothesis. This interaction is one step below the full, or saturated, model with all effects included.

three variables in the analysis could not be reproduced with a log-linear model which included only the main effects of the independent variables. Nor did the two log-linear models which allowed for 2-way interactions between intrinsic vulnerabilities and aggressive offenses only, and abusive, violent families and aggressive offenses only, fit the model. The long-linear model fit, however, when the three possible 2-way interactions, short of the saturated model (i.e., Intrinsic Vulnerabilities × Aggressive Offenses; Abusive, Violent Families × Aggressive Offenses; and Intrinsic Vulnerabilities × Abusive, Violent Families), were included. This finding suggests that there is, as supposed, not simply an additive effect, but also an interactive effect among intrinsic vulnerabilities, having been raised in an abusive, violent household, and adult aggression.

Toward a Theory of the Genesis of Violence

Nearly all violent adult criminals have histories of juvenile violence. On the other hand, as the data clearly show, all aggressive juveniles do not become violent adults. The question remains, therefore, are there ways of knowing which aggressive juveniles are most likely to make adequate nonviolent adaptations to society and which are most likely to go on to make violent criminality a career?

The data suggest that there are combinations of intrinsic vulnerabilities and environmental stressors identifiable in adolescence, and probably before then, that help to explain which delinquents will go on to commit crimes of violence as adults. It would seem that delinquent children with combinations of psychiatric, neurological, and cognitive vulnerabilities are at somewhat greater risk of continuing violence than are their more intact counterparts. Similarly, delinquent children who have been brutally abused and/or have been raised in extraordinarily violent households are at somewhat greater risk for ongoing violent adult crime than are those who have not been raised in such environments.

However, seriously intrinsically handicapped delinquents who also have grown up in violent, abusive environments are much more likely to go on to commit numerous, violent offenses as adults.

The authors found, to their surprise, that the combination of one kind of intrinsic vulnerability (a reflection of relatively minor impairment) and having been exposed to abuse and/or violence (Group IV) was not any more closely related to adult violence than having vulnerabilities only (Group II) or having been raised in an abusive, violent household only (Group III). Rather, it appeared that it was the combinations of severe impairment, as reflected in having two or three kinds of vulnerabilities, and abuse and/or family violence that were most closely associated with extreme adult aggression.

The log-linear analysis supported the initial hypothesis—that the combination of intrinsic vulnerabilities and family violence and/or abusiveness was not merely additive; rather, intrinsic vulnerabilities interacted with environmental stressors to increase the risk and severity of adult violent criminality.

How might we begin to understand this interactive effect from a clinical perspective? First and foremost, family violence and abusiveness function as a model of aggressive behavior. Children who are neuropsychiatrically and cognitively intact are better equipped than are multiply handicapped children to resist these models, choose among alternative styles, and make independent, more rational judgments regarding appropriate behavior. The intrinsically vulnerable child is more likely to react impulsively and unthinkingly when stressed.

Second, abuse engenders rage, the kind of rage that neuropsychiatrically and cognitively impaired individuals, particularly episodically paranoid individuals, find far more difficult to control than do normal, nonimpaired, healthy individuals.

Third, in many instances, when abuse involves shaking, battering, or other injury to the central nervous system, it creates the very psychiatric, neurological, and cognitive vulnerabilities that we have described.

Finally, and ironically, neuropsychiatrically impaired children, by virtue of their hyperactivity and impulsivity, often invite abuse.

Violence is possibly the most serious mental health problem confronting our society. To say that early aggression predicts later aggression leads nowhere except, perhaps, to incarceration. Furthermore, the data suggest that early aggression overpredicts adult aggression in violent delinquents about 23% of the time and underpredicts adult aggression in less violent delinquents over 60% of the time. On the other hand, within the sample of delinquents studied, a constellation of interacting clinical and environmental variables is a far better predictor of future violent behavior than is early aggression alone. More importantly, each characteristic of that constellation, unlike early aggression, carries with it very specific implications for prevention and treatment.

REFERENCES

Bender, L. (1946), *The Bender Visual Motor Gestalt Test.* New York: American Orthopsychiatric Association.

Faretra, G. (1981), A profile of aggression from adolescence to adulthood: an 18 year follow-up of psychiatrically disturbed and violent adolescents. *Am. J. Orthopsychiatry,* 51:439–453.

Halstead, W. C. & Reitan, R. M. (1979), *The Halstead-Reitan Battery.* Tucson: University of Arizona.

Hollingshead, A. B. & Redlich, F. C. (1958), *Social Class and Mental Illness—A Community Study.* New York: J. Wiley.

Kempe, C. H., Silverman, F., Steele, B., Droegmueller, W. & Silver, H. (1962), The battered child syndrome. *JAMA,* 181:17–24.

Lefkowitz, M., Eron, L. Walder, L. & Huesman, L. (1977), *Growing Up to be Violent.* New York: Pergamon.

Lewis, D. O. (1976a), Diagnostic evaluation of the juvenile offender. *Child Psychiatry, Hum. Dev.,* 6:198–213.

———Balla, D. A. (1976b), *Delinquency and Psychopathology.* New York: Grune and Stratton.

———Shanok, S. S., Pincus, J. J. & Glaser, G. H. (1979), Violent juvenile delinquents: psychiatric, neurological, psychological, and abuse factors. *J. Am. Acad. Child Psychiatry,* 18:307–319.

———Moy E., Jackson, L. D. et al. (1985), Biopsychosocial characteristics of children who later murder. *Am. J. Psychiatry,* 142:116–1167.

———Feldman, M., Jackson, L. & Bard, B. (1986), Psychiatric neurological and psycho-educational characteristics of 15 death row inmates in the United States. *Am. J. Psychiatry,* 143:838–845.

———Pincus, J. H., Lovely, R., Spitzer, E. & Moy, E. (1987), Biopsychosocial characteristics of matched samples of delinquents and nondelinquents. *J. Am. Acad. Child Adolesc. Psychiatry,* 26:744–752.

———Pincus, J. H., Bard, B. et al. (1988) Neuropsychiatric, psychoeducational and family characteristics of 14 juveniles condemned to death in the United States. *Am. J. Psychiatry,* 145:585–589.

Loeber, R. & Dishion, T. (1983), Early predictors of male delinquency. *Psychol. Bull,* 94:68–99.

Monahan, J. (1981), *Predicting Violent Behavior, an Assessment of Clinical Technique,* Vol. 14. Beverly Hills, CA: Sage Library of Social Research.

Robins, L. N. (1966), *Deviant Children Grow Up: A Sociological and Psychiatric Study of Sociopathic Personality.* Baltimore: Williams and Wilkins.

Rorschach, H. (1945), *Rorschach Test.* Switzerland: Hans Nuber Publishers.

Wechsler, D. (1974), *The Wechsler Intelligence Scale for Children (Revised).* Middleburg Heights, OH: Psychological Corporation.

Wolfgang, M. E., Figlio, R. M. & Sellin, T. (1972), *Delinquency in a Birth Cohort.* Chicago: University of Chicago Press.

———Tracy, P. E. & Figlio, R. M. (1984), *Delinquency in a birth cohort II: a summary.* A report to the Office of Juvenile Justice and Delinquency Prevention, Washington, D.C.

30

Prevention of Child Sexual Abuse: Myth or Reality

N. Dickon Reppucci and Jeffrey J. Haugaard

University of Virginia, Charlottesville

Programs to prevent child sexual abuse have proliferated as a result of increased public awareness and professional documentation of its incidence. We describe the content and format of these prevention programs in general and examine selected programs for effectiveness. Although there is limited evidence for an increase in knowledge for program participants, most evaluations suffer from basic design problems and present few results indicative of either primary prevention or detection. Overall, we argue that self-protection against sexual abuse is a very complex process for any child and that few, if any, prevention programs are comprehensive enough to have a meaningful impact on this process. Finally, we discuss several untested assumptions that guide these programs. We conclude that it is unclear whether prevention programs are working or even that they are more beneficial than harmful.

The widespread, documented incidence of child sexual abuse (Finkelhor, 1979; Russell, 1984; Wyatt, 1985) and numerous clinical reports of harm to victims (Haugaard & Reppucci, 1988) provided the impetus for the professional development of programs to prevent its occurrence. However, the recent explosion of these programs nationwide has come about in no small part because of the vast amount of publicity that this topic has received in the past five years. In 1984, the issue of child sexual abuse was dramatically brought to public awareness with the arrest in California of Virginia McMartin and six of her employees for alleged sexual abuse of 125 children over a 10-year period at her day care center. A few months later, another highly publicized case in Minnesota resulted in indictments against 24 parents and other adults for allegedly sexually abusing over 50 children. *Newsweek* and

Reprinted with permission by *American Psychologist*, 1989, Vol. 44, No. 10, 1266–1275. Copyright © 1989 by the American Psychological Association, Inc.

Life ran cover stories on child sexual abuse. *Sixty Minutes, 20-20,* and *Nightline* featured TV reports on the topic, and the Public Broadcasting System televised a four-part series on its prevention. Moreover, the pictures of missing children that appeared on milk cartons, billboards, and telephone books were and are constant reminders that untold numbers of children have disappeared, some possibly becoming victims of sexual abuse. Although charges were subsequently dismissed against all the alleged abusers in the Minnesota case, the McMartin case was still being prosecuted in March 1988, when Judge Pounders called it the "most expensive case in (USA) history" (Stewart, 1988, p. 3A), with $7.5 million spent so far. He justified the expense because "The case has benefited society as a whole, . . . because many people have become aware of a social problem that may not have been spoken about" (Stewart, 1988. p. 3A).

Recently, we (Haugaard & Reppucci, 1988) described what is and is not known about the etiology and treatment of child sexual abuse and argued strongly for increased research and action. We also noted with concern the inadequate research base for child sexual abuse prevention programs. The purpose of this article is two-fold: (a) to describe briefly the content and effects of selected sexual abuse prevention programs, and (b) to emphasize that several underlying assumptions that power these programs are frequently accepted as fact, even though they are based mainly on clinical anecdote and "best guess." Our analysis is limited to existing evaluated programs focused on teaching children vigilance either directly or indirectly through parent or teacher involvement because these are representative of the types of programs being implemented nationwide. We will not conclude, as Melton (in press) has, that the prevention of child sexual abuse is impossible, or as Finkelhor and Strapko (in press) have, that "the overwhelming and irrefutable message of the evaluation studies is that children do indeed learn the concepts that they are being taught." Rather, we will conclude that caution is warranted regarding both of these positions. We will also suggest that the reporting of sexual abuse is a complex act for the child that requires cognitive and emotional maturity and understanding that many young children may not possess.

Let us begin with a vignette from the recent evaluation of a preventive intervention.

> At the conclusion of a standard interview evaluating the use of the special *Spiderman* comic about the prevention of sexual abuse, a fourth grade boy said, "This is just what happened to me." And he proceeded to tell of being sexually molested by a teenage neighbor over a period of a year and a half starting when he was in the second grade. He was silent over that period to protect his mother from the harm the neighbor threatened to inflict upon her if he told. The boy concluded, "He said he would put soap suds in her eyes and put her in the washing machine and

he has a black belt in karate and he said he would get her." Finally the boy was asked if having had the *Spiderman* (1984) comic at the time would have made a difference. 'Yes," he replied, "I would have told my mom about it. I wouldn't have been so afraid. I would have known that it was right to tell." (Garbarino, 1987, p. 148)

THE COMPLEXITY OF SEXUAL ABUSE PREVENTION

The process that a child must go through either to repel an abusive approach or to report an occurrence of abuse is very complex. This complexity appears not to be appreciated by many of those involved in the prevention programs currently in existence, which seem to be based on the idea that children can be taught a few facts during a one- or two- shot presentation and that the children will then both understand the issues and be able to protect themselves. The extent to which the level of a child's cognitive and emotional development will affect the ways in which he or she can be self-protective often seems neglected.

Latane and Darley's (1969) paradigm for understanding the process that an individual goes through when deciding whether to react in an emergency situation can be adapted to delineate the steps that a child must go through in order to repel or report abuse. First, the child must recognize that he or she is in an abusive situation. Then the child must believe that he or she can and should take some sort of action. Finally, the child must possess and use specific self-protective skills. Each of these issues must be addressed if a child's self-protective skills are to be enhanced. For instance, a prevention program that does not provide age-appropriate, concrete instructions for how to act in an abusive situation, or a program that gives good instruction on how to act but does not help the child identify abusive situations in an age-appropriate fashion, may be of little value to the child.

Programs must first inform a child about what sexual abuse is. However, there is a lack of firm agreement as to what constitutes an abusive act (Atteberry-Bennett, 1987; Finkelhor & Associates, 1986; Haugaard & Reppucci, 1988). Although most adults can agree that certain acts always entail sexual abuse (e.g., a parent having intercourse with a child), there is considerable disagreement about other acts (e.g., whether a 10-year-old boy is experiencing sexual abuse from his mother who cleans his genitals thoroughly each night when she gives him a bath, or whether a 10-year-old girl is experiencing sexual abuse from her father when he kisses her on the lips each morning when he goes to work; Atteberry-Bennett, 1987). If children are given a broad definition of sexual abuse that they should report, many nonabusive incidents may be reported which may cause anger and suffering to those who are reported (Schultz, 1988) and may be frustrating and confusing to the children doing the reporting. If a narrow definition is provided, then acts that are abusive may go unreported. Yet, if definitions are vague, many children, especially younger children, may have no idea what is expected of them. Several prevention programs have dealt with the definitional issue of what sexual abuse is by trying to teach the concept of touches that feel good, bad, and confusing. Learning these concepts may be possible for older children, but younger children are very poor at making fine distinctions between abstract entities, for example, between good and confusing touches (Daro, 1988).

If a child is able to label a certain experience as sexual abuse, then the child must feel empowered to report or repel it. Many programs attempt to empower children by teaching them that they do not have to allow other people to touch them (under most circumstances) and that they have the right to say "no" to anyone who tries to touch them in ways that they do not want to be touched. However, children at different cognitive levels often find it more or less difficult to distinguish between times when an action should or should not be taken. Young children are much better at following broad and general rules (e.g., do not ever cross the street without a parent) than they are at following rules that require making distinctions (e.g., you can cross this street without a parent, but not this other street, and this third street can only be crossed during the daytime without a parent). We know very little about the ways that children react to such rules as "Doctors can touch you in your private parts, and your parents can touch you if they are helping you clean yourself or if you are hurt there, but no one, not even your parents, can touch you there at other times." Such rules may be incomprehensible to many children, who may simplify them so that anyone who is caring for them can touch them in certain places or that no one can touch them or make them do anything they do not want to do.

If a child comprehends that a certain act is sexual abuse and knows that he or she can and should stop it or tell someone about it, the child must have a plan for doing so. Many prevention programs teach that the child should tell a parent or other adult and keep telling adults until someone believes him or her. Although this may be a good general approach, it is questionable whether it gives the child enough information to plan and implement the reporting or repelling. Many adults have been in situations in which they know that something should be done, but without a specific plan, they chose to do nothing rather than to engage in a wrong or ineffective action. Why do we think that children, who are not as cognitively or emotionally competent as adults on most tasks (Weithorn, 1984), will be able to engage in these complex behaviors in an emotionally delicate and sometimes frightening situation?

Clearly, the process of self-protective behaviors that is being taught in prevention programs must be recognized for its complexity. Keeping this complexity in mind, we now turn to an examination of extant programs.

PROGRAMS FOR SCHOOL CHILDREN

Most of the programs to prevent child sexual abuse have been designed for use with elementary school children, although a few are for preschoolers or students in junior or senior high school. The programs tend to emphasize two goals: (a) primary prevention (keeping the abuse from ever occurring) and (b) although often mislabeled as secondary prevention, detection (encouraging disclosure of past and ongoing sexual abuse so that children can receive intervention and protection). Five years ago, Plummer (1984) suggested that nearly 500,000 children had been reached nationally by preventive education programs in schools alone. Since that time the numbers of children exposed to such programs have increased by quantum leaps.

Programs for children are generally concerned with the following themes: educating children about what sexual abuse is; broadening their awareness of the identity of possible abusers to include people they know and like; teaching that each child has the right to control the access of others to his or her body; describing a variety of "touches" that a child can experience—which are good, bad, or confusing; stressing action steps that the child can take in a potentially abusive situation, such as saying "no" to adults or leaving or running away; teaching that some secrets should not be kept and that a child is never at fault for sexual abuse; and stressing that the child should tell a trusted adult if touched in an inappropriate manner and should keep telling someone until something is done to protect the child (Conte, Rosen, & Saperstein, 1984; Finkelhor, 1986; Hazzard, Webb, & Kleemeier, 1988).

Finkelhor (1986) noted that there has been a general effort to skirt the emotionally charged topic of sexuality and sex education in prevention programs. Therefore, child sexual abuse prevention is usually approached through a protective, rather than sexual, standpoint. The concepts of good and bad touching are often approached through discussions of bullies and relatives who forcefully try to kiss a child. More intimate or long-term types of sexual abuse tend to be ignored as are specific discussions of molestation by parents. Also generally missing is the information that some "bad" touches can actually feel good. The presentations are entertaining, with occasional injections of humor. These tactics are used to increase the number of schools willing to accept prevention programs by avoiding controversy and to keep the presentations from overly frightening the children. Unfortunately, by avoiding sexuality, young children may learn that "sexuality is essentially secretive, negative, and even dangerous" (Trudell & Whatley, 1988, p. 108).

Prevention programs vary in a number of ways. Some involve only one presentation (Conte, Rosen, & Saperstein, 1984), whereas others involve as many as 38 short sessions (Committee for Children, 1983). Shorter programs generally deal with only the topic of sexual abuse prevention, whereas longer programs present a number of topics, the general theme of which is the child's right to be assertive with others in certain situations. Programs aimed at primary prevention may require more sessions than those whose major goal is case identification because some abused children will identify themselves after even brief prevention efforts (e.g., several children in Seattle identified themselves after viewing a 30-second public service announcement on television). Also, the skills and concepts for primary prevention are usually taught in the abstract and are frequently more difficult for children to grasp because they have no concrete reference point (Conte, Rosen, & Saperstein, 1984).

Prevention programs come in many formats, including slide presentations, movies, plays, discussions, and role-play situations, as well as various types of printed material such as pamphlets or comic books. Most prevention educators recommend the use of high-interest, nonthreatening formats, such as plays and puppet shows that are often the most expensive to mount (Koblinsky & Behana, 1984).

The presenters of the programs also vary (Conte, Rosen, & Saperstein, 1984). The rationale for using particular presenters includes their familiarity with the children (e.g., teachers), their expertise in the topic (e.g., specially trained volunteers or mental health professionals), or their positions in the community as authority figures who have the children's respect (e.g., police officers). Most programs take place through the schools and attempt to make use of teachers because of their ongoing contact with the children, their possible ability to deal with a sensitive topic in the best way for their class, and their role in identifying and supporting abused children. In addition, for those programs that provide follow-up discussions with the children in small groups, teachers are potentially ideal discussion leaders. However, often there is little preparation of teachers for these roles (Trudell & Whatley, 1988).

Type and length of program format and the identity of the presenter are usually determined by the resources and predilections of whatever group is most involved in bringing the program to a community. Such groups are most often composed of community members who have become part of a task force on sexual abuse or are organized by such individuals as the health coordinator of a school district. Unfortunately, there has not been any evaluation comparing the effectiveness of format, length, or presenter, either overall or for different age children.

Preventive interventions for school children have much appeal because of their potential both to reach large numbers of children in a relatively cost-efficient fashion and to reduce the number of children affected by sexual abuse. However, having positive goals is not enough. Effectiveness of intervention is critical. Yet most programs appear to continue on the strength of their positive goals rather than on a systematic evaluation of their effectiveness.

PROGRAMS FOR PARENTS AND OTHER ADULTS

Finkelhor (1986) stressed the value of prevention programs aimed at parents and professionals involved with children. Prevention programs aimed at parents, professionals involved with children, and adults in general are potentially very valuable. These programs may help parents both to identify signs indicating that their child was or is being abused and to react in a constructive manner if abuse is discovered. If parents can be encouraged to educate their children about abuse prevention, then the children may be more likely to receive repeated exposures of information from a trusted source. Moreover, a discussion about sexual abuse with a parent may make it easier for a child to talk with the parent if the child is subsequently abused. The importance of helping parents talk to their children about sexual abuse was highlighted by Finkelhor's (1984) findings. Only 29% of his random sample of 521 parents of 6- to 14-year-old children had talked with them about sexual abuse; of those parents, only 53% had mentioned that the abuser might be someone whom the child knew, and only 22% had ever suggested that a family member might be involved. In other words, only 6% of the total sample had ever suggested that a family member might be an abuser.

In spite of the possible advantages of parent education, relatively few efforts have been made to involve parents. One reason for this may be that many parents have a difficult time talking to their children about sexual topics of all sorts. In addition, Finkelhor's (1984) survey found that most parents tend to think of their own children as well supervised and able to avoid danger and that they do not want to frighten their children unnecessarily. Moreover, parents who are likely to attend such educational programs may be better informed and more likely to discuss these issues with their children anyway. For example, in the only evaluation of a parent workshop program, Porch and Petretic-Jackson (1986) found that 57% of the parents who completed pre-and postworkshop questionnaires had discussed sexual abuse with their children before the workshop took place, a percentage double that found in Finkelhor's (1984) random sample. For prevention programs to reach a broad cross-section of parents, educators may need to devise more innovative means for delivering their programs, such as providing them through places of employment or community service clubs, such as Kiwanis and Rotary. Such innovations would also have the potential advantage of reaching a greater number of men, the major perpetrators of child sexual abuse. These men might be discouraged from becoming abusers if they believed that children are more likely to tell someone of an approach (Finkelhor, 1986).

Prevention programs aimed at teachers, pediatricians, day care workers, clergy, and the police could provide information allowing these professionals to detect sexual abuse in a child more effectively and to react in a constructive manner. Although such programs exist, only three evaluations have been reported. Nevertheless, their results are encouraging. Hazzard (1984) found that elementary school teachers who participated in a six-hour training program about prevention of child abuse in general, in comparison with a control group of untrained teachers, increased significantly in knowledge about child abuse, were more likely to report talking with individual students to assess whether abuse was occurring, and discussed possible abuse situations with colleagues more often. However, they were no more likely to report cases to protective services. In a second study specifically focused on the prevention of child sexual abuse, Kleemier, Webb, Hazzard, and Pohl (1987) reported that elementary school teachers who participated in a six-hour workshop, relative to nonparticipating controls, increased in knowledge about child sexual abuse and were better able to identify behavioral indicators of abuse and to suggest appropriate interventions. Over a six-week follow-up period, they also read more about child abuse than control teachers; however, the two groups did not differ on reporting of suspected cases. In contrast, Swift (1983) found that reporting rates from 71 trained school counselors and nurses increased 500% from 10 cases during the 12-month pre-training period to 50 cases during the 12-month post-training period. Unfortunately, Swift did not distinguish the percentage of unfounded reports contained in the increased reporting rates. If there was not an increase in founded reports, was the increased reporting a benefit? Some would answer in the affirmative because such reporting may influence abusers for whom the accusations could not be founded to cease and desist. Others (such as Goldstein, Freud, & Solnit, 1979) would argue that more harm than good could be the result and that family privacy rights may have been invaded inappropriately.

OUTCOME RESEARCH FOR DAY-CARE AND SCHOOL-BASED PREVENTION PROGRAMS

Several school-based prevention programs have investigated the effectiveness with which the children learned the material presented. Before beginning the discussion, we emphasize that the investigations mentioned, regardless of their shortcomings, should be commended because they are among the very few programs that have any evaluation component at all.

Conte, Rosen, Saperstein, and Shermack (1985) evaluated a program consisting of three, one-hour presentations given by specially trained deputy sheriffs at a private day-care center. The participant group consisted of 10 four- and five-year olds, and 10 six- to ten-year olds, with a similarly composed wait-list control group. One week before the presentation and at some unspecified time after the program, each child was interviewed by a social work graduate student, most of whom were unaware of the child's group. At the postpresentation interview, children in the participating group had significantly increased their knowledge about the concepts and skills that the authors believed would help them avoid becoming victims of child sexual abuse. The older children made a larger gain than the younger children. However, although the children's knowledge increased significantly, the average number of correct responses was only 50% for the participating group on the posttest (as contrasted to 25% on the pretest).

The program presentations by the sheriffs were tape-recorded and compared with the model by which they had been trained. Analysis indicated that assault by a stranger was stressed more than had been intended and that several presenters told "horror stories" to illustrate their points even though these were not included in the training model. This information indicates the importance of ongoing monitoring to ensure that the presenter's beliefs do not unduly modify the planned presentation by altering its strength and integrity (Reppucci, 1985; Sechrest, White, & Brown, 1979).

Borkin and Frank (1986) evaluated the retention of basic information about what to do when somebody touches you in a "not okay" way with a preschool sample. The 83 three- to five-year-old children who responded had all seen an adaptation of the play *Bubbylonian Encounter* enacted by hand puppets six weeks earlier. Children were asked. "What should you do if someone tries to touch you in a way that doesn't feel good?," and answers of "say no," "run away," or "tell someone" were scored as correct. Although 43% of the four-and five-year-olds answered correctly, only one three-year-old (4%) did. Moreover, because no pretesting was done, there is no way to determine what percentage of the four- and five-year-olds would have answered correctly without ever seeing the play. These results raise the question of whether a one-time presentation is useful for teaching concepts to such young children, even when done in an interesting way.

In the most extensive study to date of the impact of sexual abuse prevention programs on preschool children, the Berkeley Family Welfare Research Group (Daro, 1988; Daro, Duerr, & LeProhn, 1987) evaluated seven representative curricula (Child Assault Prevention; Children's Self-Help; Talking About Touching; Touch Safety; Child Abuse Prevention, Intervention and Education; Youth Safety Awareness Project; and SAFE—Stop Abuse through Family Education) that ranged in duration from a one-time 15-to-30 minute session to 21 15- to 20-minute sessions over a three- to six-week period. Parents meetings of one to two hours' duration were a part of each curriculum, which apparently contributed to encouraging two thirds of the parents to discuss some of the concepts with their children following the presentation. Although a detailed reporting of this investigation is beyond the scope of this article, a few findings are worth noting. Children were more likely to interpret pictures of frequently encountered interactions such as tickling and bathing as evoking a negative affect after participation in prevention training, a result that can hardly be interpreted as positive. It appears that preschoolers were unable to comprehend the concept of a mixed-up or confusing touch. Although some of the children appeared to have a rudimentary grasp of the concept that there is a connection between the physical act of being touched and the emotion that it generates, even at posttest half the children could not provide an explanation for why they selected a particular affect in response to the pictures they were shown. Given the critical nature of this connection as a building block for the prevention programs, Daro (1988) asked, "If the children cannot explain their own response, is it possibly too much to expect that they can understand the subtle nuances and emotions described and elicited either during the prevention program or in a case of actual abuse?" In addition, children found it difficult to distinguish how touches can change or how feelings regarding touches can change. They also found the concept of differentiating between types of secrets difficult to comprehend or to accept. Even the issue of "stranger danger," one of the least ambiguous ideas presented was not internalized well enough by many children so that they could apply these teachings. In summary, this investigation clearly raises questions regarding the developmental readiness of preschoolers to grasp the concepts being taught in prevention programs in any meaningful way. Furthermore, the other two studies with preschool children also indicated that important gaps in the children's knowledge remained even after the prevention programs were presented.

Plummer (1984) evaluated a preventive program that consisted of three one-hour presentations to 112 fifth-grade students. Sixty-nine children completed pre- and posttest 23-item questionnaires that dealt with the concepts of the program. Posttest measures were given immediately after the program and two and eight months later. More students gave correct answers at the posttest immediately following the program than on the pretest. Although a majority of the concepts were still retained at the eight-month follow-up, questions about breaking promises, whether molesters were often people whom the child knew, and who was to blame if the child was touched in a sexual way were answered incorrectly significantly more often. What is particularly disturbing about the lowering of knowledge on these three items is that they are crucial concepts in any prevention program.

Ray and Dietzel (1984) evaluated a program that consisted of a slide presentation, a movie, and the distribution of a workbook that the students were encouraged to take home and discuss with their parents. One hundred ninety-one third-grade participants answered a 12-item questionnaire covering the concepts taught in the program. Half of the students saw a follow-up film two weeks after the initial presentation, which reinforced the concepts that were taught initially. Some of the students were pretested, some were posttested immediately following the presentation, and all were posttested at one and six months following the presentation.

As a group, the students answered more questions correctly on the posttest immediately after the program than on the pretest, and those students who received the follow-up movie presentation had significantly higher scores on the one-month and six-month posttests, again indicating the importance of review sessions. These findings, when combined with those of Plummer (1984), suggest that some sort of review work after the initial presentation may be an essential component for increasing retention of the material. They also indicate that prevention researchers should employ follow-up procedures to determine durability of effects.

Another noteworthy aspect of the Ray and Dietzel (1984) study was that the average number correct on the pretest was about 9 out of the 12 questions, indicating that the students already knew many of the program's concepts before it took place. Thus, although the average correct response of 11.5 on the posttest was a statistically significant increase from the pretest, it is unclear whether this small rise in absolute terms indicates a meaningful increase in knowledge. On the other hand, the children may have learned more than was revealed because of a possible ceiling effect on this limited-item questionnaire (for further discussion of this issue, see Conte, 1984; Hazzard & Angert, 1986; Kleemeier & Webb, 1986).

Only a few investigations have used a nontreatment control group. Wolfe, MacPherson, Blount, and Wolfe (1986) found that fourth- and fifth-grade children who participated in a single presentation of two five-minute skits followed by a one-hour classroom discussion showed a higher percentage of knowledge of correct actions to take in an abusive situation than a group of nonparticipating children. However, even though the differences were statistically significant, the actual percentages of children in the participating group answering each question correctly was never more than 10% higher than those in the control group.

Saslawsky and Wurtele's (1986) evaluation of the film *Touch* also used a nontreatment control group and found significant differences favoring the participating group. Again, although significant statistically, the differences between the control and participating groups were less than 2 points on both a 13-point Personal Safety Questionnaire and a 32-point scoring scale for four vignettes. It should be noted that this study did find that the gains were maintained at a three-month follow-up assessment and that these investigators were the first to report the psychometric properties of their measuring instruments, a major methodological improvement over other studies.

Swan, Press, and Briggs (1985) evaluated the effectiveness of a 30-minute presentation of the play *Bubbylonian Encounter* with a group of 63 second- through fifth-grade students. Before and soon after the play, the children were shown five videotaped vignettes depicting inappropriate and appropriate touch and were asked to identify which type of touch was in each vignette. No significant improvement was found on the posttest because of very high accuracy on the pretest for which 92% of the children correctly identified the vignettes showing sexual abuse.

Thus, the investigations by Ray and Dietzel (1984), Wolfe et al. (1986), Saslawsky and Wurtele (1986), and Swan et al. (1985) raise important cost-benefit questions. These studies present data indicating that many children had a high degree of knowledge about the concepts being taught even before the prevention programs were started and that any post-program increases, although statistically significant, were quite small in absolute terms. Given these results, the cost-benefit issue involves whether the changes in knowledge about actions to take in a hypothetical abusive situation justify the expense, time away from class, and possible negative consequences of the prevention program.

The investigation by Swan et al. (1985) is one of four that evaluated the play for possible negative effects. These investigators telephoned a separate sample of parents whose children had also seen the play within a week of the play's presentation and asked if they noticed any adverse reactions to the play in the children, such as loss of sleep or appetite, nightmares, or expression of fear, and if their children had discussed the play with them at home. Only 7% of the children had said that they did not like the play, and only 5% of the parents said that their child had shown any adverse reactions; 42% of the children had discussed the play at home.

Wurtele and Miller-Perrin (1987) asked both parents and children to fill out questionnaires measuring their fear levels before and after a prevention program. Parents also assessed frequency and severity of particular behavior problems thought to be related to program participation. No significant change in negative behaviors was found, although this may have been a function of the small sample size ($N = 25$).

In a third study that examined possible negative effects, Garbarino (1987) evaluated the impact of the widely distributed special edition of the *Spiderman* comic book that contains two stories dealing with sexual abuse. Graduate students interviewed 36 boys and 37 girls in the second, fourth, and sixth grades who had read the comic in school. More than 80% of the questions dealing with sexual abuse were answered correctly by all age groups. The children were asked how the comic made them feel in terms of arousing worry or fear. Girls in the second and sixth grades reported feeling worried or scared more than their male counterparts (35% vs. 17% in second grade and 30% vs. 17% in sixth grade). Among fourth graders, 50% of both boys and girls reported these feelings. The children were concerned that "it" might happen to them. At first glance, this result might appear to be a negative side effect; certainly Garbarino interpreted it this way. However, it could also be interpreted as positive in that the comic book may have made an impression on the children that they are less likely to forget. As with fairy tales, the most enduring have frequently been those that have been somewhat disturbing to their young audience in the process of warning them about some harmful event that could happen.

Finally, Hazzard, Webb, and Kleemeier (1988) compared the responses of 286 third and fourth grade students from four schools who participated in a three-session adaptation of the *Feeling Yes, Feeling No* curriculum with those of 113 delayed-intervention control children from two other schools, who were matched for ethnic composition and achievement level. All children were assessed before, immediately after, and six weeks after the intervention on a knowledge questionnaire. The major finding was that participating children exhibited significantly greater knowledge on the posttestings than the control group, although they showed no differences on the pretesting. In addition, parents were asked several questions about the intervention's impact on their children. Although most comments were positive, 13% of the parents noted that their children had been "more fearful of strangers," whereas less than 5% noted other negative effects, such as nightmares, fear of men, reluctance to go to school, disobedience, sleeping problems, bedwetting, and changed reactions to physical affection.

These four studies indicate that even though a sizable number of children may express some worry after a prevention program, only a small percentage of school-age children show some clear negative responses to participation. Unfortunately, we do not know whether such a small percentage change in negative behaviors would be typical in any group of children over a several-week period because no control groups were used. Recall, however, that Daro (1988) found that preschool children were more likely to interpret pictures of tickling and bathing as evoking a negative affect after participation in a prevention program. These results raise the possibility that different or more numerous negative consequences may appear in children of various ages.

The Hazzard et al. (1988) study deserves further note because it is the first report to provide evidence of substantial detection of children who revealed abuse experiences after participating in a prevention program. Eight children reported ongoing sexual abuse, and 20 others reported past occurrences. Although this result was a significant step beyond the often reported individual case of detection, the authors did not provide a definition of these disclosures nor of how many turned out to be founded cases. Given that these findings appear to be extraordinarily important, it is disappointing that Hazzard et al. concluded with the vague statement that "although follow-up information was not available on all disclosures, we were not made aware of any disclosures which were subsequently felt to be false allegations by school personnel or Protective Services" (p. 19).

A Related Study

Although they did not use sexual abuse prevention program per se, Fryer, Kraizer, and Miyoshi (1987a), 1987b) used role-play techniques to reduce susceptibility to stranger abduction. In a program consisting of eight daily 20-minute sessions, children were taught four concrete rules to follow when they were approached by a stranger and were not with a caretaking adult. Twenty-three kindergarten, first-, and second-grade students participated in the program initially and formed the experimental group, and 21 nonparticipating children from the same grades formed the control group and were given the program later. The day before and after the program, each child was sent on an errand by his or her teacher and met one of the researchers (a male stranger) who asked the child to accompany him to his car to help him carry something into the school (the in vivo abduction situation). (It should be emphasized that the researchers went to extraordinary lengths before, during, and after the program to inform parents and to protect children from any anxiety associated with meeting the stranger.)

Pretest results showed that about half of the children in each group agreed to accompany the stranger. Posttest results showed that only 22% of the participating group agreed to go and that there was no change in the control group. Six months later, participating children who had failed the posttest (four children) and the children in the control group were given the training program. Children from all groups were then subjected to a similar in vivo abduction situation. All of the participating children who had passed the original posttest, all of the control children, and two of the four "retrained" children resisted the abduction situation. The authors concluded that the testing showed that the children had developed the ability to avoid stranger abduction of the type used.

Several components that led to the success of this program may be important for developing and testing sexual abuse prevention programs. First, this program taught specific concrete rules and steps to follow. These might be easier for young children to comprehend than the less concrete "good touch/bad touch" idea (with some bad touches actually feeling good). Second, the program used active role-taking techniques rather than puppet shows or other passive learning techniques employed by most child sexual abuse prevention programs. Wurtele, Marrs, and Miller-Perrin (1987) recently provided more evidence that kindergarten children who were taught self-protective skills through modeling and active rehearsal learned them better than those in a control group who were taught the same skills by passively watching an experimenter model them. Third, the pretesting and posttesting may have served to "set up" and then reinforce the skills taught by the program. It is interesting to note that none of the control students, each of whom had been approached by a stranger two times before the program, agreed to accompany the stranger after the program. Perhaps these children were able to reflect on their own experience when taught the skills, thereby increasing their retention of them. Fourth, a few children were less able to learn the skills, and this highlights the need to assess which children may need more instruction for prevention programs to be meaningful for them. Finally, the authors showed that it is possible to provide a meaningful behavioral assessment of the effectiveness of the program. Such assessments represent the best means of estimating the strength of the behaviors being taught and should be pursued whenever appropriate.

Summary

These evaluations as a whole provide some limited support for the efficacy of sexual abuse prevention programs. The most common finding was a statistically significant, yet often slight, increase in knowledge about sexual abuse following a prevention program. The major area of knowledge gain seemed to be about the fact that family members or friends could engage in abusive activities; however, this was also the area in which the most loss of knowledge occurred on some follow-up measures. The instruments that were used to measure change often seemed to have a ceiling effect in that most children answered a high percentage of the questions accurately even before they participated in the program. Thus, it may be that the children learned more than the tests measured or that children know more of the basic concepts than the prevention educators think they do. If it is the former, better assessment instruments are needed; if the latter, the value of the programs may be questionable.

In the few studies that examined differences between older and younger children, the younger children, not surprisingly, learned significantly less. The results raise questions as to whether these programs are useful for preschool children, or whether programs that are useful for school-age children are appropriate for younger children. Review sessions seemed to increase retention of knowledge for all but the youngest age groups. In fact, without such sessions, durability of learning seems so weak that it is questionable whether there is any long-term value to prevention programs, particularly those involving only one presentation, even if there are immediate knowledge gains. The one exception to this was the Fryer et al. (1987a, 1987b) role-playing program to increase self-protective behaviors.

Most of the evaluations had basic design problems. Although a few studies did use nontreatment control groups, most did not; therefore, there is no way to indicate whether the programs were responsible for any changes that might have occurred. Other flaws included small samples, interviewers who were not unaware of the assignment of groups, lack of attention to the psychometric properties of the measuring instruments, and the lack of pretesting to establish a baseline of knowledge.

Finally, even though no investigator discussed the issue, the question of cost-benefit analysis needs to be raised. Although these programs appear to have a great deal of face validity, in general, the results are meager. More attention must be paid to the effectiveness of different types of programs for children of different ages and the relative impact of each in conjunction with their costs, both in terms of financial resources of communities and of the possible negative consequences to the participants. More sophisticated research designs are necessary before we can make any claims regarding the overall positive impact of these interventions (see also, Wurtele, 1987).

UNTESTED ASSUMPTIONS

Most prevention programs have developed from a foundation of anecdotal clinical information (Conte, 1984) and therefore are based on several untested assumptions (Reppucci, 1987). One of these assumptions is that we know what types of skills will make a child less susceptible to sexual abuse. However, research into the incidence of child sexual abuse clearly shows that sexual abuse comes in many different forms (Haugaard & Reppucci, 1988). It may be that skills useful for preventing one type of abuse might not be useful for preventing another very different type, or that some skills may be useful for children of one age but not for children of another. Clarity as to the specific skills and behaviors that prevention programs should teach is needed in order to allow researchers to develop means of measuring their acquisition. This clarity should be based on assessing what actually happens in abusive situations and the techniques that abusers use to engage their victims. However, in vivo assessment situations are very difficult to construct because of various ethical problems, not the least of which is that subjecting children to sexual abuse situations in order to assess what prevention behaviors they exhibit is not acceptable.

Another assumption is that children will be able to transfer the knowledge gained from prevention programs into effective action when needed. Prevention programs are powered by the ideas that increasing children's knowledge about abuse, providing them with action alternatives such as giving them permission to say no and get help, and bringing the dangers of abuse to their attention may be important in preventing sexual victimization, but there is no evidence to demonstrate that these ideas actually prevent abuse. In fact, Downer (1984) found that although 94% of the children in her study could define assertiveness after prevention training, only 47% could provide an example of an assertive response to an abusive situation. Furthermore, even if her children had been able to reply with an effective response, there is no evidence that in a real abusive situation they would have responded appropriately. As noted previously, most individuals, including adults, are aware of situations in which they acted quite differently from the way they knew they should act.

A third assumption is that there are no negative effects of the prevention programs or at least that the negative effects are insignificant when compared with the positive effects. It is not known whether programs about the incorrectness of some forms of touching will adversely affect the children in a number of ways, including their comfort with nonsexual physical contact between them and their parents and others and with exploratory sexual play between them and other children. Although Swan et al. (1985) and Hazzard et al. (1988) did ask parents about negative consequences seen in their children, the behaviors that they asked the parents to recall would indicate extreme and immediate negative effects. Garbarino (1987) also found that a sizable percentage of his sample did express worry and fearfulness after reading the *Spiderman* comic book. Daro's (1988) finding of increased negative affect by preschoolers to scenes of bathing and tickling also may be cause for concern. In addition, anecdotal evidence suggests that at least some children have temporary negative reactions. Conte (1984) reported that some preschool children have been afraid to ride home from school with anyone but their parents. The following vignette provides another example.

A first grade child interpreted the message that she had the right to say "no" as generalizing to all realms of behavior. For several weeks following the prevention program she frequently told her parents that she had the right to say "no" to any requests that she did not like or made her feel uncomfortable. The parents reported much anguish and frustration on their part about this behavior and about the fact that they had to punish her in order to convince her that she did not have the right to disobey them whenever she wanted to.

Neither the anecdotes nor the evaluation studies measured or provided insight into any long-term or subtle effects. Although it may be unlikely that most children are adversely affected in any way, the risk of possible negative consequences, such as increased fearfulness or disruption of children's understanding of their world, warrants their investigation.

The crux of the matter is whether any of the programs have actually achieved either of their major goals—primary prevention or detection. There is no evidence, not even one published case example, that primary prevention has ever been achieved. Often it is assumed that these programs work because well-meaning professionals and parents believe that they do. For example, Swan et al. (1985) found that over 99% of a sample of 225 parents and professionals rated the play *Bubbylonian Encounter* as a helpful tool in teaching prevention concepts, but then these investigators inappropriately concluded on the basis of these endorsements that the play "can be effective in teaching children sexual abuse prevention concepts" (p. 404). Finkelhor (1986) has also suggested that these programs may achieve primary prevention by acting as a deterrent to potential abusers who may be less likely to engage in abusive behaviors because of fear of detection. Unfortunately, no evidence exists regarding the deterrent effect of these programs. Moreover, if primary prevention is the major goal, then it may be more productive to develop prevention programs that are specifically geared to helping parents and other adults restrain from engaging in abusive sexual behaviors.

In contrast, there are some reported instances of successful detection (e.g., Finkelhor & Strapko, in press; Hazzard et al., 1988) in that individual cases of ongoing or past abuse have been discovered as a result of the interventions. In fact, Finkelhor and Strapko (in press), although they presented no data, argued that the "most important unambiguous finding" is that "prevention education encourages children to report abuse they have already suffered." However, they also point out that "researchers have not studied systematically the percentage of children who disclose the types of disclosures they make, or how these disclosures vary according to type of program, age of children or type of school context." Furthermore, no information exists on the impact of the disclosure on the child and his or her family.

We began this article with a case vignette from Garbarino's (1987) assessment of the *Spiderman* comic book intervention that uncovered a case of child sexual abuse. Such cases are often cited as justifying preventive interventions. On some sort of ethical balancing scale, the judgment that must be made is whether the possible uncovering of a small number of cases of abuse compensates for the seemingly minor negative consequences that have now been documented for up to 50% of the participants (Garbarino, 1987). Are these consequences a small price to pay in order to uncover and alleviate the possible severe abuse of a few as documented by case examples?

CONCLUSION

Without more definitive information about these untested assumptions and more thorough evaluations of ongoing prevention programs, we cannot be sure whether preventive programs are working, nor can we be sure that they are causing more good than harm. This harm may come in two forms. As mentioned, the programs may adversely affect a child's positive relationships with meaningful people in his or her life or cause the child undue worry or fear at least in the short run. However, it may also be that these programs can actually place some children at a greater risk for sexual abuse if we incorrectly assume that the children are protected because of these programs and consequently become less vigilant about the problem (Wald & Cohen, 1986). The fear is that parents, teachers, and others who work with children will abdicate their responsibility to protect to the abuse prevention programs. The complexity of the process that a child must go through to repel or report abuse, the variety of abusive situations that a child may encounter, and the short duration of most prevention programs virtually ensure that a child cannot be assumed to be protected simply because of participation in a program. Adults must be encouraged to continue and to increase their protective efforts rather than be reassured that children are learning to be self-protective.

Extensive investigations of the full range of effects of prevention programs must be undertaken. We cannot continue to assume that they accomplish their goals. Because the safety of children is the goal of these programs, we need to know much more about which ones work to teach which skills to which children. We must engage in more basic research with a goal of understanding the process that a child must go through in order to repel or report abuse and to determine how this process differs for children at various levels of cognitive and emotional development.

We have raised several questions about extant prevention programs, not to stop such efforts, but to encourage those involved to begin to ascertain by means of systematic evaluation whether they are really helping children. Without these evaluations, we risk developing programs that make adults feel better but do not protect children. Unless the usefulness of sexual abuse prevention programs can be demonstrated, the reality is that the prevention of child sexual abuse may indeed be only a myth.

REFERENCES

Atteberry-Bennett, J. (1987). *Child sexual abuse: Definitions and interventions of parents and professionals.* Unpublished doctoral dissertation. University of Virginia, Institute of Clinical Psychology, Charlottesville.

Borkin, J., & Frank, L. (1986). Sexual abuse prevention for preschoolers: A pilot program. *Child Welfare, 6*, 75–83.

Committee for Children. (1983). *Talking about touching: A personal safety curriculum.* (Available from the Committee for Children, P.O. Box 15190, Seattle, WA 98115)

Conte, J. R. (1984, August). *Research on the prevention of sexual abuse of children.* Paper presented at the Second National Conference for Family Violence Researchers, Durham, NH.

Conte, J. R., Rosen, C., & Saperstein, L. (1984, September). *An analysis of programs to prevent the sexual victimization of children.* Paper presented at the Fifth International Congress on Child Abuse and Neglect, Montreal, Canada.

Conte, J. R., Rosen, C., Saperstein, L., & Shermack, R. (1985). An evaluation of a program to prevent the sexual victimization of young children. *Child Abuse and Neglect, 9,* 319–328.

Daro, D. (1988). *Prevention programs: What do children learn.* Unpublished manuscript, University of California, Berkeley School of Social Welfare, Berkeley.

Daro, D., Duerr, J., & LeProhn, N. (1987, July). *Child assault prevention instruction: What works with preschoolers.* Paper presented at the Third National Family Violence Research Conference, University of New Hampshire, Durham.

Downer, A. (1984). *Development and testing of an evaluation instrument for assessing the effectiveness of a child sexual abuse prevention curriculum.* Unpublished master's thesis, University of Washington, Seattle.

Finkelhor, D. (1979). *Sexually victimized children.* New York: Free Press.

Finkelhor, D. (1984). *Child sexual abuse: New theory and research.* New York: Free Press.

Finkelhor, D. (1986). Prevention: A review of programs and research. In D. Finkelhor and Associates (Eds.), *A sourcebook on child sexual abuse* (pp. 224–254). Beverly Hills, CA: Sage.

Finkelhor, D., and Associates (Eds.). (1986). *A sourcebook on child sexual abuse.* Beverly Hills, CA: Sage.

Finkelhor, D., & Strapko, N. (in press). "Sexual abuse prevention education: A review of evaluation studies." In D. Willis, E. Holden, & M. Rosenberg (Eds), *Child abuse prevention.* New York: Wiley.

Fryer, G. E., Kraizer, S. K., & Miyoshi, T. (1987a). Measuring actual reduction of risk to child abuse: A new approach. *Child Abuse and Neglect, 11,* 173–179.

Fryer, G. E., Kraizer, S. K., & Miyoshi, T. (1987b). Measuring children's retention of skills to resist stranger abduction: Use of the simulation technique. *Child Abuse and Neglect, 11,* 181–185.

Garbarino, U. (1987). Children's response to a sexual abuse prevention program: A study of the *Spiderman* comic. *Child Abuse and Neglect, 11,* 143–148.

Goldstein, J., Freud, A., & Solnit, A. J. (1979). *Before the best interests of the child.* New York: Free Press.

Haugaard, J. J., & Reppucci, N. D. (1988). *The sexual abuse of children: A comprehensive guide to current knowledge and intervention strategies.* San Francisco: Jossey-Bass.

Hazzard, A. (1984). Training teachers to identify and intervene with abused children. *Journal of Clinical Child Psychology, 13,* 288–293.

Hazzard, A., & Angert, L. (1986, August). *Child sexual abuse prevention: Previous research and future directions.* Paper presented at the meeting of the American Psychological Association, Washington, DC.

Hazzard, A. P., Webb, C., & Kleemeier, C. (1988). *Child sexual assault prevention programs: Helpful or harmful?* Unpublished manuscript, Emory University School of Medicine, Atlanta, GA.

Kleemeier, C., & Webb, C. (1986, August). *Evaluation of a school-based prevention program.* Paper presented at the meeting of the American Psychological Association, Washington, DC.

Kleemeier, C., Webb, C., Hazzard, A., & Pohl, J. (1987), August). *Child sexual abuse prevention: Evaluation of a teacher training model.* Paper presented at the meeting of the American Psychological Association, New York City.

Koblinsky, S., & Behana, N. (1984). Child sexual abuse: The educator's role in prevention, detection, and intervention. *Young Children, 39,* 3–15.

Latane, B., & Darley, J. M. (1969). Bystander "apathy." *American Scientist, 57,* 244–268.

Melton, G. B. (in press). The improbability of prevention of sexual abuse. In D. J. Willis, E. W. Holden, & M. S. Rosenberg (Eds.), *Child abuse prevention.* New York: Wiley.

Plummer, C. (1984). *Preventing sexual abuse: What in-school programs teach children.* Unpublished manuscript.

Porch, T. L., & Petretic-Jackson, P. A. (1986, August). *Child sexual assault prevention: Evaluation of parent education workshops.* Paper presented at the meeting of the American Psychological Association, Washington, DC.

Ray, J., & Kietzel, M. (1984). *Teaching child sexual abuse prevention.* Unpublished manuscript.

Reppucci, N. D. (1985). Psychology in the public interest. In A. M. Rogers & C. J. Scheier (Eds.), *The G. Stanley Hall Lecture Series* (Vol 5, pp. 121–156). Washington, DC: American Psychological Association.

Reppucci, N. D. (1987). Prevention and ecology: Teen-age pregnancy, child sexual abuse, and organized youth sports. *American Journal of Community Psychology, 15,* 1-22.

Russell, D. E. H. (1984). *Sexual exploitation, rape, child sexual abuse, and work place harassment.* Beverly Hills, CA: Sage.

Saslawsky, D. A., & Wurtele, S. K. (1986). Educating children about sexual abuse: Implications for pediatric intervention and possible prevention. *Journal of Pediatric Psychology, 11,* 235–245.

Schultz, L. G. (1988). *One hundred cases of wrongfully charged child sexual abuse: A survey and recommendations.* Unpublished manuscript, West Virginia University, School of Social Work, Morgantown.

Sechrest, L., White, S. O., & Brown, E. (Eds.). (1979). *The rehabilitation of criminal offenders: Problems and prospects.* Washington, DC: National Academy of Sciences.

Spiderman and power pack. (1984). New York: Marvel Comics.

Stewart, S. A. (1988, March). Molestation trial's costs hit $7.5 M. *USA Today,* p. 3A.

Swan, H. L., Press, A. N., & Briggs, S. L. (1985). Child sexual abuse prevention: Does it work: *Child Welfare, 64,* 667-674.

Swift, C. (1983). *Consultation in the area of child sexual abuse* (NIMH Report 83–213). Washington, DC: National Institute of Mental Health.

Trudell, B., & Whatley, M. H. (1988). School sexual abuse prevention: Unintended consequences and dilemmas. *Child Abuse and Neglect, 12,* 103–113.

Wald, M. S., & Cohen, S. (1986). Preventing child abuse: What will it take? *Family Law Quarterly, 20,* 281–302.

Weithorn, L. A. (1984). Children's capacities in legal contexts. In N. D. Reppucci, L. A. Weithorn, E. P. Mulvey, & J. Monahan (Eds.), *Children, mental health, and the law* (pp. 25–55). Beverly Hills, CA: Sage.

Wolfe, D. A., MacPherson, T., Blount, R., & Wolfe, U. V. (1986). Evaluation of a brief intervention for educating school children in awareness of physical and sexual abuse. *Child Abuse and Neglect, 10,* 85–92.

Wurtele, S. K. (1987). School-based sexual abuse prevention programs: A review. *Child Abuse and Neglect, 11,* 483–495.

Wurtele, S. K., Marrs, S. R., & Miller-Perrin, C. L. 91987). Practice makes perfect? The role of participant modeling in sexual abuse prevention programs. *Journal of Consulting and Clinical Psychology, 55,* 599–602.

Wurtele, S. K., & Miller-Perrin, C. L. (1987). An evaluation of side effects associated with participation in a child sexual abuse prevention program. *Journal of School Health, 57,* 228–231.

Wyatt, G. E. (1985). The sexual abuse of Afro-American and White-American women in childhood. *Child Abuse and Neglect, 9,* 507–519.

31

Psychiatric Response to HIV Spectrum Disease in Children and Adolescents

Penelope Krener

University of California, Davis

Frank Black Miller

Duke University, Durham, North Carolina

Five clinical situations involving children and adolescents exposed to human immunodeficiency virus illustrate the psychosocial spectrum of the disease. For at-risk gay youth, anxiety and stigma complicate developing sexual practices. Children with perinatal infection may survive for years with a chronic illness, management of which is complicated by parental illness or death. Hemophiliac families must deal with the intrusion of a lethal virus into a long illness course. "Street" adolescents and substance-abusing youth pose particular challenges to public health and education. The range of child psychiatric responses described includes individual and family therapy, neuropsychological assessment, psychopharmacological management, and consultation liaison work. Key Words: HIV spectrum disease, pediatric AIDS, gay youth, vertical transmission.

Human immunodeficiency virus (HIV) infection in children and adolescents is currently a low-incidence, highly lethal disease. Its spread is related to the same risk events as in adults: sexual transmission, viral contamination of needles for intravenous drug use, blood products in medical settings, and vertical perinatal transmission to infants of infected mothers (Belfer et al., 1988). The pattern of prevalence and spread of the epidemic in the United States resembles a mosaic constructed of

Reprinted with permission from *Journal of American Academy of Child and Adolescent Psychiatry,* 1989, Vol. 28, No. 4, 596–605. Copyright © 1989 by the American Academy of Child and Adolescent Psychiatry.

Thanks are given to Elizabeth Harrison, M.D., for constructive criticisms on an earlier draft of this paper.

multiple mini-epidemics in the several population groups with different risk behaviors (Barbour, 1987; Carbine and Lee, 1988; Coffin et al., 1988; Flynn, 1988; Institute of Medicine, 1988; Krener, 1987; Parks and Scott, 1987; Perves et al., 1985; Report of Presidential Commission, 1988; Dept. of Health and Human Services [DHHS], 1986). The incubation time is long (Redfield et al, 1986; Rees, 1987) and the progression through initial stages of illness is slow (Redfield et al., 1986; Redfield and Burke, 1988). AIDS is known to be as medically devastating in child patients as in adults. The rate of spread in pediatric populations through known risk factors parallels the doubling time in adult risk groups; thus, although the prevalence is currently lower than in adult risk groups, the US Department of Health and Human Services predicts that by 1991 there will be 3000 cases of pediatric AIDS (Center for Disease Control [CDC], 1988c; Friedland et al., 1986; Black 1986; Parks et al., 1987). Seventy-eight percent of known pediatric AIDS infections occur in infants with perinatal infection (CDC, 1986), who may live for several years with chronic illness (AAP Committee on Infectious Diseases, 1986, Black 1986, CDC, 1988c, Epstein et al., 1987, Rubenstein, 1986). Risk groups are infants of mothers or fathers who use intravenous drugs, sexually abused children and adolescents whose molesters may be bisexual or IV drug users, children who have received transfusions after 1982 and before blood bank screening became routine in 1985, gay youth, and adolescents who are sexually active with multiple partners or who use intravenous drugs. Thus the spread of the epidemic in children and adolescents shows the same disproportionate increase in prevalence in poor and minority groups as that being found in the current patterns of increasing spread in adults (Report of Presidential Commission, 1988).

The greatest potential influence of the HIV epidemic may be on the psychological development of youth. As a public health issue, it is having a broad impact upon the sex and health education of children and the psychological lives of "at risk" and non-"at risk" youth. The challenge to change adolescents' behavior through education is known to be a serious one (Allen et al., 1988; Brown and Fritz, 1988; CDC, 1986; DiClementi et al., 1986; Elkins et al., 1986; Feinberg, 1988; Goodwin and Roscoe, 1988; Kegeles et al., 1988; Klein et al., 1987; Landefeld et al., 1988; Link et al., 1988; Price et al., 1985; Price, 1986; Quackenbush, 1987; Wolitski and Rhodes, 1988a, b). The problems that must be solved to change behavior through education are central to questions of learning and mastery, which are daily therapeutic issues for the practicing child psychiatrist. Psychiatric impacts and psychosocial sequelae of the HIV epidemic will be extensive and will outlast the search for a vaccine or cure.

Child and adolescent psychiatrists are likely to encounter at-risk, seropositive, or infected patients in the course of their clinical work, unless their practice excludes contact with minorities, with chronically ill children, sexually active adolescents, gay youth, and abused or molested children. The psychiatric responses required to deal with this clinical spectrum draw upon the entire range of skills currently considered part of child psychiatrists' training (AMA, 1983/84). These include pediatric liaison, family therapy, knowledge of psychotherapeutic techniques spanning common comforting to crisis intervention, familiarity with child development and neuropsychological handicaps, and competence in psychopharmacology. Required clinical skills will vary depending upon the demographic and diagnostic characteristics of the patient. Four cases from the practice of the authors illustrate this clinical spectrum and suggest indicated psychiatric treatment interventions for HIV infection in children and adolescents. A fifth consultation situation illustrates the role of the child psychiatrist in a multidisciplinary community setting where HIV spectrum disease must be dealt with. Table 1 schematizes psychiatric treatment characteristics of pediatric HIV risk groups.

CASE ILLUSTRATIONS

Case 1

A family practitioner referred a 16-year-old patient for evaluation of disturbed sleep patterns, weight loss, and dropping grades, all occurring within the previous 4 months. Physical examination was negative and a mono spot test and CBC were normal. When the parents were interviewed, they expressed surprise that their son's physician had referred him to a psychiatrist, but admitted that he had been moodier and appeared troubled during the current school year. The parents appeared to communicate fondly with each other and to corroborate each other's observations. Two younger sisters were apparently well adjusted and the family reportedly functioned well. Development history indicated that the patient had been an affectionate, apparently happy child, although he tended to be a loner with one close friend at a time, rather than to play with groups of different boys. His father, a former football player, expressed disappointment that he refused play in competitive sports, although he participated on the high-school swim team. He had not begun dating. On mental status examination he was cognitively intact but had multiple somatic concerns and numerous symptoms of anxiety. The initial interview was focused on his fears about his physical well-being, evidenced by his initial and middle insomnia, episodes of palpitation and difficulty breathing, and declining speed and stamina during his workouts in the pool. He also feared that he had begun to lose his memory and concentration. In other respects he seemed guarded, and his responses to questions about his relationships were superficial. In the second interview, the symptoms of anxiety and panic were explained to him, and he was gently confronted with the question about what might have made him anxious in the last few weeks. He confided that he was homosexual, and the previous summer he had his first sexual experiences with an older partner, aged 22, and had experienced receptive anal

TABLE 1
Psychiatric Treatment Characteristics for Pediatric HIV Risk Groups

	Gay Youth	Infants with Perinatal Infection	Transfusion Recipients	Promiscuous Adolescents	IVDA Adolescents
Developmental stage	Adolescent	Birth to school age	Birth through adolescence	Adolescents	Adolescents
Developmental resources	Age-appropriate: Identity issues	May have developmental plateauing	May be compromised by chronic illness	May be pseudomature or impulsive	May be compromised by factors that led to substance abuse
Psychiatric differential					
Axis 1	Identity, anxiety, or other	Developmental delay	Affective, anxiety, or other	Affective, anxiety, or other	Affective, anxiety, or other
Axis 2	–	Learning disorders secondary to DD	–	Character or learning disorder	Character or learning disorder
Axis 3, including neurological	STDs later, ADC	Opportunistic infections; neurological involvement	Other chronic illness if present	STDs later, ADC	Complications of drug use, later, ADC
Axis 4: stressors	Stigma	Isolation	As with other chronic illness	Homelessness or family strain	Economic or family strain
Treatment considerations	Patient may fear disclosure	Parent guilt, or death	Rage at contamination of blood	Fear, denial, impulsiveness, impede learning	Non-negotiability of addiction
Likely treatment modalities	Individual therapy; peer group support	Family support	Family support; medical liaison	Outreach, street work, affiliation with community health clinics	Outreach, drug treatment programs
Role of family	Variable, depending on youth	Important, if surviving	Important	May not be available	May not be available
Liaison	Variable	Pediatrics Day care	Pediatrics, schools	With local agencies	With local agencies
Agency type	None exist	Foster, respite, care	Hemophilia foundation and others	Youth group teen clinics alternate schools	Drug treatment programs

intercourse several times. He had tried unsuccessfully on two of these occasions to ask his partner to use a condom, and with much guilt, admitted that he had "been carried away" and had sex without protection. Since then he had lost contact with his friend but had heard that he was ill. He developed the fear that his friend might have AIDS and that he might have become infected. He insisted that his parents, particularly his father, not be told about his sexual orientation.

Treatment

The therapist was faced with difficult risk and moral calculations (Bayer et al., 1986; Dickens, 1988). She knew that the boy's chance of infection was 1 to 2% per exposure but that one exposure is sufficient to infect, and anal receptive intercourse is the most risky behavior. Antibodies can be detected in the serum of most infected persons within 6 months of infection. However, the enzyme linked immunosorbent assay (ELISA) has 1 to 3% false positives (Flynn, 1988). The western blot may also have 1 to 5% false negative results that occur in the early phases of HIV infection before all of the usual antibody responses have occurred (Flynn, 1988). A false positive result could cause unnecessary psychological trauma; a false negative result could postpone behavior changes that might protect this boy from acquiring new infections, possibly accelerating progression of his illness (Beyer et al., 1986), and that would protect his future partners from infection. If the patient is counseled to obtain antibody testing, the therapist must help him maintain confidentiality by advising that the test be obtained anonymously at an alternative testing site, and that the test not be billed to his health insurance. He must make difficult decisions about disclosure to parents (Anderson, 1987). If the patient's test result is positive, the therapist must make sure the patient understands the meaning of that result and must be prepared for crisis intervention, as up to 80% of persons who learn that they have antibodies to HIV have suicidal ideation. She must help the boy to make an alliance with a physician who can follow him for lymphadenopathy, monitor T-helper lymphocyte counts, and treat new or latent infections. If the result is negative, she must work with the boy to help him understand the need for repeated testing, and to learn methods to practice safe sex at a time in his life when sexual urges are compellingly potent, yet his sexual identity is still fragile, and his youth makes assertive behavior with older partners a difficult challenge. She must maintain her own therapeutic alliance with the boy to assist him to adjust to the challenges of being a gay youth during a stigmatizing epidemic. She might direct him to the growing popular or youth-oriented literature on the topic (De Sainte Phalle, 1987; Kerr, 1986; Langone, 1988; Preston and Swann, 1987; Reed, 1987; Shilts, 1987).

Case 2

Child psychiatric consultation was requested to deal with a difficult family situation involving an 18-month-old infant with AIDS. The infant had had failure to thrive and thrush when first seen at the 6-week checkup. The pediatric infectious disease specialist followed the infant and found hypergammaglobulinemia, a T-helper cell, count below 400, and a confirmatory ELISA test. A positive HIV antibody was subsequently found in the mother, who had a history of receiving a transfusion, and also had worked as an OR nurse in a hospital with a high proportion of patients with AIDS. With her baby she was seen subsequently in pediatric infectious disease clinic. During that time she was clinically ill. Her course was marked by successive episodes of pneumonia. She had not told her friends or parents about the HIV infection. The current hospitalization occurred when the baby was brought by his father to pediatric acute care clinic with pneumonia and was hospitalized. Father was visibly intoxicated when he visited with a flamboyantly effeminate male friend and was unable to give a clear history. The following day the maternal grandparents were discovered sitting quietly beside the crib. When the pediatrician spoke privately with them in the family room, it was learned that the infant's mother had suddenly died 3 days previously. The grandparents were acutely bereaved by the sudden death of their daughter and the discovery that their grandchild had AIDS but were ambivalent about assuming the care of the baby, saying: "We don't want *his* baby." Initially many staff were offended by the father's demeanor and expressed the view that he could not be responsible for caring for his son. During the infant's long hospitalization, the father visited daily, showed obvious responsiveness to the baby's cuing, was an attentive and competent caregiver, and spoke appropriately and openly with the nurses about his grief at losing his wife and his plans to manage as a single bisexual parent.

Treatment

The physicians have several tasks. Firstly the infant's care in the hospital will require special precautions (CDC, 1988b, 1988c). Evaluating the infant requires assessing whether neurological involvement has occurred (Detmer and Lu, 1986; Elder and Sever, 1985; Epstein et al., 1987; Janssen et al., 1988a, 1988b; Pumarola-Sune et al., 1987; Sneider et al., 1983) and planning disposition for a chronically ill child (Krener and Adelman, 1988; Loewenstein and Sharfstein, 1984; Price et al., 1985; Price 1986). Assessment by the child psychiatric consultant of the adequacy of the surviving parent to assume the infant's care is ethically awkward and tactically difficult in a pediatric setting, without a mandate for parental psychiatric assessment (Krener and Adelman, 1988). Acute family intervention is certainly indicated in this case (Krener, 1987) but is time-consuming, difficult to carry out concurrently with caring for other acutely ill children on a pediatric ward, and poorly reimbursed.

In this case, however, close communication with nursing staff allowed the physicians to greatly extend their data base. Nurses' observations of and conversations with the father supplied essential information about his strengths, the robustness of his relationship with the baby, the baby's responsiveness to him, and his support systems, particularly through his church. For children without supportive families, disposition is difficult, overtaxing agencies that were at capacity before the epidemic. The physicians need to participate in defining the child's care needs, and in dealing with ethical questions about informing prospective foster parents about the child's illness. Guidance about possible day-care placement has to be ongoing and adjusted to the current developmental capabilities and health needs of the child. Specifically, children unable to handle their secretions or who have biting behavior or open skin sores might endanger other children in a day-care or school setting, while children whose immune system is compromised might themselves be endangered by exposure to the usual infections in group settings (APA, 1987; AMA, 1983/84).

Case 3

A child psychiatrist consulting to a Regional Hemophilia program was asked to see a 14-year-old boy who was acutely distressed and refusing to attend school after learning that his serum was positive for the HIV antibody. His initial reaction of shock was immediate and stark with near-psychotic anger and denial. The emergency evaluation session included his intact family. They had developed impressive coping skills in dealing with what they termed a "medical intruder in the form of hemophilia" and had worked together and were supportive of each other and of their children. This boy had had a period of counterphobic risk-taking behavior in earlier childhood and had rebelled against some of the constraints on his activities. Until the HIV antibody was discovered in their son's serum, they felt they had conquered hemophilia, had experienced success in living with it through alliance with medical teams, and repeated transfusions, and had achieved a life-style they considered normal.

On mental status examination the boy was obviously angry and seriously depressed to a degree which made the psychiatrist consider hospitalization. Intensive outpatient intervention was begun, with two sessions per week and telephone availability offered by the psychiatrist. In his sessions the boy said he felt he had bested hemophilia only to be felled by the insertion of HIV into his blood. He had followed Ryan White's story with great interest. Issues of immortality and invulnerability rose immediately. He blamed assumed homosexual male blood donors, and voiced extreme fantasied threats of murderous retaliation and homosexual hatred. He worried that he would be classified as a junkie and fag. He said he would never be able to marry or have sex or children. He said he would be forced to become a homosexual by a quirk of fate because of contracting the virus. He ruefully wondered that this would be the only sexual avenue left to him when he dealt with the possibility that he would never have a normal heterosexual experience. He thought of having gay sex and infecting gay men in retaliation for what had befallen him.

Treatment

After the acute period, the treatment was a combination of individual, parental, and family sessions. The family lived at some distance and had to be seen for evening sessions at longer than weekly intervals, sessions which were spent partly with the boy and partly with parents, with family sessions if a crisis arose. Few physicians, psychiatrists or internists, in their region had experience with AIDS, and no local adolescent psychiatrists were practicing in their area. Adequate insurance coverage, and the family's comfort with the University Medical Center facilitated this plan. Two management crises arose in subsequent follow-up. The first occurred 1 year later when the boy required elective surgery on his knee and his parents were antagonized by an overheard comment conveying hostility toward their son because he had AIDS. Two and a half years later during his senior year in high school, he became withdrawn and apathetic, his school performance deteriorated acutely, and he had neuropsychological testing to evaluate the possibility of AIDS Dementia Complex (ADC). Mild dementia was found; however, depression was also thought to contribute to his decline in function at that time, although the patient was not actively suicidal. The psychiatrist continues to follow this boy, and the family takes comfort in knowing that he will be available. Although the course will be long (Redfield et al., 1988), the clinical picture is bound to evolve and may include a wide variety of problems (Abrams et al., 1988) associated with pre-AIDS syndromes and psychiatric and neuropsychiatric complications of the illness itself (Dilley et al., 1985; Faulstich, 1987; Forstein 1984; Nichols, 1983) until the patient's death (Kubler-Ross, 1987).

Case 4

A child psychiatrist who regularly consulted to a federally funded ambulatory health care center was asked to advise on a case which the staff found particularly difficult. A 15-year-old girl who had come to the center several times before for various medical problems was discovered to be HIV-positive and was reliably estimated to be functioning as a prostitute whose area of liveliest activity was the local high school. Clinic staff knew her fairly well; she was being raised by her mother, had an older brother in Juvenile Hall, and had never known her father. She was in a resource room in ninth grade in school, had been retained once, and planned to drop out when she turned sixteen. The staff members were perplexed about how to contain what they regarded as irresponsible and dangerous behavior. This patient was impulsive, undependable, and did not keep appointments. In the past she had been seen on walk-in basis only. The psychiatrist, therefore, joined in an outreach approach, which was part of the pattern of care delivery of this clinic: he made a home visit with the nurse. On mental status examination the patient was cooperative but flippant. She camouflaged a possible difficulty assimilating new information by offensively interrupting her visitors, which had the effect of slowing down their delivery of information to her. Very surprised by the test results, she proved to be uninformed about AIDS. Her reaction to being told that she had a virus that was infectious and dangerous was quiet denial. Since it was a lab result only and she did not feel sick, it wasn't as real to her as the gonorrhea infections she had had previously.

Treatment

Gradually an alliance was formed based on a blend of uncritical acceptance and clear limit-setting. At first the girl did not want information about her seropositivity shared with anyone and it took several trials to get her consent to inform her family. On another home visit, her mother, a single-parent, was confronted with her daughter's risky behavior and her need for regular care. Mother responded with vague concern, but her daughter's next clinic visit was broken because mother had asked her to stay with her sister's babies so that she could do something herself. On subsequent visits, the girl repeatedly was given an explanation of modes of HIV transmission and of the use of dental dams and condoms and their precarious protection. The clinic staff also informed her that they were planning to notify school personnel for the existence of an infected girl who prostitutes in the inner city school population. While never admitting her prostitution, she did not react angrily but responded with begrudging respect for the clinic's position. She continued to use the clinic as a resource for her other repeated medical problems. Continued contact with the girl was maintained: she did settle down and curbed her antisocial behaviors. She declined to attend a group but sought out certain staff members consistently to discuss her concerns.

Consultation Situation Clinical: Example 5

A child psychiatrist was invited by the staff of a community health center that ran an alternative test site to give an inservice on AIDS education for adolescent drug users. He prepared an up-to-date lecture on the neurobiologic actions of the human immunodeficiency virus and the pharmacological effects of common street drugs. Both of these were topics which he had not been taught during his residency, and he took satisfaction in extending his own psychiatric education. The inservice was planned conjointly with staff from a drug detoxification program. Certain of those workers were skeptical about the possibility of working therapeutically with these clients. They told the consultant "you are dealing with a person who'll buy a bag of stuff from someone they don't know on the street, with money that may not be theirs and take it home, cook it up, pull it into a rig that may be dirty and shoot it into what they hope is a good vein and if they don't fall over dead, they say it was good shit." The psychiatrist initially felt both ignorant and defensive.

The ensuing discussion during the inservice brought out four points to repeatedly emphasize in working with substance abusing clients of all social classes (Holmberg, 1985a, b). First, it is advisable to have a high index of suspicion for recreational drug use. Inquiry should be in plain terms; i.e., not: "Do you have a history of using street drugs?" but "What drugs do you use, who is your dealer and what do you know about how your drugs are cut?" Second, it is important not to discuss antibody test results with intoxicated clients, who may have "premedicated" themselves to "get up the courage" to come in for their test results, but who may be unable to assimilate the important information or control their reactions to it (Forstein, 1984). Third, clinicians must be aware that patients who use street medications regard themselves as proficient amateur pharmacists and need confrontation about the adverse effects of drugs on their immune systems (DHHS, 1986). Fourth, they must recall that clients who are knowledgeable about safe needles and safe sex practices when sober may not make use of that knowledge when they are stalking love or making love under the influence of alcohol or drugs, and, for example, may clean the rig the first time they use it but later in the evening when they pass the rig around they will not notice that there is blood in the barrel (McKirnan and Johnson, 1986; Mikkelson, 1988).

The psychiatrist left the inservice recognizing that he had learned more than he had taught. The social and biological information contained in his prepared remarks on pharmacological and neurological actions of substances of abuse was already known to his audience in explicit detail. The possible effects of HIV infection on the clients' functioning would occur in a context of learned and adaptive behaviors, which might threaten their treatment more than their mere ignorance of facts about the disease. He admitted that his child psychiatric residency had also not prepared him to work with patients who did not regard themselves as patients or to do psychotherapy with patients who put their impulses into action before they put their thoughts into words.

DISCUSSION

The human immunodeficiency virus is not selective; thus the cases illustrate both the wide spectrum of psychiatric symptom responses to risk and to infection, and the range of psychiatric clinical skills needed to respond to the patients' needs.

Case 1 addresses the problems of education for a particular group who are potentially alienated and for whom fear and prejudice may obstruct both information exchange and behavior change (APA, 1986b, 1987; Remafedi, 1987). Gay youth are likely to be free of infection but likely to engage in high risk behavior such as receptive anal intercourse. Homosexual youth may be rejected by family and peers and may embark on an intense search for acceptance and for physical and emotional intimacy in situations where they cannot assert themselves self-protectively. Because few gay boys would consider selecting a teenage sexual partner, and most usually seek out men in their twenties or older, they must have special preparation to develop safe practices early. Recognition that the gay teenage boy is usually vulnerable to HIV infection, and that, therefore, the window of opportunity for education is early, should be accompanied by vigorous educational efforts. Pleas for abstinence and social sanctions are not heeded. Educational efforts must not be homophobic, even implicitly. Information must be accompanied by support; AIDS neurosis, and hysterical conversation symptoms, obsessive behavior and phobic reactions may occur, as well as a fear of sex and intimacy, or a counterphobic flight into relationships. The unsolved legal problems of discrimination both for outpatients (APA, 1986a, b, 1987) and inpatients (Belfer et al., 1988; Binder, 1987) require the therapist to be a responsive, discrete, and well-informed resource, so that patients are piloted to necessary secondary prevention but weather the storms of their own emotional response to the illness and avoid the shoals of local social sanctions.

Case 2 demonstrates that multiple risk factors may be present even in patients who do not meet the expected stereotypes of substance abusing inner city minority parents of infants with AIDS (Zelnick and Kantner, 1977). The mother of an infant with AIDS may have the shock of learning that she is seropositive at the same time as learning that her infant is ill (Wofsy, 1987). Medical caregivers' judgmental feelings toward families may obstruct cooperating with them in planning for the chronic course of the illness. Families have to be helped to live with either secrecy or stigma. The usual community supports which may help a family with a chronically or terminally ill child may not be available to them. This may place extra burdens on the medical caregivers. Mothers should be counseled about the risk of future conception. It is known that successive pregnancies are likelier to lead to an infected infant in seropositive women, perhaps because of natural progression of the illness and declining T-helper cell counts, and perhaps because of factors related to the pregnancy itself (CDC, 1987s; Report of Presidential Commission 1988; Wofsy 1987). Infants have special needs for immunization, for protection against usual childhood illnesses for nutritional support and for repeated careful developmental monitoring. When neurological involvement develops, it is particularly important to try to provide a stable environment with consistent caregivers (Krener, 1987). Finally, infants who outlive their parents—so-called "border babies," residing in city hospital nurseries—pose terrible disposition problems to social services already at capacity, underlining the inadequacies of family support programs for poor clients (Institute of Medicine, 1988).

Case 3 illustrates three aspects of the care of persons with AIDS: adaptation to chronic illness, countertransference of stressed caretakers, and dementia associated with HIV infection (ADC).

Hemophilia is a chronic illness with which many productive individuals have learned to live. Ninety percent of patients with <1% factor VIII have become sero-positive in some geographic areas; the hemophilia community has responded to the epidemic early and well. Case 3 shows the impact of HIV infection in a youngster whose family is inured to chronic illness and for whom excellent psychosocial support systems are available. This patient's initial reaction of shock was acute distress and cognitive disorganization. In other families with an infected hemophiliac member, the impact is quieter and perhaps denied in spite of acknowledgment of the realities of HIV infection. Many youths and parents followed in hemophilia centers have received or sought some mental health intervention ranging from "genetic counseling" with extended length of contact to intensive individual psychotherapy or couple's therapy. The confirmation of HIV infection revives issues of immortality and invulnerability, and families who had responded before with grit and resilience may feel defeated at this point. Denial may be adaptive, if it is not accompanied by heedless behavior or medical neglect (Koocher and Berman, 1983). Early data on long survivors of HIV infection indicate that optimistic attitude, balanced life-style and stress management, a sense of control and exercise, are predictors of good course.

Surgeons and surgical staffs, particularly those caring for trauma patients, are now a risk group for HIV infection. The epidemic has catalyzed more scrupulous reverse precautions and modification of operating room practices (CDC, 1987a, b). Sharp instruments are passed more deliberately, needles are treated as dangerous, and protective wear has increased. Still, any surgeon's risk of infection with HIV is described by a formula calculating the product of risk that the patient is seropositive, the frequency of punctures (sticks/year) and the incidence of HIV positive patients upon whom he or she operates (Marcys et al., 1988). As a result, surgical staff in high prevalence areas experience erosive stress because of the constant possibility of accidental inoculation with the fatal virus. To that stress is added fatigue if their programs recruit incomplete quotas of trainees because of the prevalence of AIDS, and the personal strains of treating young dying persons. Their patients may detect these painful feelings and experience them as lack of caring, as shown in Case 3's experience during the episode when he required surgery.

AIDS dementia complex may occur at any point in the course of the illness (Price et al., 1988a, b) and becomes increasingly likely to occur with its progression. A principal aspect of the biology of HIV infection, it is currently incorporated into the definition of AIDS. The CDC definition of dementia is "clinical findings of a disabling cognitive or motor dysfunction interfering with occupational activity or loss of behavioral milestones affecting a child" (Report of Presidential Commission, 1988). It is a diagnosis of exclusion after cerebral spinal fluid examination and computerized tomography (CT) or magnetic resonance imaging (MRI). Twenty percent of patients have neurological syndromes among their initial complaint, 63% have neurological findings during the course of AIDS, and 90% of unselected autopsies have neuropathology (Price et al., 1988a). Peripheral manifestations include chronic distal symmetric polyneuropathy or inflammatory demyelinating polyneuropathy. Central manifestations are the result of direct viral infection of the brain, preferentially involving cells other than neurons, astrocytes, and oligodendrocytes. ADC is chronically progressive with subcortical dementia and a variable constellation of cognitive, motor, and behavioral disturbances. Early symptoms are impaired attention and concentration, memory loss, slowed information processing, mild frontal lobe dysfunction, and difficulty with the performance of complex sequential mental activities. Motor symptoms usually involve legs before arms, and clumsiness precedes weakness of gait. The MRI may show discrete areas of increased signal in white matter. The CT and MRI both may show cortical atrophy and ventricular dilation, but are often normal.

Diagnosis should be by neuropsychological screening, more rigorous than that done in the usual mental status examination. A careful cognitive history should probe for slowed thinking, forgetfulness, poor attention and concentration or derailment, speech problems, word finding problems, weakness, gait difficulties, and change in handwriting. Patients should be followed with annual WISC-R examinations, and semiannual tests of memory and psychomotor speed, such as the Trailmaking Test and Neurobehavioral Mental Status Examination (Northern California Neurobehavior Group, 1983). Behavioral changes may consist of apathy, loss of spontaneity, social withdrawal, and change in personality. In a minority of patients, anxiety, hyperactivity, and inappropriate behavior may occur (Price et al., 1988a). In management, discriminating between depression and dementia is important as is early identification of treatable causes of dementia (Loewenstein et al., 1984). The clinical severity of the AIDS dementia complex is correlated well with the neuropathology, which afflicts white rather than grey matter. AZT may ameliorate the course of AIDS dementia. Standard anxiolytics may be used to treat anxiety, but a delirious response to benzodiazepines may occur if an organic brain syndrome is present. High-potency neuroleptics are useful for psychosis in low doses. Psychostimulants may be palliative for psychomotor slowing.

Causes of mental status change other than HIV itself may include toxic-metabolic effects of pentamidine and AZT, hypoperfusion states, and electrolyte imbalance in very ill patients. It is important to rule out treatable causes of dementia associated with HIV infection, but not directly due to the neurotropic action of the virus. These include CNS infections or small primary CNS tumors, most commonly lymphoma, rarely Kaposi's sarcoma. Toxoplasmosis, cytomegalovirus, or tuberculosis infections may occur in immune-compromised hosts. Treponema pallidum, not responsive to the usual doses of penicillin, is a recognized fellow-traveler with HIV infection. Cryptococcosis may present as mania, but if not treated may cause irreversible damage. Clearly, close partnership between medical and psychiatric caregivers is indicated for management of this continuum of problems.

Case 4 is a representative of persons in social groups whose developmental adaptation to chaotic and deprived life circumstances had made them both vulnerable to the HIV epidemic and unlikely to be managed well medically (DHHS, 1986a, b; Rosenberg and Weiner, 1988; Roth and Bean, 1986). For children in these circumstances, the initiative and opportunism required to survive deprivation is on a continuum with impulsiveness. The flexibility and resilience required to accommodate to instability in the home is on a continuum with disorganization. Abstract understanding and verbal interactions are weak responses to physical confrontation, which may be their daily experience. Dependence may be treacherous if a child relies upon adults who may be unable to care for him or her. Learning is obstructed for hungry children in disrupted classrooms. The goal of control over one's life may be alien to a child who has never had toys, privacy, or a room of his/her own. "Just saying no" to drugs, when they are ubiquitous and integral to neighborhood power structures, may be as impractical as denying the existence of the weather. Preventive health care does not become a personal custom if one is beset by recurrent health crises; if private providers cannot "afford" to see patients with public funding, if medical caregivers in county clinics or emergency rooms are always different, and if public health-care funding is tilted toward reimbursement of acute treatment.

Thus youths labeled impulsive, disorganized, concrete, rebellious, educationally delayed, unable to say no to drugs or control their sexuality, and medically noncompliant may have successfully survived because of the very characteristics identified as pathological by the diagnostician. Recall that psychotherapeutic techniques taught in most training programs have evolved between middle-class patients and highly educated therapists. Therefore, psychotherapy with the subpopulation of Case 4 may seem impossible in the traditional sense and, perhaps, irrelevant to the adaptational tactics that they actually need for immediate coping. Therapeutic interventions should be reality-related and include clear limits and tangible services as well as interpersonal caring and understanding. As in Case 4, a plan might alternate between quasi-legal enforcement, such as reporting their infection to the state public health service for partner notification and case identification in states requiring this, and remaining available to these youth as the social service resource of firstcall when they are enveloped in an unmanageable crisis. Neighborhood based outreach programs are preferable to center-based office or clinic programs. In programs such as that serving the girl in Case 4, home visits are routine to try to overcome the expectation that health care is difficult to access, delivered by strangers, and unavailable unless illness is critical. Group interventions, appealing to health care providers because of their efficiency, may be rejected by clients because consistent early experience of competition and conflict would make the prospect of sharing's one's weaknesses among a group of peers seems ill-advised.

Interacting with the above social factors are the biological patterns of the HIV infection process. Females with sexually acquired HIV infection tend to be younger at age of diagnosis than are males with any risk factor (Allen and Curran, 1988). In different areas, the prevalence of HIV antibodies among prostitutes, significant numbers of whom are teenagers, ranges between zero and 65%, with the single most important risk factor in the United States being intravenous drug use (Rosenberg and Weiner, 1988). The present health-care delivery system, already strained by incompatibility between its middle-class social values and economic models, and the inner city utilization patterns, is unable to accommodate the disproportionate numbers of HIV infections in poor areas (Brown and Fitz, 1988; Report of Presidential Commission, 1988).

Education has been identified as the present best tactic to contain the epidemic. However, as Case 4 shows, the adolescents who are crucial targets for education may no longer be in school, so education will have to extend beyond the classroom. Education which encourages fear has been shown to have limited effectiveness (Black, 1986), and compulsory public health measures have been dubiously effective, as in premarital syphilis serologies. Review of AIDS risk behavior changes (Bayer et al., 1986) shows that in some areas knowledge is incomplete, or inconclusive. A review (Kegeles et al., 1988) of sexually active adolescents and their use of condoms showed that while adolescents may increase their knowledge concerning the prevention of sexually transmitted diseases (STDs) over time, this does not cause an increase in their condom use. The authors note that even understanding in abstract terms that condoms protect against STDs, and believing that this is of value, may not make adolescents feel personally vulnerable to contracting diseases from their sex partners. Interventions that target perceptions of personal vulnerability may be a way of increasing adolescents' motivation to use condoms.

The consultation situation in clinical Example 5 illustrates the importance of interdisciplinary cooperation and the need for greatly amplified intervention programs to respond to the problem of addiction (Report of Presidential Commission, 1988). The progression from oral or inhaled use of drugs to IV use is known, and the mechanics of HIV spread among drug abusers shows that they are markedly younger than homosexual men who have not given a history of IV drug abuse. This age skewing is particularly remarkable for females and homosexual males. The younger age of female IV drug abusers at diagnosis of AIDS could signify different patterns of drug use or a greater susceptibility to HIV infection and disease. Transmission through sharing needles, syringes, and other drug use paraphernalia has occurred since early in the epidemic in the United States (des Jarlais et al., 1987). The proportions of IV drug abuse AIDS cases vary widely; 93% of cases have been reported from 13 states, and the ratio of heterosexual to homosexual cases ranges from >5:1 in New Jersey and New York to >3:1 in California, Colorado, Texas, and Washington (DHHS, 1986b). Waiting periods for drug treatment programs in cities with high HIV prevalence are 3 to 6 months.

Public health measures such as clean needle programs have been criticized as indulging drug users. However, drug addiction is in some regard a socially contagious environmental hazard, exceedingly difficult to avoid in many situations, especially for young people. Nonetheless, victims of drug addiction are condemned more than are patients afflicted with other contagious illnesses, such as malaria, typhoid fever, or tuberculosis. Understanding local patterns of drug abuse may enable the public health community to develop more effective prevention programs for areas where a majority of the IV drug abuser population is not yet infected with HIV.

CONCLUSION

Five clinical situations illustrate the social risk spectrum of HIV infection in children and adolescents and also show that no single child psychiatric treatment technique is effective across the whole continuum. Obstacles to the effectiveness of child psychiatrists in helping youth with HIV infection and their families fall into two categories: limitations upon skills and services, and constraints upon distribution of child psychiatric expertise.

Progress is being made in overcoming resistance of some politicians, educators, and religious leaders to endorse educational efforts that acknowledge homosexuality, teenage sexual activity, and drug use. Educators are responding, however, behavior change does not follow education (DiClementi, 1986; Brandt 1988; Kegeles, 1988). Child psychiatrists have an important role in developing effective educational approaches. Case 1 shows that child psychiatrists must also help their high-risk and HIV positive patients navigate difficult straits of prejudice, and that their therapeutic alliance may be pressured by difficult ethical and confidentiality issues.

Clinical psychiatric skills are commonly taught in training settings geared to psychotherapeutic treatment of cooperative middle-class patients and psychopharmacological management of compliant patients. Comanagement by psychiatrists of patients with serious medical illness is less common. However, it is a requirement of child psychiatric training programs (AMA, 1983) to include pediatric consultation liaison training, so child psychiatrists have the skills, if not the experience, of delivering care to ill patients in medical settings. Case 2 demonstrates that the need for competence in pediatric consultation-liaison psychiatry is increasing with the spread of HIV. If child psychiatrists are not to be regarded as extraneous and unhelpful in the care of these patients, they must be prepared to work as members of a multidisciplinary team, and to follow patients over time, rather than exhibiting specialty consultation skills in single consultative episodes. How are child psychiatrists to be trained to take on this clinical burden (AMA, 1983/84)? Training programs are burdened with fiscal self-support in an era when reimbursement for poor persons' medical needs, for chronic illnesses, and for children's mental health needs is constricting to the point of strangulation of existing programs. A gravitation of training programs' clinical curricula toward reimbursable activities and insured patients results. However, reimbursement patterns curtail hospitalizations, dictate parameters of outpatient care, and deny funds for long-term treatment. Outreach may be cost-effective from an epidemiological point of view but is not adequately reimbursed on a fee-for-service basis, so it is underutilized. Case 3 is an articulate, verbal, middle-class adolescent with an intact family who endorse his therapy. Nevertheless, trainees whose clinical experience is confined to reimbursable activities may not learn the skills required to follow a patient like Case 3, who needs long-term treatment, crisis family work at times, appointments with extended and flexible hours, and liaison with other specialists for care of his evolving medical problems.

The demographics of the AIDS epidemic are orthogonal to those of health-care delivery, particularly for mental health services. Psychiatrists are likelier to see patients who are well-to-do than those who are poor, who have third party insurance, rather than those with public funding, and who have a supportive social or work system to engage with, rather than those who are isolated and without supports. Psychotherapeutic techniques are geared to serve patients who are educated, verbal, and able to enter into a treatment contract, not those whose currency for communication is action, who are seen as impulsive and unpredictable. Psychiatrists have been trained to function best in individual treatment relationships with their patients, and, with the exception of consultation liaison psychiatrists, are unlikely to be comfortable treating patients who are frequently hospitalized for medical problems and whose care is managed by a multidisciplinary team. The subcultural innuendo of complex interpersonal communication makes it difficult to do psychotherapy with a person from another class or culture; as the majority of psychiatrists in the United States are not originally from poor, black, or Hispanic backgrounds, they have not developed a familiarity with the expectations and situations of minority patients nor of merely poor patients, such as the girl in Case 4. Child psychiatrists are trained to work with families; children and adolescents whose families are unavailable to them because of death, addiction, or indifference may be regarded as too difficult to treat. Lastly, psychiatrists prefer to deal with patients who do not abuse drugs or alcohol, who are able to be helped by a therapeutic interaction with a mental health professional and who are lucid. Thus, as shown in clinical situations, patients with substance abuse disorders who have an incurable illness and who may have intermittent or progressive dementia are likely to be deprived of psychiatric support and management.

Were not these practical impediments enough, there are also countertransferential obstacles to psychiatric treatment of HIV infected patients, including value judgments negative toward persons with AIDS, feelings of helplessness in dealing with a terminal illness, ignorance of the associated complex neuropsychiatric syndromes, and financial entitlement justifying avoidance of patients with inadequate reimbursement. The psychiatric profession has made valuable contributions to understanding patient-physician relationships; expanding that understanding to absorb the ethical, sociological, neuropsychiatric, and human impact of the HIV epidemic is the next challenge.

REFERENCES

Abrams, D. I. (1988), The pre-AIDS syndromes. *Infectious Disease Clinics of North America,* 2(2).

Allen, J. R. & Curran, J. W. (1988), Prevention of AIDS and HIV infection: needs and priorities for epidemiologic research. *Am. J. Public Health,* 78,(4):381–386.

American Academy of Pediatrics Committee on Infectious Diseases (1986), School attendance of children and adolescents with human T lymphocyte virus III/lymphadenopathy—associated virus infection. *Pediatrics,* 77:430–432.

American Medical Association (1983/84), Essentials of accredited residencies in child psychiatry. In: *Director of Residency Training Program,* p. 69. Chicago: Author.

American Psychiatric Association (1986a, Dec.), *Position statement of human immunodeficiency virus (HIV) related discrimination.* Washington, DC: Author.

_____(1986b, Dec.), *Position statement on AIDS policy: confidentiality and disclosure.* Washington, DC: Author.

_____(1987), *Position statement on AIDS policy: guidelines for inpatient psychiatric units.* Washington, DC: Author.

Anderson, D. (1987), Family and peer relations of gay adolescents. *Adolesc. Psychiatry,* 14(11):162-178.

Barbour, S. D. (1987), Acquired immunodeficiency syndrome of childhood. *Pediatr. Clin. North Am.,* 34(1):247–268.

Bayer, R., Levine, C. & Wolf, S. M. (1986), HIV antibody screening. An ethical framework for evaluating proposed programs. *JAMA,* 256:1768.

Belfer, M. L., Krener, P. K. & Miller, F. B. (1988), AIDS in children and adolescents. *J. Am. Acad. Child. Adolesc. Psychiatry,* 27:147–151.

Binder, R. (1987), AIDS antibody tests on inpatient psychiatric units. *Am. J. Psychiatry,* 144:176–181.

Black, J. L. (1986), AIDS: preschool and school issues. *J. Sch. Health,* 56:93–95.

Brandt, A. M. (1988), AIDS in historical perspective: four lessons from the history of sexually transmitted disease. *Am. J. Public Health,* 78:367–371.

Brown, L. K. & Fritz, G. K. (1988), Children's knowledge and attitudes about AIDS. *J. Am. Acad. Child Adolesc. Psychiatry,* 27:505–508.

Carbine, M. E. & Lee, P. (1988), *AIDS into the 90's: strategies for an integrated response to the AIDS epidemic.* Washington, DC: National AIDS Network Centers for Disease Control American Medical Association of State and Territorial Health Officers.

Center for Disease control (1986), Additional recommendations to reduce sexual and drug-abuse related transmission of HTLV III/LAV. *MMWR,* 35:152–155.

———(1987a), Recommendations for prevention of HIV transmission in health-care settings. *MMWR,* 36(Suppl.):S3–17.

———(1987b), Human immunodeficiency virus infections in health-care workers exposed to blood of infected patients. *MMWR,* 36:285–289.

———(1987c), Public Health Service guidelines for counseling and antibody testing to prevent HIV infection and AIDS. *MMWR,* 36:509–515.

———(1988a), Condoms for prevention of STDs. *MMWR,* 37:133–137.

———(1988b), Update: Universal precautions for prevention of transmission of human immunodeficiency virus hepatitis B and other blood borne pathogens in health care settings. *MMWR,* 37:337–387.

———(1988c), Immunization of children infected with human immunodeficiency virus— supplementary ACIP statement. *MMWR,* 37(12).

Coffin, J., Haase, L., Levy, J. A. et al. (1986), Human immunodeficiency virus. *Science,* 232:697.

De Sainte Phalle N. (1987), *AIDS: You Can't Catch It Holding Hands.* San Francisco: Lapis Press.

Department of Health and Human Services (1986a), An occasional report on runaway and homeless youth data. In: *Summary Data on Youth Identified as "Possibly Suicidal."* Washington, DC: Office of Human Development Services, p. 1–7.

———(1986b), An occasional report on runaway and homeless youth data. In: *Summary Data on Alcohol and Drug Abuse Among Youth.* Washington, DC: Office of Human Development Services.

Des Jarlais, D. C., Friedman, S. R., Marmour, M. et al. (1987), Development of AIDS, HIV seroconversion and potential co-factors for T4 cell loss in a cohort of intravenous drug users. *AIDS,* 1:105–111.

Detmer, W. M. & Lu, F. G. (1986), Neuropsychiatric complications of AIDS: A literature review. *Int. J. Psychiatry Med.,* 16:21–28.

Dickens, B. M. (1988), Legal rights and duties in the AIDS epidemic. *Science,* 239:580–585.

DiClementi, R. J., Zorn, J. & Temoshok, L. (1986), Adolescents and AIDS: A survey of knowledge, attitudes and beliefs about AIDS in San Francisco. *Am. J. Public Health,* 76:1443–1445.

Dilley, J. W., Ochitill, H. N., Perl, M. & Volberding, P. A. (1985), Findings in psychiatric consultations with patients with acquired immune deficiency syndrome. *Am. J. Psychiatry,* 142:82–86.

Elder, G. A. & Sever, J. L. (1985), AIDS and neurological disorders. *Ann. Neurol.,* 23(Suppl.):S4–S6.

Elkins, T. E., McNeeley, S. G. & Tabb, T. (1986), A new era in contraceptive counseling for early adolescents. *J. Adolesc. Health Care,* 7:405–408.

Epstein, L. G., Goudsmit, J., Paul, D. A. et al. (1987), Expression of human immuno-deficiency virus in cerebrospinal fluid of children with progressive encephalopathy. *Ann. Neurol.,* 21:397–400.

Flynn, N. (1988), "HIV infection," In: *Clinical Preventative Medicine: Health Promotion and Disease Prevention,* ed. T. W. Hudson, M. A. Reinhart, S. D. Rose, & G. K. Stewart. Boston/Toronto: Little Brown and Co.

Faulstich, M. D. (1987), Psychiatric aspects of AIDS. *Am. J. Psychiatry,* 144:551–556.

Feinberg, H. F. (1988), Education to prevent AIDS: prospects and obstacles. *Science,* 239:592–596.

Forstein, M. (1984), The psychological impact of the acquired immunodeficiency syndrome. *Semin. Oncol.,* 11:77–82.

Friedland, G. H., Saltzman, B. R., Rogers, M. R. (1986), Lack of transmission of HTLV-III/LAV infection to household contacts of patients with AIDS or AIDS-related complex with oral candidiasis. *N. Engl. J. Med.,* 314:344–349.

Goodwin, M. P. & Roscoe, B. (1988), AIDSP: Students' knowledge and attitudes at a mid-western university. *JACH,* 36:214–221.

Holmberg, M. B. (1985a), Longitudinal studies of drug abuse in a fifteen year old population. 2. Antecedents and consequences. *Acta Psychiatr. Scand.,* 71:80–91.

——(1985b). Longitudinal studies of drug abuse in a fifteen year old population. 5. Prognostic factors. *Acta Psychiatr. Scand.,* 71:207–210.

Institute of Medicine, National Academy of Sciences. (1988), *Confronting AIDS: Update.* Washington, DC: Author.

Janssen, R. S., Saykin, A. J., Kaplan, J. E. (1988a), Neurological symptoms and neuro-psychological abnormalities in lymphademopathy syndrome. *Ann. Neurol.,* 23(Suppl.):S17–S18.

—— —— ——et al. (1988b), Neurological complications of human immunodeficiency virus infection in patients with lymphadenopathy syndrome. *Ann. Neurol.,* 23:49–55.

Kegeles, S. M., Adler, N. E. & Irwin, C. E. (1988), Sexually active adolescents and con-doms: changes over one year in knowledge, attitudes and use. *Am. J. Public Health,* 78:460–461.

Kerr, M. E. (1986), *Night Kites.* New York: Harper and Row.

Klein, D. E., Sullivan, G., Wolcott, D. L., Landsverk, J., Namir, S. & Fawzy, F. (1987), Changes in AIDS risk behaviors among homosexual male physicians and university students. *Am. J. Psychiatry,* 144:742–747.

Koocher, G. P. & Berman, S. J. (1983), Life threatening and terminal illness in childhood. In: *Developmental-Behavioral Pediatrics,* ed. M.D. Levine, et al. Philadelphia: W. B. Saunders, 488–520.

Krener, P. K. (1987), Impact of the diagnosis of AIDS on hospital care of an infant. *Clin. Pediatr.* (Phila.), 26:30–34.

——Adelman, R. (1988), Parent salvage and parent sabotage in the care of chronically ill children. *Am. J. Dis. Child,* 142:945–951.

Kubler-Ross, E. (1987), AIDS: *The Ultimate Challenge.* New York: Macmillan.

Landefeld, C. S., Chren, M. M., Shega, J., Sperof, T. & McGuire E. (1988), Students' sexual behavior knowledge and attitudes relating to the acquired immunodeficiency syndrome. *J. Gen. Intern. Med.*, 3:161–165.

Langone, J. (1988), *AIDS: The Facts.* Boston: Little Brown.

Link, R. N., Feingold, A. R., Charap, M. H., Freeman, K. & Shelov, S. P. (1988), Concerns of medical and pediatric house officers about acquiring AIDS from their patients. *Am. J. Public Health,* 78:455–459.

Loewenstein, R. J. & Sharfstein, S. S. (1984), Neuropsychiatric aspects of acquired immune deficiency syndrome. *Int. J. Psychiatry Med.*, 13:255–260.

Marcys, R. and the CDC Cooperative Needlesticks Surveillance Group. (1988), Surveillance of health care workers exposed to blood from patients infected with the human immunodeficiency virus. *N. Engl. J. Med.*, 319:1118–1122.

McKirnan, D. J. & Johnson T. (1986), Alcohol and drug use among "street" adolescents. *Addict. Behav.*, 11:201–205.

Mikkelson, E. J. Substance abuse in adolescents and children. *Psychiatry,* 2(35):1–6.

Nichols, S. E. (1983), Psychiatric aspects of AIDS. *Psychosomatics,* 24:1083–1089.

Northern California Neurobehavior Group (1983), *The Neurobehavioral Mental Status Examination.* Davis, CA: University of California.

Parks, W. P. & Scott, G. B. (1987), An overview of Pediatric AIDS: Approaches to Diagnosis and Outcome Assessment. In: *AIDS: Modern Concepts and Therapeutic Challenges,* ed. S. Broder. New York: Marcel Dekker.

Perves, N. K., Kleinerman, J., Kattan, M. (1985), AIDS in children: a review of the clinical, epidemiologic and public health aspects. *Pediatr. Infect. Dis. J.,* 4:230–236.

Price, J. H. (1986), AIDS, the schools, and policy issues. *J. Sch. Health,* 56(4):137–140.

———Desmond, S. & Kukulka, G. (1985), High school students' perceptions and misperceptions of AIDS. *J. Sch. Health,* 55(3):107–109.

Price, R. W., Brew, B. Sidtis, J., Rosenblum, M., Scheck, A. C. & Cleary, P. (1988a), The brain in AIDS: central nervous system HIV-1 infection and AIDS dementia complex. *Science,* 239:586–592.

———Sidtis, J. & Rosenblum, M. (1988b), The AIDS dementia complex. *Ann. Neurol.* (supplement)P:S27–S33.

Pumarola-Sune, T., Navia, B. A., Cordon-Cardo, C., Cho, E. & Price, R. W. (1987), HIV antigen in the brains of patients with the AIDS dementia complex. *Ann. Neurol.,* 21:490–496.

Quackenbush, M. (1987), Educating youth about AIDS. *Focus: A Review of AIDS Research,* 2(3).

Redfield, R. R. & Burke, D. S. (1988), HIV infection: the clinical picture. *Scientific American,* 259(4):90–99.

———Wright, D. C. & Tramont, E. C. (1986), The Walter Reed Staging Classification for HTLV III/LAV infection. *N. Engl. J. Med.,* 314:131–132.

Reed, P. (1987), *Serenity: Challenging the Fear of Aids.* Berkeley, CA: *Celestial Arts.*

Report of the Presidential Commission on the Human Immunodeficiency Virus Epidemic, June 1988. Washington, DC: Author.

Rees, M. (1987), The sombre view of AIDS. *Nature* 326:343–345.

Remafedi, G. (1987), Adolescent homosexuality: psychosocial and medical implications. *Pediatrics,* 79:331–337.

Rosenberg, M. J. and Weiner, J. M. (1988), Prostitutes and AIDS: a Health Department priority? *Am J. Public Health,* 78:418–423.

Roth, D. & Bean G. J., Jr. (1986), New perspectives on homelessness: findings from a statewide epidemiological study. *Hosp. Community Psychiatry,* 37:718–719.

Rubenstein, A. (1986). Schooling for children with acquired immune deficiency syndrome. *J. Pediatr.,* 109:301.

Shilts, R. (1987), *And the Band Played On: Politics, People and the AIDS Epidemic.* New York: St. Martin's Press.

Sneider, W. D., Simpson, D. M., Nielsen, S., Gold, J. W. M., Metroka, C. E. & Posner, J. B. (1983), Neurological complications of acquired immune deficiency syndrome: analysis of 50 patients. *Ann. Neurol,* 14;404–418.

Swann, G. & Preston, J. (1987), *Safe Sex: The Ultimate Erotic Guide.* New York: Plume/Nal.

U.S. Department of Health and Human Services. (1986), *Coping with AIDS* (DHHS Publication No. (ADM) 85-1432). Washington, DC: U.S. Government Printing Office.

Wofsy, C. (1987, April), *Drug abuse and women's medical issues.* Paper presented at the Surgeon General's Workshop on Children with HIV Infection and Their Families.

Wolitiski, R. J. & Rhodes, F. (1988a, April), *AIDS knowledge and attitudes among high school students.* Paper presented at the Western Psychological Annual Meeting, San Francisco.

_____ _____(1988b, June), *AIDS attitudes, knowledge and risk reduction in a college population.* Paper presented at the IV International Conference on AIDS, Stockholm, Sweden.

Zelnick, M. and Kantner, J. F. (1977), Sexual and contraceptive experience of young married women in the United States, 1976 and 1971. *Fam. Plann. Perspect.,* 9:55.